Injury Prevention for Children and Adolescents

Research, Practice, and Advocacy, Second Edition

Injury Prevention for Children and Adolescents

Research, Practice, and Advocacy, Second Edition

Editor

Karen DeSafey Liller, PhD

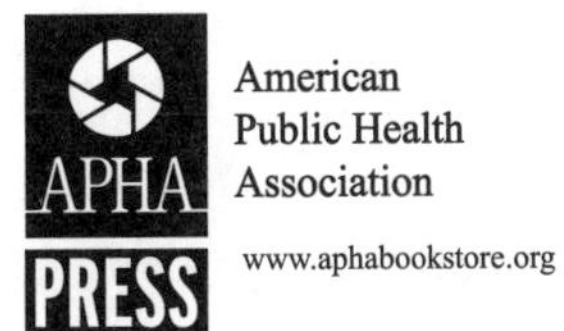

American Public Health Association
800 I Street, NW
Washington, DC 20001-3710
www.apha.org

Printed and bound in the United States of America
Typesetting: The Charlesworth Group
Cover Design: Alan Giarcanella
Printing and Binding: Victor Graphics, Inc., Baltimore, MD

Library of Congress Cataloging-in-Publication Data

Injury prevention for children and adolescents : research, practice, and advocacy / editor: Karen Liller ; foreword by Linda C. Degutis. -- 2nd ed.

p. cm.

Includes bibliographical references and index.

ISBN-13: 978-0-87553-005-5 (alk. paper)

ISBN-10: 0-87553-005-2 (alk. paper)

I. Liller, Karen DeSafey. II. American Public Health Association.

[DNLM: 1. Wounds and Injuries--prevention & control. 2. Accident Prevention. 3. Adolescent. 4. Child. WO 700]

617.1--dc23

363.34'8--dc23

2011031607

9/2011

Table of Contents

This book is again dedicated to those children and families profiled in the chapters and to all children, so that their world is free from needless injuries. I also dedicate this book to my children, Matthew and Rebecca, to my husband, Dave, who supported my long hours of work to produce this second edition, and to my parents, who provided me and my sisters love and support throughout our lives.

Great thanks go to all the chapter authors, the American Public Health Association Publications Board, and my fellow injury prevention colleagues throughout the world, who labor tirelessly to research, teach, and advocate for children so precious lives will be saved.

Foreword

During the past 50 years, we have seen progress in the field of injury prevention and intervention, particularly in the area of motor vehicle occupant protection and the development of safety standards for products that are used by infants and young children. This is the result of multiple disciplines working together to document the problem through epidemiologic research, to propose solutions through engineering and environmental strategies, to advocate for change in policy and standards, and to evaluate the effectiveness of innovations and programs once they have been put into place. Progress has been made in the treatment of injuries, through improvements in emergency medical service systems, trauma system organization, resuscitation, hospital care, and rehabilitation, with special attention paid to the unique needs of children.

Despite the progress that has been made, we still have a long way to go in decreasing morbidity and mortality due to injury in children and adolescents. Injury remains the leading cause of death and disability for children and adolescents, yet the emphasis on injury prevention and interventions, as well as funding for injury research, lags far behind that of other diseases that have lower mortality and morbidity rates. Budget issues result in cuts in funding for prevention programs and community-based interventions. Inadequate insurance coverage or lack of coverage has an impact on preventive care, acute care, and rehabilitation. Decreasing funding for program evaluation and research decreases the likelihood of advances in the field. Advocacy for injury-related efforts is challenging, because of the nature of injuries themselves and a general sense that injuries are "accidents" that happen to someone else's child.

In the second edition of this book, Dr. Liller and the chapter authors have updated their work on the problem of injury in children and adolescents and have clearly highlighted the importance of a multidisciplinary and multistrategy approach to this problem. The important examples of children who have been affected by injuries cannot be ignored, because they represent the many children and families who face the challenges that injuries present. The authors document the evidence base for various types of injury events that occur in this age group, highlight effective strategies, and describe successful advocacy efforts. The new chapters on global injury and translation of injury science into practice are important additions to the work that is presented. The book provides a framework for practitioners, program planners and evaluators, and injury researchers that is complementary to other work in this area and that fills in some gaps. This book represents the work of numerous experts in the field of injury prevention and intervention, and Dr. Liller and co-authors are to be congratulated for their success in not only highlighting the scientific aspects of injury but also linking the science to the reality of injury in children and adolescents.

Linda C. Degutis, DrPH, MSN
Director, National Center for Injury Prevention and Control
Centers for Disease Control and Prevention
Atlanta, Georgia

Prologue

Child and Adolescent Injury Prevention: A Public Health Perspective

David A. Sleet, PhD, MA, FAAHB,[1] Chester L. Pogostin, DVM, MPA,[1] Captain Stephanie Bryn, MPH,[2] Lynne Haverkos, MD, MPH,[3] Sandy Spavone, MPH,[4] Rebecca Levin, MPH,[5] Meri-K Appy, BA, and Angela Mickalide, PhD, MCHES[6]

Injuries are one of the most underrecognized public health problems facing the world today, which is why this book is so important. Causing more than five million deaths every year, violence and injuries account for 9% of global mortality and as many deaths as HIV, malaria, and tuberculosis combined (Peden et al. 2008). Young people are among the most vulnerable. Worldwide, 8 of the 15 leading causes of death for people aged 15 to 29 years are injury related, including road traffic injuries, suicides, homicides, drowning, burns, war injuries, poisonings, and falls (Krug, Sharma, and Lozano 2000).

In the United States, approximately 33 children aged 0 to 19 years die every day from an unintentional injury, and 16 young people are murdered each day. One in four children annually will be injured severely enough to miss school or require medical attention or bed rest. For every unintentional child injury death, there are approximately 19 hospitalizations, 233 hospital emergency visits, and 450 doctor visits (Borse et al. 2008).

Using a Scientific Approach to Injury Prevention

The Centers for Disease Control and Prevention, the Health Resources and Services Administration, the National Institutes of Health, the National Organizations for Youth Safety, the American Academy of Pediatrics, Safe Kids Worldwide, and our many partners are drawing attention to the devastating effects of injuries and violence, and we support efforts to develop prevention approaches that focus on addressing root causes. We encourage the use of reliable data to help determine priorities and evaluate the effectiveness of child injury prevention strategies (Borse et al. 2008). As this book emphasizes, public health strategies can and should be applied to prevent, reduce, eliminate, or reverse the trend in injuries, lessen suffering, and save children's lives.

The traditional view of child and adolescent injuries as "accidents" or random events has resulted in the historical neglect of this area of public health. Today, we recognize that most injuries, like diseases, are not accidental but predictable, preventable, and controllable.

[1]National Center for Injury Prevention and Control, Centers for Disease Control and Prevention, Atlanta, Georgia.
[2]Health Resources and Services Administration, Rockville, Maryland.
[3]Eunice Kennedy Shriver National Institute of Child Health and Human Development, National Institutes of Health, Rockville, Maryland.
[4]National Organizations for Youth Safety, Gainesville, Virginia.
[5]American Academy of Pediatrics, Elk Grove Village, Illinois. (Currently with The Injury Prevention and Research Center, Children's Memorial Hospital, Chicago, IL.)
[6]Safe Kids Worldwide, Washington, DC.

Approaches that include injury surveillance, risk factor identification, intervention development and implementation, and dissemination of effective strategies are the bedrock of public health.

Is There a Role for Public Health?

A major goal of public health is to help young people achieve healthy independence by increasing the number who are healthy, safe, and productive members of society (Centers for Disease Control and Prevention 2007). Public health professionals can contribute to reducing child and adolescent injuries by developing and evaluating injury prevention programs, supporting human and capital investments in child injury prevention, improving child injury surveillance systems, and creating comprehensive trauma care systems to improve injury outcomes and rehabilitation for injured children and youth. The chapters throughout Dr. Liller's book echo these themes.

Public health strategies can be used to encourage individual behavior change, engineer safer environments, and provide an effective and efficient emergency response system to intervene early when there is an injury. Public health can ensure that safe choices are more available in society and can be a major contributor to changing social norms—for example, by decreasing public acceptance of child maltreatment. Public health can also contribute to policy change through stricter regulations—for example, requiring helmet use for every cyclist. These opportunities to save lives result when public health works with law enforcement, product safety, and consumer advocates to raise the bar on safety (Sleet, Ballesteros, and Borse 2010).

Our organizations are committed to translation of science into effective programs and policies that prevent child and adolescent injuries and violence and minimize their consequences. The chapters in this book are fundamental to this mission because it is only through accurate data that we can make sound decisions about investing in prevention strategies.

This APHA book illustrates what is possible in child injury prevention and the best way to proceed to save more lives. As Dr. Degutis notes in her Foreword to this book, investments in childhood injury prevention are currently only a small fraction of investments made to prevent major childhood diseases, and this balance must change for us to succeed in reducing the injury problem (Hyder, Peden, and Krug 2009).

To address this problem, the Centers for Disease Control and Prevention and more than 65 of its partners are developing a National Action Plan for Child Injury Prevention (NAP). The plan, to be released in 2012, will call for specific actions in data and surveillance, research, policy and legislation, education and training, media and communications, health systems, and health care to reduce unintentional child and adolescent injuries. Planning efforts for national initiatives are also under way to prevent child maltreatment and youth violence. In addition, specific plans for the highest risk areas are also in formulation, such as Vision 20/20 (2008), a national strategy for reducing fire loss through advocacy, technologic innovation, and public education; changing the culture of the fire service; and strengthening codes and standards.

A Global Commitment to Child Injury Prevention

Many public health agencies throughout the world are making large national investments in preventing injuries, whether through research, improved road traffic safety practices, school education programs, anti-bullying campaigns, or improved trauma care systems (Peden et al. 2008). Our challenge is to ensure that these investments are used wisely and based on the best available evidence (Doll et al. 2007). For example, we still need well-designed research on theory-based interventions for children and their parents and more program evaluation to determine "what works" to prevent injuries to children and youth. We know little about effective violence prevention strategies, and what we already know is hard to adapt for application in a wide variety of settings, cultures, and communities. Nevertheless, we are committed to lowering the rates of childhood unintentional injury and violence, and we are working domestically and globally to achieve this.

Youths have galvanized support among their peers for injury prevention in the United States through the National Organizations for Youth Safety,[7] in Canada through SMARTRISK,[8] and in Europe through Youth for Road Safety.[9] In 2007, the World Health Organization organized the first World Youth Assembly for Road Safety,[10] held at the United Nations in Geneva, Switzerland, where 500 young people from more than 100 countries adopted the Youth Declaration for Road Safety. They committed to take practical measures to improve road safety and called on adults to play their part as parents and leaders.

Partnerships: The Way Forward

We recognize that the child injury crisis cannot be solved by public health alone. To address the problem comprehensively, we need families, educators, corporations, elected officials, local governments, coalitions, and nongovernmental organizations to assist. An example of an exciting partnership is *Start Safe: A Fire and Burn Safety Program for Preschoolers and Their Families,* created by the nonprofit Home Safety Council (2011) (which recently merged with Safe Kids Worldwide) in partnership with the National Head Start Association. Funded by the U.S. Department of Homeland Security, *Start Safe*[11] pairs local fire and burn safety experts with Head Start classroom teachers to deliver fire prevention lessons and safety devices to preschool-aged children (an audience at increased risk of dying in a fire) and to the parents and caregivers who can keep them safe. These are the kind of partnerships that must be built and sustained, going forward.

Engineers, social workers, health and safety professionals, developmental psychologists, and young people need to be involved in this work and in our research to uncover practical solutions. Playground and pool manufacturers, city planners, and architects can take an active interest in child injury prevention and have an important role in developing structural solutions to the problem.

Injuries to children and youths do not occur in isolation. All of us can influence the behavioral risks, design of environments, social interactions at home and school, safety of products and vehicles, construction of housing, and social norms that affect injury and violence. Risk taking and gaining independence are important parts of child development. Our goal is not to stifle growth, but rather to provide opportunities for children and adolescents to learn to make safe decisions within the context of controlled and developmentally appropriate levels of risk. Individuals and families have some responsibility for this, but so do governments and society.

What will be needed is for all civil society to partner in creating a "culture of safety." To this end, child injury prevention and safety promotion are everybody's business. The biggest obstacle to making fundamental societal changes in injury patterns is not a shortage of funds, but lack of political will; the health sector is well positioned to build the support and develop the partnerships required for change (Frieden 2010; Friel et al. 2009).

It is our hope that Dr. Liller's text will inspire public health professionals around the world to look at the potential for improving child health through injury prevention. What better future can we offer the children of the world than for them to lead healthy and productive lives without the threat of injury and violence.

[7]Web site available at http://www.noys.org.

[8]Web site available at http://www.smartrisk.ca.

[9]Web site available at http://youthforroadsafety.org.

[10]Web site available at http://www.who.int/roadsafety/week/en/index.html.

[11]Web site available at http://www.homesafetycouncil.org/startsafeprogram.

Disclaimer: The views expressed are those of the author and do not necessarily represent the official views of the Centers for Disease Control and Prevention, Health Resources and Services Administration, National Institutes of Health, Safe Kids Worldwide, and the American Academy of Pediatrics.

References

Borse N, Gilchrist J, Dellinger A, et al. 2008. CDC Childhood Injury Report: Patterns of Unintentional Injuries Among 0-19 Year Olds in the United States, 2000-2006. Atlanta, GA: Centers for Disease Control and Prevention.

Centers for Disease Control and Prevention. 2007. Goal action plan for adolescent health. Unpublished Manuscript, Version 1, October 1, 2007.

Doll L, Bonzo S, Mercy J, Sleet D, editors. 2007. *Handbook on Injury and Violence Prevention.* New York: Kluwer.

Frieden R. 2010. A framework for public health action: the health impact pyramid. *Am J Public Health.* 11:590–595.

Friel S, Bell R, Houweling T, Marmot M. 2009. Calling all Don Quixotes and Sancho Panzas: achieving the dream of global health equity through practical action on the social determinants of health. *Glob Health Promot.* (Suppl 1):9–13.

Home Safety Council. 2011. *Start Safe: A Fire and Burn Safety Program for Preschoolers and Their Families,* Washington, DC: Home Safety Council (now Safe Kids Worldwide).

Hyder AA, Peden M, Krug E. 2009. Child health must include injury prevention. *Lancet.* 373:102–103.

Institution of Fire Engineers. 2008. *Vision 20/20: National Strategies for Fire Loss Prevention.* Alexandria, VA: Institution of Fire Engineers.

Krug EG, Sharma GK, Lozano R. 2000. The global burden of injuries. *Am J Public Health.* 90:523–526.

Peden M, Oyegbite K, Ozanne-Smith J, et al., editors. 2008. *World Report on Child Injury Prevention.* Geneva: World Health Organization.

Sleet DA, Ballesteros MF, Borse NN. 2010. A review of unintentional injuries in adolescents. *Annu Rev Public Health.* 31:195–212.

List of Contributors

Editor: Karen D. Liller, PhD

Karen D. Liller, PhD, is Dean of the Graduate School and Associate Vice President for Research and Innovation at the University of South Florida (USF). She received her PhD from the USF and is also a tenured full professor specializing in public health and children's injury prevention in the College of Public Health. Dr. Liller also holds a joint academic appointment in the Department of Orthopaedics and Sports Medicine. Dr. Liller was named one of the top 15 national women scholars in health education and health promotion, has published extensively in peer-reviewed publications, edits the text *Injury Prevention for Children and Adolescents: Research, Practice, and Advocacy,* and serves on several prestigious advisory boards that focus on higher education and injury prevention. She is the co-author on several of this book's chapters and the author of the Introduction and Chapter 16.

List of Contributors

Foreword

Linda C. Degutis

Linda C. Degutis, DrPH, MSN, is the Director of the National Center for Injury Prevention and Control (NCIPC), Centers for Disease Control and Prevention (CDC).

Prologue

David A. Sleet, Chester L. Pogostin, Captain Stephanie Bryn, Lynne Haverkos, Sandy Spavone, Rebecca Levin, Meri-K Appy, and Angela Mickalide

David A. Sleet, PhD, MA, FAAHB, is the Associate Director for Science, Division of Unintentional Injury Prevention, NCIPC, CDC. He is senior advisor to the division on matters of science and policy.

Chester L. Pogostin, DVM, MPA, Former Deputy Division Director, NCIPC, CDC.

Captain Stephanie Bryn, MPH, Former Director, Injury and Violence Prevention, Maternal and Child Health Bureau, Health Resources and Services Administration (HRSA).

Lynne Haverkos, MD, MPH, Program Director, Pediatric Behavior and Health Promotion, Eunice Kennedy Shriver National Institute of Child Health and Human Development, National Institutes of Health (NIH).

Sandy Spavone, MPH, Executive Director at National Organizations for Youth Safety (NOYS).

Rebecca Levin, MPH, Senior Manager, Injury, Violence, and Poison Prevention Initiatives, Division of Safety and Health Promotion, American Academy of Pediatrics (AAP).

Meri-K Appy, BA, Former President, and Angela Mickalide, PhD, CHES, Director of Research and Programs, Safe Kids Worldwide.

Introduction

Karen D. Liller

Karen D. Liller, PhD, Dean of the Graduate School and Associate Vice President for Research and Innovation, USF.

Chapter 1: Epidemiology of Injuries Among Children and Adolescents: Focus on Unintentional Injuries

Michael F. Ballesteros and David A. Sleet

Michael F. Ballesteros, PhD, MS, is the Deputy Associate Director for Science and an epidemiologist in the Division of Unintentional Injury Prevention at the CDC's NCIPC. His work includes conducting research and developing prevention programs in the areas of child injury, global road safety, residential fires, and poisonings.

David A. Sleet, PhD, MA, FAAHB, Associate Director for Science, Division of Unintentional Injury Prevention, NCIPC, CDC.

Chapter 2: The Cost of Child and Adolescent Injuries and the Savings From Prevention

Ted R. Miller, A. Eric Finkelstein, Eduard Zaloshnja, and Delia Hendrie

Ted R. Miller, PhD, is a Senior Research Scientist and economist at the Pacific Institute for Research and Evaluation in Calverton, Maryland, with approximately 30 years of experience estimating injury costs and the savings from prevention.

A. Eric Finkelstein, PhD, MHA, Deputy Director, Associate Professor, Health Services and Systems Research Program, Duke-NUS Graduate Medical School, Singapore.

Eduard Zaloshnja, PhD, economist at the Pacific Institute for Research and Evaluation.

Delia Hendrie, MEcon, is a Senior Research Fellow and health economist at the Centre for Population Health Research at Curtin University in Australia.

Chapter 3: Hazards Associated With Common Nursery Products

Carol Pollack-Nelson and Dorothy Drago

Carol Pollack-Nelson, PhD, is a human factors psychologist, specializing in consumer product safety. As an independent consultant and researcher, she works on a wide range of product safety issues affecting children, including supervision practices and identification of hazardous juvenile products.

Dorothy A. Drago, MA, MPH, consumer product safety consultant (Drago Expert Services).

Chapter 4: Motor Vehicle and Pedestrian Injuries Among Children and Adolescents: Risk and Prevention

Bruce G. Simons-Morton and Laura J. Caccavale

Bruce Simons-Morton, EdD, MPH, is Senior Investigator and Chief of the Prevention Research Branch at the National Institute of Child Health and Human Development, where he directs a program of research on child and adolescent health behavior. His current research emphasizes the causes and prevention of motor vehicle crashes among novice young drivers.

Laura J. Caccavale, BA, Research Fellow, Prevention Research Branch, Eunice Kennedy Shriver National Institute of Child Health and Human Development.

Chapter 5: Home Injuries

Eileen M. McDonald, Deborah C. Girasek, and Andrea Carlson Gielen

Eileen M. McDonald, MS, is an Associate Scientist at the Johns Hopkins Bloomberg School of Public Health, where she is affiliated with the Johns Hopkins Center for Injury Research and Policy. Her research focuses on the application of innovative health education methods, health communication technology, and other hospital- and community-based interventions aimed at reducing pediatric injuries.

Deborah C. Girasek, PhD, MPH, Associate Professor and Director of Social and Behavioral Sciences in the Department of Preventive Medicine, Uniformed Services University of the Health Sciences.

Andrea Carlson Gielen, ScD, ScM, CHES, Professor, Director, Center for Injury Research and Policy, the Johns Hopkins Bloomberg School of Public Health.

Chapter 6: Adolescent Employment and Injury in the United States

Carol W. Runyan, Michael D. Schulman, and Lawrence E. Scholl

Carol W. Runyan, PhD, MPH, was the Director of the University of North Carolina (UNC) Injury Prevention Research Center and Professor of Health Behavior and Health Education at the Gillings School of Global Public Health and of Pediatrics in the UNC School of Medicine at the time this manuscript was prepared. She is currently Professor of Epidemiology and of Community and Behavioral Health at the Colorado School of Public Health and affiliated with the Colorado Injury Control Research Center. Her research is focused on young worker safety.

Michael D. Schulman, PhD, William Neal Reynolds Distinguished Professor and Alumni Distinguished Graduate Professor, Departments of 4-H Youth Development Family & Consumer Sciences and Sociology and Anthropology, North Carolina State University, Raleigh, and Adjunct Professor of Health Behavior and Health Education at the UNC Gillings School of Global Public Health. Dr. Schulman is also affiliated with the UNC Injury Prevention Research Center.

Lawrence E. Scholl, MPH, doctoral student, Department of Health Behavior and Health Education at the UNC Gillings School of Global Public Health, and research associate with the UNC Injury Prevention Research Center.

Chapter 7: Partnering With Schools To Prevent Injuries and Violence

Ellen R. Schmidt and Susan Frelick Goekler

Ellen R. Schmidt, MS, OT is Senior Project Director at the Education Development Center and Assistant Director for the Children's Safety Network National Injury and Violence Prevention Resource Center. She worked at the U.S. Consumer Product Safety Commission.

Susan Frelick Goekler, PhD, MCHES, Former Director of the American School Health Association and now Executive Director with the Directors of Health Promotion and Education, Washington, DC.

Chapter 8: Childhood Agricultural Injuries

Barbara C. Lee and Barbara Marlenga

Barbara C. Lee, PhD, is a senior scientist with the Marshfield Clinic Research Foundation, Marshfield, Wisconsin, where she directs the National Farm Medicine Center and the National Institute for Occupational Safety and Health-funded National Children's Center for Rural and Agricultural Health and Safety.

Barbara Marlenga, PhD, is a research scientist with the National Farm Medicine Center.

Chapter 9: Sports and Recreational Injuries

Stephen W. Marshall, Julie Gilchrist, Gitanjali Taneja, and Karen D. Liller

Stephen W. Marshall, PhD, is a Professor in the Department of Epidemiology, Gillings School of Global Public Health, at the UNC at Chapel Hill. He has co-appointments in the Departments of Orthopedics and Exercise and Sport Science and is Director of Epidemiology at the Datalys Center for Sports Injury Research and Prevention. He also is currently Interim Director of the UNC Injury Prevention Research Center.

Commander Julie Gilchrist, MD, Medical Epidemiologist, Division of Unintentional Injury Prevention, NCIPC, CDC.

Gitanjali Taneja, PhD, National Children's Study, Eunice Kennedy Shriver National Institute of Child Health and Human Development, NIH.

Karen D. Liller, PhD, Dean of the Graduate School and Associate Vice President for Research and Innovation, USF.

Chapter 10: Water-Related Injuries of Children and Adolescents

Linda Quan, Karen D. Liller, and Elizabeth Bennett

Linda Quan, MD, is Professor of Pediatrics at the University of Washington School of Medicine and a pediatric emergency medicine physician at Seattle Children's Hospital, Seattle, Washington. Her major areas of research are in pediatric drowning, pediatric cardiac resuscitation, and prehospital care of the pediatric patient.

Karen D. Liller, PhD, Dean of the Graduate School and Associate Vice President for Research and Innovation, USF.

Elizabeth Bennett, MPH, MCHES, Director of Advocacy, Partnerships and Guest Services, Seattle Children's Hospital, Seattle, Washington.

Chapter 11: Child Physical Abuse and Neglect

David DiLillo, Rosalita C. Maldonado, and Laura E. Watkins

David DiLillo, PhD, is a professor of clinical psychology at the University of Nebraska–Lincoln. His primary research interests are in the areas of child maltreatment and family violence. Within those areas, he is particularly interested in the long-term adjustment of adults who have experienced various forms of childhood trauma and maltreatment (e.g., sexual abuse, physical abuse, neglect, and exposure to domestic violence).

Rosalita C. Maldonado, MA, doctoral student in clinical psychology, University of Nebraska–Lincoln.

Laura E. Watkins, MA, doctoral student in clinical psychology, University of Nebraska–Lincoln.

Chapter 12: Firearm Injuries

Shannon Frattaroli, Katherine A. Vittes, Sara B. Johnson, and Stephen P. Teret

Shannon Frattaroli, PhD, MPH, is an Assistant Professor at the Johns Hopkins Bloomberg School of Public Health, where she is affiliated with the Johns Hopkins Center for Injury Research and Policy and the Johns Hopkins Center for Gun Policy and Research. Her research interests include understanding the role of policy in improving the health of populations, with particular attention to the effects of injury and alcohol prevention policies, the implementation of public health policies and programs, and the role of advocacy and communities in the policy and intervention processes.

Katherine A. Vittes, PhD, MPH, Research Associate, the Johns Hopkins Bloomberg School of Public Health.

Sara B. Johnson, PhD, MPH, Assistant Professor, the Johns Hopkins Bloomberg School of Public Health and the Johns Hopkins School of Medicine.

Stephen P. Teret, JD, MPH, Associate Dean and Professor, the Johns Hopkins Bloomberg School of Public Health.

Chapter 13: Youth Suicide

Lloyd Potter

Lloyd Potter, PhD, MPH, is a Professor of Applied Demography and Director of the Institute for Demographic and Socioeconomic Research at the University of Texas at San Antonio. His work focuses on conducting policy relevant research on topics related to public health and population.

Chapter 14: A Global Perspective on Injuries Among Children and Adolescents

Andrés Villaveces and Catherine Vladutiu

Andrés Villaveces, MD, PhD, MPH, is a Research Assistant Professor of Epidemiology at UNC Chapel Hill Gillings School of Global Public Health and core faculty at the UNC-Injury Prevention Research Center. He was Medical Officer at the Department of Injuries and Violence Prevention at the World Health Organization (Geneva, Switzerland) and Scientific Chief of Clinics in Quality of Care at the Geneva University Hospitals.

Catherine Vladutiu, MPH, Graduate Doctoral Student, Department of Epidemiology, UNC Chapel Hill Gillings School of Global Public Health, and Research Assistant, UNC Injury Prevention Research Center.

Chapter 15: Moving Child and Adolescent Injury Prevention and Control Research into Practice: A Framework for Translation

Michael Yonas, Shannon Frattaroli, Karen D. Liller, Ann Christiansen, Andrea Carlson Gielen, Stephen Hargarten, and Lenora M. Olson

Michael Yonas, DrPH, MPH, is an Assistant Professor in the Department of Family Medicine at the University of Pittsburgh, concentrating on the health and safety needs of children and adolescents, with a primary focus on health disparities, asthma, and the role of neighborhood stressors, such as violence.

Shannon Frattaroli, PhD, MPH, Assistant Professor, Center for Injury Research and Policy, the Johns Hopkins Bloomberg School of Public Health.

Karen D. Liller, PhD, Dean of the Graduate School and Associate Vice President for Research and Innovation, USF.

Ann Christiansen, MPH, Assistant Director, Medical College of Wisconsin, Injury Research Center.

Andrea Carlson Gielen, ScD, ScM, CHES, Professor and Director, Center for Injury Research and Policy, the Johns Hopkins Bloomberg School of Public Health.

Stephen Hargarten, MD, MPH, Professor and Chair, Medical College of Wisconsin, Department of Emergency Medicine.

Lenora M. Olson, PhD, Associate Professor, Intermountain Injury Control Research Center, Department of Pediatrics, University of Utah.

Chapter 16: Conclusions and Recommendations

Karen D. Liller

Karen D. Liller, PhD, Dean of the Graduate School and Associate Vice President for Research and Innovation, USF.

Appendix A: Selected Historical Timeline for Injury Prevention and Control

Les Fisher and Andrés Villaveces

Les Fisher, MPH, is a seasoned veteran injury researcher, practitioner, and educator and serves as a safety/management consultant and archivist for the Injury Control and Emergency Health Services Section of the American Public Health Association.

Andrés Villaveces, MD, PhD, MPH, is a Research Assistant Professor of Epidemiology at UNC Chapel Hill Gillings School of Global Public Health and core faculty at the UNC-Injury Prevention Research Center.

Appendix B: Resources

Updates by Si-won Jang, Doctoral Student in the USF College of Public Health.

Appendix C: Leading Causes of Death and Nonfatal Injury

Introduction

Karen D. Liller, PhD[1]

I am very pleased and excited to bring to you the second edition of *Injury Prevention for Children and Adolescents: Research, Practice, and Advocacy.* Within this volume, each chapter has been updated to provide you the latest data and relevant information per topic area, including incorporating research, practice, and advocacy with recommendations for future work. We have retained that all important "face of injury" component that we hope allows the injuries to become much more real to the readers. We have added new chapters that focus on the global toll of injuries on children and adolescents and translational research—two topics of paramount importance in the injury prevention field, the former in terms of the huge toll that road traffic and other injuries have on children globally and the latter in terms of the real need for injury prevention researchers to translate their findings to practice in a more far-reaching, timely, and comprehensive manner.

Also, many chapters include resources for further information, and the Appendices found in the back of the book have been updated to expand the historic timeline, resources, and data charts from the National Center for Injury Prevention and Control. We continue to define adolescence in the text (unless otherwise noted with particular ages or age groups) as the time between the onset of puberty and full maturity. As was important in the first edition, readers need to be aware that chapter authors used various reference sources to report morbidity, mortality, and other information pertaining to specific injuries and age groups. Therefore, data may vary from chapter to chapter, making it all that more important to report sources when citing data from the text. A brief description of what readers will find in each of the chapters follows.

Injuries continue to claim the lives and inflict harm on children and adolescents in the United States in proportions that are clearly unacceptable. The latest data reported from the National Center for Injury Prevention and Control show that in the United States approximately 14,000 children were killed in 2007 as the result of injuries and approximately nine million suffered nonfatal injuries. Leading causes of injury morbidity and mortality for children and adolescents continue to be motor vehicle related, violence, drownings, poisonings, falls, suffocations, and burns. But these numbers pale to what is occurring globally. According to the World Health Organization (2008) injuries and violence are responsible for over 900,000 deaths in individuals under the age of 18 each year. Most of these injuries are unintentional. Deaths are just the tip of the iceberg however as tens of millions of children are hospitalized for nonfatal inuries each year. Risk factors continue to be poverty, behaviors, the environment, and lack of access to medical care. These injuries can be prevented, and we have many of the tools to do so.

In Chapter 1, Ballesteros and Sleet review the leading causes of injury morbidity and mortality among children and adolescents, including the injury setting and effective prevention strategies. As shown in this chapter and others, alcohol continues to be a cross-cutting predisposing risk factor for injuries. No single solution will be effective. Ecologic approaches that include behavioral and environmental strategies are necessary to fully address and combat child and adolescent injuries.

[1]University of South Florida Graduate School and College of Public Health, Tampa, Florida.

An extremely important factor related to child and adolescent injury is cost and value of prevention. In Chapter 2, Miller and colleagues use analyses of national and state data sets to present data on frequency, severity, costs, and quality of life losses associated with childhood injury in the year 2000. Childhood injuries in 2000 resulted in an estimated $24 billion in lifetime medical spending and $82 billion in present and future work losses. The chapter again uses the year 2000 data because overall incidence of children's injuries in more recent years is similar and overall costs have varied only because of inflation. The savings due to several child and adolescent injury interventions have been updated in Table 2.8 and continue to show that several injury prevention strategies reviewed in this chapter are comparable or often better than the cost-effectiveness of several other widely implemented child and adolescent illness prevention measures. This chapter should be used by policymakers and others in determining how to allocate already scarce resources to those strategies that will most favorably improve the health of children and youth.

Once again, a chapter needed to be included that focuses on our youngest population—those infants and children who use nursery products. Chapter 3 begins with the story of Charlie Horn, whose tragic death caused by a tipped dresser inspired the nonprofit organization Charlie's House, whose work has saved the lives of countless children. As in the previous edition, Pollack-Nelson and Drago take a detailed look at nursery product injuries and their standards and regulations. New developments include the exciting news that, through the 2008 enactment of the Consumer Product Safety Improvement Act, mandatory standards will be required on a variety of nursery products along with the requirement of a postage prepaid registration card with the sale of these products—something long overdue. As the authors state, the work of the Consumer Product Safety Commission since the passage of the Consumer Product Safety Improvement Act will have a dramatic effect on the number of consumer injuries and fatalities. Advocacy information is also provided to help round out this very important chapter.

The leading cause of injury death for children and adolescents is motor vehicle related, including pedestrian injuries. In Chapter 4, Simons-Morton and Caccavale review the statistics surrounding these injuries, the pertinent risk factors with new information on the laws of crash causation, and the comprehensive injury prevention approaches, including technology and legislation. The authors divide this chapter into two sections—one focused on child passenger safety and one focused on young drivers. Pedestrian injuries and deaths are also covered. Important recommendations for research, practice, and advocacy are provided throughout the chapter.

Young children spend much of their time in the home environment, and this setting creates the opportunity for injuries to occur. In Chapter 5, McDonald, Girasek, and Gielen report detailed information pertaining to choking/suffocation, fire and burns, poisoning, falls, and animal bites. This information includes background statistics, risk factors, prevention and advocacy efforts, and related research. Interspersed throughout the chapter are stories of children who have suffered from these injuries. The information on animal bites is very important because these types of injuries continue to be a great public health concern. The chapter provides many updates for each of these injuries and their prevention. For example, advances in fire safety, including the use of fire-safe cigarettes and residential fire sprinklers, are described. As for the future, the authors point to the need for more research done on child supervision and improved surveillance tools, and the continued importance for organizations to address home safety for children.

In Chapter 6, Runyan, Schulman, and Scholl focus on adolescent employment and injury in the United States. They provide information not only on the settings, risk factors, and dangers of teen employment but also on the important role work plays in the life course perspective. The chapter again begins with vignettes of real teens who were injured on the job to bring home the risks associated with adolescent employment. The information provided by the authors clearly shows that teens who work often receive little safety training and poor supervision. More safety interventions are needed (both in the workplace and in schools), and they need to be evaluated for efficacy. There is a strong role for parents, community coalitions, and the media in promoting safety of the work environment for teens.

In Chapter 7, Schmidt and Frelick Goekler detail and update injuries that occur in school settings and include new information on bullying and other topics, such as behavioral and developmental factors that influence children, and resultant injuries. The chapter begins with important case profiles of school injuries. The important roles for the community, school system, and public health are highlighted. New information on child care provided to children at schools is also included. Future steps are provided that focus on the recognition that a noninjured child can learn better in school, the improvement of reporting mechanisms, the evaluation of programs, the psychosocial and physical environment changes, the policy changes, and the development of partnerships between public health and educational systems.

Many children in the United States not only work in agricultural settings but also live in this environment, increasing their potential for injuries. In Chapter 8, Lee and Marlenga begin with several actual child profiles reported in newspapers. As stated by the authors, these are "just a sampling of the tragedies that occur on the 2.2 million farms and ranches across the United States." The authors go on to report that "The fatalities have striking similarities, such as siblings working together, inadequate adult supervision, and farm machinery designed for adults who willingly choose to work in one of our nation's most dangerous occupations. Beyond the news clippings is the unreported psychologic, social, and financial toll that often reaps a devastating impact on survivors, especially parents."

We continue to include in this updated chapter information on morbidity and mortality, risk factors, research, and interventions related to the National Institute of Occupational Safety and Health initiatives, the role of the North American Guidelines for Children's Agricultural Tasks, non-work-related interventions, the need for advocacy, and future recommendations, including enhanced partnerships with agricultural organizations and businesses.

Chapter 9 focuses on child and adolescent sport and recreational injuries. Marshall and colleagues describe an all too common story of a young athlete (Tracy) suffering from a sports-related concussion that leads to a life forever changed. See this story at the You-Tube link provided in the chapter. This chapter details leading child and adolescent sport injuries in the United States, including team sports (basketball, football, baseball/softball, soccer, hockey, and cheerleading) and more individual sports (playground, bicycle, skiing/snowboarding, trampolines, all-terrain vehicles, and in-line skating/roller sports). New to this chapter is information on equestrian injuries and surveillance systems to capture injuries in high school sports. Also, because of the new information on cross-cutting topics that affect several sports and recreational activities, there are now sections on concussions, heat illness, and anterior cruciate ligament injuries. Research and effective interventions are highlighted, in addition to those groups and organizations that advocate for safer sports and recreational activities. With these groups and parent involvement, advocacy can be enhanced, thereby decreasing the number of these injuries.

Because drownings are the second major cause of unintentional injury death in children aged less than 15 years, Chapter 10 is devoted to water-related injuries. Quan, Liller, and Bennett begin the chapter again with the heartbreaking account of Preston Thomas de Ibern's death that was written by his mother, Carole Y. de Ibern. This story of Preston's life and death not only brings a "face" to this injury but also details the common risk factors, the sequelae, the long fight to survive, and the importance of advocacy efforts to pass pool safety legislation. The chapter continues with updated information pertaining to morbidity and mortality; risk factors, including diseases such as epilepsy; current research and prevention efforts; important recommendations for further research; guidelines for practice; and continued advocacy. The new definition of drowning is included along with information on the efficacy of swimming lessons and pool and spa entrapment injuries. The chapter ends again with updated information concerning personal watercraft injuries.

Three chapters of the text focus on violence-related injuries. These chapters have been grouped together on the basis of the theme of violence and not because many of the interventions and research recommendations provided in the previous chapters do not also pertain to these injuries. Although many individuals in the injury prevention field continue to divide injuries into unintentional (done without harmful intent) and violent (done with harmful intent), I believe there are many common risk factors related to both of these categories, and artificial divisions only separate those individuals and organizations who work in these areas. If risk factors such as poverty and lack of social support, and behavioral issues such as substance abuse are ameliorated, both unintentional and violence-related injuries should decrease.

In Chapter 11, DiLillo, Maldonado, and Watkins tell the very disturbing story of little Sebastian Duffek and his untimely and brutal death caused by child abuse. This chapter continues with a detailed review of morbidity/mortality and risk factor information, definitions, up-to-date research findings and prevention approaches, treatment mechanisms, and the crucial role for advocacy efforts. Recommendations for the future include the continued need for more comprehensive etiologic models of child abuse and neglect, a consensus on abuse and neglect definitions, connections between researchers and practitioners, and unrelenting perseverance in keeping the issues of abuse and neglect at the top of the policymakers' agendas.

In Chapter 12, Frattaroli and colleagues address firearm injuries. This chapter begins with the story of Anthony, who believed that his father's semiautomatic pistol was not loaded when he pointed it and fired it at his best friend, Eric, who later died as the result of the injuries. Anthony and Eric were simply playing, and Anthony thought the gun was safe after he removed the magazine or clip that held the ammunition. However, a round remained in the chamber. The authors state that, even though this story was also used in the first edition of the text, its description continues to be a "relevant and powerful example of the need for injury prevention professionals to continue to engage in research, practice, and advocacy to prevent firearm injuries." This chapter continues with a detailed examination of the nature of firearm injury in the United States, morbidity, cost figures, and risk factors. Highlighted in this chapter are the new Supreme Court rulings that reversed 125 years of case law on the interpretation of the meaning and reach of the Second Amendment to the U.S. Constitution. Now states and localities are within their legal right to enforce that the Second Amendment confers an individual right to own handguns. The authors believe that these rulings will be factors in state and local gun policy considerations now and in the future. The chapter includes up-to-date research, education, and advocacy efforts and continues to strongly support the need for injury prevention researchers, practitioners, and advocates working collaboratively to bring about sustained change.

In Chapter 13, Potter addresses the critical injury of suicide and suicidal behavior among our young population. Up-to-date information on suicide-related morbidity and mortality and risk and protective factors are provided. Individual factors, family and close relationships, and community and societal-related factors must be considered. Current and future issues related to research, practice, and advocacy are found in addition to the need for integrating research, practice, and advocacy agendas. Community-level change must be sought by public health and injury prevention professionals to effectively decrease suicide and suicidal behavior among our young adults.

The last two new chapters of the text focus on global injuries and the translation of injury research to practice. These chapters are critical because we now are a global society, and although we have made important strides in developed nations in reducing injuries and deaths, these interventions do not often translate into success in the developing world.

In Chapter 14, Villaveces and Vladutiu describe the global toll of injuries on children and adolescents. This chapter describes the sad stories of Anand, Marcela, and Leila as they confront the realities of living in impoverished settings and the dangers within. Within this chapter, the reader will learn about violence and unintentional injuries affecting children and adolescents and related strategies for intervention. Crucial to these efforts will be the knowledge transfer and training that must occur so that children worldwide can benefit.

A mission for this text is to again reach not only academicians and students but also practitioners. As we learn to better translate our injury prevention research to various population groups, we must work as a unit because our strengths and contributions as a whole greatly outweigh what we can accomplish alone.

In Chapter 15, Yonas and colleagues discuss translating research to action. The authors call attention to the need for translational research by highlighting motor vehicle injuries and violence using a proposed translational research framework. Key concepts of the framework include translation, implementation, dissemination, and diffusion. A comparison of clinical and injury prevention and control models for translational process and research is provided. The need for this type of research is paramount in the injury prevention field, and the authors report they hope the proposed framework generates much interdisciplinary discussion and the development of a common understanding to further translation of injury prevention and control to real practice. Without understanding how to most effectively translate research to action the growth and sophistication of the injury prevention and control field will be impeded.

As we move forward in the field, we will need to continue expanding on known models, such as the Haddon Matrix, the Haddon Countermeasures, the public health approach, and the role of behavior change frameworks to reach populations with tested interventions for injuries that have existed for decades and for those that will occur in the future. We will continue to recognize the importance of contributing contextual factors to injury outcomes so that an ecologic approach to injury prevention can be developed and implemented (McClure 2010; Pickett et al. 2010). The translational research movement will need to be further elucidated, tested, and used broadly, so we approach these interventions with the sophistication necessary to achieve lasting results. Then, major questions will be the following: Will our interventions be effective globally? If not, how then can we tailor them for success? How do we reach groups that have been resistant to prevention messages? Are we preparing a sufficient number of researchers and practitioners to handle future needs?

As you read this book, I hope you become intrigued with the data, research, evaluations, policies, advocacy activities, and other tangible information. However, what is important is how we focus these elements on the faces of injury—those children and adolescents who have suffered. It is for them that this work becomes that much more important and urgent. I hope you learn much from the information that lies ahead and are able to put it to exemplary use in your research, practice, and advocacy efforts now and in the future.

References

Centers for Disease Control and Prevention 2010. *Injury and Violence Prevention Control.* Available at: http://www.cdc.gov/injury/index.html. Accessed November 30, 2010.

McClure RJ. 2010. Injury risk and prevention in context. *Inj Prev.* 16:361–362. Epub 2010 Oct 24.

Pickett W, Hagel LM, Day AG,et al. 2010. Determinants of agricultural injury: a novel application of population health theory. *Inj Prev.* 16:376–382.

World Health Organization. 2008. *World Health Organization Report on Child Injury Prevention.* Available at: http://whqlibdoc.who.int/publications/2008/9789241563574_eng.pdf. Accessed August 26, 2010.

Chapter 1

Epidemiology of Injuries Among Children and Adolescents: Focus on Unintentional Injuries

Michael F. Ballesteros, PhD, MS[1] *and David A. Sleet, PhD, MA, FAAHB*[1]

A major health threat facing young people today is injury and violence. Injuries may cause temporary pain and inconvenience for some, but for others, injury can lead to disability, chronic pain, and a change in lifestyle. Understanding the public health burden, who is at risk, and the epidemiology of injury is critical to its prevention.

In 2007, injury and violence (i.e., homicide and suicide) accounted for 31.0% of all deaths to those under 20 years of age. When infants are removed, injury and violence accounted for 61.7% of all deaths, and three of the top four leading causes of death were unintentional injury, homicide, and suicide (Centers for Disease Control and Prevention 2010b).

While the focus of this chapter is on unintentional injuries, violence continues to be a public health problem for children and adolescents. In 2007, there were a total of 3320 homicides and 1665 suicides among individuals under 20 years of age; homicide and suicide were the second and third leading cause of death, respectively, for those 15–19 years of age (Table 1.1) (Centers for Disease Control and Prevention 2010b). Furthermore, in 2008, over 430,000 children and adolescents were treated in U.S. hospital emergency departments (EDs) for nonfatal assaults, and another 80,079 were treated for self-inflicted injuries (Centers for Disease Control and Prevention 2010b). Additional information on violence among children and adolescents can be found in other chapters of this book (See chapters on Firearm Injuries, Child Physical Abuse and Neglect, and Youth Suicide).

Overview of Unintentional Injuries

What were referred to for decades as "accidents" are now referred to as "injuries." Injuries are not the result of "accidents" or acts of fate; child injuries result from events that are both predictable and preventable. An *unintentional injury* is defined as "damage to the body resulting from acute exposure to thermal, mechanical, electrical, or chemical energy or from the absence of such essentials as heat or oxygen" (National Committee for Injury Prevention and Control [U.S.] 1989). Unintentional injuries include injuries from motor vehicle crashes, fires and burns, falls, drowning, poisoning, choking, suffocation, and animal bites.

Unintentional injury is responsible for almost half (42.5%) of all deaths to children between 1 and 19 years of age, killing and disabling young people in the prime of their lives (Centers for Disease Control and Prevention 2010b). In 2007, 11,560 children in the United States aged 0–19 years died from unintentional injuries—the equivalent of 32 deaths each day (Centers for

[1]Division of Unintentional Injury Prevention, National Center for Injury Prevention and Control, Centers for Disease Control and Prevention, Atlanta, Georgia

Table 1.1. The Five Leading Causes (and Number) of Childhood Deaths: United States, 2007

Rank	Age <1	Ages 1–4	Ages 5–9	Ages 10–14	Ages 15–19
1	Congenital Anomalies	Unintentional Injury	Unintentional Injury	Unintentional Injury	Unintentional Injury
	5785	1588	965	1229	6493
2	Short Gestation	Congenital Anomalies	Malignant Neoplasms	Malignant Neoplasms	Homicide
	4857	546	479	476	2224
3	SIDS	Homicide	Congenital Anomalies	Homicide	Suicide
	2453	398	196	213	1,481
4	Maternal Pregnancy Complications	Malignant Neoplasms	Homicide	Suicide	Malignant Neoplasms
	1769	364	133	180	673
5	Unintentional Injury	Heart Disease	Heart Disease	Congenital Anomalies	Heart Disease
	1285	173	110	178	346

Source: Data from National Center for Health Statistics (NCHS) Vital Statistics System for numbers of deaths; Bureau of Census for population estimates (Centers for Disease Control and Prevention 2010b).

Disease Control and Prevention 2010b). Of the five leading causes of death in ages 1–4, 5–9, 10–14, and 15–19, unintentional injury is ranked number one (Table 1.1).

Since 1999, the overall unintentional injury death rate has decreased by 10%. More substantial reductions have been seen among children aged 1–4, 5–9, and 10–14, with decreases of 22%, 31%, and 25%, respectively. In contrast, infants have seen their unintentional injury death rates increased by 35% over this same time period (Figure 1.1) (Centers for Disease Control and Prevention 2010b). As described later in this chapter, these differences across age groups are due to different trends in death rates by injury cause and age group.

Deaths only represent the most severe injuries that occur. In 2008, there were almost 8.8 million children and adolescents seen in U.S. EDs for an unintentional injury. Of these, 2.6% were either hospitalized or transferred to another health care facility for additional treatment. Almost 1.7 million more male children were seen in EDs than females, and ED rates were highest for the youngest and oldest age groups (Centers for Disease Control and Prevention 2010b).

Among children younger than 15, the most common injuries treated in EDs were for *falls* and *struck by or against* (being struck by, hit, or crushed or striking against a human, animal, or inanimate object other than a vehicle or machinery). Other leading injuries for younger children were *bites/stings* (a poisonous or nonpoisonous bite or sting through the skin, other than a dog bite) and *foreign body* (entrance of a foreign body into or through the eye or other natural body opening that does not block an airway or cause suffocation [asphyxia]). For 15- to 19-year-olds,

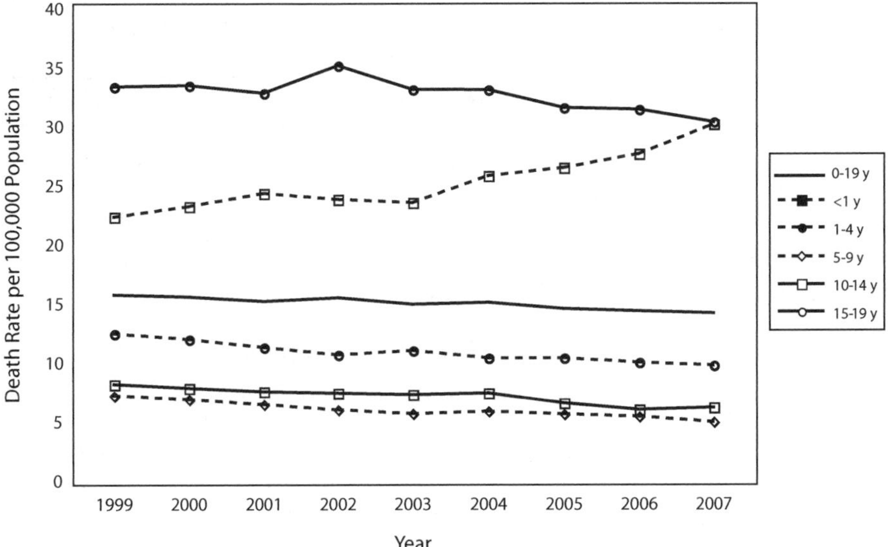

Figure 1.1. Trends in Unintentional Injury Death Rates Among Children 0–19 Years, by Age and Year: United States, 1999–2007

the most common injuries were *struck by or against, falls, overexertion, motor vehicle occupant,* and *cut or pierce* (see Table 1.2) (Centers for Disease Control and Prevention 2010b).

Costs

The total lifetime costs for unintentional injuries to children and adolescents were over $87 billion in 2000. These costs include direct medical costs, other resource costs (e.g., police, fire department, litigation), and work-loss costs (includes victims and family and friends who care for the injured). The cost per case was, on average, $5743. This varied depending on age, with the cost being $5278 for children ages 0–4 years, $4870 for 5–9, $5348 for 10–14, and $7266 for 15–19 (Miller et al. 2006).

Disparities in Morbidity and Mortality

Injury risk differs by gender and age. Regardless of age, more male children are killed from unintentional injuries than female. This difference is particularly striking for those ages 15–19, for whom the death rate for males is more than twice the rate for females. Injury death rates for infants and the oldest adolescents are over six times the rate for those ages 5–9 (Table 1.3) (Centers for Disease Control and Prevention 2010b).

Racial and ethnic disparities in injury are pronounced. Among all children, American Indians and Alaska Natives (AIs/ANs) and Blacks consistently had higher total injury death rates than Whites, Asia/Pacific Islanders, and Hispanics. These differences are most pronounced among infants. Among children less than 12 months old, unintentional injury death rates for Blacks and AIs/ANs are over twice the rate for Whites, over three and a half times the rate of Hispanics, and over six times the rate for Asian/Pacific Islanders. For the oldest adolescents (15- to 19-year-olds), whereas death rates for AIs/ANs are still the highest, the rate for Blacks is less than Whites and Hispanics (Figure 1.2) (Centers for Disease Control and Prevention 2010b).

Table 1.2. Five Leading Causes of Nonfatal Unintentional Injuries Treated in Emergency Departments, 0–19 Years of Age, All Races, Both Sexes: United States, 2008

Rank	Age <1	Ages 1–4	Ages 5–9	Ages 10–14	Ages 15–19
1	Fall	Fall	Fall	Fall	Struck by/against
	125,097	878,612	639,091	607,365	614,858
2	Struck by/ against	Struck by/ against	Struck by/ against	Struck by/ against	Fall
	37,010	371,404	399,995	583,948	479,934
3	Bite/Sting	Bite/Sting	Cut/Pierce	Overexertion	Overexertion
	13,092	134,920	106,907	293,813	386,442
4	Foreign Body	Foreign Body	Bite/Sting	Cut/Pierce	MV Occupant
	11,035	123,369	83,107	135,610	357,374
5	Fire/Burn	Cut/Pierce	Pedal Cyclist	Pedal Cyclist	Cut/Pierce
	9101	81,571	80,743	108,016	198,643

Source: Data from National Electronic Injury Surveillance System All Injury Program operated by the U.S. Consumer Product Safety Commission (Centers for Disease Control and Prevention 2010b). MV, motor vehicle.

The leading causes of unintentional injury death also vary by age group. More infants died from *suffocation* than all other injury causes combined. *Drowning* was the leading cause for children ages 1–4, followed by *motor vehicle traffic injuries*, *fire/burn*, and *suffocation*. *Motor vehicle traffic injuries* were the leading cause for those ages 5–9, 10–14, and 15–19. *Drowning* and *fire/burn* were also leading causes for these age groups, and among 15- to 19-year-olds, *poisoning* was the second leading cause of unintentional injury death (Table 1.4) (Centers for Disease Control and Prevention 2010b).

Developmental factors play an important role in injury during adolescence (Mercy, Sleet, and Doll 2006). The high incidence of adolescent traffic-related injury is due in part to lack of experience, as well as lack of maturity. Many months or even years of experience may be needed for adolescents to become proficient in driving (Lonero, Clinton, and Sleet 2006). Young drivers may also lack experience to recognize, assess, and respond to hazards, and they may be willing to accept higher levels of risks while walking, riding a bike, or driving a car or motorcycle (Irwin, Burg, and Uhler Cart 2002).

In addition, adolescence is a stage of development characterized by increased independence from parents, social pressure from peers, and risk-taking behavior (Sleet and Mercy 2003). Adolescent alcohol use simply exacerbates these problems.

Distracted driving, the use of cell phones while driving, in-vehicle Internet, and onboard navigation systems place additional demands on the adolescent driver's attention (World Health Organization 2011; Madden and Lenhart 2009). Research has determined that the crash risks are four times higher when using mobile communication devices such as mobile phones, and as

Table 1.3. Unintentional Childhood Injury Deaths and Rates per 100,000, All Races, by Sex: United States, 2007

Age Group	Sex	Number of Deaths	Population	Crude Rate
<01	Males	715	2,187,030	32.69
	Females	570	2,086,513	27.32
	Both	1285	4,273,543	30.07
01-04	Males	987	8,419,134	11.72
	Females	601	8,037,539	7.48
	Both	1588	16,456,673	9.65
05-09	Males	572	10,142,052	5.64
	Females	393	9,694,878	4.05
	Both	965	19,836,930	4.86
10-14	Males	774	10,388,301	7.45
	Females	455	9,903,611	4.59
	Both	1229	20,291,912	6.06
15-19	Males	4542	10,990,585	41.33
	Females	1951	10,455,025	18.66
	Both	6493	21,445,610	30.28
00-19	Males	7590	42,127,102	18.02
	Females	3970	40,177,566	9.88
	Both	11,560	82,304,668	14.05

Source: Data from NCHS Vital Statistics System for numbers of deaths; Bureau of Census for population estimates (Centers for Disease Control and Prevention 2010b).

much as 20 times higher when using texting devices while driving (Ranney 2008). This presents special risks to adolescents, whose skills managing the driving task are already hampered by lack of experience (Pratt 2003).

Global Implications

Unintentional injuries are also recognized as a global health problem, with road traffic injuries being the leading cause of death for youth around the world (World Health Organization 2007). To draw attention to the growing problem of child and adolescent injuries and effective prevention strategies, the World Health Organization (WHO), together with UNICEF, released the *World Report on Child Injury Prevention* in 2008 (Peden et al. 2004). To complement the

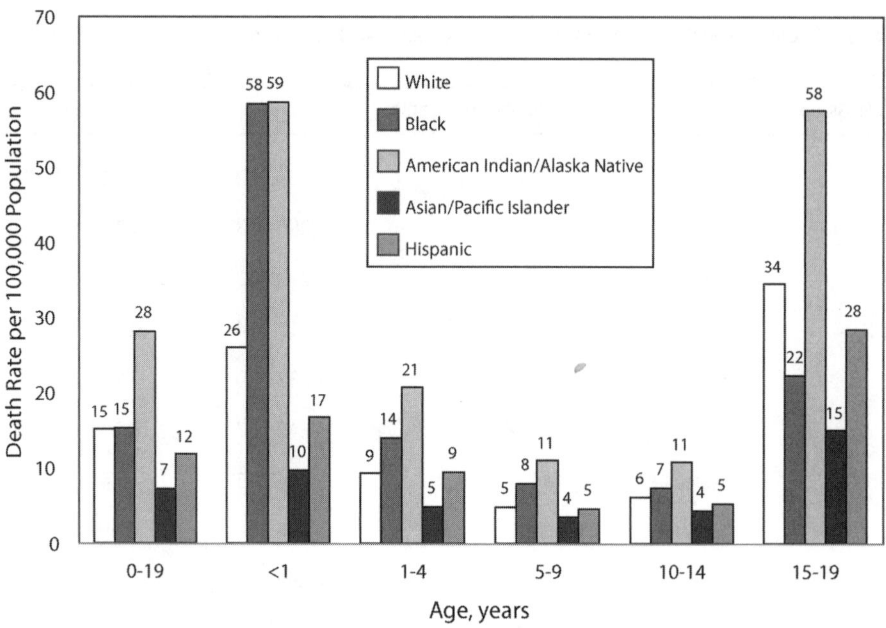

N.B., Hispanics are not included in any racial categories

Figure 1.2. Unintentional Injury Death Rates Among Children 0–19 Years, by Age and Race/ Ethnicity: United States, 2005–2007

WHO report, the Centers for Disease Control and Prevention (CDC) released the *CDC Childhood Injury Report* (Borse et al. 2008), which describes patterns of unintentional injuries among 0- to 19-year-olds in the United States from 2000 to 2006.

Alcohol and Injuries

Alcohol is the most commonly used drug among adolescents, and the prevalence and toll of underage drinking in America is widely underestimated. More young people drink alcohol than smoke tobacco or use marijuana (Bonnie and O'Connell 2004). Overall in 2001, there were 40,933 injury-related deaths associated with excessive alcohol use or binge drinking among all ages. Of these, over half were unintentional deaths (13,878 traffic deaths and 12,233 nontraffic deaths) (Centers for Disease Control and Prevention 2004a).

In 2007, 75% of students in grades nine through twelve had ever consumed alcohol in their lifetime, and 44.7% reported having at least one drink on at least one occasion during the past month. Twenty-six percent of students engage in episodic heavy drinking—consuming five or more drinks on a single occasion (Community Guide Branch 2010). Underage drinking is not just a problem among older teens: almost one in five eighth graders age 13–14 report alcohol use (Bonnie and O'Connell 2004).

Alcohol's pathway to impairment leading to injury can be biological and psychological, directly affecting adolescent performance by slowing the decision making process, reducing visual acuity and adaptation to brightness and glare, dividing one's attention, changing perceptions, increasing reaction time, increasing the sense of confidence, inhibiting self-control, and reducing perception of hazards (Lunetta and Smith 2005). These changes can be particularly pronounced

Table 1.4. Five Leading Causes of Unintentional Injury Deaths, 0–19 Years of Age, All Races, Both Sexes: United States, 2007

Rank	Age <1	Ages 1–4	Ages 5–9	Ages 10–14	Ages 15–19
1	Suffocation	Drowning	MV Traffic	MV Traffic	MV Traffic
	959	458	456	696	4593
2	MV Traffic	MV Traffic	Fire/Burn	Drowning	Poisoning
	122	428	136	102	838
3	Drowning	Fire/Burn	Drowning	Other Land Transport	Drowning
	57	204	122	80	317
4	Fire/Burn	Suffocation	Suffocation	Fire/Burn	Other Land Transport
	39	149	42	78	133
5	Fall	Pedestrian	Other Land Transport	Poisoning	Fire/Burn
	24	124	40	69	87

Source: Data from NCHS Vital Statistics System for numbers of deaths; Bureau of Census for population estimates (Centers for Disease Control and Prevention 2010b). MV, motor vehicle.

during adolescence, when the brain has yet to fully mature, and experiences in adapting to the effects of alcohol are limited.

Alcohol use is associated with 48% of motor vehicle fatalities among those aged 15–20 years, and with 33% of motor vehicle fatalities among children less than 15 years of age (Centers for Disease Control and Prevention 2001). Alcohol use is a factor in more than 30% of all drowning deaths (Cummings and Quan 1999), 14% to 27% of all boating-related deaths (Logan et al. 1999), 34% of all pedestrian deaths (Centers for Disease Control and Prevention 1999), and 51% of adolescent traumatic brain injuries (Kraus, Rock, and Hemyari 1990). Alcohol is implicated in deaths due to falls, fire, hypothermia, occupational work, poisoning, and water transport (Centers for Disease Control and Prevention 2004a).

Alcohol use is also associated with drug use and delinquency (Wechsler et al. 1995), weapon carrying and fighting (Presley et al. 1997), and motor vehicle crashes (S. Liu et al. 1997; Sleet et al. 2009). In 2007, 10.5% of high school students reported driving a motor vehicle after drinking alcohol, and 29.1% reported they rode in a car in the past 30 days with a driver who had been drinking alcohol (Community Guide Branch 2010; Jones and Shults 2009).

Road Traffic Injuries

Road traffic injuries include injuries to passengers and drivers of automobiles, pedestrians, bicyclists (i.e., pedal cyclists), and riders of motorcycles. Traffic injuries are the leading cause of death for children and adolescents in the United States, accounting for 58% of all unintentional injury-related deaths (Centers for Disease Control and Prevention 2010b). In 2007, 6683 children and adolescents died in motor vehicle-related crashes (Centers for Disease Control and Prevention 2010b). Motor vehicle occupants represented 2887 of these deaths. In 2008, 1.1 million children and adolescents were treated in hospital EDs for traffic injuries. Of these, about half were drivers or passengers whereas the rest were largely bicyclists, motorcyclists, and pedestrians (Centers for Disease Control and Prevention 2010b).

The likelihood that children and adolescents will be injured in traffic crashes increases when

- Drivers and passengers don't use seat belts
- A driver transporting children or adolescents has been drinking (Quinlan et al. 2000)
- New and inexperienced drivers transport other teenage passengers (Chen et al. 2000)
- Drivers are distracted by other passengers, cell phone use, and texting while driving

Road traffic injuries are also a global problem among youth and the leading cause of death for youth aged 10–24 years. Of the 1.2 million people who lose their lives in road traffic crashes each year, almost a third of them are youth under the age of 25 years (Peden et al. 2004).

The comprehensive costs of motor vehicle occupant, pedal cyclist, and pedestrian injury, including monetized Quality Adjusted Life Years lost among children of all ages, were over $60 billion in 2000 (Miller et al. 2006). Recent findings put the costs at over $99 billion in 2005 (Naumann et al. 2010).

Motor Vehicle Occupants (Passengers and Teen Drivers)

In 2007, 2887 children and adolescents were killed as occupants in unintentional motor vehicle crashes in traffic. Over 75% of these deaths are among those 15 to 19 years old. For children under 10, the death rates are approximately the same for males and females; however, for those 15 and older, the death rate for males is 80% higher than the rate for females (Figure 1.3a). From 1999 to 2007, the number of occupant fatalities among all children and adolescents decreased by 17% (Centers for Disease Control and Prevention 2010b), perhaps due to increases in use of safety seats and seat belts, as well as stronger graduated licensing laws.

In 2008, an estimated 529,372 children and adolescents were injured and treated at an ED for injuries sustained as an occupant in a motor vehicle crash. Sixty-seven percent of those injured were adolescents (15–19 years), and 56% were female (Centers for Disease Control and Prevention 2010b).

The use of age-appropriate restraints, such as child safety seats, booster seats, and seat belts, can greatly reduce the number of fatal and nonfatal injuries among child occupants in motor vehicle crashes. Unfortunately, child restraint use decreases as children get older. Restraint use is 99% for children under 1 year, but only 85% for those 8 to 12 years old when children are transitioning from riding in a child safety seat to a booster seat or adult size safety belt.

In addition, although safety seat use is high for infants, 14% are not riding rear-facing in the vehicle as recommended for best protection from injury. Improper use of child safety restraints, such as loose harnesses or incorrect attachment of the safety seat in the seat of the car, also continues to be a problem. Additionally, only 43% of 4- to 7-year-olds are riding in booster seats, despite research showing that the use of booster seats among this age group can dramatically reduce the risk of injury compared with use of seat belts alone (National Highway Traffic Safety Administration 2009b; Winston et al. 2000). Many states have now mandated booster seat use for children who are not yet able to use an adult seat belt or who have outgrown their child safety seat.

Young drivers account for 6.4% (13.2 million) of all licensed drivers in the United States (National Highway Traffic Safety Administration 2009h). Although teenagers drive less than most other drivers, they are involved in a disproportionately high number of crashes. The fatal

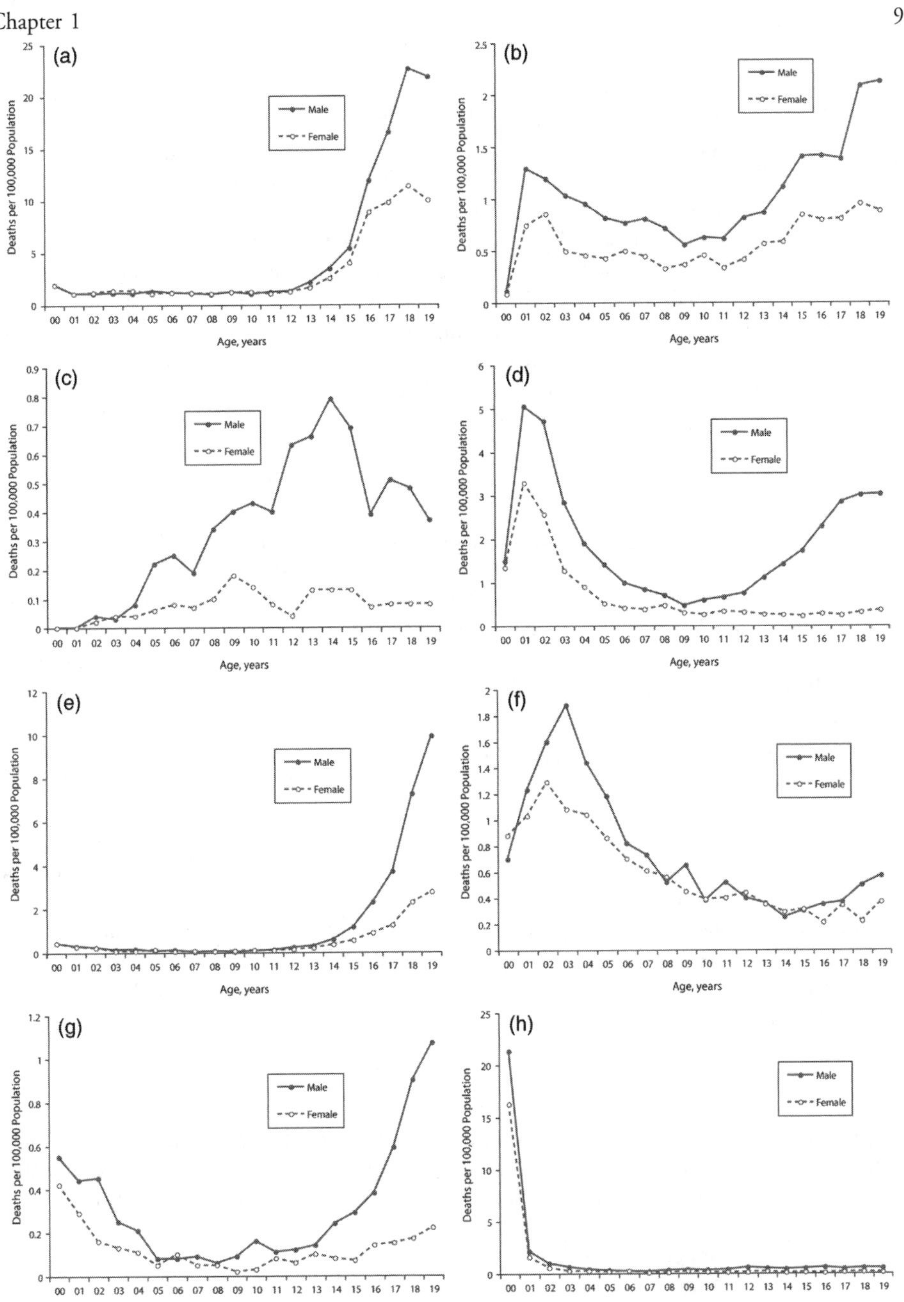

Figure 1.3. (a) Unintentional Motor Vehicle Occupant Traffic Death Rates Among Children 0–19 Years of Age: United States, 2003–2007. (b) Unintentional Pedestrian Traffic Death Rates Among Children 0–19 Years of Age: United States, 2003–2007. (c) Unintentional Bicyclist Traffic Death Rates Among Children 0–19 Years of Age: United States, 2003–2007. (d) Unintentional Drowning Death Rates Among Children 0–19 Years of Age: United States, 2003–2007. (e) Unintentional Poisoning Death Rates Among Children 0–19 Years of Age: United States, 2003–2007. (f) Unintentional Fire and Burn Death Rates Among Children 0–19 Years of Age: United States, 2003–2007. (g) Unintentional Fall Death Rates Among Children 0–19 Years of Age: United States, 2003–2007. (h) Unintentional Suffocation Death Rates Among Children 0–19 Years of Age: United States, 2003–2007.

crash rate per mile driven for younger drivers (from ages 16 to 19) is four to six times the risk for older drivers (ages 30–59), and the fatal crash risk is highest at age 16; the crash rate per mile driven is twice as high for 16 year olds as it is for 18- through 19-year-olds (Insurance Institute for Highway Safety 2010c). Young drivers are less likely than adults to drive after drinking alcohol, but their crash risk is substantially higher when they do (Peck et al. 2008).

Crash risk for both males and females is particularly high during the first months of driving and drops as young drivers accumulate more experience behind the wheel. Graduated licensing systems are designed to delay full licensure while allowing young drivers to gain experience under lower risk conditions (e.g., limits on night driving and teenage passenger restrictions) (Hartling et al. 2004; Williams and Shults 2010). Research suggests that the most strict and comprehensive graduated driver licensing (GDL) systems are associated with reductions of 38% and 40% in fatal and nonfatal injury crashes, respectively, of 16-year-old drivers (Baker, Chen, and Li, 2007).

Pedestrians

In 2007, there were 854 pedestrian fatalities among children and adolescents. Of these, 31% were children 0 to 4 years old, 14% were 5 to 9, 15% were 10 to 14, and 40% were 15 to 19 years old. Sixty-four percent of the deaths were males. Death rates in traffic are highest among 19 year olds (Figure 1.3b). From 1999 to 2007, the number of pedestrian fatalities among all children and adolescents decreased by 18% (Centers for Disease Control and Prevention 2010b), perhaps due to less walking (decreased exposure) and changes in the built environment to reduce vehicle speed and improvements in pedestrian crossing environments.

In 2008, an estimated 57,644 children and adolescents were injured and treated at an ED as pedestrians. Almost 70% of those injured were older children (10 to 19 years), and 60% were males (Centers for Disease Control and Prevention 2010b).

Fatalities to pedestrians less than 15 years of age most often occur between 4:00 P.M. and 7:59 P.M. and between 8:00 P.M. and 11:59 P.M. (43% and 21% of deaths, respectively), and 76% of deaths in this age group occurred at nonintersection locations (National Highway Traffic Safety Administration 2009c), indicating many pedestrian fatalities occur when children "dart-out" into traffic, mid-block. Additionally, 34% of pedestrian deaths to adolescents had some alcohol involvement either on the part of the driver or the pedestrian (National Highway Traffic Safety Administration 2009g).

Bicyclists

In 2007, there were 148 bicyclist fatalities among children and adolescents (includes other pedal cycles, such as tricycles and unicycles). Of these deaths, 78% were 10 to 19 years of age; and 80% were males. Death rates in traffic for males increase until age 14, then decrease at older ages (Figure 1.3c). This may be due to younger children riding bicycles more than adolescents. From 1999 to 2007, the number of bicycle fatalities among all children and adolescents decreased by 42% (Centers for Disease Control and Prevention 2010b), possibly because of greater use of bicycle helmets and changes in the cycling environment to make it safer.

In 2008, an estimated 276,020 children and adolescent bicyclists were injured and treated at an ED. Approximately two thirds (68%) of those injured were children 5 to 14 years old, and 73% were males (Centers for Disease Control and Prevention 2010b).

Among all ages, deaths to bicyclists occur more frequently in urban areas (69%), at nonintersection locations (64%), between the hours of 5:00 P.M. and 9:00 P.M. (28%), and during the months of June (9%) and September (12%) (National Highway Traffic Safety Administration 2009a). These differences can be attributed to increased exposure of children and adolescents during these times and seasons.

In 2008, alcohol involvement (either for the driver or bicyclist) was reported in more than one third of incidents that resulted in a bicyclist death (National Highway Traffic Safety Administration 2009a). Severe head injuries are responsible for 64% to 86% of bicycle-related fatalities (Sosin, Sacks, and Webb 1996). Research has shown that bicycle helmets reduce head and facial injuries for bicyclists of all ages involved in all types of crashes (Thompson, Rivara, and Thompson 2000), yet only 35% of riders report wearing a helmet for all or most trips (Royal and Miller-Steiger 2008). In 2008, 91% of individuals killed were not wearing a helmet (Insurance Institute for Highway Safety 2010a).

Over the past decade, the number of states that mandated bicycle helmet use for children has increased (Bicycle Helmet Safety Institute 2011), which may partially explain the overall decrease in bicycle fatalities over the past several years. Bicycle helmet legislation appears to be effective in increasing helmet use and decreasing head injury rates in the populations for which it is implemented (Macpherson and Spinks 2008).

Motorcyclists

In 2007, there were 249 motorcyclist fatalities to children and adolescents. Eighty-eight percent were among those 15 to 19 years old, and two thirds were 18 or 19 years old. From 1999 to 2007, the number of motorcycle fatalities among all children and adolescents increased by 84% (135 deaths in 1999) (Centers for Disease Control and Prevention 2010b).

In 2008, an estimated 57,967 children and adolescents were injured and treated at an ED as motorcyclists. Almost 60% of those injured were older children (10 to 19 years), and 90% were males (Centers for Disease Control and Prevention 2010b).

Among all ages, per vehicle mile traveled, motorcyclists are about 37 times more likely than passenger car occupants to die in a motor vehicle traffic crash and nine times more likely to be injured (National Highway Traffic Safety Administration 2009e). Approximately half of all motorcycle deaths occur in single-vehicle crashes and 35% of motorcycle riders were speeding (Insurance Institute for Highway Safety 2010b; National Highway Traffic Safety Administration 2009e). Injury rates are nearly 1.5 times higher during weekends than on weekdays (based on number of hours) and two thirds of injuries occur during the daytime (National Highway Traffic Safety Administration 2009f).

In 2009, use of Department of Transportation-compliant motorcycle helmets for all ages was 67% (National Highway Traffic Safety Administration 2009d). Helmet use has been shown to reduce the risk of head injury by 69% and reduce the risk of death by 42% (B. C. Liu et al. 2008).

Home and Recreation Injuries

Child and adolescent injuries occurring in the home and in recreation represent a significant burden in health care costs, injuries, and deaths. Research has demonstrated that many interventions directed at the home and recreational environments work to prevent injuries; however, many of these strategies have not gained wide acceptance and use. This section describes the epidemiology of injuries due to drowning, poisoning, fires and burns, falls, and suffocation.

Drowning

Drowning is defined as "... respiratory impairment from submersion/immersion in liquid" (van Beeck et al. 2005). In 2007, there were 1056 fatal unintentional child and adolescent drownings in the United States, averaging approximately 20 incidents per week (Centers for Disease Control and Prevention 2010b). Almost half of these deaths were among children less than 5 years of age.

Most of the drowning deaths occur from May through August, on Saturdays and Sundays, and between noon and 8:00 P.M. (Brenner 2003).

In 2008, an additional 3856 children were treated in EDs for nonfatal drownings. These incidents can cause brain damage that may result in long-term disabilities including seizures, motor deficitis, learning disabilities, and permanent loss of basic functioning (a permanent vegetative state) (Meyer, Theodorou, and Berg 2006).

For children older than 1 year of age, males are at greater risk than females. Drowning death rates for both sexes peak at 1 to 2 years of age, but for males, there is a second peak among adolescents (Figure 1.3d). African American youth had the highest rate of drowning (1.73 per 100,000) in 2006, whereas White youth had the lowest (0.87 per 100,000). Between 2001 and 2007, the fatal unintentional drowning rate for Blacks aged 10–19 years was 2.29 times the rate for Whites. For AIs/ANs and Asian/Pacific Islanders, the rates were 1.53 and 1.58 times the rate for Whites, respectively (Centers for Disease Control and Prevention 2010b).

Almost 80% of infant drownings occur in the home setting primarily in bathtubs (55%) and buckets (12%); children 1–4 years are most likely to drown in swimming pools (56%); and most adolescents drown in natural bodies of water (Brenner et al. 2001; Centers for Disease Control and Prevention 2004b).

Among all those injured in drowning incidents, 71 children and adolescents died from incidents related to recreational boating, and 669 were treated for nonfatal boating-related injuries in 2008, with most of these deaths and injuries occurring to those over 13 years of age (U.S. Coast Guard 2009).

Alcohol involvement (among either the adolescents or an adult who is present) was the leading contributing factor in fatal boating accidents, contributing to about one in five reported boating deaths (Howland et al. 1995; U.S. Coast Guard 2009). Factors such as the physical environment (access to swimming pools) and a combination of social and cultural issues (developing swimming skills and choosing safe water recreation) may contribute to the racial differences in drowning rates (Branche et al. 2004). In survey research, men of all ages, races, and educational levels consistently reported greater swimming ability than women (Gilchrist, Sacks, and Branche 2000). Formal swimming lessons have been shown to be protective against drowning risk for children of all ages, including those 1 to 4 years old (Brenner et al. 2009).

Poisoning

A poison is any substance harmful to the body when ingested (eaten), inhaled (breathed), injected, or absorbed through the skin. Any substance can be poisonous if enough is taken. Unintentional poisoning includes the use of drugs or chemicals for recreational purposes in excessive amounts, such as an "overdose." It also includes lead and carbon monoxide poisoning and the excessive use of drugs or chemicals for nonrecreational purposes.

In 2007, 29,846 (75%) of the 40,059 overall poisoning deaths in the United States were unintentional. Among children and adolescents, there were 972 unintentional poisoning deaths in 2007. In 2008, there were an estimated 109,767 ED visits (Centers for Disease Control and Prevention 2010b); there are also approximately 1.6 million exposures reported to poison control centers each year (Bronstein et al. 2009). While most deaths (86%) occur among those 10 to 19 years of age (Figure 1.3e), children under 5 years account for most of the calls to poison control centers (80%).

This is a growing problem with the number of poisonings almost tripling since 1999 (n = 346), with those 15 to 19 years of age accounting for 76% of the increase in deaths. Among this age group, poisoning was second only to motor vehicle crashes as a cause of unintentional injury death in 2007 (Table 1.4), and male death rates were over three times higher than females (5.84 versus 1.87) (Centers for Disease Control and Prevention 2010b).

Young children are especially vulnerable to inadvertent exposure to prescription and over-the-counter medications, especially when these items are not stored securely (Centers for Disease Control and Prevention 2006; Schillie et al. 2009). Other substances, such as household cleaners and products used for laundry and personal care, also pose risks to young children (Franklin and Rodgers 2008). The reason for the rise in poisoning deaths among adolescents is unclear. While rising poisoning death rates among older age groups are related to increases in the use and availability of prescription narcotics (Paulozzi, Budnitz, and Xi 2006), the Substance Abuse and Mental Health Services Administration (SAMHSA) reports that nonmedicinal use of prescription-type drugs has decreased among adolescents (Substance Abuse and Mental Health Services Administration 2008).

Fires and Burns

In 2007, unintentional fires and burns killed 544 children and adolescents. In 2008, more than 130,000 children and adolescents were burned severely enough that they required a visit to an ED; 94% of the deaths were due to residential fires (Centers for Disease Control and Prevention 2010b). The number of deaths has declined dramatically over the past 20 years (1289 deaths in 1987), perhaps due to safer consumer products and reductions in home fires.

Home fire deaths occur disproportionately in the South, among populations at the lowest income levels. More than one third of house fires occur December through February (U.S. Fire Administration 2004, 2005). Death rates are highest for children 2 to 3 years old (Figure 1.3f). Among all ages, death rates for Blacks are almost three times higher than the rate for Whites (1.60 vs 0.57, respectively) (Centers for Disease Control and Prevention 2010b). The most common causes of residential fires are cooking and heating equipment, and the most common cause of fire-related deaths is cigarette smoking (Ahrens 2003). Alcohol contributes to approximately 40% of deaths in house fires (Smith, Branas, and Miller 1999).

Fire and burn injury rates are highest in the youngest children because of their natural curiosity, impulsiveness, and lack of experience in assessing danger and risk (Lindblad and Terkelsen 1990). Additionally, younger children are incapable of escaping from a residential fire on their own. Infants and children have limited awareness and mobility to safely exit a house during a fire, particularly without the assistance of an adult.

Young children are vulnerable to scald burns because their thinner skin burns at a lower temperature. Because young children also have a larger body surface area-to-mass ratio, a typical scald burn can be more severe since it results in a greater percentage of the body being burned (Ring 2007). Hot tap water and liquids, steam, and grease from cooking are particular risks for young children (Allasio and Fischer 2005; Drago 2005; Katcher 1981; Lowell, Quinlan, and Gottlieb 2008).

Falls

In 2007, 178 children and adolescents died from falls. Males accounted for 72% of these deaths. Death rates are highest for males 18 and 19 years old. Children under 3 years old are also at higher risk (Figure 1.3g) (Centers for Disease Control and Prevention 2010b).

In 2008, over 2.7 million children and adolescents were seen at an ED because of a fall injury. Sixty percent were children under the age of 10, and 57% were males (Centers for Disease Control and Prevention 2010b).

Among all ages, more than half of all fall deaths occur at home (Runyan et al. 2005). Fall injuries to younger children may be associated with falls from buildings and structures (Pressley and Barlow 2005), playground equipment (Vollman et al. 2009; Phelan et al. 2001), bunk beds

(Mack, Gilchrist, and Ballesteros 2007), and activities such as sports and recreation (Conn, Annest, and Gilchrist 2003).

Suffocation

In 2007, 1263 children and adolescents died from suffocation. Data include any threat to breathing, including strangulation in bed, and inhalation of gastric contents, food, and other foreign bodies.

Of these deaths, 76% were among infants less than 1 year of age, which resulted in dramatically higher death rates (Figure 1.3h), and 60% were males. From 1999 to 2007, the number of suffocation deaths among all children and adolescents increased by 52%; all of the additional deaths have been in infants (Centers for Disease Control and Prevention 2010b).

In 2008, an estimated 14,021 children and adolescents were seen at an ED because of a suffocation/inhalation injury. Seventy-five percent were children under the age of 10, and 35% were infants. Over half (57%) were males (Centers for Disease Control and Prevention 2010b).

Food, coins, and toys, including latex balloons, are commonly associated with choking among children. Young children have narrower airways; their chewing and swallowing coordination is immature; and they are more likely than older children to put nonfood items in their mouths (Committee on Injury, Violence, and Poison Prevention 2010).

A topic of special concern for infants is safe sleep. Risk factors include sleeping with soft bedding materials, sleeping in the prone position, co-sleeping with an adult or sibling, and sleeping in environments in which the infant's head can become trapped between two objects, such as the mattress and crib/wall/bed frame, or between the slats of the crib (Scheers, Rutherford, and Kemp 2003).

Work-Related Injuries

From 1998 to 2007, the Centers for Disease Control and Prevention (CDC) National Institute for Occupational Safety and Health identified a total of 5719 fatal injuries among younger workers, averaging 572 per year. An estimated 10-year decline of 14% was observed in the rate of deaths, as well as an estimated 19% decline in the rate of nonfatal work injuries among younger workers.

Among younger workers, the highest nonfatal injury rates were experienced by workers aged 18 and 19 years of age. For the younger worker, the nonfatal injury rate was twofold higher than the rate for older workers. Younger Hispanic workers had a fatality rate that was significantly higher than the rate for non-Hispanic White workers and non-Hispanic Black workers. Transportation-related deaths, largely highway crashes, were the most frequently recorded events in all age groups.

For nonfatal injuries, contact with objects or equipment was the most common event and accounted for a larger proportion of injuries among younger workers (49%) compared with older workers (40%). Younger workers experienced the highest rates of fatal injury in mining (36.5 per 100,000 full-time equivalent workers [FTEs]), agriculture (21.3 per 100,000 FTEs), and construction (10.9 per 100,000 FTEs) (Centers for Disease Control and Prevention 2010a).

Summary and Conclusions

Unintentional injuries are the largest source of premature morbidity and mortality among children and adolescents and the leading cause of death. Transportation is the largest source of these injuries to young people, primarily due to motor vehicle injuries suffered as drivers and passengers, but also as bicyclists and pedestrians. Other major causes of unintentional injuries related to the home and recreation include drowning, poisoning, fires and burns, falls, and suffocation. Risk is related to age and sex, and varies depending on the specific cause of injury. While the overall death rate from unintentional injury has decreased slightly over the past several years, the overall public health burden remains high, and the number of deaths from motorcycles, poisoning, and infant suffocation has been increasing.

Understanding the epidemiology of unintentional injury among young people, including trends and patterns in morbidity and mortality, as well as the identification of high-risk groups, is critical to prevention. Many effective and promising prevention interventions exist (Doll et al. 2007; Sleet, Ballesteros, and Borse 2010), and several chapters in this book discuss key aspects of these strategies. Despite the existence of effective interventions, children and adolescents remain among the highest risk populations. Numerous lifestyle factors such as risk-taking behavior, sensation seeking, nonuse of seat belts and child restraints, insufficient protection in sports and recreation, alcohol use, and exposure to hazards and hazardous environments directly influence the likelihood of injury (Sleet, Ballesteros, and Baldwin 2010). Injury epidemiology can help us understand and explain contributing factors, identify groups at high risk, and target interventions to affect change in both environments and behaviors to improve the health of children and adolescents.

Disclaimer: The views expressed are those of the authors and do not necessarily represent the official opinions of the Centers for Disease Control and Prevention.

References

Ahrens M. 2003. The U.S. Fire Problem Overview Report: Leading Causes and Other Patterns and Trends. Quincy, MA: National Fire Protection Association, Fire Analysis and Research Division.

Allasio D, Fischer H. 2005. Immersion scald burns and the ability of young children to climb into a bathtub. *Pediatrics.* 115:1419–1421.

Baker SP, Chen L, Li G. 2007. Nationwide *Review of Graduated Driver Licensing.* Washington, DC: AAA Foundation for Traffic Safety.

Bicycle Helmet Safety Institute. 2011. Helmet Laws for Bicycle Riders. Available at: http://www.helmets.org/mandator.htm. Accessed July 10, 2011.

Bonnie RJ, O'Connell ME, and National Research Council. 2004. *Reducing Underage Drinking: A Collective Responsibility.* Washington, DC: National Academies Press.

Borse NN, Gilchrist J, Dellinger AM, et al. 2008. CDC Childhood Injury Report: Patterns of Unintentional Injuries Among 0–19 Year Olds in the United States, 2000–2006. Atlanta, GA: Centers for Disease Control and Prevention, National Center for Injury Prevention and Control.

Branche CM, Dellinger AM, Sleet DA, et al. 2004. Unintentional injuries: the burden, risks and preventive strategies to address diversity. In: Livingston IL, editor. *Praeger Handbook of Black American Health: Policies and Issues Behind Disparities in Health.* Westport, CT: Praeger. 317–327.

Brenner RA. 2003. Prevention of drowning in infants, children, and adolescents. *Pediatrics.* 112:440–445.

Brenner RA, Taneja GS, Haynie DL, et al. 2009. Association between swimming lessons and drowning in childhood: a case-control study. *Arch Pediatr Adolesc Med.* 163:203–210.

Brenner RA, Trumble AC, Smith GS, et al. 2001. Where children drown, United States, 1995. *Pediatrics.* 108:85–89.

Bronstein AC, Spyker DA, Cantilena LR Jr, et al. 2009. 2008 Annual Report of the American Association of Poison Control Centers' National Poison Data System (NPDS): 26th Annual Report. *Clin Toxicol (Phila)* 47:911–1084.

Centers for Disease Control and Prevention. 1999. Pedestrian fatalities—Cobb, DeKalb, Fulton, and Gwinnett counties, Georgia, 1994–1998. *MMWR Morb Mortal Wkly Rep.* 48:601–605.

Centers for Disease Control and Prevention. 2001. Alcohol involvement in fatal motor-vehicle crashes—United States, 1999–2000. *MMWR Morb Mortal Wkly Rep.* 50:1064–1065.

Centers for Disease Control and Prevention. 2004a. Alcohol-attributable deaths and years of potential life lost—United States, 2001. *MMWR Morb Mortal Wkly Rep.* 53:866–870.

Centers for Disease Control and Prevention. 2004b. Nonfatal and fatal drownings in recreational water settings—United States, 2001–2002. *MMWR Morb Mortal Wkly Rep.* 53:447–452.

Centers for Disease Control and Prevention. 2006. Nonfatal, unintentional medication exposures among young children—United States, 2001–2003. *MMWR Morb Mortal Wkly Rep.* 55:1–5.

Centers for Disease Control and Prevention. 2010a. Occupational injuries and deaths among younger workers—United States, 1998–2007. *MMWR Morb Mortal Wkly Rep.* 59:449–455.

Centers for Disease Control and Prevention. 2010b. Web-Based Injury Statistics Query and Reporting System (WISQARS). Atlanta, GA: Centers for Disease Control and Prevention, National Center for Injury Prevention and Control. Available at: http://www.cdc.gov/ncipc/wisqars. Accessed April 29, 2010.

Chen LH, Baker SP, Braver ER, Li G. 2000. Carrying passengers as a risk factor for crashes fatal to 16- and 17-year-old drivers. *JAMA.* 283:1578–1582.

Committee on Injury, Violence, and Poison Prevention. 2010. Prevention of choking among children. *Pediatrics.* 125:601–607.

The Community Guide Branch, Epidemiology Analysis Program Office. *Preventing Excessive Alcohol Consumption*, Guide to Community Preventive Services, The Community Guide. May 10, 2010 [cited July 1, 2010]. Atlanta, GA: Centers for Disease Control and Prevention, Office of Surveillance, Epidemiology, and Laboratory Services. Available at: http://www.thecommunityguide.org/alcohol/index.html. Accessed August 7, 2011.

Conn JM, Annest JL, Gilchrist J. 2003. Sports and recreation related injury episodes in the US population, 1997–99. *Inj Prev.* 9:117–123.

Cummings P, Quan L. 1999. Trends in unintentional drowning: the role of alcohol and medical care. *JAMA.* 281:2198–2202.

Doll LS, Bonzo SE, Mercy JA, Sleet DA, editors. 2007. *Handbook of Injury and Violence Prevention.* New York: Springer.

Drago DA. 2005. Kitchen scalds and thermal burns in children five years and younger. *Pediatrics.* 115:10–16.

Franklin RL, Rodgers GB. 2008. Unintentional child poisonings treated in United States hospital emergency departments: national estimates of incident cases, population-based poisoning rates, and product involvement. *Pediatrics.* 122:1244–1251.

Gilchrist J, Sacks JJ, Branche CM. 2000. Self-reported swimming ability in US adults, 1994. *Public Health Rep.* 115:110–111.

Hartling L, Wiebe N, Russell K, et al. 2004. Graduated driver licensing for reducing motor vehicle crashes among young drivers. *Cochrane Database Syst Rev.* no. 2:CD003300.

Howland J, Mangione T, Hingson R, et al. 1995. Alcohol as a risk factor for drowning and other aquatic injuries. In: Watson RR, editor. *Alcohol and Accidents. Drugs and Alcohol Abuse Reviews.* Totowa, NJ: Humana Press. 85–104.

Insurance Institute for Highway Safety (IIHS). 2010a. *Fatality Facts: Bicycles.* Arlington, VA: IIHS.

Insurance Institute for Highway Safety (IIHS). 2010b. *Fatality Facts: Motorcycles.* Arlington, VA: IIHS.

Insurance Institute for Highway Safety (IIHS). 2010c. *Fatality Facts: Teenagers.* Arlington, VA: IIHS.

Irwin CE Jr, Burg SJ, Uhler Cart C. 2002. America's adolescents: where have we been, where are we going? *J Adolesc Health.* 31(6 Suppl):91–121.

Jones SE, Shults RA. 2009. Trends and subgroup differences in transportation-related injury risk and safety behaviors among US high school students, 1991–2007. *J Sch Health.* 79:169–176.

Katcher ML. 1981. Scald burns from hot tap water. *JAMA.* 246:1219–1222.

Kraus JF, Rock A, Hemyari P. 1990. Brain injuries among infants, children, adolescents, and young adults. *Am J Dis Child.* 144:684–691.

Lindblad BE, Terkelsen CJ. 1990. Domestic burns among children. *Burns.* 16:254–256.

Liu BC, Ivers R, Norton R, et al. 2008. Helmets for preventing injury in motorcycle riders. *Cochrane Database Syst Rev.* no. 1:CD004333.

Liu S, Siegel PZ, Brewer RD, et al. 1997. Prevalence of alcohol-impaired driving: results from a national self-reported survey of health behaviors. *JAMA.* 277:122–125.

Logan P, Sacks JJ, Branche CM, et al. 1999. Alcohol-influenced recreational boat operation in the United States, 1994. *Am J Prev Med.* 16:278–282.

Lonero LP, Clinton KM, Sleet DA. 2006. Behavior change interventions in road safety. In: Gielen AC, Sleet DA, DiClemente RJ, editors. *Injury and Violence Prevention: Behavioral Science Theories, Methods, and Applications.* San Francisco, CA: Jossey-Bass. 213–233.

Lowell G, Quinlan K, Gottlieb LJ. 2008. Preventing unintentional scald burns: moving beyond tap water. *Pediatrics.* 122:799–804.

Lunetta P, Smith GS. 2005. The role of alcohol in injury deaths. In: Preedy VR, Watson RR, editors. *Comprehensive Handbook of Alcohol Related Pathology.* New York: Academic Press. 147–164.

Mack KA, Gilchrist J, Ballesteros MF. 2007. Bunk bed-related injuries sustained by young children treated in emergency departments in the United States, 2001–2004, National Electronic Injury Surveillance System—All Injury Program. *Inj Prev.* 13:137–140.

Macpherson A, Spinks A. 2008. Bicycle helmet legislation for the uptake of helmet use and prevention of head injuries. *Cochrane Database Syst Rev.* no. 3:CD005401.

Madden M, Lenhart, A. 2009. *Teens and Distracted Driving.* Pew Internet and American Life Project. Washington, DC: Pew Research Center.

Mercy JA, Sleet DA, Doll L. 2006. Applying a developmental and ecological framework to injury and violence prevention. In: Liller KD, editor. *Injury Prevention for Children and Adolescents: Research, Practice, and Advocacy.* Washington, DC: American Public Health Association. 1–14.

Meyer RJ, Theodorou AA, Berg RA. 2006. Childhood drowning. *Pediatr Rev.* 27:163–168.

Miller TR, Finkelstein AE, Zaloshnja E, Hendrie D. 2006. The cost of child and adolescent injuries and the savings from prevention. In: Liller KD, editor. *Injury Prevention for Children and Adolescents: Research, Practice, and Advocacy.* Washington, DC: American Public Health Association. 15–64.

National Committee for Injury Prevention and Control (U.S.). 1989. *Injury Prevention: Meeting the Challenge.* New York: Oxford University Press.

Naumann RB, Dellinger AM, Zaloshnja E, et al. 2010. Incidence and total lifetime costs of motor vehicle-related fatal and nonfatal injury by road user type, United States, 2005. *Traffic Inj Prev.* 11:353–360.

National Highway Traffic Safety Administration. 2009a. Bicyclists and Other Cyclists. *Traffic Safety Facts 2008 Data.* Washington, DC: National Center for Statistics and Analysis, NHTSA.

National Highway Traffic Safety Administration (NHTSA). 2009b. Booster Seat Use in 2008. *Traffic Safety Facts Research Note.* Washington, DC: National Center for Statistics and Analysis, NHTSA.

National Highway Traffic Safety Administration (NHTSA). 2009c. Children. *Traffic Safety Facts 2008 Data.* Washington, DC: National Center for Statistics and Analysis, NHTSA.

National Highway Traffic Safety Administration (NHTSA). 2009d. Motorcycle Helmet Use in 2009–Overall Results. *Traffic Safety Facts Research Note.* Washington, DC: National Center for Statistics and Analysis, NHTSA.

National Highway Traffic Safety Administration (NHTSA). 2009e. Motorcycles. In *Traffic Safety Facts 2008 Data.* Washington, DC: National Center for Statistics and Analysis, NHTSA.

National Highway Traffic Safety Administration (NHTSA). 2009f. Motorcyclists Injured in Motor Vehicle Traffic Crashes. *Traffic Safety Facts Research Note.* Washington, DC: National Center for Statistics and Analysis, NHTSA.

National Highway Traffic Safety Administration (NHTSA). 2009g. Pedestrians. *Traffic Safety Facts 2008 Data.* Washington, DC: National Center for Statistics and Analysis, NHTSA.

National Highway Traffic Safety Administration (NHTSA). 2009h. Young Drivers. *Traffic Safety Facts 2008 Data.* Washington, DC: National Center for Statistics and Analysis, NHTSA.

Paulozzi LJ, Budnitz DS, Xi Y. 2006. Increasing deaths from opioid analgesics in the United States. *Pharmacoepidemiol Drug Saf.* 15:618–627.

Peck RC, Gebers MA, Voas RB, Romano E. 2008. The relationship between blood alcohol concentration (BAC), age, and crash risk. *J Safety Res.* 39:311–319.

Peden M, Scurfield R, Sleet D, et al, editors. 2004. *World Report on Road Traffic Injury Prevention.* Geneva: World Health Organization.

Phelan KJ, Khoury J, Kalkwarf HJ, Lanphear BP. 2001. Trends and patterns of playground injuries in United States children and adolescents. *Ambul Pediatr.* 1:227–233.

Pratt SG. 2003. Work-Related Roadway Crashes: Challenges and Opportunities for Prevention. Cincinnati, OH: Centers for Disease Control and Prevention, National Institute for Occupational Safety and Health.

Presley CA, Meilman PW, Cashin JR, Leichliter JS. 1997. *Alcohol and Drugs on American College Campuses: Issues of Violence and Harassment.* Carbondale: Southern Illinois University Core Institute.

Pressley JC, Barlow B. 2005. Child and adolescent injury as a result of falls from buildings and structures. *Inj Prev.* 11:267–273.

Quinlan KP, Brewer RD, Sleet DA, Dellinger AM. 2000. Characteristics of child passenger deaths and injuries involving drinking drivers. *JAMA.* 283:2249–2252.

Ranney TA. 2008. Driver Distraction: A Review of the Current State-of-Knowledge. Washington, DC: National Highway Traffic Safety Administration.

Ring LM. 2007. Kids and hot liquids—a burning reality. *J Pediatr Health Care.* 21:192–194.

Royal D, Miller-Steiger D. 2008. National Survey of Bicyclist and Pedestrian Attitudes and Behavior, Volume II: Findings Report. Washington, DC: U.S. Department of Transportation, National Highway Traffic Safety Administration, Office of Behavioral Safety and Research.

Runyan CW, Casteel C, Perkis D, et al. 2005. Unintentional injuries in the home in the United States Part I: mortality. *Am J Prev Med.* 28:73–79.

Scheers NJ, Rutherford GW, Kemp JS. 2003. Where should infants sleep? A comparison of risk for suffocation of infants sleeping in cribs, adult beds, and other sleeping locations. *Pediatrics.* 112:883–889.

Schillie SF, Shehab N, Thomas KE, Budnitz DS. 2009. Medication overdoses leading to emergency department visits among children. *Am J Prev Med.* 37:181–187.

Sleet DA, Ballesteros MF, Baldwin GT. 2010. Injuries: an underrecognized lifestyle problem. *Am J Lifestyle Med.* 4:8–15.

Sleet DA, Ballesteros MF, Borse NN. 2010. A review of unintentional injuries in adolescents. *Annu Rev Public Health.* 31:195–212.

Sleet DA, Howat P, Elder R, et al. 2009. Interventions to reduce impaired driving and traffic injury. In: Verster JC, Pandi-Perumal SR, Ramaekers JG, de Gier JJ, editors. *Drugs, Driving and Traffic Safety.* Boston: Birkhäuser. 436–456.

Sleet DA, Mercy JA. 2003. Promotion of safety, security, and well-being. In: Bornstein MH, Davidson L, Keyes CLM, Moore KA, editors. *Well-Being: Positive Development Across the Life Course.* The Crosscurrents in Contemporary Psychology Series. Mahwah, NJ: Lawrence Erlbaum Associates. 81–98.

Smith GS, Branas CC, Miller TR. 1999. Fatal nontraffic injuries involving alcohol: a metaanalysis. *Ann Emerg Med.* 33:659–668.

Sosin DM, Sacks JJ, Webb KW. 1996. Pediatric head injuries and deaths from bicycling in the United States. *Pediatrics.* 98:868–870.

Substance Abuse and Mental Health Services Administration (SAMHSA). 2008. The National Survey on Drug Use and Health (NSDUH) Report, Trends in Substance Use, Dependence or Abuse, and Treatment Among Adolescents: 2002 to 2007. Rockville, MD: SAMHSA, Office of Applied Studies.

Thompson DC, Rivara FP, Thompson R. 2000. Helmets for preventing head and facial injuries in bicyclists. *Cochrane Database Syst Rev.* no. 2:CD001855.

U.S. Coast Guard. 2009. Recreational Boating Statistics 2008. Washington, DC: U.S. Department of Homeland Security, U.S. Coast Guard, Office of Auxiliary and Boating Safety.

U.S. Fire Administration (USFA). 2004. Fire Risk. *Topical Fire Report Series.* Emmitsburg, MD: U.S. Department of Homeland Security, USFA, National Fire Data Center.

U.S. Fire Administration (USFA). 2005. Fatal Fires. *Topical Fire Report Series.* Emmitsburg, MD: U.S. Department of Homeland Security, USFA, National Fire Data Center.

van Beeck E, Branche CM, Szpilman D, et al. 2005. A new definition of drowning: towards documentation and prevention of a global public health problem. *Bull World Health Org.* 83:853–856.

Vollman D, Witsaman R, Comstock D, Smith GA. 2009. Epidemiology of playground equipment-related injuries to children in the United States, 1996–2005. *Clin Pediatr (Phila).* 48:66–71.

Wechsler H, Dowdall GW, Davenport A, Castillo S. 1995. Correlates of college student binge drinking. *Am J Public Health.* 85:921–926.

Williams AF, Shults RA. 2010. Graduated driver licensing research, 2007–present: a review and commentary. *J Safety Res.* 41:77–84.

Winston FK, Durbin DR, Kallan MJ, Moll EK. 2000. The danger of premature graduation to seat belts for young children. *Pediatrics.* 105:1179–1183.

World Health Organization (WHO). 2007. *Youth Declaration for Road Safety.* Geneva: WHO. Available at: http://www.who.int/roadsafety/week/activities/global/youth/youth-declaration-lowres_en.pdf. Accessed July 1, 2010.

World Health Organization (WHO). 2011. *Mobile Phone Use: A Growing Problem of Driver Distraction.* Geneva: WHO. Available at: http://www.who.int/violence_injury_prevention/publications/road_traffic/en/index.html. Accessed August 7, 2011.

Chapter 2

The Cost of Child and Adolescent Injuries and the Savings From Prevention[1]

Ted R. Miller, PhD,[2] A. Eric Finkelstein, PhD, MHA,[3] Eduard Zaloshnja, PhD,[2] and Delia Hendrie, MEcon[4]

Cost-of-illness data are useful in comparing magnitudes of various health problems, assessing risks, setting research priorities, and selecting interventions that most efficiently reduce health burdens. With analyses of national and state data sets, this chapter presents data on the frequency, costs, and quality-of-life losses associated with child and adolescent injury in 2000. The frequency, severity, and costs of injury—unintentional and intentional—make it a leading child and adolescent health problem. Child and adolescent injuries in 2000 resulted in an estimated $24 billion in lifetime medical spending and $82 billion in present and future work losses, including caregiver losses. These injuries killed approximately 18,000 children and left approximately 160,000 children and adolescents with permanent work-related disabilities. Because Medicaid and other government sources paid for 29% of the days children spent in hospitals because of injury, the government has a financial interest in, and arguably a responsibility for, ensuring the safety of disadvantaged children.

Many proven child safety interventions cost less than the medical and other resource costs they save. Thus, governments, managed care companies, and third-party payers could save money by increasing the routine use of selected child safety measures, such as functional family therapy for juvenile offenders, booster seats, bicycle helmets, smoke alarms, and graduated driver licensing. Yet these and other proven injury prevention interventions are not universally implemented. Possible barriers to adoption include the following: (1) savings may be split across multiple payers, (2) the payback period may be too long, (3) safety device subsidizers would have to subsidize parents who would buy the devices anyway as well as parents who would not, and (4) intervention may be a risky departure from proven practice or prove politically difficult.

Injury is a common and costly childhood affliction, accounting for approximately 15% of medical spending among those aged 1–19 years (Miller, Romano, and Spicer 2000). Indeed, for children and adolescents 5–19 years of age, injury rivals the common cold in frequency (Bureau of the Census 1997). Injuries, however, are much more likely than colds to have lasting effects. Injury has long been the leading mechanism of death among those aged 1–19 years (Rice et al. 1989). In 2000, approximately 18,000 children and adolescents died of injuries. Another 160,000 children and adolescents were permanently disabled as a result of an injury. This estimate comes from the analyses reported in this chapter.

[1]This chapter was adapted, in part, from Miller TR, Romano EO, Spicer RS. 2000. The cost of unintentional childhood injuries and the value of prevention. *Future Child.* 10:137–163 (by permission of the David and Lucile Packard Foundation, Los Altos, CA).

[2]Pacific Institute for Research and Evaluation, Calverton, Maryland.

[3]Health Services and Systems Research Program, Duke-NUS Graduate Medical School, Singapore.

[4]School of Public Health, Curtin University, Perth, Australia.

Coupled with its high death rate, the frequency and severity of nonfatal injury make it a costly childhood health problem. Quantifying the costs associated with childhood injuries is important. Cost estimates translate different injuries—deaths, broken legs, dog bites, even rapes—to a common metric and allow injuries to be compared with other prevalent health conditions. This makes cost data a useful element in gauging the relative size of various problems, assessing risks, setting research priorities, and selecting interventions that most efficiently reduce the burden of injury. For example, injury costs by diagnosis can inform a decision between spending a playground improvement budget to fix swings (estimated to prevent seven broken arms at a total medical cost of $14,300) or slides (estimated to prevent two broken legs at a total medical cost of $11,200). Measuring the benefit of interventions in dollars also helps planners and evaluators to estimate the "net cost" of a safety investment (i.e., the total cost of the investment minus the benefits accrued). On a broader scale, comparably measured costs of injury and illness provide insight into the relative magnitude of these problems and inform resource allocation. Finally, cost data can be used for advocacy purposes by conveying risk reductions in a way that captures the attention of politicians, the media, and the public. For example, a car safety seat give-away program targeting Medicaid recipients may reduce an infant's risk of death by 1% and yield net government savings of $15 per seat (Miller, Demes, and Bovbjerg 1993). Although both risk reduction and government savings are important, communicating the benefit in monetary terms may be more informative for policy makers concerned with overall state or federal budgets.

The widely quoted report *Incidence and Economic Burden of Injuries in the United States, 2000* (Finkelstein et al. 2006) and its predecessor *Cost of Injury in the United States, 1989: A Report to Congress* (Rice et al. 1989) estimated medical spending and other costs resulting from child and adolescent injuries. They provided cost of injury estimates that helped draw recognition to the role of injury as a major public health threat. They did not differentiate injuries by intent, however, combining unintentional injuries with intentional harm, such as child abuse and homicide, although costs of intentional injury have been published separately (Corso et al. 2007; Miller, Cohen, and Wiersema 1996). They omitted sexual assault. Their age categories for children and adolescents were coarse: 0–4, 5–14, and 15–24 years. They also grouped costs by relatively few mechanisms. Their groupings fail to distinguish among important subcategories of motor vehicle injuries (occupant, pedestrian, and pedalcycle) and do not capture other important injury categories, such as bites/stings and overexertion.

This chapter defines the costs associated with child and adolescent injuries and briefly reviews the concepts used in estimating injury costs. It then reports estimates of the lifetime costs of childhood injury in the year 2000 that are based on more mechanism-specific and child-specific data than are available elsewhere. This information allows us to assess the trend since 1985 and compare the costs of injuries and other child and adolescent health problems. To more fully address the issue of injury's priority in child preventive health, the chapter closes with a review of cost-effectiveness estimates for selected child and adolescent injury prevention interventions and comparisons with similar estimates for other child and adolescent health measures.

Injury Costs and Quality of Life Losses

Defining Costs

Injuries among children and adolescents impose a financial burden on many segments of society. Parents and health insurers, for example, assume responsibility for a myriad of medically related expenses resulting from injury. Parents may be forced to stay home from work to care for an injured child, affecting both the family's income and their employer's profit. Children and adolescents disabled from an injury may be unable to work in the future. Deciding which of these costs to include in cost of injury estimates is critical, because the decision can influence the estimated monetary burden of injuries by orders of magnitude. As recommended by the Panel on Cost-Effectiveness in Health and Medicine (Gold et al. 1996), we adopt a *societal perspective* that attempts to estimate all costs associated with child and adolescent injuries—costs to victims, families, government, insurers, and taxpayers. Other perspectives would constrain the analysis to, for example, government expenditures or health care payer expenditures, which include only a subset of total injury costs.

We separate injury costs into resource and productivity costs. *Resource costs* are associated with caring for injury victims and managing the aftermath of injury incidents. Medical costs dominate them. *Productivity costs* value wage work and housework that children and adolescents will be unable to do because of their injury, as well as the work that parents or other adults forego to care for injured children. Box 2.1 more fully describes the cost of injury concepts used in this chapter.

Because injuries sustained during childhood and adolescence may affect the productivity (and quality of life) of both children and their caregivers over time, accounting for losses to both parties is critical. For example, an employed adolescent temporarily disabled from an injury may lose wages in the near term. Likewise, an injury that keeps a child or adolescent home from school for a few days may force a parent to stay home to act as a caregiver. Because injuries are relatively frequent among children, total work losses by adult family members while caring for injured children and youth also are a major cost. Of course, the most extreme impact on productivity occurs when a child or adolescent is killed or permanently disabled by an injury. In such instances, a lifetime of work is lost.

Defining Quality of Life Losses

This chapter primarily focuses on *resource and work loss costs* associated with child and adolescent injuries. However, these costs do not fully capture the burden of these injuries. Injuries also reduce the quality of life of children and families. Losing a child unnecessarily to injury can cause a lifetime of mental anguish. Children and youth who are permanently disabled by injury may experience lifelong pain or have permanent loss of motor or cognitive functioning. To capture these less quantifiable consequences of child and adolescent injuries, we report quality of life losses, valued in nonmonetary terms as quality-adjusted life years (QALYs) (see Box 2.2). Both monetary costs and quality of life measures should be considered when allocating resources, and both should be incorporated into cost-effectiveness analyses that weigh "net costs" against quality of life improvements.

Estimating Costs and Quality of Life Losses

The next two sections report findings from an analysis that estimated the incidence and present and future costs of child injuries (including poisonings and medically treated child neglect) that occurred during 2000. We included injuries that affected children and youth aged 0–19 years and resulted in a physician office visit, a hospital outpatient visit, an emergency department visit, a hospitalization, or a death. We used youth and provider survey data to add interpersonal violence that resulted only in a mental health care visit. We lacked the data needed to include other injuries treated only in the mental health care system, except possibly for suicide acts; as documented below, the literature on untreated post-traumatic stress disorder (PTSD) after childhood injury suggests those cases are rare. Cost of injury estimates were computed by multiplying the *number* of injury victims in 2000—stratified by age group, sex, place of treatment/survival, and mechanism—times the corresponding *costs* per victim (in 2000 dollars). Data for these estimates were extracted from the literature and 11 national and 3 state data sets.

Box 2.1

Cost-of-Injury Concepts

Incidence-Based Versus Prevalence-Based Costs

Incidence-based costs are the present value of the lifetime costs that may result from injuries that occur during a single year. For example, the incidence-based cost of head injuries in 2000 estimates total lifetime costs associated with all head injuries that occurred in 2000. Incidence-based costs measure the total savings over one's lifetime that prevention could yield and are the appropriate costs for cost-effectiveness analysis. Present value shows the amount that would be invested today to pay future costs when they come due. It is computed using a discount rate, essentially an inflation-free interest rate. We discount because (1) money deposited today will earn interest, so less than $1 needs to be deposited today to pay $1 in the future; and (2) the future is uncertain; in 10 years, we may be able to regrow injured nerve tissue, ending the quality of life loss from an injury, or a catastrophe could shorten average life span, unexpectedly truncating lives and with them the losses caused by permanently disabling prior injury. This chapter uses the 3% discount rate recommended by the Panel on Cost-Effectiveness in Health and Medicine (Gold et al. 1996).

Prevalence-based costs measure all injury-related expenses during 1 year, regardless of when the injury occurred. For example, the prevalence-based cost of head injuries in 2000 measures the total health care spending on head injuries during 2000, including spending on victims injured many years earlier. Prevalence-based costs are needed to project health care spending and evaluate cost controls.

Resource Versus Productivity Costs

Resource costs are broken down into medical costs and other resource costs. Productivity costs include immediate and future work losses due to a childhood injury.

Medical costs include emergency medical services, physician, hospital, rehabilitation, prescription, and related treatment costs, as well as ancillary costs (e.g., crutches, physical therapy, home health aides, long-term care) and coroner/medical examiner expenses for fatalities. Except for victims of interpersonal violence, lack of data forced us to omit the costs of mental health care for the injured and their family and friends traumatized by an injury incident. Our rape costs also omit the costs of treating associated sexually transmitted diseases and substance abuse.

Other resource costs include police, child welfare, and fire department costs; costs of processing compensation for injury losses through litigation, insurance, or public programs such as Medicaid, food stamps, and Supplemental Security Income; plus the travel delay for uninjured travelers that results from transportation crashes and the injuries they cause. We excluded other resource costs from our costs per injury.

Work loss costs include victims' lost wages and the value of lost household work and fringe benefits. Work losses by family and friends who care for injured children and adolescents also are included. We excluded productivity losses of employers of injured adolescents (e.g., investigating an injury at work, shuffling schedules or hiring and training a replacement for a youth who misses work because of an injury) and of parents who are temporarily or permanently diverted from work when their offspring have disabling injuries.

We report total and per-injury costs and QALY losses by age group, sex, intent, mechanism, and cost category. We discuss the QALY losses more selectively because of space limitations and the greater uncertainty surrounding these estimates. Appendix 2.1 more fully describes the methods used to estimate injury frequencies, costs, and QALY losses.

Box 2.2

Quality-Adjusted Life Years

Estimating QALYs is one way to value the good health lost to an individual who has a health problem, is disabled, or dies prematurely. A QALY is a measure based on individual preferences for states of health that assigns a value of "1" to a year of perfect health and "0" to death (Gold et al. 1996). QALY losses are affected by the duration and severity of a health problem. To estimate QALY losses, years of potential life lost to a fatal injury are added to the number of years spent with an injury-related disability times a "weighting factor" that represents the severity of the disability. Per the recommendations of the Panel on Cost-Effectiveness in Health and Medicine (Gold et al. 1996), QALY losses in future years are discounted to present value at a 3% discount rate as they are summed. Such "weighting factors" can be estimated by using rating scales (Hirsch et al. 1983) or tradeoff methods that elicit individual preferences between death and various health states (Drummond et al. 1997; Miller et al. 1995).

We based our QALY loss estimates on physician ratings of the functional losses resulting from injury by diagnosis that are routinely used in regulatory analysis by the National Highway Traffic Safety Administration (Blincoe et al. 2002). The ratings, although the best available, are not fully validated and more than 20 years old. Thus, our QALY loss estimates indicate only the order of magnitude of the losses.

For sexual assault, we instead used QALY estimates derived from jury awards for noneconomic damages by Miller, Cohen, and Wiersema (1996). Their estimates are consistent with the QALYs we used for physical injury. Had we used their QALY estimates for physical assault, our QALY loss per physical assault would have been 0.169 instead of 0.163, a 3.7% difference.

This chapter uses 2000 incidence and cost data throughout. As Figure 2.1 shows, the incidence of fatal and serious medically treated childhood injuries has remained essentially flat since 2000. Indeed, the estimated number of injury-related deaths, admissions to hospital through the emergency department, and emergency department transfers to another facility (typically for admission or access to specialty care) was 313,493 in 2000 and 315,912 in 2007. Thus, although serious injury rates per thousand children have declined, overall incidence in more recent years should be similar to the 2000 level and overall costs should vary only because of inflation.

Incidence

Approximately 18,000 children and youth aged 0–19 years died and 17 million were medically treated as the result of injuries in 2000. Approximately 250,000 survivors were admitted to hospitals (Table 2.1, left). The right panel of Table 2.1 shows injury rates per 10,000 children and youth in the noninstitutionalized U.S. population. In 2000, 21% of U.S. children and youth had medically treated injuries. The injury rate at ages 0–9 years combined was 70% of the rate at ages 10–19 years combined. The lowest injury rate was at ages 5–9 years.

The left panel in Table 2.2 shows injury incidence by intent (i.e., unintentional, suicide act, assault, undetermined, or legal/military action) and mechanism (the process causing the injury, e.g., cut/pierce, poisoning, submersion). The overwhelming majority of child and adolescent injuries (89%) were unintentional. Sexual assaults accounted for 6% of cases, physical assaults accounted for 4% of cases, and suicide acts and cases with undetermined intent accounted for

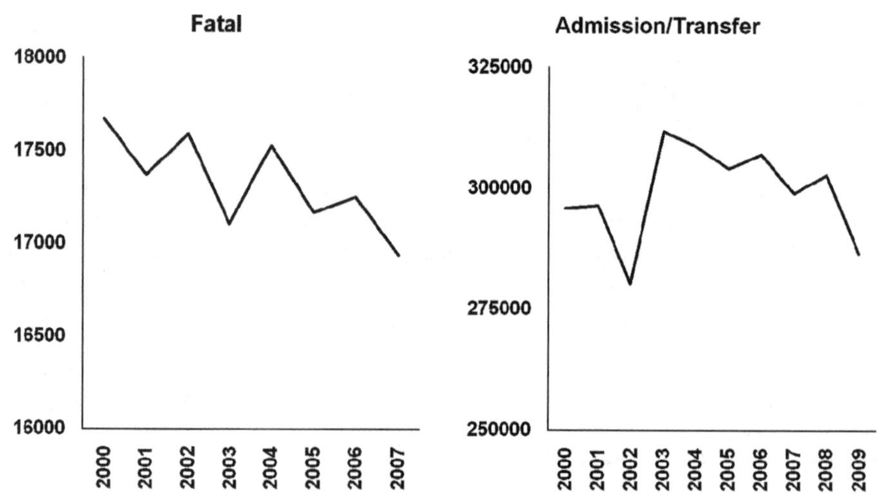

Source: WISQARS on-line query system, http://www.cdc.gov/injury/wisqars/index.html; accessed October, 2010.

Figure 2.1. Time Trends in Child Fatalities and Child Hospital Admissions or Transfers From the Emergency Department

approximately 0.5% each. Assaults increased in importance at ages 15–19 years, accounting for 17% of the injuries.

Variations in the leading mechanisms across age groups suggest it may be appropriate to target select prevention practices to specific ages. Among unintentional injuries, the leading mechanisms were falls (28% of all injuries) and struck by/against (22%). The pattern was markedly different at ages 15–19 years than younger ages, with falls decreasing from 33% to 15%, motor vehicle occupant injuries increasing from 4% to 15%, overexertion injuries increasing from 5% to 12%, bites and stings decreasing from 9% to 2%, and struck by/against injuries increasing slightly from 21% to 24%. Burns, poisonings, and submersions primarily occurred at ages 0–4 years, and unintentional firearm injuries (including BB gun injuries) and struck by/against injuries occurred at ages 10–14 years. Pedalcyclist injuries peaked at ages 5–9 and 10–14 years, whereas motor vehicle occupant injuries started increasing at ages 10–14 years. The incidence of falls declined more than 600,000 cases (>50%) between ages 10–14 and 15–19 years.

In terms of frequency, poisonings dominated the suicide acts and sexual assaults dominated the assaults. Physical assault injuries most often resulted from being struck by another person or a weapon or pushed into something. Most injuries of undetermined intent lacked external cause codes in the source data, and consequently lacked data on both intent and mechanism.

Boys were 1.2 times as likely as girls to have medically treated injuries, as the right panel in Table 2.2 shows. Their excess risk was highest at ages 0–4 years and lowest at ages 15–19 years. Boys were the victims in only 15% (0.18/1.18) of child sexual assaults. They were half as likely as girls to have fatal or medically treated suicide acts, but 1.3 times as likely to have physical assaults or unintentional injuries. Their risks were especially high for all types of firearm injuries, 5 to 15 times the risks for girls. Their pedalcycle and unintentional suffocation risks also were substantially elevated, as were their burn risks at ages 0–4 and 15–19 years. Girls generally were at higher risk of bites and stings, motor vehicle occupant injury at ages 10–14 and 15–19 years, and overexertion injuries at ages 0–4 and 5–9 years (although some of these differences may not be statistically significant). Boys aged 5–9 and 10–14 years were at the greatest added risk of assault compared with girls. Physical assault rates equalized at ages 15–19 years, perhaps because of dating violence. Some of the risk differentials reflect differences between boys and girls in terms of activities and behavior. Others are hard to explain and warrant exploration.

Child and Adolescent Injury Costs

The estimated lifetime medical and productivity costs of injuries experienced by U.S. children and youth aged 0–19 years during 2000 totaled $106 billion (Table 2.3). The bulk of this financial burden (77%) resulted from future work losses experienced by injured children and youth and current work losses by their caregivers. Current and future losses of earnings and fringe benefits accounted for 63% ($67.1 billion) of the total lifetime childhood injury costs. Household work loses accounted for 14% ($14.8 billion). Medical costs made up the remainder, accounting for 23% ($24.4 billion) of lifetime costs. Thus, although injuries may be viewed appropriately as a *health* problem, from a cost perspective, injuries are even more an *economic* problem. Each year injuries kill or disable approximately 160,000 otherwise healthy children and youth before they have a chance to enter the workforce and maximally contribute to society. The current workforce is affected, too, as many adult caregivers are forced to stay home to tend to injured offspring.

Injuries in 2000 cost an average of $1320 per U.S. resident aged 0–19 years (as shown in the right panel of Table 2.3). Averaged across injured and uninjured children and youth, medical spending on injury averaged $300 per child. Future work losses and parental work losses due to injury averaged $1020 per child. By comparison, a middle-income household with two parents spent $590 per child on clothing and $1590 per child on food in 2000 (Figure 2.2) (Lino 2001).

Costs by Injury Severity

Table 2.4 differentiates costs among fatalities, hospital-admitted survivors, and other medically treated survivors. The most severe child and adolescent injuries, those that result in death, disproportionately contributed to lifetime injury costs. Fatal injuries represented 0.1% of all child and adolescent injuries in 2000, but produced 23% of injury-related costs. By contrast, the least severe injuries, nonfatal injuries where the child was not hospitalized, accounted for 93% of all child and adolescent injuries, yet produced only 55% of the estimated lifetime costs. Thus, although the rare injury fatalities contributed disproportionately to the financial burden of child and adolescent injuries, the most common and least severe injuries still accounted for more than half of total injury costs.

The severity of child and adolescent injuries also affected the relative contribution of medical costs versus productivity losses to total injury costs. Medical spending accounted for 93% of the cost of sexual assaults that require only mental health treatment. In contrast, when a child or adolescent had a medically treated nonfatal injury, caregiver work losses typically cost much more than medical treatment. Although hospital care is expensive, medical costs still accounted for a smaller proportion of hospitalized injury costs (21%) than work loss of caregivers and permanently disabled children and youth (79%). For children and youth killed as a result of an injury, the overwhelming cost (99%) was the future work that they will never do. Medical costs accounted for less than 1% of the total injury costs for these victims.

Per injured child, costs averaged $6200, including $1430 in medical spending and $4770 in work losses. Costs averaged $1.35 million per fatality, $71,900 per hospital-admitted injury, $3700 per injury treated without hospitalization, and $5670 per sexual assault injury resulting in only mental health treatment.

Costs by Age

As children grow, their motor skills and cognitive skills develop and their environment changes. Therefore, their injury risks shift. Critical milestones that affect injury risk may include starting

Table 2.1. Incidence and Rates per 10,000 Residents of Fatal and Medically Treated Injury Cases, by Age Group and Gender, 0–19 Years: United States, 2000

	Incidence					Rate per 10,000 Residents				
	0–4 y	5–9 y	10–14 y	15–19 y	Total	0–4 y	5–9 y	10–14 y	15–19 y	Total
					Total					
Fatal	3532	1561	2180	10,505	17,778	1.8	0.8	1.1	5.2	2.2
Admitted	47,200	37,200	51,300	112,600	248,300	25	18	25	56	31
Not admitted	3,437,900	3,261,600	4,728,500	4,441,000	15,869,000	1793	1587	2303	2196	1972
Mental health only	26,500	160,000	350,600	464,200	1,001,300	14	78	171	230	124
Total	3,515,100	3,460,400	5,132,600	5,028,300	17,136,400	1833	1684	2500	2487	2129
					Male					
Fatal	2059	923	1474	7891	12,347	2.1	0.9	1.4	7.6	3.0
Admitted	27,300	23,200	33,400	70,000	153,900	28	22	32	67	37
Not admitted	2,067,800	1,814,000	2,759,400	2,577,200	9,218,400	2108	1724	2623	2480	2235
Mental health only	8800	40,200	81,200	31,600	161,800	9	38	77	30	39
Total	2,106,000	1,878,300	2,875,500	2,686,700	9,546,500	2147	1785	2733	2586	2315

(*continued on next page*)

Table 2.1. *(continued)*

	Incidence					Rate per 10,000 Residents				
	0–4 y	**5–9 y**	**10–14 y**	**15–19 y**	**Total**	**0–4 y**	**5–9 y**	**10–14 y**	**15–19 y**	**Total**
					Female					
Fatal	1473	638	706	2614	5431	1.6	0.6	0.7	2.7	1.4
Admitted	19,900	14,000	17,900	42,600	94,400	21	14	18	43	24
Not admitted	1,370,100	1,447,600	1,969,100	1,863,800	6,650,600	1463	1444	1968	1896	1695
Mental health only	17,700	119,800	269,400	432,600	839,500	19	119	269	440	214
Total	1,409,200	1,582,000	2,257,100	2,341,600	7,589,900	1505	1578	2255	2382	1935

Note: Totals and rates were computed before rounding.

Table 2.2. Injury Incidence and Relative Risk, by Gender, Age Group, and Mechanism, Ages 0–19 Years: United States, 2000

	Incidence					Relative Risk, Male Rate/Female Rate				
	0–4 y	5–9 y	10–14 y	15–19 y	Total	0–4 y	5–9 y	10–14 y	15–19 y	Total
					Unintentional					
Cut/pierce	127,428	166,324	301,375	295,522	890,649	1.70	1.64	2.65	1.36	1.80
Submersion	3209	864	573	747	5393	1.73	2.06	0.98	2.31	1.73
Fall	1,375,414	1,052,670	1,221,752	603,439	4,253,275	1.36	1.25	1.34	1.21	1.30
Burn	138,887	27,649	22,833	100,902	290,271	1.87	0.90	1.05	4.48	2.13
Firearm	499	1913	18,765	7644	28,821	2.42	5.95	24.55	10.87	15.01
Motor vehicle occupant	89,041	83,191	219,624	596,883	988,739	2.06	1.06	0.43	0.78	0.77
Pedalcyclist	36,281	200,948	171,248	75,538	484,015	2.50	1.77	3.65	8.56	2.78
Pedestrian	8363	17,140	28,370	19,910	73,783	1.59	1.71	0.83	1.22	1.16
Bites and stings	436,957	312,100	304,213	99,917	1,153,187	0.78	1.03	0.59	0.70	0.77
Overexertion	77,099	102,444	335,912	488,193	1,003,648	0.76	0.64	1.33	1.99	1.43
Poisoning	170,430	103,766	55,267	61,281	390,744	1.10	1.42	2.66	0.91	1.28
Struck by/against	501,879	624,122	1,265,662	990,638	3,382,301	1.84	1.38	2.57	1.47	1.83

(*continued on next page*)

Table 2.2. *(continued)*

	Incidence					Relative Risk, Male Rate/Female Rate				
	0–4 y	5–9 y	10–14 y	15–19 y	Total	0–4 y	5–9 y	10–14 y	15–19 y	Total
Suffocation	66,059	2277	1660	1250	71,246	8.52	1.74	2.84	2.88	7.33
Other specified	225,157	292,636	269,962	307,009	1,094,764	1.27	1.14	0.37	1.71	1.00
Unspecified	143,525	209,640	363,156	406,378	1,122,699					
Total	3,400,228	3,197,684	4,580,372	4,055,251	15,233,535	1.42	1.17	1.34	1.37	1.33
					Suicide					
Cut/pierce		140	1891	12,663	14,694			0.09	0.59	0.51
Firearm		6	239	1156	1401			7.17	7.80	7.70
Poisoning		404	10,465	39,004	49,873			0.21	0.43	0.38
Suffocation		16	399	676	1091			7.30	4.43	5.30
Other specified		216	1748	4673	6637			0.79	1.23	1.16
Unspecified		121	38	181	340					
Total		903	14,780	58,353	74,036		1.16	0.29	0.55	0.49

(continued on next page)

Table 2.2. *(continued)*

	Incidence					Relative Risk, Male Rate/Female Rate				
	0–4 y	5–9 y	10–14 y	15–19 y	Total	0–4 y	5–9 y	10–14 y	15–19 y	Total
					Assault					
Cut/pierce	452	2898	6268	22,931	32,549	0.81	1.46	1.46	2.30	1.98
Firearm	146	543	2048	10,505	13,242	2.44	1.91	1.56	9.22	5.43
Struck by/ against	32,885	66,147	147,007	310,678	556,717	0.87	1.64	1.85	1.23	1.39
Suffocation	53	14	418	208	693	0.92	0.95	2.08	2.13	1.93
Sexual only	26,496	159,917	350,659	464,263	1,001,335	0.47	0.32	0.29	0.07	0.18
Other specified	6983	31,479	13,649	17,655	69,766	1.68	11.36	1.46	0.72	2.30
Unspecified	826	315	556	40,023	41,720					
Total	67,841	261,313	520,605	866,263	1,716,022	0.75	0.73	0.56	0.37	0.48
Undetermined[a]	46,817	298	15,176	38,507	100,798				0.74	1.57
Legal/military	236	121	1607	9976	11,940			8.09	5.13	4.52
Grand total	3,515,122	3,460,319	5,132,540	5,028,350	17,136,331	1.43	1.13	1.21	1.09	1.20

Note: We did not test whether relative risks differed significantly from 1.0.

[a]Seventy-four percent of the cases of undetermined intent also had unspecified mechanisms.

Table 2.3. Costs of Injury, Total and per Child, by Cost Category and Age Group, Ages 0–19 Years: United States, 2000

	Total Cost, Millions of 2000 Dollars					Cost per Child, 2000 Dollars				
	0–4 y	5–9 y	10–14 y	15–19 y	Total	0–4 y	5–9 y	10–14 y	15–19 y	Total
Medical	4051	4285	6850	9248	24,433	211	209	334	457	304
Wage work[a]	12,794	10,620	17,830	25,813	67,057	667	517	869	1277	833
Household work	2533	2359	3604	6297	14,792	132	115	176	311	184
Total	19,378	17,263	28,283	41,357	106,282	1010	841	1379	2045	1321

[a]For children aged <15 years, includes parental work loss and child work loss to permanent disability and death.

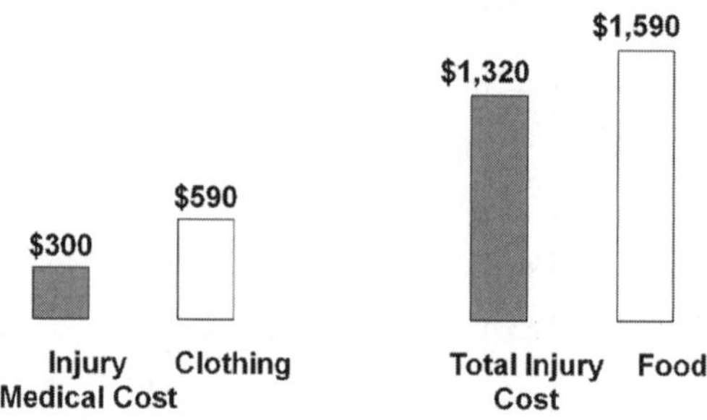

Figure 2.2. Annual Spending Per U.S. Child

to crawl, walk, attend school, ride a bicycle, drink alcohol, and drive a car, as well as developing an ability to recognize and make decisions about dangerous situations. Thus, injury rates, mechanisms, and severity vary with age.

We examined injury rates and costs in 5-year age groups. Adolescents aged 15–19 years experienced higher rates of injuries that were fatal or required hospitalization compared with children in younger age groups (Table 2.1). Similarly, injury costs were higher among adolescents than among children of other ages. We estimated the total lifetime medical and productivity costs of injuries that teenagers aged 15–19 years experienced in 2000 at $41 billion (Table 2.3). Among younger and school-aged children, costs were considerably less ($19 billion among 0- to 4-year-olds, $17 billion among 5- to 9-year-olds, and $28 billion among 10- to 14-year-olds). Adolescents also had higher lifetime costs per child due to injury ($2040 per injury) (but slightly lower average costs compared with the $2240 average for young adults aged 20–24 years).

The higher total injury costs among adolescents reflected the greater absolute number of hospitalized and fatal injuries that occurred in this age group. More than 10,500 adolescents aged 15–19 years died of injuries that occurred in 2000—more than the number of deaths from injuries among all children aged 0–14 years combined (7273 deaths). The higher number of adolescent fatalities translated into higher total injury costs in this age group, because youth who were killed lost a lifetime of future work. The mechanisms of injuries sustained by adolescents also tended to result in the most costly injuries per victim. For example, as shown in Table 2.5, intentional firearm injuries and suffocation (suicide or assault) were among the most costly mechanisms of child and adolescent injury per victim. Although rare, these injuries occurred more frequently among adolescents than children in any other age group (Table 2.2). The injury surge in adolescence probably resulted from increased exposure to risk, with 30% of ninth- to twelfth-grade students binge drinking and many starting to drive (estimated from the 2001 Youth Risk Behavior Surveillance System, Centers for Disease Control and Prevention, 2003).

Costs by Intent

Unintentional injury costs were the dominant factor in child and adolescent injury. They accounted for 93% of injury costs at ages 0–4 years, 90% of injury costs at ages 5–9 years, and 87% of injury costs at ages 10–14 years, but only 71% of injury costs at ages 15–19 years. Unintentional injury costs increased rapidly starting at ages 10–14 years, increasing approximately $9 billion (57%) over their costs at ages 5–9 years ($15.5 billion; Table 2.5). They increased again, by $5 billion, at ages 15–19 years.

In adolescence, intentional injury costs tripled. They jumped from $3.7 billion at ages 10–14 years to $11.5 billion and accounted for 28% of injury costs at ages 15–19 years. Suicide acts accounted for 7% ($2.8 billion), physical assaults (physical assaults are computed as total assaults

Table 2.4. Total and Unit Costs and Quality-Adjusted Life Year Losses of Injury, by Severity, Ages 0–19 Years: United States, 2000

	Total Cost, Millions of 2000 Dollars					Cost/Case, 2000 Dollars				
	Medical	Wage Work	House Work	Total	Total QALYs	Medical	Wage Work	House Work	Total	QALYs / Case
Fatal	134	19,615	4322	24,071	501,434	7548	1,103,316	243,131	1,353,996	28.2
Admitted	3698	11,779	2371	17,848	386,293	14,894	47,440	9548	71,882	1.6
Not admitted	15,308	35,662	7712	58,683	593,165	965	2247	486	3698	0.04
Mental health	5293	317	70	5679	666,140	5286	316	70	5672	0.67
Total	24,433	67,373	14,475	106,282	2,147,033	1426	3913	863	6202	0.13

QALY = quality-adjusted life year.

Table 2.5. Total and Unit Costs of Injury, by Age Group and Mechanism, Ages 0–19 Years: United States, 2000

	Total Cost, Millions of 2000 Dollars					Cost per Injury Case, 2000 Dollars				
	0–4 y	5–9 y	10–14 y	15–19 y	Total	0–4 y	5–9 y	10–14 y	15–19 y	Total
					Unintentional					
Cut/pierce	360	450	658	709	2177	2826	2706	2183	2398	2444
Submersion	824	315	303	663	2105	256,679	364,789	528,958	886,949	390,229
Fall	6821	6563	6947	3318	23,649	4959	6235	5686	5498	5560
Burn	965	392	220	579	2157	6949	14,186	9631	5742	7430
Firearm	31	35	127	333	527	63,124	18,276	6793	43,536	18,275
Motor vehicle occupant	1377	1027	1853	11,665	15,922	15,465	12,341	8437	19,543	16,103
Pedalcyclist	136	1028	1404	773	3341	3752	5116	8198	10,229	6902
Pedestrian	442	520	529	825	2316	52,899	30,327	18,637	41,439	31,389
Bites and stings	694	460	640	365	2159	1589	1473	2104	3658	1873
Overexertion	358	317	1904	1345	3923	4646	3090	5667	2755	3909
Poisoning	244	107	87	620	1058	1434	1027	1569	10,117	2707
Struck by/ against	2750	2025	6400	4366	15,540	5479	3244	5056	4407	4594

(continued on next page)

Table 2.5. *(continued)*

	Total Cost, Millions of 2000 Dollars					Cost per Injury Case, 2000 Dollars				
	0–4 y	**5–9 y**	**10–14 y**	**15–19 y**	**Total**	**0–4 y**	**5–9 y**	**10–14 y**	**15–19 y**	**Total**
Suffocation	847	69	121	123	1160	12,822	30,272	72,942	98,249	16,279
Other specified	1173	1282	1518	2206	6179	5210	4380	5624	7185	5644
Total	17,945	15,572	24,497	29,465	87,479	5278	4870	5348	7266	5743
					Suicide					
Cut/pierce			32	154	189			16,853	12,146	12,829
Firearm			159	1418	1577			664,328	1,226,274	1,125,393
Poisoning			52	275	330			5013	7047	6612
Suffocation		12	251	802	1065		727,018	629,280	1,186,438	975,937
Other specified			20	178	201			11,408	38,184	30,299
Total		20	517	2839	3376		22,482	34,974	48,644	45,508
					Assault					
Cut/pierce	26	34	70	462	591	56,719	11,685	11,161	20,134	18,162
Firearm	49	69	241	2899	3259	336,915	127,869	117,784	275,935	246,077
Sexual only[a]	151	914	1985	2629	5679	5714	5714	5662	5662	5672

(continued on next page)

Table 2.5. *(continued)*

	Total Cost, Millions of 2000 Dollars					Cost per Injury Case, 2000 Dollars				
	0–4 y	**5–9 y**	**10–14 y**	**15–19 y**	**Total**	**0–4 y**	**5–9 y**	**10–14 y**	**15–19 y**	**Total**
Struck by/ against	212	424	676	2025	3336	6436	6408	4598	6518	5993
Suffocation	51	15	24	57	146	957,802	1,039,716	57,027	273,572	210,765
Other specified	453	162	140	237	992	64,876	5160	10,255	13,417	14,223
Total	1208	1639	3167	8650	14,663	17,803	6273	6082	9985	8545
Undetermined	224	32	90	318	665	4801	106,350	5958	8271	6604
Legal/military				85	99				8542	8276
Grand total	19,378	17,263	28,283	41,357	106,282	5513	4989	5511	8225	6202

Note: A few numbers were deleted because they were based on fewer than five cases. Estimates <50 million generally were based on relatively small samples and should be used with caution.

[a]Two male and 56 female rape-murders were classified by the mechanism causing death.

minus sexual assaults) accounted for 15% ($6.0 billion), and sexual assaults accounted for 6% ($2.6 billion). The data suggest that effective violence prevention programs targeting adolescents should be a priority and might offer significant savings.

Costs by Mechanism of Injury

Five primary mechanisms of unintentional injury accounted for approximately 75% of total lifetime unintentional injury costs among children and youth aged 0–19 years. As shown in the left side of Table 2.5, these mechanisms included falls, occupant injury in motor vehicle crashes, pedestrian and pedalcyclist injury combined, being struck by/against an object or person, and overexertion injuries (e.g., strains, sprains, and muscle tears). These five mechanisms of unintentional injuries contributed substantially to overall injury costs because the combination of the *frequency* of the injury in the population and *average cost per victim* was exceedingly high. The relative importance of frequency versus cost per case, however, varied by type of injury. For example, although falls were relatively low in cost ($5600 per victim, as shown in the right side of Table 2.5), they were the most prevalent injuries. As a result, they were the largest contributor to total child and adolescent unintentional injury costs (Table 2.2). In contrast, although motor vehicle crashes that injured children and adolescents occurred less frequently than falls, the resulting injuries were often severe and costly (averaging $16,100 per victim). It was primarily the severity of such injuries that made motor vehicle crashes the second leading contributor to total unintentional injury costs among children and youth. Injury prevention efforts ideally would include a mix of interventions that greatly reduce the prevalence of less costly injuries and that more modestly reduce severe injuries.

The relative cost per injury case varied greatly across mechanisms (Table 2.5, right). The data fell into two clusters, with costs per case either more than $200,000 or less than $35,000. Suicide acts with a firearm or by suffocation/hanging were most costly at $1,125,000 and $976,000 per case, respectively, including medical and work loss costs. Drowning or submersion caused the most expensive unintentional injuries at $390,000 per case. Among assaults, the most costly involved firearms ($246,000) or suffocation ($211,000). Although high-cost mechanisms occurred less frequently among children and adolescents than most injury mechanisms, the severity of the injuries and the long-term disability and deaths that often resulted made them extremely expensive when they did occur. The last three columns in Table 2.6 illustrate this clearly, showing that fatality probabilities exceeded 13% (130 per thousand) for every high-cost category but decreased to less than 1.5% (15 per thousand) for every remaining injury category.

Unintentional pedestrian injuries and all categories of intentionally self-inflicted injuries involved a hospital admission or death in at least 10% of cases. The admitted suicide acts, however, tended to involve short hospital stays that may result more from the need to provide temporary protection from repeat injury than from treatment of physical effects. Indeed, many were coded as psychiatric admissions.

The most costly unintentional injury mechanisms were fairly consistent across the child and adolescent age categories, although their relative importance differed (Table 2.5). Through age 14 years, falls were the most costly mechanism of unintentional injury, struck by/against was second, and motor vehicle occupant injury was third or fourth. Among 15- to 19-year-olds, however, motor vehicle crashes and struck by/against displaced falls as the most costly injury mechanisms. Some mechanisms only showed up as leading contributors for one or two age groups. Burns, suffocation, and drowning/submersion were the fourth to sixth leading mechanisms of injury costs at ages 0–4 years, but not a leading mechanism at other ages. Pedalcyclist injury tied for third place at ages 5–9 years and was in fifth place at ages 10–14 years. Overexertion injury was in the top five at ages 10–14 and 15–19 years. Pedestrian injury was in fifth place at ages 5–9 years and again at ages 15–19 years.

Table 2.6. Quality-Adjusted Life Years Lost per Year, by Age Group and per Case, and Other Severity Measures, by Mechanism, Ages 0–19 Years: United States, 2000

	Total QALYs Lost					QALYs Lost per Case	Total Medical, Millions of 2000 Dollars	Fatal per 1000 Cases	Fatal or Admitted per 1000 Cases	Fatalities
	0–4 y	5–9 y	10–14 y	15–19 y	Total					
Unintentional										
Cut/pierce	1336	1036	2707	2899	7978	0.01	697	0.007	8	6
Submersion	17,267	5985	5019	10,545	38,815	7.20	39	246.8	580	1331
Fall	155,755	115,481	102,903	48,095	422,236	0.10	4827	0.04	12	184
Burn	11,837	6046	3062	3077	24,021	0.08	397	2.4	23	685
Firearm	765	747	1799	5162	8473	0.29	58	6.7	79	193
Motor vehicle occupant	35,703	23,840	30,915	202,713	293,172	0.30	2401	6.7	46	6589
Pedalcyclist	4310	21,721	19,668	8662	54,360	0.11	631	0.5	24	227
Pedestrian	12,298	12,898	10,204	13,279	48,679	0.66	344	14.2	139	1047
Bites and stings	959	978	1370	3311	6618	0.01	610	0.2	6	200
Overexertion	1013	1406	29,210	13,266	44,896	0.04	1233	0.001	4	1
Poisoning	1794	666	903	9729	13,092	0.03	295	1.1	32	442

(*continued on next page*)

Table 2.6. *(continued)*

	Total QALYs Lost					QALYs Lost per Case	Total Medical, Millions of 2000 Dollars	Fatal per 1000 Cases	Fatal or Admitted per 1000 Cases	Fatalities
	0–4 y	5–9 y	10–14 y	15–19 y	Total					
Struck by/against	10,651	18,562	56,313	33,979	119,506	0.04	3039	0.03	5	108
Suffocation	20,444	1326	2076	1982	25,828	0.36	52	12.1	43	865
Other specified	15,063	15,707	21,866	53,472	106,109	0.10	1298	0.5	21	516
Total	305,133	241,521	316,607	432,547	1,295,808	0.09	16,887	0.8	14	12,532
Suicide										
Cut/pierce			94	607	709	0.05	28	0.4	261	6
Firearm			3137	24,789	27,929	19.93	13	718.8	827	1007
Poisoning			518	3550	4068	0.08	131	2.5	471	126
Suffocation		203	4754	14,134	19,092	17.50	6	632.4	806	690
Other specified			220	3061	3321	0.50	17	14.2	119	94
Total		253	8754	46,314	55,321	0.75	197	26.0	408	1930

(continued on next page)

Table 2.6. *(continued)*

	Total QALYs Lost					QALYs Lost per Case	Total Medical, Millions of 2000 Dollars	Fatal per 1000 Cases	Fatal or Admitted per 1000 Cases	Fatalities
	0–4 y	5–9 y	10–14 y	15–19 y	Total					
					Assault					
Cut/pierce	636	455	928	8822	10,841	0.33	99	6.4	90	208
Firearm	1374	1701	4851	51,210	59,135	4.47	202	134.2	500	1777
Sexual only[a]	21,380	129,037	221,915	293,809	666,140	0.67	5293	0[a]	0[a]	[a]
Struck by/against	1310	1662	1824	7675	12,471	0.02	1319	0.1	8	41
Suffocation	1565	383	548	1183	3678	5.31	2	181.8	215	126
Other specified	12,349	1572	1669	3164	18,755	0.27	231	7.1	39	493
Total	46,313	135,283	232,405	368,692	782,692	0.46	7245	1.7	11	2999
Undetermined	5520	690	1543	4256	12,009	0.12	89	2.9	49	287
Legal/military				1063	1203	0.10	15	2.5	8	30
Grand total	356,974	377,754	559,433	852,871	2,147,033	0.13	24,433	1.0	16	17,778

QALY = quality-adjusted life year.

Note: A few numbers were deleted because they were based on fewer than five cases. Estimates <1000 QALYs generally were based on relatively small samples and should be used with caution.

[a]Two male and 56 female rape-murders were classified by the mechanism causing death.

A more detailed breakdown of injuries by mechanism and age group (results available on request) revealed that the nature of fall risks varied by age. Falls caused an estimated 25% of injuries at ages 0–4, 5–9, and 10–14 years and 15% of injuries at ages 15–19 years, resulting in an estimated 27% of lifetime unintentional childhood injury costs. They accounted for 34% of costs at ages 0–4 years, 41% at ages 5–9 years, 24% at ages 10–14 years, and 13% at ages 15–19 years. At ages 0–4 years, the largest factors were falls from furniture, stairs, and slipping. At ages 5–9 years, fall risks shifted to playgrounds, trees, and slipping incidents, and to pedalcycles, slipping, and sports at ages 10–14 years. Even though total falls decreased precipitately after age 14 years, falls in sports (and related overexertion and striking injuries) remained important through age 19 years. Although Rice et al. (1989) identified fall injuries as a major childhood risk factor in 1985, few effective approaches, with notable exceptions of window guards, stair gates, improved stairway and baby walker design, and protective sporting gear such as helmets and kneepads, have been developed to prevent them. The high frequency and cost of fall injuries in 2000 strongly support the need to identify cost-effective strategies to reduce the incidence of falls among children.

Motor vehicles and other vehicles ranging from pedalcycles to trains to Jet Skis pose risks to child and adolescent passengers and pedestrians. Bicycles are typically the first vehicles that children drive. At ages 5–14 years, pedestrian and pedalcycle injuries together outranked injuries to motor vehicle occupants in cost. Motor vehicle crash costs increased steadily throughout childhood and took a noticeable leap when girls aged 10–19 years and boys aged 15–19 years began riding with friends and siblings and subsequently reached driving age. The increase in motor vehicle injury costs for girls aged 10–14 years is a target for exploration and intervention. We speculate it occurred because socializing with older teenagers who have cars may be more common among girls. Crashes imposed by far the largest injury costs for adolescents aged 15–19 years, comprising 28% of total injury costs for this age group.

Unintentional struck by/against injuries are an ill-defined mix that includes sports injuries, people hit by falling objects, people bumping into furniture and closing doors on fingers, and people tripping and striking hard objects as they land, among other things. Better epidemiology is needed to understand this injury mechanism, which accounted for 15% of total costs and 21% of injuries, but only 1% of fatalities and 7% of hospital admissions. Although unintentional struck by/against injuries are a major contributor to child and adolescent injury costs, outside of sports, we know too little about these injuries to develop preventive interventions.

Quality of Life Losses

Injuries among children impose more than monetary costs on society. They reduce the quality of life among injured children and their families. We measured those losses in units of quality-adjusted life year (QALY). A QALY is a year of healthy life and functioning (see Box 2.2). The QALY losses were estimated from physicians' estimates by diagnosis of the effects that a childhood injury has on mobility, cognition, bending/grasping/lifting, sensory function, pain, and appearance (e.g., scarring or prostheses), as well as on the ability to work and the value people place on those functional losses. In total, children and adolescents fatally and nonfatally injured in 2000 lost the equivalent of 2.1 million years of life (Table 2.4), a loss comparable to 75,000 child and adolescent deaths. To compute the number of equivalent deaths, we divided the QALY loss by 29, which is the present value (at a 3% discount rate) of the 66 years of life that the average 11-year-old child has remaining.

The QALYs lost were concentrated in three groups of injuries. Injury fatalities accounted for 23% of QALYs lost, although only 0.1% of all childhood injuries in 2000 resulted in death (not shown). Hospital admissions were 1.5% of cases but accounted for 18% of QALYs lost. Another 28% of the QALYs lost were associated with medically treated nonfatal injuries that did not require hospitalization. The losses for these injuries resulted from short-term disability and from long-term disability that arose when complications developed or a nonfatal injury, such as a facial laceration or arm fracture, scarred a child or permanently restricted range of motion.

Sexual assault accounted for 31% of all QALY losses (Figure 2.3). Sexual assault resulted in substantial economic and personal losses, and was responsible for 30% to 40% of girls' QALY losses in every age group from 5–19 years and for approximately 16% of boys' QALY losses at ages 5–9 and 10–14 years. The average sexual assault victim's loss was 0.67 QALYs. Policy discussion and preventive effort on this dominating problem are too modest. Child and adolescent sexual assault is a national tragedy. We should do more.

Similar to the patterns observed for injury frequency and costs across age groups, total estimated QALY losses were highest among adolescents aged 15–19 years (853,000 QALYs, a loss comparable to 30,700 child deaths) and lowest among children aged 0–4 years (357,000 QALYs, a loss comparable to 11,900 child deaths). The number of children in each 5-year age group was similar. The differences in QALY losses resulted from the same injury frequency and severity differences that caused teenagers to have higher resource and productivity loss costs.

Because children develop rapidly early in life, the 0- to 4-year age group lumps evolving risks. Therefore, we examined QALY losses by detailed mechanism and individual year of age (not shown). For infants, the largest losses came from suffocation; other breathing threats, including submersion, assaults, and other maltreatment; and falls from beds, on stairs, and of unspecified nature. Fatalities dominated QALY loss at this age. Drownings, house fires, assaults, and falls were the largest threats at ages 1 to 2 years. Motor vehicle pedestrian and occupant incidents also began to emerge as risks by age 2 years, a pattern that strengthened at ages 3 to 4 years.

Choosing a Burden Measure to Guide Resource Allocation

Decisions on how to allocate injury surveillance, research, and prevention resources among injury mechanisms should be made with full information on the societal burden imposed by each injury mechanism. The gold standard measures, because they capture the burden most completely, are total costs and QALY losses. Ideally, the easiest comparisons would result if these measures were combined into a single comprehensive measure, but the methods currently available to combine them are controversial (Kenkel 2001; Krupnick 2004; Miller 2000; Sunstein 2003). Furthermore, these measures rarely are available below the national level, but resource allocation decisions often must be made locally. Comparing the injury mechanisms that create the largest burden according to different measures is helpful in understanding the relative degree of resource misallocation that is likely to result if local decision-makers base policies on different second-best measures.

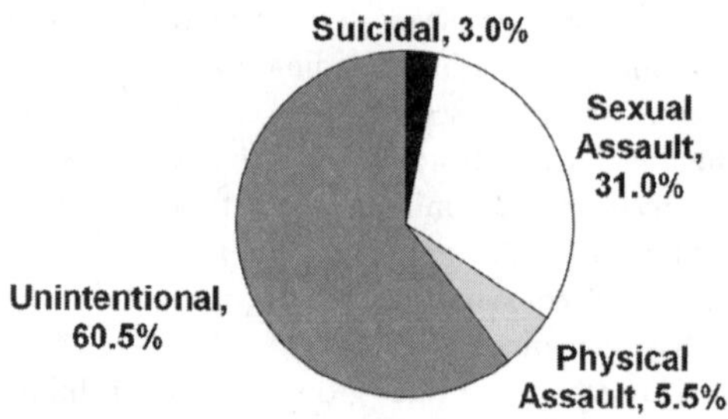

Figure 2.3. QALYs Lost to Iinjury, by Type, Among Children and Youth aged 0–19 years: United States, 2000

Tables 2.5 and 2.6 display a range of measures that could be used to set prevention priorities. Sexual assault dominated QALY loss to child and adolescent injury. It cost only slightly fewer QALYs than unintentional falls and motor vehicle occupant injuries combined. The three leading mechanisms contributing to medical and productivity costs and the next three contributors to QALY loss were identical (Table 2.6): unintentional falls, motor vehicle occupant injuries, and injuries from being struck by or against an object. Because their fatality rate was low, struck by/against injuries, nevertheless, were a far larger contributor to total costs than to QALY losses. Notable incongruities between total costs and total QALY losses also arose for unintentional cut/pierce injuries, unintentional bites and stings, and firearm suicide acts. Again, high or low fatality rates for these mechanisms drove the differentials. Priority decisions about these injuries may be clearer if a dollar value is placed on the QALYs.

Because mortality data by injury mechanism have been readily available at the state and county levels for decades, fatal counts traditionally have been used in injury priority-setting. The fatal burden ranking differed markedly from rankings based on the gold standard measures (total costs and QALYs). Fatal counts, however, differed only modestly in rank ordering from three other measures: QALYs lost per case (except for sexual assaults), total cost per case, and fatalities per thousand medically attended or fatal injury cases. Fatalities and these related burden and severity measures are unwise choices to guide resource allocation and program planning.

Counts of live hospital discharges for injury (Table 2.6) or the sum of discharges and fatalities (data not shown) yielded rankings that more closely matched the rankings on the gold standard measures than fatality counts did. However, they undervalued the total burden of sexual assault. The magnitude of sexual assault was only identified by measures that incorporated total QALY losses or by a total medical cost measure. For other mechanisms, live discharge counts tracked total medical costs reasonably closely, although firearm suicide acts were a more important contributor to discharges than to medical costs. Summed counts of hospital discharges and fatalities also tracked reasonably well with total costs, although poorly with total QALYs lost. When available, hospital discharge data are better guides for local planning than fatality data.

Rankings for suicide acts based on incidence measures differed markedly from rankings based on costs or QALYs. The cost and QALY measures increased the importance of suicide acts involving firearms or suffocation and decreased the emphasis on poisoning suicide acts (which ranked 3rd as a cause of admission but 23rd as a factor in total costs or QALY losses). These biases need to be factored into suicide prevention decision-making that is based on incidence measures.

Table 2.7 combines the QALY and cost measures by placing a dollar value on a QALY. Although monetized QALYs have been criticized for methodological reasons (Kenkel 2001; Krupnick 2004), we attached a monetary value to the QALY estimates to allow for a better understanding of the relative burden of QALYs vis-a-vis total medical and productivity losses. The dollar value was derived in the same controversial way that the U.S. Department of Transportation and the U.S. Food and Drug Administration, as well as a variety of peer-reviewed publications (Cutler and Richardson 1998; French et al. 1996; Miller and Hendrie 2005; Miller and Levy 2000; Tolley, Kenkel, and Fabian 1994), derive it. They divide the value of a statistical life (the amount that a group of people are collectively willing to pay, and actually do pay, to save one life) by the present value of the expected number of years of life saved. We used a conservative value of statistical life of $3.4 million (in 2000 dollars), which came from a systematic review (Miller 1990) and is used in regulatory analyses at the U.S. Department of Transportation and U.S. Department of Justice. The corresponding value per QALY, net of the value of productivity, is $98,851.

The monetized QALYs reveal that QALY losses accounted for two thirds of total childhood injury costs. Although much of the preceding discussion focused on quantifying the economic burden of injuries, this finding reveals that the noneconomic burden, including pain and

Table 2.7. Comprehensive Costs of Injury Including Monetized Quality-Adjusted Life Years, by Age Group and Mechanism, Total and for Females, Ages 0–19 Years: United States, 2000

	Total Cost, Millions of 2000 Dollars					Total for Females, Millions of Dollars					%
	0–4 y	5–9 y	10–14 y	15–19 y	Total	0–4 y	5–9 y	10–14 y	15–19 y	Total	Female
					Unintentional						
Cut/pierce	492	552	925	995	2965	174	216	195	210	794	27
Submersion	2531	907	799	1705	5941	878	282	192	151	1503	25
Fall	22,218	17,979	17,119	8072	65,388	9295	7850	7262	1992	26,399	40
Burn	2135	990	523	884	4531	827	408	229	190	1654	36
Firearm	107	109	305	843	1364	36	16	28	87	167	12
Motor vehicle occupant	4906	3383	4909	31,703	44,902	1546	1531	2128	10,719	15,923	35
Pedalcyclist	562	3175	3348	1629	8714	64	1459	577	114	2213	25
Pedestrian	1658	1795	1537	2138	7128	586	587	545	600	2318	33
Bites and stings	789	556	775	693	2814	440	267	310	214	1231	44
Overexertion	458	456	4791	2656	8361	253	271	484	868	1876	22
Poisoning	422	172	176	1582	2352	165	65	71	349	652	28
Struck by/against	3803	3860	11,966	7725	27,353	1190	1736	1546	2296	6769	25

(continued on next page)

Table 2.7. *(continued)*

	Total Cost, Millions of 2000 Dollars					Total for Females, Millions of Dollars					% Female
	0–4 y	5–9 y	10–14 y	15–19 y	Total	0–4 y	5–9 y	10–14 y	15–19 y	Total	
Suffocation	2868	200	326	319	3713	1112	77	47	54	1289	35
Other specified	2662	2834	3680	7492	16,668	824	1181	1334	1661	5001	30
Total	45,611	36,969	51,180	68,434	202,194	18,046	17,854	17,504	20,813	74,216	37
Suicide											
Cut/pierce			41	214	259			27	87	116	45
Firearm			469	3868	4337			81	413	494	11
Poisoning			104	626	732			62	263	327	45
Suffocation		32	721	2199	2952			132	392	528	18
Other specified			42	481	529				111	125	24
Total		45	1377	7388	8809			318	1280	1605	18
Assault											
Cut/pierce	88	79	162	1334	1663	38	31	65	249	383	23
Firearm	185	238	721	7961	9104	59	97	126	782	1064	12
Sexual only[a]	2265	13,669	23,922	31,672	71,528	1514	10,237	18,380	29,513	59,644	83

(continued on next page)

Table 2.7. *(continued)*

	Total Cost, Millions of 2000 Dollars					Total for Females, Millions of Dollars					% Female
	0–4 y	5–9 y	10–14 y	15–19 y	Total	0–4 y	5–9 y	10–14 y	15–19 y	Total	
Struck by/against	341	588	856	2784	4569	97	84	165	680	1026	22
Suffocation	206	52	78	174	510	103	27	47	134	311	61
Other specified	1674	318	305	550	2846	663	103	115	214	1095	38
Total	4759	14,944	26,044	44,474	90,220	2891	10,608	18,942	31,853	64,293	71
Undetermined	770	100	243	739	1852	246	26	41	195	508	27
Legal/military				190	218					11	5
Grand total	51,141	52,059	78,867	121,225	303,293	21,184	28,497	36,805	54,147	140,633	46

Note: Cost for Male equals Total Cost minus Cost for Females. A few numbers were deleted because they were based on fewer than five cases. Estimates <100 million generally were based on relatively small samples and should be used with caution.

[a]Two male and 56 female rape-murders were classified by the mechanism causing death.

suffering, is what truly drives the burden. Clearly, these noneconomic factors need to be considered when allocating scarce health care resources toward injury prevention activities. For example, for sexual assault, 92% of the total burden results from QALY losses. Sexual assaults account for 7% of female injury costs at ages 0–4 years, 36% at ages 5–9 years, 50% at ages 10–14 years, and 54% at ages 15–19 years.

Summary of Cost and Quality of Life Losses

We estimate that injuries in 2000 to U.S. children and youth aged 0–19 years imposed $106 billion in lifetime medical and productivity costs and cost 2.1 million QALYs. Injuries left approximately 18,000 children and youth dead and 160,000 with permanent disabilities that restricted their ability to work and reduced their quality of life. Costs per injured person aged 0–19 years averaged $6200. Costs per injury were higher at ages 15–19 years than at younger ages, suggesting adolescents' injuries were more severe. Although unintentional falls, motor vehicle crashes, and injuries resulting from striking by/against people or objects dominated the costs, sexual assaults were the leading cause of QALY loss. Injury costs increased as children passed age 10 years and especially age 15 years. Beginning at age 10 years, violence (assaults and suicide acts) emerged as a major cost factor. The limitations of these estimates are discussed in Appendix 2.1.

Trend Over Time

The medically treated or fatal injury rate per 100,000 children and youth aged 0–19 years declined 26% between 1985 and 2000 (from 26,600 per 100,000 to 20,100 per 100,000). To compare with 1985 injury rates from Rice et al. (1989), we re-ran their nonadmitted injury counts from the 1984–1986 National Health Interview Survey, excluding cases that were not medically treated. The decline was fairly uniform across ages, with injury rates in 2000 22% lower than in 1985 at ages 0–4 years, 31% lower at ages 5–14 years, and 28% lower at ages 15–19 years.

The important question is why injury rates declined. To gain insight, we probed the trend by cause. Injury rates declined for most of the causes Rice et al. (1989) analyzed (Figure 2.4). They decreased by 25% for burns, 14% for falls, 22% for firearm injuries, 40% for poisoning, and 29% for other non-motor vehicle injuries. One major factor was the implementation of 21-year

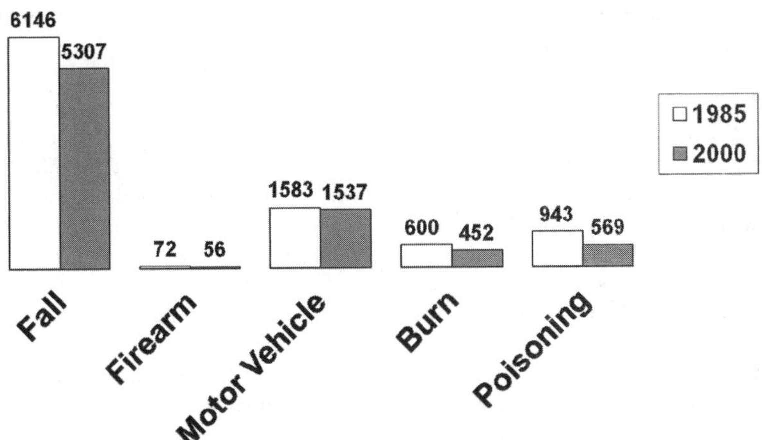

Figure 2.4. Injury Rates, by Cause, Among Children and Youth aged 0–19: United States, 1985 and 2000

minimum drinking age laws in 19 states during 1986 to 1988 (Alcohol Policies Project 1998). The largest declines were for burns and poisonings, both areas where the nation mounted aggressive intervention campaigns in the 15-year interval. In fire and burn prevention, the U.S. Consumer Product Safety Commission (2006) mandated that cigarette lighters have "childproof" dual catches, cigarette smoking declined, smoke alarms continued to spread, building codes gradually shifted homes away from dual-faucet plumbing (reducing scalds), and use of electric rather than flammable-fuel home heating increased dramatically between 1980 and 2000 (from 18% to 30% of all homes) (U.S. Census Bureau 2005). Table 2.8 presents estimates of the savings from these and other measures listed. Poisoning measures included expanded coverage by poison control centers, which triage poisoning treatment, allowing many exposures to be handled without outside medical intervention; sustained media-based parent education about safe storage; and increased unit dose packaging, for example, of iron supplements starting in 1997 (Tenenbein 2005). In contrast with a 47% decline through age 14 years, the medically treated poisoning rate increased by 5% at ages 15–19 years, possibly suggesting a lack of progress in reducing suicide acts and drug overdoses. The decline in firearm injuries may have resulted in part from laws and education campaigns that have promoted safe firearm storage in homes with children (Grossman et al. 2005).

There was one glaring exception. The motor vehicle injury rate was virtually unchanged between 1985 and 2000. The critical factor was exposure. Daily miles of travel increased by 50% at ages 0–15 years (from 16.2 miles to 24.5 miles) from 1983 to 2001 (Hu and Reuscher 2004), with an even larger increase at ages 16–20 years (from 22.2 to 38.1 miles). Overall, motor vehicle injuries per mile traveled decreased by more than 36%. Important factors in this gain included numerous state safety laws, among them zero alcohol tolerance for youth, a 0.08 maximum blood alcohol level for all drivers, graduated licensing with a driving curfew, the 21-year minimum drinking age, and safety belt use mandates, as well as the spread of airbags. Repeal of the 55 miles per hour national speed limit had an offsetting effect.

Implications of Injury Costs for Investing in Safety Behaviors and Practices

The first part of this chapter examined the lifetime costs and quality of life losses associated with child and adolescent injuries that occurred during 2000. The following sections explore the implications of these costs for decisions about policy investments in safety behaviors and practices. We examine how the medical costs and lost productivity of child and adolescent injuries compare with the costs of other child and adolescent health problems, with emphasis on a payer's perspective. That analysis points to the government as a major player in child and adolescent injury prevention and control. Funding priorities should be influenced by the relative magnitude of the burden of child and adolescent injuries compared with illnesses and how much of the burden is financed by the public sector. Our research raises the question of whether the level of government funding for injury prevention is consistent with the magnitude of the problem. A second, and arguably more important factor in determining appropriate resource allocation, concerns the percent of the burden that could be eliminated through allocation of additional resources. The last part of this chapter considers that issue.

Comparing Costs and Sources of Payment for Childhood Injury and Illness

The estimated medical costs of child and adolescent injury exceed the costs associated with low birth weight, an important health problem afflicting children in the United States (Miller, Romano, and Spicer 2000). The annual productivity losses are comparable to those resulting from high school dropout (Biglan et al. 2004). In 2000, child and adolescent injuries accounted for 11% of hospital discharges, 42% of nonadmitted emergency department visits, and 11% of physician office visits. The visit counts come from the National Ambulatory Medical Care Survey

(NAMCS), National Hospital Ambulatory Medical Care Survey (NHAMCS), and Healthcare Cost and Utilization Project Nationwide Inpatient Sample (HCUP-NIS) incidence data sets used to estimate injury incidence.

As Figure 2.5 shows, injury was responsible for 15.7% of medical spending for ages 0–19 years in 2008 (exclusive of spending on uncomplicated live births). Our analysis of 2008 Medical Expenditure Panel Survey (MEPS) data shows injury ranked third in spending behind mental conditions (24.5%) and asthma (18.2%). Injury accounted for more medical spending for ages 0–19 years (15.7%) than all infectious diseases combined (12.6%).

In terms of lost productivity, child and adolescent injuries are approximately twice as costly as child and adolescent illnesses. In 2000, 45% of all deaths and related future work loss costs among children and youth aged 1–19 years resulted from unintentional injury, 18.5% resulted from intentional injury, and only 36.5% resulted from illness.

Given the tremendous financial burden of child and adolescent injuries, in terms of both medical and future productivity costs, continued investment in effective injury prevention makes sense. Who should invest in prevention, however, largely depends on who pays the costs associated with child and adolescent injuries. The remainder of this section describes the payment sources for injury-related medical costs and lost productivity costs.

Payment Sources for Medical Costs

Private insurers paid most of the medical bill for child and adolescent injury. Health and auto insurers combined paid 80% of the bill in 2000, according to MEPS. Government paid 10% of the bill, and the remaining 10% was paid by uninsured families (Miller, Romano, and Spicer 2000). The government's Medicaid and Child Health Insurance programs paid a larger share of the hospital bills. Tabulating 2007 HCUP-NIS data reveals that private insurers only paid for approximately half of child injury discharges and associated costs, with 40% paid by government, 5% paid by auto insurance and other sources, and only 5% paid by charity care and self-pay.

Payment Sources for Lost Productivity

Work loss costs fall heavily on victims and their families, with modest contributions from property-casualty insurance and public welfare programs, including Supplemental Security Income and food stamps. Government loses the associated income taxes. Presumably property-casualty insurance (workers' compensation or auto insurance) partially covers work loss costs for the 5% of adolescent injury victims whose medical costs it pays. The financial burden of short-term work losses by parents of injured children and youth fall on parents and their employers.

How Cost-Effective Are Child and Adolescent Injury Prevention Strategies?

Estimating the cost-effectiveness of injury prevention strategies relative to the cost-effectiveness of efforts aimed at mitigating other child and adolescent health problems is useful to inform decisions about the allocation of scarce resources. For example, the costs and outcomes of one intervention (e.g., child safety seat use) can be compared with the costs and outcomes of another intervention (e.g., immunizations or drug abuse prevention) when the outcomes measured are the same. In health-related studies, the outcome most frequently considered is good health measured in QALYs. Decision-makers may decide to invest only in interventions that cost less than a specified amount per QALY saved. Alternatively, they may decide to invest in one intervention over another because it has a more favorable cost-effectiveness ratio (i.e., the cost per QALY is lower).

Table 2.8. Unit Costs, Cost Savings, and Costs/Quality-Adjusted Life Year Saved for Childhood/General Injury Prevention Measures, Child Development, and Substance Abuse Prevention Measures That Indirectly Target Injury, and Selected Other Child Preventive Health Measures (in 2009 Dollars, Computed at a 3% Discount Rate)

	Unit Cost	Medical Cost Savings	Productivity and Other Savings	QALY Savings[a]	Benefit–Cost Ratio	Cost/QALY[a]
1. Road Safety Personal Protection						
Pass child safety seat law, ages 0–4 y	$58/new user	$160	$530	$1500	38	<0
Child safety seat distribution, ages 0–4 y	$52/seat provided	$160	$530	$1500	42	<0
Child seat misuse check-up	$6/seat in use	$57	$220	$300	81	<0
Pass booster seat law, ages 4–7 y	$39/new user	$360	$790	$1300	63	<0
Booster seat, distribution, ages 4–7 y	$35/seat	$360	$790	$1300	71	<0
Pass/upgrade safety belt law	$340/new user	$290	$1900	$3900	18	<0
Enhanced belt law enforcement	$360/new user	$290	$1900	$3900	17	<0
Pass motorcycle helmet law	$1500/new user	$240	$1700	$2900	3.1	39,000
Voluntary motorcycle helmet use	$270/helmet	$240	$1700	$2900	18	<0
Pass bicycle helmet law, ages 3–14 y (Miller, Zaloshnja, and Hendrie 2009)	$13/new user	$59	$210	$310	44	<0
Pass bicycle helmet law, ages ⩾15 y (Miller, Zaloshnja, and Hendrie 2009)	$110/new user	$36	$80	$160	2.5	40,000

(continued on next page)

Table 2.8. *(continued)*

	Unit Cost	Medical Cost Savings	Productivity and Other Savings	QALY Savings[a]	Benefit–Cost Ratio	Cost/QALY[a]
Bicycle helmet distribution, ages 3–14 y (Miller, Zaloshnja, and Hendrie 2009)	\$12/helmet	\$59	\$210	\$310	48	<0
Voluntary bicycle helmet use, ages ⩾15 y (Miller, Zaloshnja, and Hendrie 2009)	\$19/helmet	\$36	\$80	\$160	15	<0
Voluntary all-terrain vehicle helmet use	\$150/helmet	\$11	\$140	\$430	3.9	38,000
Child pedestrian safety program	\$1900/child/y	\$900	\$4300	\$11,700	9.0	<0
2. Impaired Driving Prevention						
0.08% driver blood alcohol limit	\$3.60/driver	\$3	\$19	\$32	14	<0
Zero alcohol tolerance, drivers aged <21 y	\$39/driver	\$61	\$310	\$590	25	<0
Sobriety checkpoints	\$12,000/checkpoint	\$5400	\$22,000	\$55,000	6.8	<0
Administrative License Revocation	\$3500/ALR	\$3700	\$16,000	\$40,000	17	<0
Administrative License Revocation with Per Se Law	\$3300/ALR	\$4500	\$19,000	\$47,000	21	<0
Alcohol-testing ignition interlock	\$1200/vehicle	\$300	\$1800	\$4800	6.6	<0

(continued on next page)

Table 2.8. *(continued)*

	Unit Cost	Medical Cost Savings	Productivity and Other Savings	QALY Savings[a]	Benefit–Cost Ratio	Cost/QALY[a]
3. Other Road Safety						
Painting lines on roads	$270/mile	$1000	$2700	$14,000	67	<0
Post-mounted reflectors	$370/reflector	$1600	$14,000	$27,000	113	<0
Flashing beacons on hazardous curves	$21,000/beacon	$20,000	$106,000	$213,000	16	<0
Flatten crest vertical curves	$320,000/curve	$24,000	$66,000	$144,000	0.7	231,000
Install bridge-end guardrail	$11,000/bridge	$6000	$105,000	$313,000	38	<0
Install median barrier (1–12 ft. median)	$236,000/mile	$26,000	$180,000	$394,000	2.5	56,000
Install median barrier (>13 ft. median)	$236,000/mile	$5600	$39,000	$88,000	0.6	310,000
Livestock control, Native America	$9/grate	$1	$14	$1	1.8	<0
Provisional licensing + midnight driving curfew	$84/driver	$43	$250	$390	8.1	<0
Change driving curfew to 10 P.M.	$160/driver	$26	$150	$230	2.5	38,000
55 mph speed limit	$9/added travel hour	$2	$13	$19	3.7	23,000
Mobile speed camera (Chen 2005)	$740,000/camera-y	$1,600,000	$5,600,000	$6,800,00	19	<0

(continued on next page)

Table 2.8. *(continued)*

	Unit Cost	Medical Cost Savings	Productivity and Other Savings	QALY Savings[a]	Benefit–Cost Ratio	Cost/QALY[a]
Red light camera (Council et al. 2005)	$11,500/camera-y	$7,000	$26,000	$16,000	4.3	<0
4. Fire Prevention and Control						
Childproof cigarette lighter	$0.05/lighter	$0.40	$1.40	$1.80	72	<0
Less porous cigarette paper	$0.0001/pack	$0.005	$0.008	$0.061	747	<0
Pass smoke alarm law (Miller and Lawrence 2010)	$49/new user	$9	$150	$660	17	60
Alkaline-battery smoke alarm voluntary use (Miller and Lawrence 2010)	$44/home	$9	$150	$660	18	<0
Lithium-Battery SAIFE program (Miller and Lawrence 2010)	$310/home	$17	$280	$1220	4.9	22,000
Sprinkler system: Colonial (Butry et al. 2007; Miller and Lawrence 2010)	$2300/home	$100	$1110	$4000	2.5	52,000
Sprinkler system: Townhouse (Butry et al. 2007; Miller and Lawrence 2010)	$2100/home	$100	$1110	$4000	2.7	46,000
Sprinkler system: Ranch House (Butry et al. 2007; Miller and Lawrence 2010)	$900/home	$100	$1110	$4000	6.2	13,000

(continued on next page)

Table 2.8. *(continued)*

	Unit Cost	Medical Cost Savings	Productivity and Other Savings	QALY Savings[a]	Benefit–Cost Ratio	Cost/QALY[a]
Mattress flammability standard (U.S. Consumer Product Safety Commission 2006)	$26/mattress	$0.65	$10	$60	2.8	47,000
5. Other Targeted Injury Prevention						
Harlem Hospital Safe Communities Program	$75/child	$220	$800	$2800	51	<0
American Academy of Pediatrics TIPP Injury Prevention Counseling, Ages 0–4 y	$11/child	$8	$19	$71	8.9	6000
Baby walker redesign to prevent stairway falls (Rodgers and Leland 2008)	$3.60/walker	$17	$20	$150	46	<0
Impact-absorbing playground surfacing (Ball 2004)	$14,000/playground	$3300	$25,000	$100	2.0	36,000
Youth suicide prevention, Native America	$215/youth	$44	$1100	$6400	35	3300
Winter coats that float drowning prevention, Native Alaska	$0.12/person	$0	$64	$190	2100	<0

(continued on next page)

Table 2.8. *(continued)*

	Unit Cost	Medical Cost Savings	Productivity and Other Savings	QALY Savings[a]	Benefit-Cost Ratio	Cost/QALY[a]
6. Non-Offender Violence Prevention Programs (also address substance abuse risk, suicide, and so forth)						
Perry preschool and home visits	$20,000/child	$1800	$49,000	$47,000	4.9	<0
Nurse–family partnership 2-y home visits	$10,700/child	$1400	$23,000	$27,000	4.8	<0
Syracuse 5-y home visits	$66,000/child	$1080	$31,000	$28,000	0.9	171,000
Parent training	$4600/child	$640	$3700	$14,000	3.9	28,000
Big Brothers/Big Sisters mentoring	$4800/child	$190	$4800	$3500	1.8	<0
Graduation incentives	$24,000/child	$400	$4900	$6600	0.5	351,000
7. Youth Offender Programs with Multi-Risk Orientation (address interpersonal violence, suicide, substance abuse, and so forth)						
Multisystemic therapy	$6550/client	$6600	$133,000	$114,000	39	<0
Functional family therapy	$3000/client	$2500	$50,000	$42,000	32	<0
Multidimensional treatment foster care	$2800/client	$4700	$95,000	$81,000	65	<0
Drug courts	$2900/client	$260	$6900	$4600	4.1	<0

(continued on next page)

Table 2.8. *(continued)*

	Unit Cost	Medical Cost Savings	Productivity and Other Savings	QALY Savings[a]	Benefit–Cost Ratio	Cost/QALY[a]
8. Narrowly Targeted Crime Prevention and Youth Offender Programs (address interpersonal violence only)						
Monitored burglar and fire alarms	$910/home/y	$2	$490	$490	1.1	122,000
Youth offender aggression replacement training	$580/client	$1400	$28,000	$24,000	90	<0
Lansing adolescent diversion	$2200/client	$1900	$46,000	$37,000	39	<0
Intensive probation supervision, youth	$2200/client	$250	$5000	$4400	4.4	<0
Scaring young offenders straight	>$0	$0	$0	$0	0	Infinite
Young offender boot camp	$2800/client	−$810	−$16,000	−$14,000	−0.1	Infinite
9. Programs that Protect Youth from Adult Offenders						
20-bed domestic violence shelter (Chanley et al. 2001)	$18,000/bed	$12,360	$34,100	$153,000	11	<0
Moral reconation therapy	$410/client	$360	$6100	$6200	31	<0
Reasoning and rehabilitation	$430/client	$100	$2200	$1700	9.4	<0
Cognitive-behavioral sex offender treatment	$9300/client	$1020	$3200	$15,000	2.1	30,000

(continued on next page)

Table 2.8. *(continued)*

	Unit Cost	Medical Cost Savings	Productivity and Other Savings	QALY Savings[a]	Benefit–Cost Ratio	Cost/QALY[a]
10. Youth Development through Integrated Family or Community and School Programs (reduce injury related to substance abuse and other violent behavior)						
Across Ages	$2100/pupil	$240	$810	$1600	1.2	119,000
Adolescent Transitions	$1500/pupil	$470	$3280	$8500	8.2	10,100
CASAstart	$6900/pupil	$340	$1600	$2400	0.6	261,000
Child Development Project	$280/pupil	$130	$550	$810	5.2	<0
Guiding Good Choices (formerly Preparing for the Drug-Free Years)	$870/family	$220	$1000	$1600	3.2	18,000
SOAR Social Development-Parent/Teacher Training	$3700/child	$770	$9300	$13,000	6.4	<0
Social Competence Promotion	$430/pupil	$250	$820	$1600	6.3	2000
Strengthening Families	$1100/family	$650	$3600	$7500	11	<0

(continued on next page)

Table 2.8. *(continued)*

	Unit Cost	Medical Cost Savings	Productivity and Other Savings	QALY Savings[a]	Benefit–Cost Ratio	Cost/QALY[a]
11. School- or Community-based Life Skills (prevent substance abuse and related injury)						
All Stars	$170/pupil	$240	$1690	$4400	36	<0
Family Matters	$190/family	$230	$1660	$4400	32	<0
Good Behavior Game	$75/pupil	$49	$770	$2200	41	1300
Keepin' It Real	$160/pupil	$300	$1270	$2800	28	<0
Life Skills Training	$270/pupil	$140	$1680	$4300	22	1300
Project Alert	$140/pupil	$50	$310	$300	4.4	<0
Project Northland	$490/pupil	$320	$2590	$6200	19	0
Project STAR (aka Midwest Prevention Program)	$490/pupil	$190	$1550	$3400	11	4400
Project Toward No Drugs	$220/pupil	$100	$410	$630	5.1	<0
STARS for Families	$150/family	$110	$230	$800	7.6	<0

(*continued on next page*)

Table 2.8. *(continued)*

	Unit Cost	Medical Cost Savings	Productivity and Other Savings	QALY Savings[a]	Benefit–Cost Ratio	Cost/QALY[a]
12. Environmental Alcohol Interventions (reduce alcohol-related injury)						
21-y minimum legal drinking age	$200/youth 18–20 y	$43	$240	$450	3.6	23,000
20% alcohol tax	$11/drinker/y	$4	$36	$62	9.3	<0
30% alcohol tax	$21/drinker/y	$6	$46	$81	6.3	8400
Mandatory server training	$58/driver	$11	$69	$116	3.4	20,000
Enforce serving intoxicated patron law	$0.44/driver	$3	$12	$16	71	<0
13. Post-Event Injury Control						
Poison Control Center Services	$43/call	$320	$0	$0	7.4	<0
Regional Trauma System Services	$1850/admit	$2200	$510	$2300	2.7	<0
Tetanus-diphtheria-pertussis vaccination, ages 0–6 y (Ortega-Sanchez and the Working Group on Leading Economic Issues on New Vaccines for Adolescents 2005)	$90/child	$500	$1780	$0	25	<0

(continued on next page)

Table 2.8. *(continued)*

	Unit Cost	Medical Cost Savings	Productivity and Other Savings	QALY Savings[a]	Benefit–Cost Ratio	Cost/QALY[a]
14. Tobacco Prevention and Control						
Know Your Body (smoking)	$175/pupil	$130	$2100	$6100	47	800
Minnesota Smoking Prevention Program	$120/pupil	$120	$2000	$5700	67	<0
Project TNT	$220/pupil	$60	$1040	$3000	19	5500
Youth Anti-smoking Mass Media Campaign	$450/pupil	$70	$1200	$3500	11	11,000
Stop Smoking Mass Media Campaign	$1300/quitter	$1400	$22,000	$63,000	68	<0
Reduce Cessation Program Prices	$260/quitter	$1400	$22,000	$63,000	329	<0
Brief Tobacco Counseling	$6700/quitter	$1400	$22,000	$63,000	13	9000
Add Nicotine Patch	$4800/quitter	$1400	$22,000	$63,000	18	5800
Instead Add Nicotine Gum	$8450/quitter	$1400	$21,800	$62,800	10	12,000
Full Tobacco Counseling	$3300/quitter	$1400	$21,800	$62,800	26	3300
Add Nicotine Patch	$3100/quitter	$1400	$21,800	$62,800	27	3000
Instead Add Nicotine Gum	$4900/quitter	$1400	$21,800	$62,800	18	6000

(*continued on next page*)

Table 2.8. *(continued)*

	Unit Cost	Medical Cost Savings	Productivity and Other Savings	QALY Savings[a]	Benefit-Cost Ratio	Cost/QALY[a]
15. Other Child Preventive Health						
Hepatitis B vaccination of newborns (Graham et al. 1998)						5100– 80,000
Pneumococcal vaccination of infants (Ortega-Sanchez and the Working Group on Leading Economic Issues on New Vaccines for Adolescents 2005)	\$300/person					9000
Varicella vaccination, 18 mo (Goldsmith, Hutchison, and Hurley 2004)	\$46/person				5.4	25,000–49,000
Measles/mumps/rubella immunization (Tengs et al. 1995)	\$58/person				26	<0
Hepatitis A vaccination of college freshmen (Ortega-Sanchez and the Working Group on Leading Economic Issues on New Vaccines for Adolescents 2005)	\$57/person					<0
Screening + human papilloma vaccination, females age 12 y (Ortega-Sanchez and the Working Group on Leading Economic Issues on New Vaccines for Adolescents 2005)	\$530/person					18,000–32,000
Meningococcal vaccination, ages 11–17 y (Ortega-Sanchez and the Working Group on Leading Economic Issues on New Vaccines for Adolescents 2005)	\$110/person					97,000

(continued on next page)

Table 2.8. *(continued)*

	Unit Cost	Medical Cost Savings	Productivity and Other Savings	QALY Savings[a]	Benefit–Cost Ratio	Cost/QALY[a]
Cereal fortification with folic acid to improve pregnancy outcomes (Kelly et al. 1996)						<0
Water fluoridation (Goldsmith, Hutchison, and Hurley 2004)						<0
Phenylketonuria screening of newborns (Tengs et al. 1995)						<0
Neonatal intensive care, weight 500–999 g (Boyle et al. 1983)						34,000
Neonatal intensive care, weight 1000–1499 g (Boyle et al. 1983)						20,000

QALY, quality-adjusted life year; SAIFE, Smoke Alarm Installation and Fire Education; SOAR, Skills, Opportunities, and Recognition; TIPP, The Injury Prevention Program; TNT, Toward No Tobacco.

(a) Cost/QALY = QALYs saved/(intervention cost − resource cost savings).

(b) To determine the number of QALYs saved, divide the QALY savings by $125,379. Total savings are the sum of the Medical Cost, Productivity, and QALY savings. The benefit–cost ratio equals total savings divided by the unit cost.

(c) Includes three alarms per home.

Source: Price-adjusted from Miller and Hendrie (2005) or Miller and Levy 2000 unless another citation is shown.

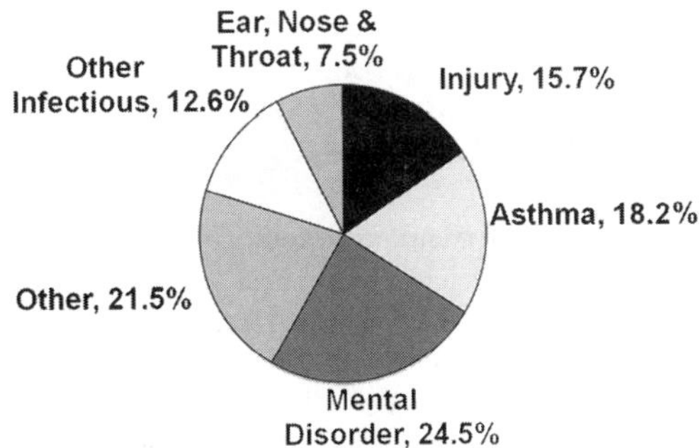

Source: Medical Expenditure Panel Survey 2008 on-line analysis system. Excludes normal birth.

Figure 2.5. Medical Spending by Condition Among Children and Youth aged 0–19: United States, 2008

By drawing primarily on four related systematic reviews (Aos et al. 2004; Miller and Hendrie 2005; Miller and Hendrie 2009; Miller and Levy 2000), this section summarizes the cost-effectiveness and return on investment of a diversity of child, adolescent, and all-age injury prevention measures that published studies have demonstrated to be effective. Table 2.8 summarizes results for 11 categories of injury prevention measures, with most of the measures targeting road crashes, youth violence, or substance abuse and the injuries it causes. These areas have the richest literature with respect to the cost-effectiveness of select interventions. All the analyses reported in Table 2.8 use a 2.5% or 3% discount rate and take a societal perspective. They use the status quo as a comparator group unless otherwise indicated. The estimates assume that program effectiveness levels observed in demonstration programs would decline by 25% in replication. The estimates for unintentional injury and suicide all were recomputed for the systematic reviews using the same QALY loss estimates used in this chapter, except that the losses for physical assaults come from the same source we used for sexual assaults (Miller, Cohen, and Wiersema 1996). The benefit–cost analyses in Table 2.8 monetized QALYs with the method used to construct Table 2.7. Because Table 2.8 is in 2009 dollars, the estimated number of QALYs saved by any prevention measure can be computed by dividing its quality of life cost saving estimate from Table 2.8 by $125,379. This value is the same as the $98,851 used in Table 2.7, but inflated from 2000 dollars to 2009 dollars. Again, we emphasize that the QALY estimates are approximate and that monetizing them is controversial.

The cost-effectiveness of the injury prevention strategies is compared with published cost-effectiveness estimates for measures that address other important neonatal and childhood problems, including drug and alcohol abuse, smoking, various vaccinations, nutritional additives, phenylketonuria screening, and neonatal intensive care. The data presented suggest that many child and adolescent injury prevention strategies have similar cost-effectiveness ratios compared with other well-accepted strategies to prevent child and adolescent illnesses.

Many measures in Table 2.8 appear cost-effective, and some even offer the potential for long-term savings. If the medical and other resource costs saved by an intervention exceed its implementation and maintenance costs, the intervention offers *net cost savings* (cost/QALY < $0 in Table 2.8). Society as a whole will save money if the program is implemented, although the savings may be spread across many payers. We label measures that offer net cost savings or cost less than $100,000 per QALY as cost-effective, which is consistent with North American literature (Clement et al. 2009; Lee, Chertow, and Zenios 2009). Even counting the value of the QALYs saved, some interventions, although effective, do not offer a positive return on investment. Their benefit–cost ratio is less than 1.0. Other interventions work but may not offer a high enough return to merit widespread adoption.

Cost-Savings Estimates for Injury Interventions

This section discusses the injury interventions by topic. Fuller descriptions and citations for most of the measures appear in the systematic reviews (Aos et al. 2004; Miller and Hendrie 2009; Miller and Levy 2000). Others, noted in Table 2.8, come from recent reports. Footnotes in the text describe our adjustments to make the recent published estimates comparable to the estimates from the systematic reviews. Most commonly we reduced benefits by 25% because the effectiveness came from an unreplicated demonstration program, we applied a 3% discount rate, or we recomputed the benefits with the injury costs given here or used in the systematic reviews.

Road Safety Personal Protection

Personal protection in road safety encompasses motor vehicle, pedalcyclist, pedestrian, and all-terrain vehicle safety mandates and personal choices. Of 15 interventions in this area, 12 offer net cost savings. That means the medical and other resource costs they save exceed the intervention cost. Child occupant protection and bicycle helmet laws pay for themselves, as do safety belt use laws and enforcement. Voluntary use of the mandated safety devices yields the same benefits per user as use induced by a law but costs less because laws are costly to pass and implement and laws that force adults to use safety equipment cost personal freedom and impose discomfort and inconvenience.[5]

Impaired Driving

Such measures as zero alcohol tolerance for drivers under the legal drinking age and blood alcohol limits for other drivers may reduce alcohol consumption and associated harms, including crime, high-risk sex, and suicide acts. However, only their impact on impaired driving has been evaluated (Miller and Hendrie 2005). Even with that narrow evaluation, all six impaired driving measures in Table 2.8 offer net cost savings. These interventions have both a specific deterrence effect and a general deterrence effect. Sobriety checkpoints, for example, apprehend some impaired drivers who would otherwise have crashed, but fear of getting caught in sobriety checkpoints also deters people from driving after drinking. This general deterrence effect typically dominates (Hingson and Howland 1990).

Other Road Upgrading and Rules of the Road

Table 2.8 shows a small sampling of the road upgrades that highway engineers have in their arsenal. These improvements range widely in cost and expected return, with many offering net cost savings but some only worth implementing on the riskiest roads. Passage and passive enforcement of safety laws tend to offer net cost savings. Although red light cameras are much less expensive than mobile speed cameras, speed cameras offer a larger return on investment because drivers speed far more frequently than they run red lights (Chen, 2005; Council et al., 2005).[6] Provisional or graduated youth driver licensing with a nighttime driving curfew and

[5]To cost a bicycle helmet law for ages 15 and over, we assumed the ratio of helmet cost to costs of associated discomfort, inconvenience, and loss of personal freedom would be proportional to those for a motorcycle helmet law.

[6]In the red light camera calculation, we substituted more recent effectiveness data from Insurance Institute for Highway Safety (2011) for the effectiveness data in Council et al. (2005).

passenger restrictions for novice drivers probably offers benefits beyond the road safety benefits shown here. Getting youth home sooner, especially in conjunction with zero alcohol tolerance laws for young drivers, is likely to reduce heavy drinking, risky sex, and violence.

Fire Prevention and Control

National adoption of childproof cigarette lighters already is providing net cost savings and reducing smoking-related injuries. Less porous cigarette paper will self-extinguish if left to smolder, thus reducing deadly cigarette fires, many of which also involve alcohol (Istre et al. 2001). Mattress flammability standards also address these risks. Smoke alarm laws, fire department or community smoke alarm installation and maintenance programs, and sprinkler systems in new construction address these risks and broader fire risks. Both a mandated shift to less porous paper and voluntary smoke alarm use would offer net cost savings.

Other Targeted Injury Prevention

The Harlem Hospital Childhood Safe Communities Program organized a community response to unintentional childhood injury in a low-income neighborhood. It adopted approaches ranging from traffic calming to school playground renovation by local residents to after-school programs. This program, which offers net cost savings, has been replicated by Children's Hospitals in several cities (Spicer et al. 2004).

Evaluation of physician counseling by pediatricians through The Injury Prevention Program (TIPP) of the American Academy of Pediatrics suggests that it produces good health at a cost of $6000 per QALY (Miller and Galbraith 1995). Baby walker redesign to prevent stairway falls offered net cost savings (Rodgers and Leland 2008). More forgiving playground surfacing is cost-effective, but seems to lose much of its potential effectiveness by increasing child risk-taking and decreasing parent supervision (Ball 2004).[7] The only economic analyses of suicide and drowning prevention that we found were for programs in Native American communities (Zaloshnja et al. 2003). The programs were cost effective in these settings.

Violence Prevention

Nonoffender Violence Prevention Programs

Some violence prevention measures try to prevent children from becoming troubled. They aim to address the root causes of crime and could reduce multiple risky behaviors associated with injury, including binge drinking and drug abuse. Except for home visitation programs for infants and toddlers, however, these measures have been evaluated solely in terms of their impact on violence or crime more broadly. That makes their costs/QALY conservative. Three of the six listed programs in Table 2.8 targeting nonoffenders offer net cost savings, but two others are not cost-effective. Intensive home visitation, possibly coupled with preschool enrichment, can reduce infant/toddler abuse and a range of problems as the targeted low-income toddlers reach adolescence and adulthood, although the return on these costly investments takes decades and has not always appeared. That makes them difficult to recommend when resources are tight. Integrated youth development programs (discussed below) may be more cost-effective.

[7]Because the injury reductions achieved in randomized trials were not achieved in scale up, we reduced the effectiveness estimate by 75%. Costs per hospital-treated playground fall were computed using the U.S. Consumer Product Safety Commission's injury cost model (Miller, Lawrence, Jensen, et al. 1998).

Youth Offender Programs With Multi-Risk Orientation

The four youth offender programs identified all intensively treat troubled youth aged 12 to 17 years and yield net cost savings. These interventions address the causes of delinquency and related substance abuse. They seek to improve family and school/community functioning. Multisystemic therapy costs more per youth than functional family therapy or treatment foster care, but also has a greater impact on problem behaviors. Treatment foster care also appears cost-effective, but in addition to financial resources, it requires trained, dedicated foster parents for each child.

Narrowly Targeted Crime Prevention and Youth Offender Programs

Three of the narrowly targeted crime prevention measures assessed are not cost-effective, and three offer net cost savings. Intensive probation supervision for young offenders yields net cost savings primarily because it is less expensive than incarceration, not because it improves outcomes. Only two youth measures in this group are strong candidates for widespread implementation: aggression replacement training and diversion of low-risk first offenders from juvenile court to a service-oriented system. These interventions are less costly than the multi-risk approaches to violence prevention, but they also yield narrower benefits.

Programs That Protect Youth From Adult Offenders

A domestic violence shelter protects women and children from victimization, yielding net cost savings (Chanley, Chanley, and Campbell 2001; National Center for Injury Prevention and Control 2003).[8] Moral reconation therapy and the Reasoning and Rehabilitation program achieve net cost savings by preventing a return to violence postrelease. Cognitive-behavioral therapy treatment for sexual offenders also cost-effectively reduces repeat offending. These programs are more effective than other violent offender programs (Miller and Levy 2000).

Youth Development Through Integrated Family or Community and School Programs

Eight youth development programs integrate family, community, and school efforts to strengthen families or adolescents; evaluations suggest they may reduce violence and delay initiation of alcohol, tobacco, or other drug use. Reduced alcohol use should reduce impaired driving, interpersonal violence, suicide acts, and unintentional falls, burns, drownings, and pedestrian injuries. The youth development programs are comprehensive and often expensive. Meta-analysis (Aos et al. 2004; Hansen, Derzon, and Dusenbury 2004) suggests the greatest impacts on alcohol initiation, and consequently on injury, will result from the Strengthening Families Program (16.7%), followed by Social Competence Promotion (10.8%); Skills, Opportunities, and Recognition (8.1%, plus a verified violence reduction); and Guiding Good Choices (also known as Preparing for the Drug-Free Years, 7.9%). The proven benefits of CASAstart are smaller than its costs. Across Ages offers a minimal proven return. Some of these interventions, the Strengthening Families Program and Guiding Good Choices, have been replicated successfully. Others are one-time demonstrations, so their effectiveness is especially uncertain. An important limitation of these programs is that they generally require a large parental commitment. Their reach is limited because many parents will not commit the time, and financial incentives to increase parental participation make them expensive.

[8]We recomputed the annualized capital costs at a 3% discount rate and used the actual wages of paid staff even though they reportedly were below market. We substituted data from the National Criminal Victimization Survey and two published studies (Finkelstein et al. 2006; National Center for Injury Prevention and Control 2003) on the costs and risk of death per domestic violence victimization and on the average victimizations per victim.

Substance Abuse Prevention

School- and Community-Based Life Skills Programs

Six of the ten school-based and community-based life skills training programs offer net cost savings, and three more cost less than $10,000 per QALY saved. The Good Behavior Game improves early elementary school classroom order in the short term and seems to reduce violence in the long run (Substance Abuse and Mental Health Services Administration 2010). Among the middle-school programs, the greatest effects on alcohol initiation, and thus on injury, have been achieved with Keepin' It Real (10.9%), STARS for Families (8.3%), All Stars (7.0%), Project Northland (6.9%), and Family Matters (6.9%).

Environmental Alcohol Interventions

Two of the five environmental alcohol interventions in Table 2.8 offer net cost savings. Increasing alcohol excise taxes to 20% of the pre-tax selling price is cost-effective, especially against alcohol-related youth injury, but politically difficult. The review suggests that the national 21-year minimum drinking age reduces the number of adolescent injuries. Passing and enforcing laws against serving intoxicated (and underage) patrons and training servers to recognize impairment and terminate service without excessive confrontation may be cost-effective strategies to reduce adolescent injuries, but these need wider evaluation before moving to national implementation.

Postevent Injury Control Through Medical Intervention

Health services improve trauma outcomes. Establishing regional hospital specialties in trauma care, then triaging serious injuries to these hospitals, increases the costs of initial treatment but improves survival and ultimately reduces the medical care costs required to achieve maximum medical recovery (Miller and Levy 1995). Regional or phone-in poison control centers advise on poisoning response 24 hours a day. They greatly reduce poisoning treatment costs and may improve outcomes by advising on whether treatment is needed, supervising home treatment of minor poisonings without more costly medical intervention, more quickly linking serious cases to appropriate treatment, and providing toxicologic consultation to hospital staff (Institute of Medicine Committee on Poison Prevention and Control 2004). Tetanus-diphtheria-pertussis vaccination reduces possible bacterial complications of wounds (Ortega-Sanchez and the Working Group on Leading Economic Issues on New Vaccines for Adolescents 2005). This combination vaccination protects against three diverse conditions, only one of which is associated with injury. The vaccines were combined to reduce delivery costs. The measures discussed in this paragraph all offer net cost savings.

Comparison With the Cost-Effectiveness of Other Child and Adolescent Health Risks

To further interpret the cost-effectiveness analyses of child and adolescent injury prevention efforts, we examined similar estimates of cost per QALY saved for other neonatal and child health risks (categories 14 and 15 in Table 2.8). These examples were selected because the cost-effectiveness studies (1) were of good quality; (2) used a 3% discount rate (which makes them comparable to the injury cost-effectiveness estimates) or could readily be recomputed at that discount rate (because discounting only was needed to compute the QALYs lost to mortality); and (3) represented diverse approaches to child and adolescent risk reduction (Boyle et al. 1983; Graham et al. 1998; Kelly et al. 1996; Ortega-Sanchez and the Working Group on Leading

Economic Issues on New Vaccines for Adolescents 2005; Tengs et al. 1995).[9] Tobacco prevention and control measures (category 14) had low costs per QALY saved. The health effects they addressed were far enough in the future, however, that they rarely achieved net cost savings, although their costs/QALY saved were reasonably low. Of the remaining measures (category 15), 42% offered net cost savings, including measles-mumps-rubella vaccination, hepatitis A vaccination of college freshmen, cereal fortification with folic acid, water fluoridation, and newborn screening for phenylketonuria. Assorted vaccinations and neonatal intensive care were less cost-effective but within the $100,000 per QALY implementation threshold.

Summary of Cost-Effectiveness Estimates

This section summarizes the cost-effectiveness of child and adolescent injury prevention interventions in the literature and compares the results with other child and adolescent interventions. Thirty-two of 48 unintentional injury prevention measures (67% of the unintentional injury measures in categories 1–5 of Table 2.8) and 13 of 20 child and adolescent intentional injury prevention measures (65% of measures in categories 6–9) offer net cost savings, as do all three injury control measures (category 13). Of the 23 youth substance abuse prevention measures, 12 (52% of measures in categories 10–12) offer net cost savings. These 23 measures often reduce youth alcohol use and related injuries.

The cost-effectiveness of child and adolescent unintentional injury prevention strategies reviewed is comparable to or better than the cost-effectiveness of several other widely implemented child and adolescent illness prevention measures. Only 3 of 12 tobacco prevention and control programs (25%) offered net cost savings, as did 5 of the other 12 child and adolescent health interventions (42%). These findings should be interpreted cautiously because the studies are not completely comparable, especially in their methods for estimating QALY savings, and standard errors are not available to gauge the reliability of the estimates.

Despite the substantial uncertainty about the cost-effectiveness estimates reported in this chapter, these findings suggest that society may benefit from the implementation of many child and adolescent safety measures and that more widespread use of these measures may be warranted. Third-party payers, such as managed care organizations, other health insurers, and auto insurers, may save money by advocating for, subsidizing, or paying to promote routine use of some safety measures, such as child safety seats, booster seats, and smoke alarms. Yet these and other proven injury prevention interventions are not universally implemented.

Many barriers hamper adoption, as follows:

- Savings may be split across multiple payers. Even interventions that would save government more than they cost may be difficult to implement if the savings are split across insular departments or multiple levels of government.
- The payback period may be too long. Governments concerned with annual budgets sometimes demand even shorter payback periods than the private sector.
- The expected return is uncertain and situational. The estimates shown are averages. They will vary with local risk levels and prevention efforts.
- Health care payers may be intimidated by prevention. They know how to profit by managing and predicting treatment costs, but tread risky ground when investing in and trying to manage the unfamiliar area of prevention.

[9] The estimate for neonatal intensive care in Table 2.8 was recomputed at a 3% discount rate and omitted expected earnings gains (an indirect cost) from the calculation of net costs to avoid double counting. This estimate unavoidably reflects 1978 treatment capabilities so it may not accurately measure current cost-effectiveness.

- Safety device subsidizers would have to subsidize parents who would buy the devices anyway, as well as parents who would not. That can dilute their return on investment.
- Affordability is an issue. Low-income families may not be willing or able to purchase safety equipment (e.g., child safety seats, bicycle helmets) that protects their children against injuries and related financial and functional losses. Absent government and charitable intervention, therefore, children from low-income families may be at greater risk for injuries. For example, low-income parents are less likely to own a child safety seat than other parents, but those who do own child safety seats use them at the same rate as other parents (Mayer and LeClere 1990).
- Intervention may be politically difficult. Interference with the personal freedoms of adults is unacceptable in some political circles. Moreover, legislation often imposes discomfort and inconvenience costs for new safety device users, mobility loss costs when legal driving conditions are restricted, or delay costs at enforcement checkpoints. Some interventions may not be culturally acceptable.
- Investment dollars are scarce. Although injury prevention may be an inexpensive way to buy good health, financially pressed investors may hesitate to pay to achieve gains in quality of life, even for children. In addition, even if injury prevention produces good health at a lower price than existing health interventions, unless resources are growing, increasing injury prevention requires shrinking those entrenched interests.

Policy makers selecting injury prevention interventions should apply a series of filters. The estimates in this chapter provide the first filter, allowing elimination of interventions that offer a questionable return on investment. This financial information also should be used to guide choices between interventions that score comparably on other criteria. Additional filters might include political feasibility, local priorities, appropriateness for the target population, aggregate impact on the injury problem, affordability, unmeasured spillover benefits (e.g., shifting drinking to residential settings may reduce impaired driving and barroom brawling but also could increase domestic violence; a designated driver or free taxi home may dangerously increase intoxication levels), immediacy of the impacts (weeks to implement an education program versus years to pass a law), and reductions in effectiveness due to prior or planned implementation of measures with overlapping impacts.

Many other injury prevention measures merit careful evaluation and, if effective, cost-effectiveness analyses. Among others, possible candidates include youth suicide prevention; readily grasped, small-diameter handrails without sharp edges; window guards; pool fencing ordinances; learn-to-swim programs; and home safety inspections that incorporate low-tech interventions, such as childproof cabinet latches and plastic plug covers for electric outlets. Particularly for safety measures that are expensive, widespread adoption should be informed by cost-effectiveness analyses.

Conclusions

In 2000, injuries were by far the most prevalent and expensive health risk faced by children and adolescents aged 1–19 years. Child and adolescent injuries that occurred in 2000 resulted in $26 billion in lifetime medical spending and $82 billion in present and future work losses. Injuries permanently disabled 160,000 children and youth; they cost the same number of QALYs as 75,000 child and adolescent deaths would cost. In aggregate, the most costly risks were falls, motor vehicle crashes, and incidents where someone unintentionally was struck by or struck against an object. Despite their relatively small numbers, deaths and hospitalized injuries accounted for 40% of the costs and QALY losses. Sexual assaults accounted for 31% of the QALY losses.

Most injuries are, in theory, preventable, and proven strategies exist to reduce the injury toll. Indeed, the child and adolescent injury toll declined 26% between 1985 and 2000. Moreover, from a societal perspective, the cost of preventing injuries often is less than the cost of treating them. The studies reviewed reveal that providing child safety seats, booster seats, and bicycle helmets to infants and children enrolled in Medicaid would save tax dollars. Equipping homes with working smoke alarms and intensive sobriety and safety-belt use checkpoints would reduce insurance bills. Further restricting child gun access would reduce firearm injuries (Grossman et al. 2005). Aggression replacement training and functional family therapy for youthful offenders are saving taxpayers money in Washington state and could elsewhere. Yet these and other proven injury prevention interventions often are not widely implemented, and injury remains the leading cause of child and adolescent death from ages 1 to 19 years.

Although the data and methods we used to quantify the burden have many limitations, this chapter presents policy makers with the clearest picture available of the economic and noneconomic burden of child and adolescent injuries and compares this burden with that of other child and adolescent problems. It also presents the most promising strategies for reducing this burden. As a result, this chapter provides a road map that can be used when determining how best to allocate scarce health care resources in efforts to improve the health of children and youth in this country.

Appendix

Methods of Estimating Incidence-Based Childhood Injury Costs and Quality of Life Losses

The incidence-based costs reported estimate the present value of all expected costs over the child's life span. The present value of future costs depends on how many years in the future the costs are borne and on the discount rate.

Estimating the costs and quality of life losses associated with child and adolescent injuries required separately estimating the frequency of injuries, the present and future costs (medical and productivity) of the injuries, and the QALYs lost because of injury.

The subsections below summarize the data sources and limitations of the methods used to estimate each component of injury frequency, cost, and quality of life losses in this analysis. Details on the methods used to estimate incidence, medical costs, and productivity losses have been published by Finkelstein et al. (2006). Their book excludes sexual assault.

Estimating Injury Occurrence

Injury Frequency, Diagnosis, Mechanism, and Intent

Fatal injury counts were derived from the 2000 National Vital Statistics System fatality census (National Center for Health Statistics 2010b) with supplemental information about on-the-road crash deaths from the Fatality Analysis Reporting System census of deaths involving motor vehicles on public roads. We used the 2000 HCUP-NIS data file to estimate hospitalized nonfatal injury episodes. HCUP-2000 contains data on 8 million inpatient stays from 1000 hospitals (Agency for Healthcare Research and Quality 2010a). We removed readmissions from the HCUP-NIS counts using readmission rates by primary diagnosis group derived from pooled 1997–1998 hospital discharge census data for Maryland, Vermont, and New Jersey, a choice driven by necessity; no other readily accessible data exist about readmission rates. HCUP-NIS identifies mechanisms for 83% of injury incidents. Under the assumption that these cases were representative, we inferred missing external cause codes by applying the mechanism distribution by age group, sex, and primary diagnosis for cases with known mechanism.

We estimated injury survivors treated in the emergency department and released from the 2001 National Electronic Injury Surveillance System (NEISS) All Injury Program (AIP) (National Center for Injury Prevention and Control 2010), which details all injuries at a national probability sample of 66 hospitals. We validated the NEISS counts against counts from the 1999–2000 NHAMCS, which surveys a representative sample of 500 emergency departments (National Center for Health Statistics 2010a). The comparison revealed the AIP incidence and NHAMCS emergency department visit counts agree to within 2.5%, suggesting the NEISS-AIP counts are sound incidence estimates. We estimated the number of injuries resulting in medical treatment without hospitalization or emergency department treatment from parallel provider surveys in the NHAMCS family, the 1999–2000 NAMCS of office visits, and the 1999–2000 NHAMCS hospital outpatient department sample (National Center for Health Statistics 2010a).

NHAMCS and NAMCS detail injury mechanism and diagnoses but count visits, not incidents. Thus, NAMCS might report three office visits that resulted from a single dog bite. To estimate incident counts, we compared these data with data from data sets that counted incidents but had other information gaps that precluded their use as the primary incidence data sets. We compared the outpatient and office visit counts with incidence and visit counts by broad mechanism from the 1999 MEPS (Agency for Healthcare Research and Quality 2010b). MEPS tracks all health care for a national sample of noninstitutionalized residents over a 2-year period. The comparison confirmed that the other data sets include many follow-up visits. We reduced the NHAMCS and NAMCS visit counts to match the MEPS victim counts by sex within each 5-year age group. We first removed NHAMCS and NAMCS cases within each age-sex strata where mechanism information was missing or coded as "unspecified" (~19% of cases from each file). Next, within the seven broad mechanism categories in MEPS, we multiplied the weights of all remaining visits within each strata times the ratio of the MEPS victim count to the NHAMCS or NAMCS visit count. This procedure reduced the weighted NHAMCS and NAMCS counts by age group, sex, and broad mechanism so that they matched the corresponding MEPS incidence estimates.

Sexual assault incidence, net of cases that also involved physical assault, came from the 1995 National Survey of Adolescents in the United States (Kilpatrick and Saunders 2000). From the survey data on victimization history, we reconstructed the percentage of children and youth who were sexually assaulted by age and sex and removed those cases that also involved medically treated physical assault. We applied the percentages to U.S. resident population counts for 2000 to estimate the number of children sexually assaulted. Mental health provider survey data suggest that virtually all victims of child sexual assault and sexual abuse eventually will receive mental health treatment to deal with their victimization (Cohen and Miller 1998).

These data sets provide nationally representative estimates, but have methodological limitations that may lead to an undercounting or overcounting of injuries. For example, HCUP-NIS does not clearly distinguish initial hospitalizations from transfers and follow-up hospitalizations, so some injuries may have been counted more than once, even though we tried to remove transfers and follow-ups from the analyses. Basing our count of poisonings treated in doctors' offices on MEPS self-report rather than diagnosis codes caused us to classify 90,000 poisonings in other mechanism categories. (Classifying these cases as poisonings would mean poisonings in the 0–14-year age groups decreased by 53% rather than 71% between 1985 and 2000. The count for ages 15–19 years would not change.)

Estimating Injury Costs

We estimated lifetime costs that result from a fatal or nonfatal injury. The costs fit into two categories: (1) medical and (2) work loss. We discounted future costs (and QALYs) to present value at a 3% discount rate and defined costs from a societal perspective that includes all costs: costs to victims, families, government, insurers, and taxpayers. Estimates were price-adjusted to 2000 dollars (or 2009 dollars in the cost-effectiveness estimates) using the Employment Cost Index and Consumer Price Indices by medical care component (e.g., hospital). Mental health care costs for sexual and physical assault/abuse by age group came from Cohen and Miller (1998) and Miller, Cohen, and Wiersema (1996), as did associated, largely treatment-related parental work losses for sexual assault. These studies derived their mental health care costs from a survey of providers that collected the number of visits per episode of care by crime type, as well as average payments per visit. All other costs were estimated using the methods used by the Centers for Disease Control and Prevention in updating the 1989 report (Rice et al. 1989). These methods are documented in detail by Finkelstein et al. (2006).

Medical Costs

In summary, by diagnosis group, we used HCUP-NIS charge data adjusted with cost-to-charge ratios developed for use with HCUP-NIS by Agency for Healthcare Research and Quality, data from MEDSTAT's MarketScan database on the ratio of professional fee payments to hospital payments, inpatient rehabilitation cost estimates from Miller et al. (2004), 1999 National Nursing Home Survey data on nursing home payments for patients who were discharged to nursing homes according to HCUP-NIS, and MEPS data (five longitudinal interviews over a 2-year period) about other postdischarge costs. By combining these estimates, we derived short- to medium-term medical costs (on average, through month 18 postinjury) for injuries resulting in hospitalizations with live discharges. We used MEPS data to quantify short- to medium-term unit medical costs for injuries not requiring a hospitalization. To compute lifetime costs, we divided the estimates by the percentage of lifetime medical costs that occur in the first 18 months by diagnosis group and whether admitted to the hospital. The lifetime percentages were computed from 1979–1988 National Council on Compensation Insurance Detailed Claims Information (DCI) data on more than 450,000 nonelderly adult injury victims (Miller et al. 1995). Although these data are old, more recent data on this percentage were not available. Moreover, the DCI and MEPS showed similar percentages of costs in months 0–6 versus 7–18, which suggests the aged DCI percentages remain reasonably accurate and are appropriate for childhood injuries.

For fatalities, we obtained the distribution of place of injury death by mechanism and age group from 2000 National Vital Statistics System data. We computed costs separately for six different places of death (death-on-scene, death-on-arrival to the hospital, death at the emergency department, death at the hospital after inpatient admission, death at home, and death at a nursing home). The medical costs incurred, depending on place of death, include coroner/medical examiner, emergency or nonemergency medical transport, emergency department treatment, inpatient hospitalization, and nursing home care.

Productivity Costs

Productivity cost estimates paralleled the Consumer Product Safety Commission's injury cost model (Miller et al. 1998), in which those estimates were tailored to children. Work loss and QALY loss per injury by diagnosis and age/gender adapt published estimates (Miller et al. 1998; Zaloshnja et al. 2004) by substituting a refined cost per day of household work lost from Haddix et al. (2003). For nonfatal injuries, the work loss cost is the sum of the lifetime loss due to permanent disability (averaged across permanently disabling and nondisabling cases) plus the loss due to temporary disability. We assumed the lower-earning parent would stay home with an injured child on each day that an adult with a comparable injury would have been unable to work. For fatal injuries, the work loss cost is the present value of expected lifetime earnings, fringe benefits, and household work. The work loss days are built from 1993 Bureau of Labor Statistics data on days lost per injury with work loss; 1986–1992 National Health Interview Survey data on the probability an injury to an employed person will cause work loss; and DCI data on the percentage of injuries that result in permanent total and permanent partial disability, as well as the percentage of earning power lost for partial disabilities.

Limitations of the Incidence and Cost Estimates

This chapter provides up-to-date and comprehensive estimates of the incidence and cost of childhood injuries in the United States. The estimates are gleaned from myriad data sources; their limitations unavoidably apply to our estimates. For example, our physician's office visit count is limited to the civilian noninstitutionalized population. Although we used the best data available, some of our sources are old, some extrapolate values for children from data on working-age populations, some are based on nonrepresentative samples, and all are subject to reporting and measurement error. Some data sets lacked complete coding information and required imputation of missing data. These factors may have incorporated significant bias into the cost estimates. Our approach was designed to minimize the potential bias. However, more current and nationally representative data would have been preferable.

Our tables that break the data into detailed categories especially are challenged by small samples of cases. The detailed estimates have great uncertainty. Readers are cautioned that the actual incidence and costs for any given injury mechanism category could be substantially higher or lower than the estimates reported in this chapter. Moreover, because we used multiple data sets and assumptions to generate estimates, we could not compute standard errors.

This chapter excludes many injuries and does not capture all the costs of the injuries it does include. It excludes injuries treated only by dentists, chiropractors, acupuncturists, and other alternative medicine healers, as well as injuries that, although potentially severe, did not receive medical attention. It focuses on medical and work loss costs. It excludes other resource costs (e.g., for property damage, police services, fire services, victim services, cost recovery through tort litigation, and adjudication and sanctioning for criminal behavior). Including those costs would increase the proportion of total costs associated with highway crashes and physical and sexual assaults. It also ignores PTSD associated with unintentional injury. Three studies (Daviss et al. 2000; de Vries et al. 1999; Schreier et al. 2005) found that at least 25% of samples of children hospitalized for injury had diagnostic PTSD; however, these children rarely were treated for even persistent symptoms. For lack of data, we excluded the costs and QALY losses resulting from their PTSD. Similarly, we excluded the costs and QALY losses that often result when the psychologic trauma of assault victimization causes victims to become violent or abuse substances (Kendler et al. 2000; Nelson et al. 2002; Widom, Schuck, and White 2006).

Our tables report intent as recorded by the medical system. Comparison of our estimates for ages 15–24 years (which includes cases not shown in this chapter) with contemporaneous 1999–2000 data from the National Crime Victimization Survey suggests the medical system captured cases not requiring hospitalization, including child physical abuse and domestic violence. It recorded 135,000 more treated assaults than the National Crime Victimization Survey. Unlike the nonhospitalized cases, where the federal government asks and sometimes pays a sample of providers to code intent, the hospital counts are derived from administrative data systems. They capture only 60% of the 46,000–49,000 hospitalizations estimated from National Crime Victimization Survey data for ages 15–24 years. Correcting this coding shift from assault to unintentional (or rarely, to undetermined) would increase our physical assault incidence estimate by only 3% but increase physical assault costs by 10% and the associated medical costs by 22%. Also, our medically treated physical assault estimates assume that all mental health treatment was for victims who also were medically treated. Although this procedure captures total medical costs of assault correctly, it undercounts medically treated physical assaults, omitting ones treated only by mental health providers. We also excluded the costs and QALY losses from sexually transmitted diseases that resulted from sexual assault.

Although the hospitalization and mental health cost estimates used in this analysis are age-specific, other data are not. Specifically, the permanent disability cost estimates associated with productivity account for the longer life span of children, but are not child-specific in other respects. Work loss cost estimates in this analysis have other drawbacks too. Because women and minorities are paid less than White men for comparable work, productivity costs undervalue their lives (Rice et al. 1989). For example, by using a 3% discount rate, at age 7 years the present value of lifetime wage and household work loss resulting from the death of a girl is $949,000 compared with $1,363,000 for the death of a boy. Because children's earnings are in the future, their present value also is less than the present value earnings losses of young adults, even though more years of future work are lost (Rice et al. 1989). Some of the minor cost contributors in this analysis, notably coroner costs, also have limitations, in that data used to estimate them are 10 to 25 years old. Inflating these old estimates to current dollars may introduce some inaccuracy, but they contribute too little to total costs to justify the expense of collecting new estimates.

For all these reasons, our estimates should be interpreted with caution. They are, however, the best available estimates of childhood injury incidence and costs in the United States today. Future studies will improve on the methodology and results.

Estimating Lost Quality of Life: Methods and Limitations

Quality of life losses were estimated as the present value of the sum of years of potential life lost to fatal injury, plus the QALY losses resulting from nonfatal injury. For each death and for paralyzing injuries that shorten the life span, the years of life lost were estimated from a life expectancy table (Arias 2002; Berkowitz et al. 1992). QALY loss per child sexual assault came from Miller, Cohen, and Wiersema (1996). For QALY losses associated with physical injury that caused temporary or permanent disability, estimates by injury diagnosis and victim age were taken from a previous study (Miller et al. 1995). Although that study's estimates are routinely used in regulatory analysis by the National Highway Traffic Safety Administration, they rely on physician ratings of functional outcomes in the 1980s that were never fully validated. The estimates combined physician ratings of the impact of injuries over time on the ability to think, see, walk, and so forth, and on pain (Hirsch et al. 1983; Miller et al. 1995) with diagnosis-specific National Council on Compensation Insurance data on the probability that injury would permanently reduce earning capacity or prevent the victim from working and on the percentage earnings reduction (National Council on Compensation Insurance 1998). The rating scales used were not tailored to children, although the physicians were asked to rate probable impairment levels and durations separately for children. The estimated impairment impacts were translated into QALY losses using a systematic review of survey data that weighed the relative importance that respondents placed on different dimensions of impact (Miller et al. 1995). Most of these weights were specific to a child and adolescent population, but reflect the views of adults rather than children of the value of temporary and permanent functional losses by children. The uncertainty in our QALY loss estimates, nevertheless, is large.

For sexual assault, we started with the nonmonetary losses per rape and per sexual abuse case that Miller, Cohen, and Wiersema (1996) derived from 361 jury verdicts for sexual assault, most of them against bars that served drunken patrons, public places with unsafe parking lots, improperly secured hotels, or employers that poorly screened or supervised staff who were working with children. We summed the average noneconomic loss and wage loss per sexual assault. We divided the sum by the amount Cohen and Miller (2003) estimate juries were willing to award for a lifetime of QALY loss. They derived that estimate from regressions on jury awards for physical assault and the QALY loss estimates by diagnosis used in the present chapter. This calculation showed that the mean loss for all sexual assaults was 2.36% of lifetime QALYs, with slightly higher percentage losses when the victims were children aged less than 11 years. By comparison, had we used survey-based estimates of what people are willing to pay to reduce their risk of a rape or a homicide (Cohen et al. 2004), the lifetime loss would have been 2.44% of QALYs. Thus, our estimates are conservative. Multiplying the percentage loss times the present value of lifetime QALYs implicit in the willingness to award estimate, the estimated loss is 0.807 QALYs per sexual assault victim aged less than 11 years and 0.633 QALYs per sexual assault victim aged more than 11 years.

Acknowledgments

The research reported was supported in part by a contract from the National Center for Injury Prevention and Control, Centers for Disease Control and Prevention, National Institute on Mental Health Grant R01 MH60622, and a Children's Safety Network contract from the Maternal and Child Health Bureau, Health Resources, and Services Administration. Participating in the International Collaborative Effort on Injury Statistics, sponsored by the National Center for Health Statistics with funding from the National Institute of Child Health and Development, also contributed critically to this research. The authors thank Ian Fiebelkorn at Research Triangle Institute and Bruce Lawrence at the Pacific Institute for Research and Evaluation for assistance in computing the numbers reported. The authors are especially grateful to our Project Officer at the Centers for Disease Control and Prevention, Phaedra Corso, for insightful advice, comments, and hard work, helping us to develop and document the medical and work loss cost estimates for physical injury presented in the first half of this chapter. The sexual assault estimates, QALY-related work, and cost-savings analyses were not funded by the Centers for Disease Control and Prevention. Nothing in this chapter should be construed as the official position of the funding agencies.

References

Agency for Healthcare Research and Quality. 2010a. *Healthcare Cost and Utilization Project—Nationwide Inpatient Sample.* Rockville, MD: Agency for Healthcare Research and Quality. Available at: http://www.hcup-us.ahrq.gov/nisoverview.jsp. Accessed October 15, 2010.

Agency for Healthcare Research and Quality. 2010b. *Medical Expenditure Panel Survey.* Rockville, MD: Agency for Healthcare Research and Quality. Available at: http://www.meps.ahrq.gov/mepsweb. Accessed October 15, 2010.

Alcohol Policies Project. 1998. *Fact Sheet: Lowering the Minimum Drinking Age Is a Bad Idea.* Center for Science in the Public Interest. Available at: http://www.cspinet.org/booze/mlpafact.htm. Accessed June 7, 2005.

Aos S, Lieb R, Mayfield J, et al. 2004. *Benefits and Costs of Prevention and Early Intervention Programs for Youth.* Olympia, WA: Washington State Institute for Public Policy.

Arias E. 2002. *United States Life Tables, 2000.* National Vital Statistics Reports. 53:6. Hyattsville, MD: National Center for Health Statistics.

Ball DJ. 2004. Policy issues and risk-benefit trade-offs of 'safer surfacing' for children's playgrounds. *Accid Anal Prev.* 36:661–670.

Berkowitz M, Harvey C, Greene CG, Wilson SE. 1992. *Economic Consequences of Traumatic Spinal Cord Injury.* New York: Demos.

Biglan A, Brennan PA, Foster SL, Holder HD. 2004. *Helping Adolescents at Risk: Prevention of Multiple Problem Behaviors.* New York, NY: Guilford.

Blincoe LJ, Seay A, Zaloshnja E, et al. 2002. *The Economic Impact of Motor Vehicle Crashes, 2000.* Washington, DC: U.S. Department of Transportation, National Highway Traffic Safety Administration.

Boyle MH, Torrance GW, Sinclair JC, Horwood SP. 1983. Economic evaluation of neonatal intensive care of very-low-birth-weight infants. *N Engl J Med.* 308:1330–1337.

Bureau of the Census. 1997. *Statistical Abstract of the United States 1997.* 117th ed. Washington, DC: U.S. Government Printing Office.

Butry DT, Brown MH, Fuller SK. 2007. *Benefit-Cost Analysis of Residential Fire Sprinkler Systems.* Gaithersburg, MD: National Institute of Standards and Technology.

Centers for Disease Control and Prevention (CDC). 2003. *2001 National School-Based Youth Risk Behavior Survey: Public-Use Data Documentation.* Atlanta, GA: CDC. Available at: ftp://ftp.cdc.gov/pub/data/yrbs/2001/yrbs2001.pdf. Accessed June 16, 2011.

Chanley SA, Chanley JJ Jr, Campbell HE. 2001. Providing refuge: the value of domestic violence shelter services. *Public Adm Rev.* 31:393–413.

Chen G. 2005. Safety and economic impacts of photo radar program. *Traffic Inj Prev.* 6:299–307.

Clement FM, Harris A, Li JJ, et al. 2009. Using effectiveness and cost-effectiveness to make drug coverage decisions: a comparison of Britain, Australia, and Canada. *JAMA.* 302:1437–1443.

Cohen MA, Miller TR. 1998. The cost of mental health care for victims of crime. *J Interpers Violence.* 13:93–110.

Cohen MA, Miller TR. 2003. Willingness to award non-monetary damages and the implied value of life from jury awards. *Int Rev Law Econ.* 23:165–181.

Cohen MA, Rust R, Steen S, Tidd S. 2004. Willingness-to-pay for crime control programs. *Criminology.* 42:86–106.

Corso P, Mercy J, Simon T, et al. 2007. Medical costs and productivity losses due to interpersonal and self-directed violence in the U.S. *Am J Prev Med.* 32:474–482.

Council FM, Persuad B, Eccles K, et al. 2005. *Safety Evaluation of Red-Light Cameras.* McLean, VA: Federal Highway Administration.

Cutler DM, Richardson E. 1998. The value of health: 1970–1990. *Am Econ Rev.* 88:97–100.

Daviss WB, Mooney D, Racusin R, et al. 2000. Predicting posttraumatic stress after hospitalization for pediatric injury. *J Am Acad Child Adolesc Psychiatry.* 39:576–583.

de Vries AP, Kassam-Adams N, Cnaan A, et al. 1999. Looking beyond the physical injury: posttraumatic stress disorder in children and parents after pediatric traffic injury. *Pediatrics.* 104:1293–1299.

Drummond MF, O'Brien B, Stoddart GL, Torrance GW. 1997. *Methods for the Economic Evaluation of Health Care Programmes.* 2nd ed. Oxford, England: Oxford University.

Finkelstein EA, Corso PC, Miller TR, et al. 2006. *Incidence and Economic Burden of Injuries in the United States, 2000.* New York: Oxford University.

French MT, Mauskopf JA, Teague JL, Roland J. 1996. Estimating the dollar value of health outcomes from drug abuse interventions. *Med Care.* 34:890–910.

Gold MR, Siegel JE, Russell LB, Weinstein MC, editors. 1996. Cost-Effectiveness in Health and Medicine: Report of the Panel on Cost-Effectiveness in Health and Medicine. New York, NY: Oxford University.

Goldsmith LJ, Hutchison B, Hurley J. 2004. *Economic Evaluation Across the Four Faces of Prevention.* Hamilton, Ontario: Centre for Health Economics and Policy Analysis, McMaster University.

Graham JD, Corso PS, Morris JM, et al. 1998. Evaluating the cost-effectiveness of clinical and public health measures. *Annu Rev Public Health.* 9:125–152.

Grossman DC, Mueller BA, Riedy C, et al. 2005. Gun storage practices and risk of youth suicide and unintentional firearm injuries. I 293:707–714.

Haddix AC, Teutsch SM, Corso PS. 2003. *Prevention Effectiveness, A Guide to Decision Analysis and Economic Evaluation.* 2nd ed. New York: Oxford University.

Hansen WB, Derzon JH, Dusenbury L. 2004. *Analysis of Magnitude of Effects of Substance Abuse Prevention Programs Included in the National Registry of Effective Programs through 2003: A Core Components Analysis.* Washington, DC: Center for Substance Abuse Prevention, Substance Abuse and Mental Health Services Administration.

Hingson R, Howland J. 1990. Use of laws to deter drinking and driving. Alcohol *Health Res World.* 14:36–43.

Hirsch A, Eppinger R, Shame T, et al. 1983. *Impairment Scaling from the Abbreviated Injury Scale.* Washington, DC: National Highway Traffic Safety Administration.

Hu PS, Reuscher TR. 2004. *Summary of Travel Trends, 2001 National Household Travel Survey.* Washington, DC: Federal Highway Administration.

Institute of Medicine Committee on Poison Prevention and Control. 2004. *Forging a Poison Prevention and Control System.* Washington, DC: National Academies.

Istre GR, McCoy MA, Osborn L, et al. 2001. Deaths and injuries from house fires. *N Engl J Med.* 344:1911–1916.

Insurance Institute for Highway Safety. 2011. Web page: Q & As: Red light cameras. Arlington, VA: Insurance Institute for Highway Safety. Available at: http://www.iihs.org/research/qanda/rlr.html. Accessed June 22, 2011.

Kelly AE, Haddix AC, Scanlon KS, et al. 1996. Cost-effectiveness of strategies to prevent neural tube defects. In: Gold MR, Siegel JE, Russell LB, Weinstein MC, editors. *Cost-Effectiveness in Health and Medicine.* New York: Oxford University. Note 4.

Kendler KS, Bulik CM, Silberg J, et al. 2000. Childhood sexual abuse and adult psychiatric and substance use disorders in women: an epidemiological and cotwin control analysis. *Arch Gen Psychiatr.* 57:953–959.

Kenkel DS. 2001. Using estimates of the value of a statistical life in evaluating regulatory effects. In: Kuckler F, editor. *Valuing the Health Benefits of Food Safety: A Proceedings.* Washington, DC: U.S. Department of Agriculture. 2–13.

Kilpatrick DG, Saunders BE. 2000. *National Survey of Adolescents in the United States (1995).* Charlestown, SC: Medical University of South Carolina. Available at: http://dx.doi.org/10.3886/ICPSR02833. Accessed May 18, 2011.

Krupnick AJ. 2004. *Valuing Health Outcomes: Policy Choices and Technical Issues.* Washington, DC: Resources for the Future.

Lee C, Chertow G, Zenios S. 2009. An empiric estimate of the value of life: updating the renal dialysis cost-effectiveness standard. *Value Health.* 12:80–87.

Lino M. 2001. *Expenditures on Children by Families, 2000 Annual Report.* Washington, DC: U.S. Department of Agriculture, Center for Nutrition Policy and Promotion.

Mayer M, LeClere FB. 1990. *Injury Prevention Measures in Households With Children in the United States, 1990.* Hyattsville, MD: National Center for Health Statistics.

Miller TR. 1990. The plausible range for the value of life: red herrings among the mackerels. *J Forensic Econ.* 3:17–39.

Miller TR. 2000. Assessing the burden of injury: progress and pitfalls. In: Mohan D, Tiwari G, editors. *Injury Prevention and Control.* New York, NY: Taylor & Francis, 49–70.

Miller TR, Cohen MA, Wiersema B. 1996. *Victim Costs and Consequences—A New Look.* Washington, DC: National Institute of Justice.

Miller TR, Demes J, Bovbjerg R. 1993. Child seats: how large are the benefits and who should pay? In: *Child Occupant Protection.* Malvern, PA: Society for Automotive Engineers.

Miller TR, Galbraith MS. 1995. Injury prevention counseling by pediatricians: a benefit-cost comparison. *Pediatrics.* 96:1–4.

Miller TR, Hendrie D. 2005. How should governments spend the drug prevention dollar: a buyer's guide. In: Stockwell T, Gruenewald P, Toumbourou J, Loxley W, editors. *Preventing Harmful Substance Use: The Evidence Base for Policy and Practice.* West Sussex: John Wiley & Sons. 415–431.

Miller TR, Hendrie D. 2009. *Substance Abuse Prevention Dollars and Cents: A Cost-Benefit Analysis.* Rockville, MD: Center for Substance Abuse Prevention, Substance Abuse and Mental Health Services Administration.

Miller TR, Langston EA, Lawrence BA, et al. 2004. *Rehabilitation Costs and Long-Term Consequences of Motor Vehicle Injury.* Washington, DC: National Highway Traffic Safety Administration.

Miller TR, Lawrence BA. 2010. *Cost-Effectiveness Analysis of Residential Fire Masks. Final Report.* Calverton, MD: U.S. Consumer Product Safety Commission.

Miller TR, Lawrence BA, Jensen A, et al. 1998. *Estimating the Cost to Society of Consumer Product Injuries: The Revised Injury Cost Model.* Bethesda, MD: U.S. Consumer Product Safety Commission.

Miller TR, Levy DT. 1995. The effect of regional trauma care systems on costs. *Arch Surg.* 130:188–193.

Miller TR, Levy DT. 2000. Cost-outcome analysis in injury prevention and control: eighty-four recent estimates for the United States. *Med Care.* 38:562–582.

Miller TR, Pindus NM, Douglass JB, Rossman SB. 1995. *Nonfatal Injury Costs and Consequences: A Data Book.* Washington, DC: Urban Institute.

Miller TR, Romano EO, Spicer RS. 2000. The cost of childhood unintentional injuries and the value of prevention. *Future Child.* 10:137–163.

Miller TR, Zaloshnja E, Hendrie D. 2009. Cost of traumatic brain injuries in the United States and the return to helmet investments. In: Jallo J, Loftus, C, editors. *Brain Trauma and Critical Care.* New York: Thieme. 445–459.

National Center for Health Statistics. 2010a. *Ambulatory Health Care Data.* Hyattsville, MD: National Center for Health Statistics. Available at: http://www.cdc.gov/ncipc/wisqars/nonfatal/datasources.htm. Accessed October 15, 2010.

National Center for Health Statistics. 2010b. *Mortality Data, Multiple Cause-of-Death Public-Use Data Files.* Hyattsville, MD: National Center for Health Statistics. Available at: http://www.cdc.gov/nchs/products/elec_prods/subject/mortmcd.htm. Accessed October 15, 2010.

National Center for Injury Prevention and Control. 2003. *Costs of Intimate Partner Violence Against Women in the United States.* Atlanta, GA: Centers for Disease Control and Prevention.

National Center for Injury Prevention and Control. 2010. *National Electronic Injury Surveillance System All-Injury Profile.* Atlanta, GA: Centers for Disease Control and Prevention, National Center for Injury Prevention and Control. Available at: http://www.cdc.gov/ncipc/wisqars/nonfatal/datasources.htm. Accessed October 15, 2010.

National Council on Compensation Insurance. 1998. *Detailed Claims Information Special Tabulation.* Boca Raton, FL: National Council on Compensation Insurance.

Nelson EC, Heath AC, Madden PA, et al. 2002. Association between self-reported childhood sexual abuse and adverse psychosocial outcomes: results from a twin study. *Arch Gen Psychiatry.* 59:139–145.

Ortega-Sanchez I and the Working Group on Leading Economic Issues on New Vaccines for Adolescents. 2005. *An Inquiry into the Projected Cost-Effectiveness of New Vaccines and Other Health Interventions for Adolescents.* Atlanta, GA: Centers for Disease Control and Prevention.

Rice DP, MacKenzie EJ, Jones AS, et al. 1989. *Cost of Injury in the United States: A Report to Congress.* San Francisco, CA: Institute for Health and Aging, University of California, and Injury Prevention Center, The Johns Hopkins University.

Rodgers GB, Leland EW. 2008. A retrospective benefit-cost analysis of the 1997 stair-fall requirements for baby walkers. *Accid Anal Prev.* 40:61–68.

Schreier H, Ladakakos C, Morabito D, et al. 2005. Posttraumatic stress symptoms in children after mild to moderate pediatric trauma: a longitudinal examination of symptom prevalence, correlates, and parent-child symptom reporting. *J Trauma.* 58:353–363.

Spicer RS, Miller TR, Durkin MS, Barlow B. 2004. A benefit-cost analysis of the Harlem Hospital Injury Prevention Program. *Inj Control Saf Promot.* 11:55–57.

Substance Abuse and Mental Health Services Administration. 2010. *Model Programs: Good Behavior Game*. Washington, DC: U.S. Department of Health and Human Services. Available at: http://modelprograms.samhsa.gov/textonly_cf.cfm?page=effective&pkProgramID=84. Accessed October 15, 2010.

Sunstein CR. 2003. *Lives, Life-Years and Willingness to Pay*. Washington, DC: AEI-Brookings Joint Center for Regulatory Studies.

Tenenbein M. 2005. Unit-dose packaging of iron supplements and reduction of iron poisoning in young children. *Arch Pediatr Adolesc Med*. 159:557–560.

Tengs TO, Adams ME, Pliskin JS, et al. 1995. Five hundred life-saving interventions and their cost-effectiveness. *Risk Anal*. 15:369–390.

Tolley G, Kenkel D, Fabian R, editors. 1994. *Valuing Health for Policy: An Economic Approach*. Chicago, IL: University of Chicago.

U.S. Census Bureau. 2005. *Historical Census of Housing Tables, House Heating Fuel*. U.S. Census Bureau, Housing and Household Economic Statistics Division, December 2, 2004. Available at: http://www.census.gov/hhes/www/housing/census/historic/fuels.html. Accessed June 7, 2005.

U.S. Consumer Product Safety Commission. 2006. 16 CFR Part 1633, Final rule: standard for the flammability (open flame) of mattress sets. *Federal Register*. 71:13472–13523.

Widom CS, Schuck AM, White HR. 2006. An examination of pathways from childhood victimization to violence: the role of early aggression and problematic alcohol use. *Violence Vict*. 21:675–690.

Zaloshnja E, Miller TR, Galbraith MS, et al. 2003. Reducing injuries among Native Americans: five cost-outcome analyses. *Accid Anal Prev*. 35:631–639.

Zaloshnja E, Miller TR, Romano EO, Spicer RS. 2004. Crash costs by body part injured, fracture involvement, and threat-to-life severity, United States, 2000. *Accid Anal Prev*. 36:415–427.

Chapter 3

Hazards Associated With Common Nursery Products

Carol Pollack-Nelson, PhD[1] and Dorothy Drago, MA, MPH[2]

Charlie Horn was one of a set of triplets. He was more laid back than his siblings, Will and Brigit, content to sit, play, and turn the pages of a book. On November 1, 2007, when he was 2.5 years old, he and his triplet brother, Will, went down for a nap in their room. At first check, Charlie was asleep on the floor at the foot of Will's bed. At the final check, Charlie was on his knees, his head and shoulders trapped in a drawer of a tipped dresser. He asphyxiated.

Charlie's parents, Brett and Jenny Horn, had secured taller pieces of furniture they thought could tip, but they never expected a 30-inch–tall child's dresser to tip. Now they know that appearances of stability can be misleading. Hoping to spare other parents their kind of tragedy, Brett and Jenny Horn turned their grief into advocacy. They have worked with the Missouri State Senate to achieve stricter guidelines for furniture and have engaged in public speaking to increase awareness of furniture tip-over and the devastating consequences. They encourage the use of furniture straps and have distributed more than 25,000 of them free as a means of improving awareness.

The Horns have elicited the assistance of their local Safe Kids USA, Children's Mercy Hospital staff, and other experts to create a nonprofit organization, Charlie's House, named after their son. Ultimately, Charlie's House will be a model home that people can walk through and learn ways to reduce hazards to make homes safer for young children. They have already helped raise more than $150,000 in cash and pledges to buy land for Charlie's House, which will be centrally located in Kansas City, near Children's Mercy Hospital. They also have a Web site (at http://www.charlieshouse.org) that educates about home safety, and in particular makes people more aware of the tragedy that can be associated with furniture tip-over.

The Consumer Product Safety Commission

In 2008, an estimated 63,700 children aged 5 years and younger were treated for injuries associated with nursery products in emergency departments throughout the United States (Chowdhury 2009). The U.S. Consumer Product Safety Commission (CPSC) is the government agency responsible for overseeing the safety of consumer products, including nursery items. The Commission is an independent federal regulatory agency created in 1972 by Congress under the Consumer Product Safety Act. The agency's mission is to protect the public from unreasonable risks of serious injury or death involving a wide variety of consumer products. To accomplish its mission, the Commission collects data and information relating to injury and death associated with approximately 15,000 different consumer products. The Commission maintains four different databases:

[1]Independent Safety Consulting, Rockville, MD.
[2]Drago Expert Services, Plymouth, MA.

1. The National Electronic Injury Surveillance System (NEISS). The NEISS system is composed of a sample of approximately 100 hospital emergency departments that are statistically representative of hospital emergency departments nationwide. These emergency departments record data (in accordance with a CPSC coding manual) pertaining to cases that involve consumer products. These data are transmitted to the CPSC once a day. The CPSC uses these data to estimate the number of injuries occurring nationwide. A NEISS record includes product code(s), treatment date, age, sex, diagnosis, body part injured, disposition (e.g., released or hospitalized), location where the incident occurred (e.g., school or home), and a brief description of the event.
2. Death Certificate File (DTHS). In cases in which a death was associated with a consumer product, the CPSC purchases the death certificates from the state health departments. A DTHS record includes date of death, age, sex, race, external cause of death (E-Code), product code(s), location, and a brief description of the circumstances of the death. Not all states participate in this program, so the number of deaths reported through the CPSC should always be considered a minimum number.
3. Injury/Potential Injury Incident File (IPII). The IPII database contains summaries of product-related reports from a variety of sources, including the agency's toll-free "hotline," newspaper accounts, reports from medical examiners, letters to CPSC, and referrals from other government agencies. An IPII record includes product code(s), incident date, age, sex, hazard, disposition (e.g., released or hospitalized), city and state, and a brief description of the event.
4. In-Depth Investigations File. This file contains summaries of follow-up investigations of certain cases originally reported through one of the other databases. In-depth investigation reports are based on interviews with the victim, a parent, or a witness. The reports provide details about incident sequence, human behavior, and product involvement. A fifth, publicly searchable, database will be available in early 2011. This new database consists of "reports of harm" submitted by consumers, government agencies, health care professionals, child service providers, and public safety entities. It will also include all recall notices. It has its origins in the Consumer Product Safety Improvement Act (CPSIA) (Consumer Product Safety Commission [CPSC] 2008), which requires the CPSC to establish and maintain a product safety information database that is available to the public. The database will be available and searchable through the CPSC Web site at http://www.saferproducts.gov. The new database is described at 16 CFR part 1102 (2011).

On the basis of the data collected, the CPSC may pursue a variety of options to address hazards. The CPSC can (1) develop mandatory standards (which may be based to some extent on a voluntary standard); (2) work with industry to develop voluntary standards; (3) "defer" to an existing voluntary standard, lending it the status of a quasi-mandatory standard; (4) ban products from the marketplace; or (5) require that products be recalled and "fixed" so they no longer pose a hazard.

Standards can potentially be helpful in ensuring the quality and safety of nursery products. Of the nursery items discussed in this chapter, there has been a long-standing mandatory standard only for cribs. There have been voluntary standards for other nursery products, but no mandatory standards. That is now changing. In 2008, Congress enacted the CPSIA (CPSC 2008). One of the primary purposes of the Act is to establish consumer product safety standards and other safety requirements for children's products. The Act requires the CPSC to assess the effectiveness of voluntary standards and develop mandatory safety standards for the following infant and toddler products: cribs (including full-size and non-full-size cribs, portable cribs, play yards (playpens), cribs used in hotels and child care facilities, and places where cribs are offered for use or lease); toddler beds; high chairs, booster chairs, and hook-on chairs; bath seats; gates and other enclosures for confining a child; stationary activity centers; infant carriers; strollers; walkers; swings; and bassinets and cradles.

According to the CPSIA, the CPSC must make existing voluntary safety standards for these products mandatory (assuming that the Commission is satisfied with the voluntary standard's requirements) or develop a stricter mandatory safety standard. Once the Commission has issued these mandatory safety standards, it will be illegal for any company to manufacture, sell, or import a product that fails to comply. To date, the Commission has issued mandatory standards for four nursery products: baby walkers, bath seats, toddler beds, and cribs. The mandatory baby walker standard is consistent with the voluntary standard with some additional and more stringent requirements, including adding a parking brake test for walkers equipped with parking brakes. Although baby walkers and toddler beds are not reviewed in this chapter, the passage of the mandatory rules is worth noting. The bath seat standard likewise essentially adopts the voluntary standard, adding stricter requirements for stability/tip-over, tighter leg-opening requirements, and a larger permanent on-product warning label alerting that bath seats are not safety devices and that infants should never be left unattended in a bath seat. The new mandatory crib standards (for full-size and non-full-size cribs) incorporate the voluntary standards and add some new requirements. The new standard is discussed further in the section "Cribs."

In addition to developing mandatory standards for nursery products, the CPSIA also requires manufacturers to provide a postage prepaid registration card with the sale of each of these infant and toddler products (16 CFR part 1130 2009). The purpose of the registration card is to enable the manufacturer or retailer of the product to contact consumers with recall or other safety information. As of June 28, 2010, registration cards are required for full-size cribs and non-full-size cribs, toddler beds, high chairs, booster chairs, hook-on chairs, bath seats, infant carriers, strollers, walkers, swings, bassinets, cradles, play yards, stationary activity centers, and gates and other enclosures for confining a child. As of December 29, 2010, registration cards are required for children's folding chairs, changing tables, infant bouncers, infant bath tubs, bed rails, and infant slings.

One of the most significant effects of the CPSIA is restrictions in the amount of dangerous chemicals, most notably lead and phthalates, that can be present in toys and child care articles. A "children's toy" means a product primarily intended for use of a child aged 12 years or younger when playing; a "child care article" means a product that a child aged 3 years or younger would use for sleeping, feeding, sucking, or teething. This includes cribs, play yards, and high chairs.

Lead is known to affect brain development, and high lead levels are associated with severe cognitive impairment. The limits on the amount of lead in children's products are being phased in over the course of 3 years. Children's articles with more than 300 parts per million total lead content by weight are banned in the United States. In the future, that limit may be reduced to 100 parts per million. There are also stricter limits on the amount of allowable lead in paint and other surface coating materials. Whereas the original ban on lead in paint (16 CFR part 1303 1977) limited the amount of lead to 0.06% of the weight of the total nonvolatile content of the paint, the new limit is 0.009%.

Phthalates are chemicals that are added to plastic to increase its flexibility, transparency, durability, and longevity. In other words, phthalates can make plastic objects softer and more pliable. Phthalate exposure in children may be related to asthma and allergies, endocrine disruption, birth defects, and autism. The effects of phthalate exposure continue to be studied. The CPSIA bans three phthalates—di-(2-ethylhexyl) phthalate, dibutyl phthalate, and benzyl butyl phthalate—in concentration of more than 0.1% in toys and child care articles.

The work of the CPSC, particularly since the passage of the CPSIA in 2008, will likely have a dramatic effect on the number of consumer product injuries and fatalities. However, its effect is not likely to be seen for a number of years since preexisting products linger in the marketplace for some time. Also, there is a lag in data reporting to the CPSC.

Nursery Product Safety

The word "nursery" conjures up an image of a peaceful environment for an infant or toddler. However, as Charlie Horn's death demonstrates, that is not always the reality. Each year thousands of children are injured, some fatally, by nursery products. Consumers are often surprised by dangerous nursery products, and many consumers expect that products intended for use by a baby are tested and their safety assured. However, there is no premarket safety clearance procedure for nursery products (or any other consumer products) in the United States.

The passage of the CPSIA ensures that there will be mandatory standards for nursery products. Once a mandatory standard is in place, it becomes illegal to manufacture or sell a noncompliant nursery product in the United States. However, consumers must keep in mind that, to date, most nursery products are not regulated by a mandatory standard. Further, although standards are an important method for bolstering product safety, they do not eliminate all hazards. Standards typically attempt to address the most frequent and serious hazards associated with a product, but other risks may not be addressed. Furthermore, standards apply to a class of products and do not necessarily address hazards unique to any particular manufacturer's product.

Nursery Product Injury and Fatality Data

Although mandatory and voluntary standards have led to a decline in nursery product injuries and fatalities, incidents do still occur. This chapter examines injury and fatality data associated with ten common nursery items. The data cited in this chapter were obtained from the National Injury Information Clearinghouse at the CPSC. Records from the death certificate database (DTHS), incident investigations database (In-Depth Investigations File), and reported incidents database (IPII) for the period 2004–2009 were reviewed; NEISS records from 2008 were reviewed to determine nationwide injury rates for that year.

The CPSC's data are available to anyone upon request. Depending on the type and extent of request, there may be a charge for the data. Typically, data are purged of manufacturer and brand names. Consumers can check NEISS estimates on the CPSC Web site at http://www.cpsc.gov.

Bassinets and Cradles

Bassinets and cradles are used as sleep environments for newborns and very young infants. A typical bassinet is a basket-like container on freestanding legs with wheels. These classic-style bassinets make it convenient to push an infant from room to room. Co-sleeper/bedside bassinets are (or can be) open on one side, allowing them to attach to the parents' bed, keeping the baby separate, but nearby, during the night. In addition to the freestanding models, bassinets are sometimes included as accessories on play yards.

Cradles typically have a stationary frame, but rock side-to-side or front-to-back. Like bassinets, cradles are sometimes included as accessories on play yards.

Other products that are sold as sleep environs for very young infants include baby hammocks and Moses baskets. Moses baskets are legless bassinets. Some designs have carrying handles. Baby hammocks are less common but are used in a manner similar to cradles.

The most common cause of fatality associated with bassinets, cradles, baby hammocks, and Moses baskets is mechanical suffocation, usually associated with pillows or other soft bedding that was placed inside. Between 2004 and 2009, 118 bassinet/cradle deaths—an average of 20 per year—were reported to the CPSC. Many of these infants were found face down on soft bedding. Thus, objects placed in the sleep environment, rather than the product, were the primary cause of death.

Parents may be enticed to purchase plush bedding and pillows for an infant, believing that these items will make the sleep environment cozier. Given that mattresses typically provided with bassinets are thin (the voluntary standard for bassinets and cradles limits mattress depth to 1 ½ inches; American Society for Testing and Materials [ASTM] 2010g), this behavior is foreseeable. Unfortunately, babies can suffocate in plush bedding and pillows. The voluntary standard for bassinets requires labeling warning about the dangers of adding pillows and soft bedding. Astonishingly, some Moses baskets found for sale on-line included pillows and comforters! Including such products will likely cause some parents to mistakenly believe that these plush items are safe for use with a sleeping baby. However, selling pillows and comforters with any sleep environment for a baby is a dangerous practice.

Other patterns of asphyxia occur when the baby becomes entrapped between the mattress and the sidewall in a bassinet, between structural components, such as drop rails on bassinets designed as co-sleepers, or by being pressed against a side or end of a cradle that comes to rest at an angle, rather than level.

There have also been reports of fatal entrapment involving "sleep positioners" used in bassinets and cribs. A sleep positioner is intended and marketed as a product that prevents a baby from rolling onto his or her stomach. These products seem to have been developed as a reaction to the American Academy of Pediatrics advice to place babies to sleep on their backs to reduce the likelihood of sudden infant death syndrome (SIDS) (American Academy of Pediatrics 2005). However, a baby placed on its side can roll onto its stomach or into another unsafe orientation. For example, the baby's head can roll off a positioner, but the baby lacks the muscle control to bring the head back to a neutral position. In September 2010, the CPSC issued a joint Press Release with the Food and Drug Administration advising consumers to stop using sleep positioners (CPSC 2010a). The CPSC reported that 12 infants aged 1 to 4 months have died when they suffocated in sleep positioners or became entrapped and suffocated between a sleep positioner and the side of a crib or bassinet. Most of the infants had rolled from the side to the stomach position.

An estimated 500 to 600 bassinet and cradle-related injuries are treated yearly in emergency departments. Approximately half of the injuries are associated with the baby falling out of the bassinet. Infants aged 6 months or younger make up the majority of cases, with head injuries common. When children older than the intended user age use these products, they can fall while trying to climb out. Other severe, but less common, injuries are associated with product collapse or tip-over. Minor to moderate injuries are associated with sharp points, sharp edges, or splinters.

Since 2004, there have been three bassinet recalls. One involved an entrapment hazard and two involved the creation of uneven sleep surfaces.

- In 2008, the entrapment deaths of a 6 ½-month-old Kansas girl and a 4-month-old Missouri girl between the rails of a convertible bassinet-co-sleeper prompted the recall of 900,000 Simplicity 3-in-1 and 4-in-1 convertible bassinets. The bassinets contained metal bars covered by an adjustable fabric flap that attached by Velcro. The fabric got folded down when the bassinet was converted into a bedside co-sleeper. If the Velcro was not properly resecured when the flap was adjusted, an infant could slip through the opening and become entrapped in the metal bars and suffocate.
- In May 2008, Eddie Bauer Soothe & Sway portable play yards were recalled because the rocking bassinet accessory could come to rest at an angle. No deaths were reported, although there were ten reports of infants rolling to one side, six of whom were found with their faces pressed against the side or bottom of the bassinet.
- In 2009, another Eddie Bauer product (Complete Care Play Yard) and a Safety 1st product were recalled by the Dorel Juvenile Group, Inc., because a support bar in the floor board of the

bassinet accessory for the play yard could become detached from its sleeve, creating an uneven sleep surface. No injuries were associated with this problem.

Originally published in 2002, the American Society for Testing and Materials (ASTM) Standard Consumer Specification for Bassinets and Cradles (ASTM 2010g) was developed to address the hazards of suffocation, tip-over, and collapse. The standard now also applies to bassinets that are accessories on play yards. The standard requires performance criteria to, among other things, preclude unintentional folding and tip-over, limit mattress thickness, and limit the space between the mattress and sidewall. It also requires warnings addressing falls and suffocation.

As part of its responsibilities under CPSIA, the CPSC is required to create a mandatory standard for bassinets and cradles. The new proposed standard (16 CFR part 1218 2010) would adopt the ASTM voluntary standard (F2194) for bassinets and cradles but with added requirements, including an additional performance requirement and test procedure for maximum allowable rocking and rest angles of the sleep surface, and maximum allowable flatness angle. Additional requirements are noted in Table 3.1.

The current proposed mandatory standard for bassinets and cradles excludes Moses baskets, which means they may not be covered by the final mandatory requirements. Consumers are not typically knowledgeable about the content of standards or incident data on consumer products. They are likely to presume that a nursery product, such as a Moses basket, is safe for use with their infant. Neonatal and obstetric nurses and pediatricians are an important source of information for parents of new babies. They can and must reinforce the notion that soft bedding is unsafe for babies.

Bath Seats or Rings

In 2005, it was estimated that approximately 42% of new mothers owned a baby bath seat (CPSC 2010b). Bath seats (also called "bath rings") are plastic devices used to support an infant during bathing. Bath seats are typically attached to the tub surface by suction cups. Most bath seats are recommended for children beginning at 6 months of age, the age at which the average infant can sit unsupported (Bukatko and Daehler 1992). The upper age limit for using a bath seat depends on the particular product (e.g., its size) and is normally stated on the packaging. However, it has been suggested that consumers cease using bath seats when a child reaches 8 or 9 months, the time at which an infant can pull to a stand, because infants who try to get out of the bath ring may be at risk for drowning (Rauchschwalbe, Brenner and Smith 1997). As such, the useful life of a bath seat is only a few months.

Although there are relatively minor injuries reported with bath seats (e.g., contusion, abrasion), drowning is the major hazard pattern associated with these products. From 2004 through 2007, more than a dozen bath seat fatalities were reported annually to the CPSC. In 2008 and 2009, there were a total of 13 deaths reported. It is important to know that fatality records for 2008 and 2009 are not yet complete, so it is likely that additional fatal incidents will come to light in the future. Victims ranged in age from 2 to 22 months. The mean age was approximately 8 months.

In nearly all of the drowning incidents reported to the Commission, a lapse in direct, adult supervision was noted. In most cases, the parent or caregiver reportedly had left the bathroom where the baby was being bathed. In many cases, the baby had been left in the bath seat with an older sibling in the tub. In those cases, the older sibling was between 2 and 4 years of age. Parents typically reported that they had left the bathroom for only a few minutes, to get a towel or to answer the phone. However, because drowning can occur in as little as 3 to 5 minutes and in as little as an inch of water (Rauchschwalbe, Brenner, and Smith 1997), even a few minutes away can prove fatal.

Researchers have suggested that some parents erroneously believe that children who can sit unassisted and pull themselves up will be capable of lifting their heads out of water or otherwise save themselves from drowning (O'Carroll, Alkon, and Weiss 1988; Pearn et al. 1979). However, as the incident data demonstrate, infants and toddlers are not necessarily capable of lifting their heads and chests out of the water, particularly when a bath seat is involved, because it may trap the baby's legs or chest.

Another erroneous belief apparently held by some parents is that an older child is capable of "watching" the infant in the tub (Jensen et al. 1992). In Rauchschwalbe, Brenner, and Smith's (1997) parental survey about bath seats, some respondents reported feeling more comfortable leaving a child unattended "for a moment in the bath" if the infant was contained in a bath seat or there was an older child present. However, as the data demonstrate, older siblings may not recognize the risk or be capable of responding to and rescuing a drowning baby (Thompson 2003).

Incident data demonstrate that older children cannot be relied on to protect an infant from drowning, even when the infant is situated in a bath seat. An incident in Laurel Bay, South Carolina, exemplifies this point. In this case, a 9-month-old girl drowned while in a bath seat and with her 2-year-old sister in the tub. The mother left the children unattended for an estimated 2 to 5 minutes. When she returned, the baby was outside of the bath seat and submerged in the water. It was not known how the baby got out of the bath seat. In another case in Rexburg, Idaho, a 5-month-old girl drowned after she was able to roll out of a bath sling/recliner seat. The victim's mother had left her in the tub with her 3-year-old sister for an estimated 1 to 2 minutes to retrieve items from another room.

Many incidents involving bath seats report that the child was found unresponsive in the water. In a number of these cases, the victim was found out of the bath seat. The incident report typically states that parents did not know how the child got out of the seat. In a few other cases, infants were found in the bath seat, slumped over with their faces in the water.

Reducing the likelihood of injuries and fatalities associated with bath rings requires effort by both consumers and manufacturers. Since December 6, 2010, manufacturers have had to comply with the mandatory safety standard for bath seats (16 CFR part 1215 2010). The standard incorporates the voluntary standard for bath seats and bath rings (ASTM F1967 2010d) with modifications for stricter requirements, such as a more stringent leg opening based on a modified torso probe more analogous to a baby in a wet environment, more realistic test conditions, and a larger warning label, effectively doubling the size of the previously required label.

Consumers are advised to purchase only bath seats that meet the new standard. This may mean passing up a used or handed-down bath ring. Furthermore, consumers are advised to follow the manufacturers' instructions for the appropriate uses for the product, including limitations for the types of tubs where the seat can be used. This is important because some bath seats cannot be safely installed in certain types of tubs. In 2005, a manufacturer recalled 250,000 bath seats after learning that the seats could break and tip over (causing the child to fall into the water) when installed in a nontraditional or sunken bathtub. According to the recall notice, these types of seats should not have been used with nontraditional bathtubs.

Most important, parents must maintain constant supervision when their baby is in the bath seat. Bath seats that look sturdy and securely mount to the tub give a false sense of security. Bath seats should never be trusted to keep a baby's head out of the water or to prevent a baby from submerging or climbing out of the seat. It is hard for parents to appreciate that their baby can drown in a product that is designed to keep the baby upright during bath time. The data are clear: leaving an infant in a bath seat for a few minutes, even when in the company of an older sibling, can be a fatal mistake.

Table 3.1. Regulations and Standards for Nursery Products

Nursery Product	Regulations and Standards	Year Originally Approved	Current Version Published	Key Provisions Relevant to Salient Hazards
Bassinets	ASTM F 2194	2002	2010	Tests for unintentional collapse
				Tests for tip-over
				Limits mattress thickness
				Limits space between mattress and sidewall
				Limits inter-slat spacing
				Limits corner post extensions
Bath seats	16CFR1215 (M)[1]	2010	2010	Tests for suction cup detachment from tub
				Tests for suction cup detachment from seat
				Limits size of leg openings
				Tests for stability
				Warns about drowning potential
Bedding (infant)	ASTM F 1917	1999	2008	Limits string lengths to minimize strangulation risk
				Tests bumper guards for attachment in all corners
				Warns about suffocation on pillows
				Warns about strangulation on wall hangings, sheets
Bed rails	ASTM F 2085	2001	2010	Tests for entrapment within bed rail
(portable toddler)				Tests for entrapment between bed rail and mattress
				Requires 9-inch minimum space between end of rail and end of mattress

(*continued on next page*)

Table 3.1. *(continued)*

Nursery Product	Regulations and Standards	Year Originally Approved	Current Version Published	Key Provisions Relevant to Salient Hazards
				Warns to not put infants in adult beds
Bouncy seats	ASTM F 2167	2001	2010	Requires waist and crotch restraint
				Tests for tip-over
				Tests for significant slippage on a surface
Carriers (hand-held)	ASTM F 2050	2000	2009	Tests for handle breakage or unlatching
				Tests for significant slippage on a surface
				Requires restraint system
Carriers (worn)	ASTM F 2236	2003	2009	Limits size of leg openings
				Tests for fasteners breaking or disengaging
				Tests for seam separation
				Tests for slippage of adjustable straps of >1 inch
				Must support test weight
Changing tables	ASTM F 2388	2004	2009	Tests structural integrity
				Tests for tip-over
				Tests that barrier minimizes fall risk
				Tests for entrapment
Chests and dressers	ASTM F 2057	2000	2009	Tests for stability/tip-over
				Requires tip-over restraints to be sold with product
				Warns about injuries from tip-over

(*continued on next page*)

Table 3.1. (*continued*)

Nursery Product	Regulations and Standards	Year Originally Approved	Current Version Published	Key Provisions Relevant to Salient Hazards
				Instructs on how to fill/open drawers
				Warns to not put TVs on top of dressers
Cribs (full size)	16CFR1219 (M)[2]	2011	2011	Defines dimensions of crib and mattress
				Limits inter-slat spacing
				Bans drop-side design
				Prescribes hardware; restricts use of wood screws
				Tests for head entrapment in cut-outs
				Tests for entrapment in gaps in mattress support
				Requires dynamic impact testing for mattress support system, side rails, slat strength
				Requires testing to simulate long-term shaking
				Minimizes potential for mis-assembly
Cribs (non-full size)	16CFR1220 (M)[3]	2011	2011	Defines dimensions of crib and mattress
				Limits inter-slat spacing
				Bans drop-side design
				Prescribes hardware; restricts use of wood screws
				Tests for head entrapment in cut-outs
				Tests for entrapment in gaps in mattress support

(*continued on next page*)

Table 3.1. *(continued)*

Nursery Product	Regulations and Standards	Year Originally Approved	Current Version Published	Key Provisions Relevant to Salient Hazards
				Requires dynamic impact testing for mattress support system, side rails, slat strength
				Requires testing to simulate long-term shaking
				Minimizes potential for misassembly
Cribs (full size)	ASTM F 1169 (M)	1988	2010	See entries for 16CFR1219
Cribs (non-full size)	ASTM F 406 (M)[4]	1977	2010	See entries for 16CFR1220
Crib corner posts	ASTM F 966	1990	2000[5]	Limits corner post extensions
Durable infant or toddler products	16CFR1130 (M)[6]	2010	2010	Requires manufacturers to:
				provide postage-paid consumer registration form;
				keep records of consumers who register; and
				permanently place on each product the manufacturer
				name, model number, contact information, and date of manufacture
Gates and enclosures	ASTM F 1004	1986	2009	Tests for entrapment in openings
				Tests for positional strangulation in openings
				Tests gate push-out force
				Prescribes gate height
High chairs	ASTM F 404	1975	2008	Requires waist and crotch restraint
				Limits size of leg openings
				Tests for unintentional tray detachment

(*continued on next page*)

Table 3.1. (*continued*)

Nursery Product	Regulations and Standards	Year Originally Approved	Current Version Published	Key Provisions Relevant to Salient Hazards
				Tests overall chair stability
				Tests overall chair integrity
				Warns that restraint must be used
				Warns that tray is not substitute for restraint
Play yards	ASTM F 406[7]	1977	2010	Tests for unintentional folding
				Tests for "V" formation on collapse
				Tests automatic latches/locking devices
				Tests for finger/button mesh-entrapment
				Tests for body entrapment in mesh-sided pens
				Limits length of attached cords/straps to 7.4 inches
				Tests for entrapment with accessory changing table/bassinet
				Limits size of loop formed by changing table restraint
Swings (infant)	ASTM F 2088	2001	2009	Requires waist and crotch restraint
				Limits incline angle to <5 degrees
				Tests for tip-over
				Tests for unintentional folding
				Tests for hardware detachment due to vibration
				Requires containment of electrolyte if battery leaks

(*continued on next page*)

Table 3.1. *(continued)*

Nursery Product	Regulations and Standards	Year Originally Approved	Current Version Published	Key Provisions Relevant to Salient Hazards
Strollers	ASTM F 833	1983	2010	Tests for adequate brake performance Tests for tip-over Tests for unintentional collapse/folding Requires waist and crotch restraint Tests for pinch/scissor/shear injury Tests for entrapment in leg openings

M = mandatory (otherwise, voluntary); ASTM = American Society for Testing and Materials; CFR = Code of Federal Regulations.

[1]Effective December 6, 2010; incorporates previous voluntary standard, ASTM F 1967-08a, with enhancements.

[2]16CFR1219 incorporates the original crib regulation, 16CFR1508, and ASTM F 1169-10.

[3]16CFR1220 incorporates the original non-full-size crib regulation, 16CFR1509, and ASTM F406-10a.

[4]Previously, non-full-size cribs were addressed in a separate standard, ASTM F 1822, originally published in 1988, withdrawn in 2006. They are now addressed in the same standard as Play Yards, ASTM F 406. The crib-related requirements of F 406 are incorporated into 16CFR1220.

[5]Withdrawn in 2009. Requirements are incorporated into other relevant standards.

[6]This is a registration rule affecting 18 categories of products, including every product in this table, except chests and dressers.

[7]The play yard-related requirements of this standard are excluded from 16CFR1220 and are still voluntary.

Carriers and Seats (Not Including Child Safety Seats)

Parents have a wide range of baby carriers and infant seats to choose from today. Some carriers are worn by the parent, as a front-carrier, backpack, or sling. Others are handheld carriers or bouncer seats that provide a place for the baby to sit independently from the parent. In 2008, a CPSC report estimated that more than 5000 injuries to children younger than 5 years were associated with infant seats (including bouncer seats) or carriers (Chowdhury, 2009).

Front and Back Carriers

For front and back carriers, most injuries were caused by falls that resulted when a defective component broke or separated. For example, a buckle or lock opened up, webbing or straps slipped open, or fabric ripped or detached. In most cases, the parent was able to catch the baby before she or he hit the ground and the child was not hurt. However, there were a few cases where the child sustained a head injury (e.g., skull fracture) as a result of falling from a carrier. Other incidents associated with front and back carriers include the infant slipping through a leg opening, pinching of the baby's skin by a plastic clip, and blood flow restriction in the leg hole of the carrier. There were no fatalities associated with front or back carriers between 2004 and 2009.

Since 2004, all of the recalls involving front and back infant carriers were for potential component failure. For example, in 2005, BabySwede recalled its Baby Bjorn carriers after learning that the back support buckle could detach from the shoulder straps, posing a fall hazard to the baby. At the time of the recall, the manufacturer had received 93 reports of the back support buckle detaching from the shoulder straps. No injuries were reported.

Other front and back carriers recalled since 2004 for component failures include the Playtex Hip Hammock (in 2005), Baby Trend Back Pack Carriers (in 2007), Beco Baby Butterfly Carriers (in 2008), Optave Action Baby Carriers (in 2008), and Regal Lager CYBEX Infant Carriers (in 2010).

Slings

Slings are carriers that are worn across the front of the caregiver. As was the case with front and back carriers, slings can and do detach as the result of component failure, posing a fall risk to the infant. Of the approximately 200 estimated sling-related injuries occurring in 2008, nearly all were associated with a fall, and many involved slings that had detached. Falls also occurred when the parent fell while wearing the sling. In some instances, the baby was injured after falling from a sling when a parent bent over.

Infant slings have been recalled in the last several years because of the risk of component breakage. For example, in 2005, a company called ZoloWear recalled its infant carriers/slings because of the potential breakage of stitching on the sling. Other slings recalled because of possible component failure since 2004 include Infantino SlingRider Infant Carriers (in 2007) and Ellaroo Ring Sling Baby Carriers (in 2008).

One of the most serious and potentially fatal risks posed by any infant carrier is positional asphyxiation. This hazard has been reported to occur in various types of baby seats and carriers, and occurs when the baby's air supply is restricted because of his or her position within the carrier. This hazard pattern typically affects the youngest infants, those younger than 6 months of age, although the hazard pattern also has been seen in somewhat older infants.

Six sling-related fatalities were reported between 2004 and 2009. In all cases, the baby was found nonresponsive by the parent after being in the sling for a period of time. In one case, a 3-month-old baby girl was being carried by her mother. She was found unconscious and not breathing after 10 minutes. In another case, a mother was attending a La Leche class at a church. Her 26-day-old son was in a cloth sling and breastfeeding. He stopped nursing, and the mother believed he was sleeping. Approximately 10 minutes later, she noticed that he was not breathing. The cause of death was asphyxiation.

In 2010, two companies recalled their baby slings because of concerns for positional asphyxiation. Infantino, LLC, announced a recall and free replacement program for its "SlingRider" and "Wendy Bellissimo" infant slings after learning of three fatalities in 2009 involving infants ranging from 6 days to 3 months of age. The CPSC advised consumers not to use these slings for infants aged less than 4 months because of a risk of suffocation. Sprout Stuff also recalled its baby slings in 2010 after a 10-day-old infant died.

The voluntary standard for carriers that are worn on the body, ASTM F2236, was last updated in 2009 (ASTM 2009e). In addition to requiring that carriers support a certain amount of weight, the standard also limits the size of leg openings in an effort to prevent babies from slipping through. The standard has requirements for components that are aimed at preventing fasteners from breaking or disengaging, seams from separating, and straps from slipping. Note that this standard specifically excludes slings. ASTM is currently developing a standard for slings.

To minimize the risk of injury with front and back carriers and slings, parents are advised to use carriers that are matched to the infant's size and weight. This is particularly important for slings, because the fatality data indicate that very young infants are at greater risk of suffocation because of positional asphyxiation when in a sling. Parents must monitor their baby while she or he is in a carrier to make sure that the head is not bent forward, restricting the airway in the neck, and that the nose and mouth are not blocked in a way that prevents the infant from breathing freely, because young infants cannot signal for help if in trouble. The condition of a carrier should be checked before use, including latches, straps, and buckles, to make sure they are not cracked or broken, they can hold securely, and they will not open easily or unexpectedly. Also, with back carriers, it is important to make sure that the baby is restrained and seated far enough down in the seat to reduce the likelihood that he or she will topple out.

Handheld Baby Carriers and Bouncer Seats

Handheld baby carriers and bouncer seats have also been associated with infant fall injuries. In 2008, there were an estimated 2200 injuries associated with infant bouncer seats and more than 1000 injuries associated with handheld baby carriers.

Falls were the primary cause of injuries for both handheld baby carriers and bouncers. For bouncer seats, 77% of injuries seen in U.S. emergency departments were fall-related.

Approximately half of those expressly mentioned that the baby or carrier fell from an elevated surface, such as a counter, washing machine, or chair. Many carrier falls also resulted when the carrier toppled off an elevated surface. Parents often place a baby in a carrier on an elevated surface where they are working (e.g., kitchen table, counter, dining room table, washing machine) to stay engaged with the baby while doing chores. A combination of factors, namely, the bouncing or rocking feature of the seat, the baby's movements, and the placement on an elevated surface, come together to pose a very serious fall risk that typically results in injuries to the head and face, as well as to the rest of the body. Babies who are secured in restraints may flip off of an elevated surface with the seat. Unrestrained babies may be ejected out of the seat and onto the floor.

Other falls associated with handheld carriers and bouncer seats resulted from the seat tipping or coming apart, or the parent falling or tripping while holding the baby in the seat. In some cases, the parent and baby fell down stairs.

Although falls from bouncer seats and handheld carriers can lead to serious injuries, fatalities are rare. Fatalities are more likely to occur if the baby's airway is compromised. From 2004 to 2009, there were six fatalities reported in bouncer seats. In all cases, the babies were found unresponsive in the seats. Several cases specifically mentioned that the death was due to positional asphyxiation. This is what happened in the case of a 4-month-old baby girl who was found slumped over to the side of her bouncer seat after having been put in the seat for a nap.

Two additional fatalities were reported between 2004 and 2009 that resulted when the babies became suspended over the side of the seat. One case involved a 2-month-old baby girl from Spokane, Washington, who was found suspended over the side of a bouncer chair in which she was sleeping. The infant was strapped into the seat. Another fatality involved a 3-month-old baby who had been put to sleep on his back, but apparently rolled over and pushed his way to the top of the seat where his head fell over the top.

Two other potentially fatal hazards that did not show up in the 2004–2009 data are (1) strap entanglement and (2) overturn of the carrier on plush surfaces. An infant who becomes entangled in restraint straps can strangle as the result of the straps being too loose on the body and the baby's movement in the carrier while sleeping or trying to get out of the carrier. Also, a carrier that is placed on a soft or plush surface, such as a bed or couch, is at risk of overturning. If the seat overturns and the baby lands face-down on a plush surface, she or he can suffocate because of limited air flow (Pollack-Nelson 2000). Some parents place infant seats and carriers on plush surfaces, such as beds or waterbeds, under the mistaken impression that such surfaces provide a soft landing in the event that the seat overturns.

Voluntary standards for handheld carriers and bouncer seats have incorporated design and testing requirements aimed at addressing hazards such as strap entanglement, falls from carriers, and overturn. For example, the bouncer seat standard, ASTM F2167 (ASTM 2010f), which was last updated in 2010, requires waist and crotch restraints to help retain the baby securely in the seat. The standard also has provisions that minimize the risk of tip-over and prevent significant slippage on a surface. These aspects of the standard are intended to reduce the likelihood of a bouncer seat overturning or falling, particularly from an elevated surface.

The ASTM standard for handheld carriers, ASTM F2050 (ASTM 2009c), was last updated in 2009. This standard also has requirements that are intended to prevent significant slippage on a surface. In addition, the standard has requirements for handles to prevent them from breaking or unlatching.

Parents are urged to purchase only handheld infant carriers and bouncer seats that comply with voluntary standards. However, even a carrier that complies can still present a risk to a baby. Carriers should not be placed on elevated surfaces, because they can fall off simply because of the child's own activity while in the seat. Parents must be vigilant in securing provided waist and crotch restraints, per the manufacturers' instructions. Parents must pay close attention to the baby's position in the carrier or bouncer seat to ensure that the airway is clear and the baby is breathing. Also, blankets and pillows should not be used to snuggle a baby in a carrier, because these can impede breathing.

Changing Tables and Dressers

A changing table is a basic nursery accessory found in many homes with infants. These products can be used from birth to approximately 3 years, depending on the weight specifications of the particular product. Stand-alone changing tables typically consist of three levels with the changing table on top and storage shelves below. These products typically have a guard rail around the perimeter of the changing table to help contain the baby. Some changing tables are built onto the top of a dresser. These may or may not have a guard rail around the perimeter. Sometimes changing tables are incorporated as accessories on play yards. See the section "Play Yards (Playpens)" in this chapter for injury and fatality data and recalls relating to such accessory changing tables.

In 2008, there were an estimated 3282 changing table injuries nationwide. This number is substantially higher than the national estimate in 2003, which was 1800, but approximately the same as the estimate in 2000 (3170). These estimates are still relatively small and subject to greater variation than estimates based on larger absolute numbers. Thus, care must be taken to not necessarily interpret the fluctuations as statistically significant.

A fall is the predominant hazard pattern associated with changing tables, representing 94% of estimated injuries in 2008. Most of these falls occurred when the child tumbled off of the table and onto the floor. In some cases, this happened when the parent left the baby's side, even if only momentarily (e.g., to get a diaper). In other cases, the fall occurred when the infant or toddler suddenly squirmed away from the parent's control. Using a safety restraint can lessen the chances of a fall. However, even when straps are in use, parents must attend to their child closely, because straps may not adequately restrain the child and may pose an entanglement and strangulation hazard.

Aside from falls resulting from an active or unattended baby, falls can also occur if the changing table is defective and breaks. Between 2004 and 2008, the CPSC investigated a number of incidents that resulted when a changing table broke. In one case, a 15-month-old was standing on a changing table and fell to the second level of the table when the top level he was on folded. There were no injuries in that incident. In another case, a 2-month-old boy was having his diaper changed by his mother on a changing table that was attached to a bassinet when the changing table collapsed. This caused his head to roll and strike part of the changing table. In these cases, the close proximity and attention of parents prevented any serious consequence.

Recalls of changing tables since 2004 have all been because of concern for failure that could lead to a fall. For example, in 2006, Scandinavian Child recalled its Cariboo Folding Changing Tables and Cariboo Bassinet Changers because the cloth surface could come apart, posing a fall hazard to the baby. In 2010, Child Craft reissued an older (2001) recall notice for changing tables that may have had joints that were not properly glued and could separate, presenting a fall hazard to babies.

Although falls accounted for the majority of incidents reported with changing tables, there were also reports of limb and finger entrapment. Entrapment of limbs can occur between the side rails of a changing table. Most do not lead to serious injury. However, there is one report of a 2-month-old girl who had a fractured leg after her foot became entrapped several times between the slats of a decorative railing surrounding a baby changing table.

There have been two fatalities associated with changing tables that are part of a play yard between 2004 and 2009. In one case, a 7-week-old girl asphyxiated after being put to sleep on the changing table that was attached to the top of her play yard. Within a few hours, the baby was discovered face-down and unresponsive in a V-shaped form in the changing table. Another fatality involved a 2-month-old girl who was sleeping in the changing table portion of portable play yard. She was found unresponsive and face down in the changing table with her face pushed against one of the ends of the table.

The CPSC will be reviewing the ASTM standard for changing tables, ASTM F2388 (ASTM 2009f), as part of its responsibility under the CPSIA. In the future, the CPSC will issue a mandatory standard for changing tables that could be more stringent than the current industry standard.

Dressers are often incorporated into a nursery as a stand-alone product, or in many cases, with a changing table on top. What may be surprising is that dressers are associated with thousands of childhood injuries each year and a number of deaths. In 2008, the CPSC estimated that there were more than 17,000 such injuries to children younger than 5 years. Two thirds of these injuries resulted when the child ran into the dresser and struck his or her head or other body part. In some cases, the child was jumping on the bed and struck the dresser after falling off the bed. Most injuries associated with impacting a dresser are relatively minor (contusions or lacerations), but head injuries can also occur.

The next most frequently reported hazard pattern, associated with approximately 21% of injuries, involved the dresser or television being pulled down on top of the child. This typically occurs when a child is climbing on the dresser or its drawers. Children are avid climbers and can be highly motivated to seek out objects placed on top of a dresser.

Dresser tip-over often leads to severe injuries and has resulted in death in many cases. Between 2004 and 2009, 55 dresser-related deaths were reported to the CPSC. Many more incidents resulted in hospitalization of the child. Most of the fatalities involved a child being crushed by a fallen dresser or television. Victims ranged in age from 8 months to 4 years. Tip-over typically resulted when infants and young children pulled to a standing position using the dresser or when older children climbed on the dresser. For example, an 8-month-old boy in Columbia, South Carolina, died after he crawled to a dresser and attempted to pull himself up. The dresser tipped forward, and the television toppled off onto the child's face.

When older children are involved in dresser or television tip-over incidents, it is usually the result of climbing on the dresser in an effort to get to something on top (e.g., a video or television). The instability caused by their climbing can cause the dresser or television to topple over and kill them. For example, a 3-year-old from Mazomanie, Wisconsin, was climbing on a dresser to reach a DVD player that was on top of a television. The television tipped off the dresser and landed on her head. In another fatal incident, a 2-year-old opened the lower dresser drawer and stood on it in an effort to reach the top drawer where her pajamas were. Her mother, in a nearby bathroom, heard a loud noise and discovered that a 26-inch television had fallen from the dresser onto her child.

Dresser and television-related crush injuries and deaths have been studied by the CPSC (Gipson 2009) and covered in the news media and medical literature. In 2009, the Center for Injury Research and Policy at Nationwide Children's Hospital found that from 2000 to 2007, there was a more than 40% increase in the number of injuries resulting from tip-over (Gottesman et al. 2009). Most incidents resulted from a television on a dresser tipping over onto the child.

To stem the hazard, the voluntary standard (ASTM F2057) (ASTM 2009d) requires manufacturers to include a tip restraint with each chest, door chest, and dresser taller than 30 inches. The tip restraint allows the dresser to be attached to the wall, and this should prevent it from overturning if a young child climbs on the drawers or dresser. Parents are advised to use these restraints to anchor dressers that are situated in children's rooms or rooms of the home where children play. Tip restraints will not necessarily prevent a television or other objects that are positioned on top of the dresser from falling over. To inhibit children from climbing on furniture that might result in tip-over, parents are advised to install drawer stops on children's furniture and not to place items that are attractive to children, such as toys or the remote control, on top of a dresser.

The second most prevalent fatal hazard pattern associated with dressers is entrapment and wedging between the dresser and another object in the room. Six such incidents (11% of the fatalities) occurred between 2004 and 2009. The victims ranged in age from 6 to 14 months. The hazard pattern typically resulted when an infant had been placed on a bed and rolled off the bed, becoming wedged between the bed (or mattress) and an adjacent dresser. Parents may not recognize that even young infants can scoot and move around, and this puts them at risk of falling off the bed and possibly becoming wedged. Infants should sleep in a crib or bassinet, not an adult bed.

Since 2004, there have been three dresser recalls—some children's dressers, others not. None of these recalls relate to the hazard patterns identified in the incident data, but they are relevant nonetheless. In 2006, Hold Everything recalled plastic hardware covers that were easily removable and could present a choking hazard to young children. Also in 2006, The Land of Nod recalled Antique White Furniture from its Cottage Collection because of the presence of lead paint. In 2008, IKEA recalled its KVIBY chests after learning that the glass drawer knobs on the chest could break during assembly or use, posing a laceration hazard.

Cribs

Cribs constitute the sleeping environment for infants and young children, usually to approximately 3 years of age. Cribs are approximately 28 × 52 inches, with a rail height of approximately 26 inches when measured from the top of the rail in its highest position to the top of the mattress support in its lowest position. Mattresses should not exceed 6 inches in thickness.

There were an estimated 11,500 crib/mattress-related injuries treated in emergency departments in 2008. Most of the incidents involved children aged 12 to 23 months. Contusions, abrasions, and internal injuries associated with climbing or falling out of the crib were the most frequent injuries represented in the data, and most of these injuries affected the head and face.

In the 3-year period from 2004 to 2006, there were at least 93 deaths involving cribs and another 153 deaths from November 2007 to July 2010. A frequent cause was entrapment, primarily between the mattress and the side rail, but also between slats when slat failure occurred. Many deaths involved bedding (pillows, blankets, quilts, comforters, sheets).

The types of hazards to which children are most susceptible relate to their phase of physical and cognitive development. Young infants, until approximately 5 or 6 months of age, who do not have well-developed muscle and movement control, are at highest risk for crib-related suffocation deaths simply because they cannot move out of harm's way by themselves. Their heads are relatively larger than at any other age and the neck muscles are weaker. The smaller bifrontal diameter (compared with the bitemporal diameter) gives the head a wedge shape and makes it more likely to fit into a small space and remain entrapped.

At this age, infants cannot move away from pillows or soft bedding, which are frequent culprits in mechanical suffocation. In crib fatalities involving bedding, infants were primarily found face-down in pillows, quilts, or blankets. As with bassinets/cradles, it seems that the message about the hazard of soft bedding, especially pillows, needs to be made more effectively. Also, several crib deaths that may in fact be mechanical suffocations get classified as SIDS. These two mechanisms of death essentially present identically at autopsy. Efforts need to be focused on on-site investigation and reenactment of such deaths to minimize the likelihood that they will be erroneously classified as SIDS.

As infants get older and more mobile, injuries associated with entrapment and climbing out of the crib become more common than suffocation. Entrapment can result in asphyxia from compression, strangulation, or hanging; falls can result in head injury, bruises, and fractures. Entrapment incidents reported in the injury and fatality data typically mentioned that hardware (drop-side tracks and hardware, side rail bolts, and mattress supports) was missing or loose, allowing a larger than normal space to be created between the frame and the mattress. Of approximately 1200 crib-related incidents reported to the CPSC between 2004 and 2009, hardware or structural failure was noted in approximately 45%. For example, one report stated that the crib's side rail snapped off from the frame when a 15-month-old girl was jumping in the crib; another stated an 8-month-old boy died from entrapment when the side of his crib detached as the spring-loaded safety pegs failed; and another reported that after hearing a loud pop, a grandparent found that several slats had detached from a crib and fallen to the floor while his 5-month-old grandson slept. The most important thing parents can do is to check their cribs regularly for integrity. All sides must be firmly connected, and the mattress supports should all be intact.

An unusual entrapment scenario involved a product called a "crib tent," manufactured by Tots in Mind. The product is a dome-shaped enclosure intended to be attached to the crib to prevent a child from getting out on his own. The dome shape is held in place by crisscrossing tension rods. In 2007, a 23-month-old became entrapped between the crib rail and a tension rod of the crib tent after the dome suddenly and forcefully inverted. The child was permanently disabled as the result of asphyxia. Tots in Mind made similar products for play yards. Those tents were recalled because of a different entrapment hazard, but apparently the recall did not include the crib tent. Refer to the "Play Yards (Playpens)" section of this chapter for injury, fatality, and recall information related to the use of tents with these products.

Whenever a crib's structural integrity is compromised, there is the potential for a hazardous gap to be created in which a child can become entrapped and asphyxiate. Drop-side cribs have taken center stage as the most hazardous cribs on the market because of the numerous incidents involving hardware failure. As a result of such failures, the drop side can pull away from the frame, creating an entrapping gap, or the drop side can suddenly and unexpectedly release, leading to falls from the crib.

An astounding approximately 5 million drop-side cribs were recalled between November 2007 and December 2009 because of hardware failure. By June 2010, the CPSC had issued 40 recalls of more than 11 million cribs (all types) for product defects, not for violation of the crib standard.

A few recalls were related to violations of the standard. For example, in 2005, Pottery Barn recalled Spindle cribs because the spindles could detach, creating an entrapment space. In 2006, Orbelle Trade, Inc., recalled cribs because the space between the mattress and the side rail was larger than the standards allowed. In addition, the cribs were missing instructions and warnings. In 2008, Baby Appleseed and Mother Hubbard's Cupboards recalled cribs whose mattress support system for the lowest mattress position did not provide the full 26 inches required height to the rail. Children could therefore fall out of the crib.

There have been mandatory standards in place for full-size cribs (16 CFR part 1508 1973) and non-full-size cribs (16 CFR part 1509 1976) since the 1970s. The standards set requirements for side rail height, slat spacing, type of hardware, locking drop-sides, surface finishing, mattress size and thickness, and assembly instructions. In 1982, the Commission amended the rules to address the hazard of head and neck entrapment in head/footboard cutouts. The new amendment included a test where a "headform" probe is placed in any partially bounded opening along the upper edges of the crib end or side panel, and then rotated to evaluate the potential for entrapment.

In 1988, the ASTM voluntary standard supplemented the mandatory federal requirements for cribs by including requirements for mattress supports, glued or bolted connections, drop-side latches, and specifications to prevent dislodgement of teething rails (ASTM F1169 for full-size cribs) (ASTM 2010c). At the same time, similar hazards were addressed for non-full-size cribs in ASTM F1822 (ASTM 1988). One particular test incorporated (from the Canadian Standard) into the 2010 version of the voluntary full-size crib standard was a test to simulate lifetime shaking of the crib. There has been no test that simulates the effect on the crib of years of jumping and tugging by a child. Cribs endure a lot of stress, especially when they are used for multiple children. This kind of testing should go a long way toward ensuring crib integrity, which is so essential to crib safety.

The hazard presented by tall finials was addressed by another ASTM standard in 1990, ASTM F966 (ASTM 2000). Tall finials (corner posts) acted as clothing or necklace catch points. When children attempted to climb out of a crib or lean over a finial, their loose clothing or necklace would catch on the finial, creating a noose that strangled them. The standard limited the height of any finial to 0.06 inches above the upper edge of an end or side panel, unless the corner post extended 16 inches above the uppermost surface of the side rail in its highest position. Although the ASTM F966 standard was withdrawn in 2009, its essence has been incorporated directly into other standards, where relevant.

This long history of mandatory rules and voluntary standards has come to an end. Under its new regulatory responsibilities under the CPSIA, the CPSC has promulgated new mandatory standards for full-size cribs (codified at 16 CFR part 1219) and non-full-size cribs (codified at 16 CFR part 1220), effective June 28, 2011. These new standards incorporate the original mandatory regulations and incorporate by reference the requirements of the respective voluntary standards (ASTM F406 2010a; ASTM F1169 2010c). The new mandatory standard will be the agency's first across-the-board overhaul of regulations for infant beds in almost three decades. At the same time, the CPSC is revoking the original mandatory crib standards at 16 CFR parts 1508 and 1509 to eliminate confusion and to allow all crib-related requirements to be together. In addition, the regulation will be strengthened by new requirements to more effectively address the hazards, in particular entrapment, evidenced in the data (Table 3.1).

No doubt the recent problems with drop-side cribs fueled one of the major changes. Drop-side cribs have been popular because they allow convenient access to the baby. Apparently the shift away from traditional wood-and-metal construction to cheaper, plastic hardware and fittings is responsible for drop-side parts wearing down and failing. In its new regulations, the CPSC essentially bans this design by requiring that crib sides be fixed in place and have no movable segments less than 20 inches from the top surface of the mattress.

A second major change is that the new regulations apply not only to manufacturers, distributors, and retailers, but also to owners and operators of child-care facilities, including in-home child care, and public accommodations, such as hotels and motels. This means that it will be unlawful to sell, lease, or otherwise provide a crib that does not meet the standard. Although the effective compliance date for manufacturers, retailers, and distributors is June 28, 2011, the effective compliance date for this additional group of child care entities is December 28, 2012.

Although there is no change to the original slat spacing requirements in the new standards, it is interesting that among the 1200 crib-related reported incidents there were more than 300 cases of children getting legs—mostly knees and thighs—trapped between slats. Most resulted in bruises, but there were occasional fractures. In some cases, slats had to be sawed to free the child. Maximum slat spacing allowed is 2.375 inches. Average knee breadth for 2-year-olds, the youngest age for which data were available, was reported as 2.44 inches (Steenbekkers 1993) and 2.48 inches (Snyder et al. 1977), but the third and fifth percentiles from the respective studies were 2.2 inches and 2.12 inches, so some portion of the user population is at risk. The Commission recognizes this issue, but believes that this hazard cannot be adequately addressed by changes in slat spacing because making the space smaller will still place some infants at risk, and making the space larger is not acceptable.

Because bedding has been involved in sleep-related suffocation and strangulation incidents, the ASTM published a standard for infant bedding and related accessories (ASTM F1917) originally in 1999, with a current version published in 2008 (ASTM 2008b). The standard addresses strangulation hazards presented by decorative ribbons, bumper guard ties, wall hangings, fitted sheets, and unraveling threads. For example, it limits string length to 7 inches, except for strings on bumper and headboard guards, which are limited to 9 inches. The 7-inch limit is based on the neck circumference of a fifth percentile 0- to 3-month-old (7.2 inches). The 9-inch allowance for bumper and headboard guards ensures that these products can be tied securely to crib rails. The standard also has labeling requirements for infant bedding items. Decorative pillows are required to carry a label informing of the suffocation potential and advising against the use of a pillow in the crib. Fitted crib sheets must be labeled to remind users that the sheet must fit securely to avoid entanglement or strangulation.

Gates, Enclosures, and Bed Rails

Gates, enclosures, and bed rails are devices used to contain a child in a given space. Gates serve as barriers intended to be installed in an opening such as a doorway to keep young children out of certain areas. A common use for gates is to block the top of stairs. Enclosures are self-supporting barriers intended to completely surround an area and create a space where the child can be placed to play, for example. Gates and enclosures are typically used for children aged 6 to 24 months. Bed rails are intended to be installed on adult beds as a means of preventing a child from rolling off the bed and onto the floor. Because it is not advisable to place a child younger than 2 years in an adult bed, bed rails are intended for use with children aged 2 to 5 years, that is, children who can get in and out of bed without assistance.

Most of the 2230 estimated emergency department-treated injuries in 2008 associated with gates and enclosures were sustained by children 8 months to 2 years old, corresponding to the primary intended users' ages. Most of the injuries were contusions, abrasions, lacerations, or internal injury to the head. At the time of injury, children fell into the gate, fell while climbing the gate, or pushed/pulled the gate down. In an estimated 335 cases, the child and the gate fell down stairs. In some cases, children were able to defeat latches or bypass the gate altogether.

Four deaths associated with baby gates were reported in the 6-year period from 2004 to 2009. In one case, which was deemed negligent care of a child, a baby gate had been placed on top of a play yard as a barrier to prevent a 16-month-old from climbing out. Heavy containers were then placed on top of the baby gate. The toddler got trapped between the gate and the play yard and asphyxiated. In two cases, 2-year-olds were able to bypass baby gates and reach a pool and pond, respectively, and drown. In the fourth case, the baby gate was being used to cover a window. A 12-month-old girl was able to get between the gate and the window frame and fell three stories to her death. Although the first death described is a clear example of child abuse, the other deaths suggest that a gate was used appropriately in the sense that it was "erected as a barrier in an opening" just as the standard defines the intended use. However, the choice of a baby gate to prevent access to pools, ponds, and open windows is not recommended. Other, more permanent, barriers would be more appropriate for such openings. For example, doors with alarms and fencing are more reliable than a baby gate for preventing access to backyard water, and window fall prevention guards are specifically designed to minimize access to open windows.

Since 2004, two brands of gates have been recalled because of concerns for component failure. Safety 1st gates were recalled in 2009 for hinge failure that could create a fall hazard. In March 2010, Evenflo recalled gates because of slats breaking or detaching, again, creating a fall hazard.

Historically, head entrapment in diamond- and V-shaped openings of accordion-style gates or enclosures was the major hazard. Head entrapment after a foot-first entry was also reported in the injury data. In 1986, the ASTM published a voluntary standard, ASTM F1004 (ASTM 1986), for expansion gates and expandable enclosures, to address head entrapment and the ability of the gate to resist "push-out" force exerted by a child. For example, the voluntary standard limits the size of completely bounded openings to essentially less than 3 × 5.5 inches (the size of a small child's torso) to prevent entrapment. The standard was updated in 2009 (ASTM 2009a).

The standard has been effective in eliminating entrapment deaths, yet it does not appear to limit the potential for children to climb up and over gates (other than requirements pertaining to forces necessary to dislodge gates). Most toddlers have a natural inclination to climb. Climbing is a skill that most children develop before 2 years of age. A gate is a natural challenge to this budding motor skill, so it is foreseeable that children would attempt to scale a barrier. Openings in gates could function as foot/hand holds for climbing. The fifth percentile foot breadth of 13- to 18-month-olds was reported as 1.57 inches; the 95th percentile foot breadth of 19- to 24-month-olds was reported as 2.36 inches (Snyder et al. 1975). Eliminating the potential for climbing on gates could reduce gate-related injuries by up to approximately 20%.

With regard to bed rails, an estimated 3000 young children were treated in emergency departments in 2008, primarily for lacerations and bruises associated with bumping, falling into, or running into the rails. Many of these children were younger than 2 years, and inasmuch are younger than the intended age of bed rail users. The most serious hazard pattern associated with bed rails is entrapment. From 2004 to 2009, at least 20 infants died after becoming entrapped in bed rails or between the bed rail and the bed or bedding. Almost all (19) were aged less than 2 years, including 16 who were younger than 1 year—again, too young for this type of product.

ASTM F2085 (ASTM 2010e), a voluntary standard for bed rails, addresses entrapment potential, including entrapment between bed rail components and between the bed rail and where it attaches to a mattress. It also addresses entrapment between the ends of the bed rail and the ends of the bed. On the basis of the injury and fatality data, the current standard evaluates entrapment potential using a probe that simulates children as young as 3 months old. However, when the standard was first published in 2001, there were no performance requirements for openings that could pose potential entrapment areas. Therefore, a possible explanation for the deaths reported is that the bed rails were made before 2003, the year the standard included a test procedure for entrapment of young children. It is also possible that the bed rails involved in the fatal incidents were not fully or properly attached to the bed or were used on a bunk bed or other type of bed for which bed rails are not recommended. There were no bed rail recalls between 2004 and 2009.

High Chairs

High chairs are freestanding chairs that elevate the child to a standard dining table height to facilitate eating or feeding. They are intended for infants who can sit up unassisted, which is usually at approximately 8 to 9 months of age, until 3 years of age.

There were an estimated 7976 emergency department-treated injuries associated with high chairs in 2008, and an additional 2300 injuries associated with attachable high chairs. Most high chair injuries involved children aged 2 years and less, and occurred when the child fell out of the chair (68%) or the child and chair tipped (14%). The head and face were most often injured, suggesting the fall was head-first. Few injuries required hospitalization. Injuries associated with attachable chairs were similar in pattern and injury site. Children primarily fell out (80%) or the child pushed off from the table to which the chair was attached, falling backward along with the chair (15%). Head and face injuries were most common. Only one child was reportedly hospitalized, and that was for a skull fracture.

The other databases showed similar hazard patterns, including incidents where a child was able to undo the restraint or kick off or unlatch the tray. Multi-position chairs showed some unique hazard patterns, including sudden collapse, and structural failure. Arm entrapment between the seat and leg frame was also reported. This hazard is understandable if one looks at current styles of stand-alone high chairs. Many appear to sit on "A"-frame legs, rather than the "traditional or old fashioned" four separate legged chairs.

Six deaths involving stand-alone high chairs were reported to the CPSC between 2004 and 2009. Cause of death was asphyxia by entrapment in three cases (12 months, 14 months, and 3 years old), strangulation by the restraint in one case (18 months old), strangulation by clothing catching on the chair in one case (13 months old), and head trauma from falling backward with the chair in one case (2 years old). No deaths were associated with attachable chairs. One death was associated with a booster. In that case, a father strapped a 7-month-old baby into the booster seat and set it in the bath tub. When he left her unattended for a few minutes, the seat overturned, and she drowned.

Historically, high chair injuries occurred when children fell out of the chair, and deaths occurred when children slipped under the tray table and either were strangled by the safety belt or suffered compression asphyxia by the tray. Falls were associated with children not being strapped into the chair and with product tip-over. Children who were able to stand on the chair seat could fall over a side. Head and face injuries were most common.

In 1975, the first ASTM standard for high chairs was published, ASTM F404. The current version of this standard was published in 2008 (ASTM 2008a). Two key portions of the standard address restraints and tray performance. A restraint system must be provided and must include a waist and crotch restraint, designed such that the crotch restraint's use is mandatory when the restraint is in use. Leg openings must not be large enough to allow passage of a baby's lower torso. The standard also states that tray latch releases should not be accessible to the child's feet (or else the child might inadvertently contact the latch, causing the tray to fall) or even be visible to the child. The tray must not become disengaged from its original position when subjected to horizontal and vertical pull tests. The standard also tests for chair stability, simulating situations with a seated and climbing child.

According to the primary pattern of injuries reported in this chapter, one can only conclude that restraints were not used or were not effective in these incidents. Despite the ASTM standard's requirement that the chair carry a warning advising consumers that the tray table is not designed to hold the child in the chair, it is understandable that consumers might hold the misconception that the tray table acts as a barrier to the child's getting out, and thus the restraint is unnecessary. This belief, along with the time and inconvenience associated with fastening the restraint, may cause some consumers not to secure a child in a high chair restraint.

Further, although the ASTM standard requires restraint system retention testing of a high chair that includes horizontal and vertical pull tests on a restrained test dummy that simulates the weight, proportions, and center of gravity of a young child, the actual motion of a child struggling to get out of the chair might be different. As a result, a high chair may pass the ASTM restraint test; however, a child who is squirming or attempting to exit the high chair might successfully defeat the restraint.

The voluntary standard does not address hanging by clothing while attempting to climb out. As noted earlier, this hazard pattern was the cause of the death of a 13-month-old in recent years. Catch points and protrusions that present hanging hazards are addressed in many other standards that cover children's safety issues. The CPSC should ensure that this hazard is adequately addressed when it considers adopting the ASTM high chair standard as a mandatory regulation.

There were a number of high chair recalls from 2005 to 2010, all related to a fall hazard associated with structural failures. In 2005, Cosco reissued a recall of "Options 5" high chairs because of concerns that the seats could separate from the frame and fall to the floor or suddenly collapse. In 2007, Graco also reissued an earlier recall that involved Contempo high chairs with a collapse hazard.

In 2008 and 2009, Evenflo recalled its Majestic and Environ high chairs because of the potential for hardware on both sides of the chair to loosen and fall out, causing the back of the seat to suddenly fall back or detach. The loose caps and screws posed an additional choking hazard.

Fisher-Price and IKEA also recalled high chairs in 2009. Fisher-Price recalled its 3-in-1 High Chair to Booster because of concerns about seat collapse. IKEA recalled its LEOPARD high chairs because the snap locks used to secure the seat to the frame could break, allowing the seat and child to drop through the frame. The loose snap locks posed an additional choking hazard.

Most recently, in 2010, Graco recalled approximately 1.2 million high chairs because the screws holding the front legs could loosen and fall out or the plastic bracket on the rear leg could crack, causing the chair to become unstable and tip over unexpectedly. The frequency with which high chairs are recalled underscores the importance of parents checking their children's high chairs before use and being on the lookout for component defects or failures.

Infant Swings (Portable Baby Swings for Home Use)

Infant swings are used to calm a crying baby and to otherwise free up a caregiver's hands. Some infant swings are configured as a baby seat between two sets of tall legs. Others are portable, floor-type swings. These consist of a baby seat between shorter legs and with a carrying handle.

In 2008, the CPSC estimated that there were approximately 1600 infant swing injuries nationwide that year. Approximately three quarters of those resulted from the baby falling out of the swing. In some cases, the fall was precipitated by the action of an older sibling, typically a preschooler. For example, falls associated with swings resulted when older siblings tried to remove a baby from an infant swing or while interacting with the baby in such a way that it caused the baby and swing to fall over. For example, a 2-month-old baby's head was contused when her 2-year-old sibling pulled the baby out of the swing. The swing fell with the baby in it. In other cases, the fall was due to component failure that caused the swing to come apart or the infant to fall to the ground. In Sharon, Pennsylvania, a parent reported that a 1-month-old baby girl fell to the ground when the bar that connects the swing's legs became detached.

Another hazard pattern noted in the data involved the baby being restrained in a swing, but found hanging upside down. In Tallahassee, Florida, a 6-month-old boy was found swinging upside down from the waist in an infant swing and gasping for air. The metal latch on the lower back of the seat had unlocked by itself, causing the seat to tip over. In Somerset, New Jersey, parents found their 3-month-old boy with his head to the floor and his body still strapped into the swing. No injury was reported in these incidents. However, other incidents have resulted in harm to the baby. A 7-month-old boy from McDonough, Georgia, was found hanging upside down with his face down on the hardwood floor during infant swing use. He received a bump on his forehead and suffered a mild concussion.

Another hazard pattern reported with infant swings stems from the baby's hand or head striking the legs if the baby leans to one side. One parent reported that a 2-month-old boy leaned over to the side, striking his head on the swing's side legs. He received a bruise to the head. Other parents have reported entrapment in the seat components. For example, a 4-month-old baby girl in Dalmatia, Pennsylvania, reportedly got her head stuck on one side of a baby swing, receiving a bruise to her temple. A similar incident was reported in Inwood, West Virginia, where a 5-month-old baby girl's head got trapped between the swing's side rail and the back of the swing.

Infant fatalities have also been reported in baby swings. From 2004 to 2009, there were 13 baby swing deaths reported to the CPSC. Victims ranged in age from two-weeks to 10-months; all but two victims were six-months old or younger. In eight incidents, it was stated that the baby died of positional asphyxiation or was found unresponsive in the seat. This hazard pattern results from a combination of the swing's movement and movements of the baby that cause the baby's position to shift from how he or she was originally placed in the swing. This shift can prove fatal if the baby's head bends forward in such a way that the chin rests on the chest, causing airway impairment. Because parents may not remain with the baby the entire time he or she is in the swing, particularly once the baby falls asleep, the parent may not be aware of the danger.

The remaining fatalities were due to the following circumstances: a swing folding up on the baby; the baby falling from the swing and landing in a prone position on a futon; the swing falling over when twin babies were placed inside and one baby landing on top of the other; a baby falling out of a swing and onto a bed; and a house fire.

Since 2004, there have been two recalls of floor-mounted, portable infant swings. In 2007, the Fisher-Price Rainforest swing was recalled because of concern that infants can shift to one side of the swing and become caught between the frame and the seat, posing an entrapment hazard and causing minor injuries (e.g., bruising, redness to the skin). In 2004, Graco recalled their Travel-Lite swing after learning that the swing's carrying handle could fail to stay in place properly and drop or be pushed down, hitting a child in the head. In addition, the three-point seatbelt could fail to prevent a child from leaning forward or to either side, posing a risk that the child could fall forward and strike his or her head on the floor or the swing's frame. At the time of the recall, Graco had received approximately 28 reports of incidents involving the handle falling down on young children and approximately 100 reports of children falling forward or to the side. Injuries resulting from these incidents included bloody or swollen lips, red marks, bumps, and bruises.

In 2009, Amby Baby USA recalled their Baby Motion Beds. These hammock-like products are not exactly swings, but might be used similarly. The Amby Motion beds were recalled because the side-to-side shifting or tilting of the hammock could cause the infant to roll and become entrapped or wedged against the hammock's fabric or mattress pad, resulting in a suffocation hazard. The manufacturer was aware of two infant suffocation deaths involving a 4-month-old girl and a 5-month-old boy in the Amby Baby hammock.

The ASTM Standard F2088 (2009b), originally drafted in 2001 and updated in 2009, addresses hazards associated with infant swings, such as tip-over, unintentional folding, and hardware detachment caused by vibration.

Play Yards (Playpens)

Portable play yards (or playpens) are enclosures intended to provide a sleep or play environment for children who are shorter than 35 inches in height, that is, essentially the same age child for whom a crib is intended. Play yards often incorporate accessories, such as bassinets or changing tables, for additional convenience.

Exploring their surroundings is a primary function for young children. It is not surprising that they do not like to be limited or restrained, because it interferes with their desire to discover and experience. Thus, it is also not surprising that children attempt to climb out of play yards just as they attempt to climb out of cribs and over gates.

In 2008, there were an estimated 1411 emergency department-treated injuries associated with play yards. Those injured ranged in age from 7-months to 4-years; most were 18-months of age or younger. Approximately half (48%) of the injuries were related to the child climbing out of the play yards, and injuries were associated with falling. One fourth of play yard-related injuries resulted from the child falling and hitting the side of the play yard. These injuries typically involved the head or face.

There have been a number of fatalities associated with play yards. Since 2004, there has been an average of 16 deaths each year. Many incidents resulted from suffocation on soft bedding that was placed in the play yard, such as adult-sized and baby pillows, comforters, and plush toys. In other cases, the infant died of positional asphyxiation after becoming wedged between a mattress or mattress pad and the side of the play yard. The infant asphyxiates when his head and face become entrapped in the gap between the pad and the side of the play yard. Positional asphyxiation also can occur when a child is outside the play yard and becomes wedged between the play yard and another structure. For example, a number of cases reported that a child had been placed on a bed to sleep, slipped off, and became wedged between the bed and the nearby play yard. This hazard pattern was described in the death of a 5-month-old girl from Waianae, Hawaii. In this case, the baby became entrapped between the head of an adult bed and an adjacent play yard after her father put her to sleep on his queen-sized adult bed. The baby appeared to have slid off the bed when she became trapped.

A number of fatalities were associated with strings or straps that were accessible to the child while in the play yard. This includes cases where the play yard was positioned close to window blinds with the cords within reach of the child. In these cases, the child strangled on a loop of the cord or the long cord became entangled around the baby's neck. This pattern occurred in the death of a 12-month-old girl from Greenwich, Connecticut. She was placed in a play yard for a nap. The play yard was positioned near a Roman shade. The baby apparently accessed the cord, and she was found with it wrapped twice around her neck. Any cord can pose a fatal threat to an infant or young child. Other strangulation fatalities occurring in play yards involved toy straps (i.e., used to suspend a toy from the top rail), straps hanging down from a changing table that was incorporated above a play yard, and the cord from a computer mouse.

Another hazard pattern noted in the fatality data resulted from the practice of placing a weight on top of the play yard in an effort to retain the child who might otherwise try to climb out. In some cases, parents use a mesh cover that serves as a lid. In other cases, they improvise, using handy objects to cover the play yard. Regardless of the type of cover used, the hazard pattern is the same: The infant lifts the weighted cover, gets his head over the top rail of the play yard, and the weighted lid falls back down to exert pressure on the back of the head. The mechanism for this type of asphyxiation caused the fatality of a 12-month-old boy in Midlothian, Virginia. In this case, the infant's father placed cardboard and a metal dog cage on top of the baby's play yard. The baby was found with his head and neck over the top rail and the cardboard and dog cage behind his head.

An ASTM standard for play yards (ASTM F406) was first published in 1977 and most recently updated in 2010 (ASTM 2010a). The standard addresses hazard patterns, including climbing out of the play yard; entrapment between the rails of the play yard and accessories, such as bassinets and changing tables; falls onto play yard parts; entrapment of fingers, body parts, and buttons in mesh; and finger pinching/shearing as a result of scissor action. The standard also has requirements intended to prevent the play yard from unintentionally folding. If it were to inadvertently fold, the top rail must not create a "V" formation, historically associated with strangulation and crushing injuries.

Consumers are advised to purchase play yards that comply with voluntary standards. That alone, however, is not sufficient to ensure the safety of an infant while in a play yard. Consumers must be aware of hazardous objects in the home that might be accessible to a child while she or he is in a play yard, such as plastic bags and window cords. The most inconspicuous objects can be attractive to a curious child. Play yards should be kept at least 2-feet from window coverings that have cords, desks, or dressers, and from other hazardous objects, such as plastic bags.

If a child has demonstrated the ability to climb out of a play yard, be sure there are no items in the play yard the child could use to stand on and that would facilitate climbing out. Under no circumstances should any cover be placed over the top of the play yard. As the data demonstrate, covering a play yard presents a risk of mechanical asphyxiation or strangulation.

Parents are advised to use only the mattress pad that is designed for the particular play yard because it will fit to the edges of the play yard without leaving gaps that could entrap a child's head and face. It is advised to keep plush bedding and toys out of the play yard. Pillows should never be used. Finally, caregivers should check the hardware and structure of the play yard to ensure that there are no loose components and that the bottom structure does not sag or tilt because either of these conditions can contribute to wedging and suffocation.

Because play yards can have a long life, associated hazards can remain in consumers' homes and day care centers for many years. Consumers and day care operators need to be aware of recalls affecting play yards, even those that are many years old. Since 2004, millions of play yards have been recalled. Most of the recalls involve serious hazards, such as the risk of entrapment and suffocation.

In 2007, Kolcraft recalled portable play yards after a 10-month-old boy strangled on the accessory changing table's restraint strap that was hanging down into Kolcraft's "Sesame Beginnings" Travel Play Yard. Twelve different Kolcraft play yards were included in this recall. All had raised changing tables with a restraint strap that formed a loop beneath the changing table, posing a strangulation hazard to a child in the play yard.

In addition to the strangulation hazard associated with the changing table restraint strap, one play yard (the Contours 3-in-1 model) also had a raised cradle that rocked back and forth. This design posed a suffocation hazard, because a child could roll and get trapped against the side of the cradle. Kolcraft received 45 reports of children rolling to the side of the rocking cradle attachment.

In 2009, PlayKids USA issued a recall of its convertible cribs (cribs/playpens/bassinets/beds) because of entrapment and suffocation hazards. The sides of the convertible cribs were made of a mesh that expands, creating a gap between the mattress and the side through which an infant could slip. This posed suffocation and entrapment hazards for young children. In 2008, a 5-month-old baby suffocated after becoming entrapped between the mattress and the stationary side rail of the convertible crib.

Numerous other brands of play yards were also recalled in 2009. Fisher-Price recalled its Rainforest Portable Play Yards manufactured by Simplicity Inc., and SFCA Inc., because one or more rails could collapse unexpectedly, posing a fall or entrapment hazard to young children. This same hazard pattern prompted the recall of Simplicity Travel Tender Play Yards by various retailers, including Babies "R" Us, Target, Kohl's, and Burlington Coat Factory stores. Kolcraft recalled its Carter's Sesame Street, Jeep, Contours, Care Bear, and Eric Carle Play Yards because of concern that the play yard's side rail could fail to latch properly. If that happened and a child pushed against the rail, it could unlatch unexpectedly, posing a fall hazard. The company received 347 reports of the play yard sides collapsing unexpectedly, resulting in 21 injuries to young children, including bumps, scrapes, bruises, and one concussion.

Dorel Juvenile group issued two recalls in 2009. First, Eddie Bauer Soothe & Sway Play Yards were recalled due to a risk of suffocation. This action was prompted by reports of infants rolling to one side of the play yard and their faces becoming pressed against the side or bottom of the bassinet. Additionally, Dorel recalled its Safety 1st Disney Care Center Play Yard and Eddie Bauer Complete Care Play Yard. Both products have a bassinet feature that can come apart, creating an uneven sleeping surface, posing a risk of suffocation or positional asphyxiation.

Kolcraft recalled over 1 million play yards in 2009 due to a potential fall risk. This recall, which affected 21 product models, was a response to a product defective rail latch that could open unexpectedly, posing a fall hazard to children.

In 2010, a portable play yard accessory, the Tots in Mind Cozy Indoor Outdoor Portable Play Yard Tent, was recalled. The dome-shaped white-colored mesh tent is designed to fit over play yards, similar to the crib tent discussed earlier in this chapter. This product is intended to prevent children from climbing out of the play yard. The tent has a zippered side that opens and closes for putting in and taking out the child. Clips that attach the tent to the top of the play yard can break or be removed by a child. A child can lift the tent and become entrapped at the neck between the rigid play yard frame and the metal base rod of the tent, posing a strangulation hazard.

In December 2008, a 2-year-old boy from Vinalhaven, Maine, was found hanging with his neck entrapped between the play yard frame and the metal base rod of the tent that had been partially tied by pieces of nylon rope and partially attached by clips. The tent was tied to the play yard because the child was able to pop off the clips. Apparently, the child became entrapped while attempting to climb out of the play yard. In three other incidents involving this product, children were able to remove one or more clips and place their necks between the tent and the play yard. The children were not injured. As noted in the section "Cribs" in this chapter, Tots in Mind also made a crib tent similar to the play yard tent. However, the crib tent was not recalled.

Incidents involving tents, changing tables, and bassinets attached to play yards highlight the hazards that can be introduced by accessories.

Recalls of play yards continue in 2011. AOSOM recalled its wooden play yards after learning of structural failures causing the wood to break, split and/or crack at points where screws and other hardware are located. Another company, Arms Reach Concepts, recalled its Bed-Side Sleepers after receiving reports of infants falling from the raised mattress into the bottom portion or becoming entrapped between the edge of the mattress and the side of the play yard.

Strollers

Baby strollers are a staple for most parents with young children. Today's strollers are associated with fewer injuries than in years past; however, thousands of injuries are still being treated in emergency departments each year. In 2008, the CPSC estimated that there were more than 12,000 such injuries that year, down from approximately 15,000 in 2000.

Stroller injuries decline in frequency as the child ages. Nonetheless, across age groups, the most common hazard pattern involves the child falling or climbing out of the stroller. More than half of all stroller injuries involve falls, which often are due to the child not being restrained or the child getting out of the restraint by unbuckling or wiggling out of it. Injuries to the head, neck, and face are typical. Most are treatable contusions, abrasions, and lacerations. Some are more serious fractures or internal injuries.

Falls from strollers are often associated with how the stroller is being used. For example, approximately 10% of injuries result from the stroller falling down stairs or being dropped when someone tried to carry the stroller on stairs. Another 10% of injuries are associated with the stroller tipping over. In many cases, tip-over results from the stroller hitting something, such as a curb, or after the stroller rolled away from the parent. In other cases, the stroller tipped over after the child stood in the stroller. Many tip-overs are associated with a sibling pushing the stroller.

Other stroller injuries result from being struck by a motor vehicle while in the stroller, tripping on or otherwise running into the stroller, and fingers or appendages being trapped, pinched, or cut in moving components of the stroller.

Deaths in strollers are not common. A total of ten stroller-related deaths were reported to the Commission from 2004 to 2009. Four of the fatalities were asphyxiations related directly to entrapment in the product. In three incidents, the victims (aged 6–8 months) became entrapped between the seat and the tray. The fourth entrapment resulted when a 4-year-old boy's head and chest were compressed in a stroller that collapsed. Another stroller-related fatality resulted from mechanical suffocation. In this case, a 2-month-old boy in Clearwater, Florida, was found face-down in bedding. He had been placed to sleep on his side in the stroller.

The remaining fatalities involving strollers were related to factors external to the product. For example, two children died when they were struck by a motor vehicle while in the stroller. The remaining three fatalities resulted from drowning or fire.

The ASTM voluntary standard, F833 (ASTM 2010b), is intended to mitigate stroller injuries and fatalities. The standard has provisions to reduce the likelihood of tip-over and unintentional collapse or folding. Also, the standard addresses adequate brake performance and prevention of pinch/scissor/shearing injuries. It also has specifications that prevent lower torso entrapment in leg openings.

Although the ASTM standard is intended to prevent injuries by designing safety into the stroller, recalls issued by manufacturers and the CPSC are intended to prevent injuries after the product is already on the market. Since 2004, there have been 21 stroller recalls. Fourteen of these recalls were the result of component failure that could cause the stroller to collapse or the user to fall. Component failures that prompted these recalls included detachment of handlebars or locking clips, seat detachment, wheel detachment, brake failure, and restraint failure. Five recalls were for the potential of finger pinch, laceration, or amputation. The other recalls were for the potential of (1) choking on a toy from an activity bar and (2) abrasion on (because of proximity to) rear tires when a child is seated in the add-on seat. Strollers affected by these recalls include the following brands: Baby Trend, Simplicity, Maclaren, Regal Lager, Dorel Juvenile Group's Cosco strollers, Graco, Sycamore Kids Inc., Kelty, Stokke, International Playthings, Bugaboo, Baby Jogger, and Britax. It is interesting that the recall of approximately one million Maclaren strollers was for fingertip amputation or laceration that occurred while the product was being opened or unfolded, that is, the child was a bystander and not inside the stroller. (For complete information on each of these recalls, go to http://www.cpsc.gov and click on the link for Recalls.)

To prevent stroller injuries and fatalities, consumers are urged to directly supervise their child while in a stroller or carriage. Although stroller-related fatalities are relatively rare, they do occur, particularly if a child is left to sleep in the stroller and becomes repositioned in a way that compromises the airway or causes entrapment or entanglement. Stroller injuries are relatively common, and most are related to falls. By being close and attentive to their child in a stroller, parents can prevent some hazard patterns that lead to falls, such as children attempting to exit the stroller or stand in the stroller, and sibling actions that can cause tip-over. In addition to ensuring that children use a stroller carefully, parents also must exercise caution, particularly around stairs.

The Role of Supervision in Injury Prevention

Product-related injuries and fatalities stem from a number of factors, including product design, child's age and personality, play environment, and presence of others in the play environment. Another factor, one that is widely cited in incident reports, is the lack of supervision. Although "appropriate" supervision may not prevent injuries from occurring, it can produce a rapid response to an injury, thereby mitigating its effects.

Defining the adequacy of supervision is difficult to do because there are many ways of conceptualizing supervisory behaviors. Saluja et al. (2004) proposed a theory of supervision that provides a template for investigating the relationship between supervision and injury risk. According to their model, supervision is evaluated on three dimensions: attention, proximity, and continuity. As these variables increase, so does supervision.

The research on supervision demonstrates that supervision practices vary as a child gets older. Peterson, Ewigman, and Kivlahan (1993) found that for young children and high hazard situations, parents, medical professionals, and social workers agree that vigilant supervision is needed. However, as children get older and the environment less hazardous, there is greater variability in the amount of time a child can be left unsupervised.

Pollack-Nelson and Drago (2002) studied supervision of parents with children aged 2 to 6 years. Results were consistent with the findings of Peterson et al. (1993). In particular, parents professed greater supervision of younger children. For example, when children are playing out of sight, most parents with 2- and 3-year-old children reported checking on them every 5 to 15 minutes, whereas most parents with 4- and 5-year-old children reported checking on them every 15 to 30 minutes, and those with children aged more than 5 years reported checking on them approximately 30 minutes to 1 hour.

Although parents reported checking on their young children with some frequency, a contradiction in behavior and perceived risk was noted in the study. Approximately three quarters of respondents stated that their children get up in the morning before they do. Yet, the overwhelming majority (95%) perceived that this posed no or slight risk to their child. This may be due to the perception that their home is relatively safe, whether or not it actually is. Eighty percent of respondents reported that their homes were moderately to very "childproof." Yet, the only "childproofing" measures taken with some frequency were the use of outlet covers, locks on cabinets and drawers, and baby gates. Further, with the exception of outlet covers, these other safety measures were used by only approximately one third of respondents. Thus, the perception of safety may not be objectively correct and may exceed the actual level of safety in the home.

Research by Chen and colleagues (2007) found that parents supervise 4- and 5-year-old children less frequently than younger children, despite the fact that injuries among children aged 4 to 5 years is nearly as high as that of younger age groups. This study also found that parents supervise less frequently when children play in the company of older siblings, compared with playing alone. The perception by parents that an older sibling can prevent or adequately respond to a dangerous situation is false as demonstrated in the injury data (e.g., bath seats, strollers). The researchers concluded that many caregivers have an inadequate understanding of injury mechanisms and that caregiver education could be beneficial.

Morrongiello et al. (2004) studied parental strategies for managing toddlers' in-home injuries and found that parental strategies, including close supervision, along with environmental strategies (i.e., modification of the environment to control access to hazards), significantly reduced children's risk of in-home injuries. Further, these strategies were found to be more effective in managing injury risk than child-based strategies (teaching rules to young children). Young children cannot be relied on to learn and self-regulate their behavior because they simply are not ready to do so. Toddlers and preschoolers are curious about the world around them. They are motivated to explore and test things for themselves. This can prompt them to climb on furniture to access objects of interest that may be dangerous. It also means trying out appliances and other objects that they have observed their parents using. Even the most obedient 4-year-old is still too young to self-regulate.

Parents cannot be expected to have their eyes on each of their children at all times. However, as the research by Morrongiello et al. (2004) demonstrates, close supervision can reduce injury risk in the home. This, along with protective devices or barriers to prevent access to dangerous objects and situations, should be used by parents. Although teaching children about safety is important, it should not be relied on as the primary injury prevention strategy, especially for preschoolers, because young children are not yet capable of self-regulation.

Advocacy/Practice/Future Research

There are a number of different means by which individual consumers and professionals in the field of consumer health and safety can be involved and have an impact on the safety of nursery products, such as (1) working with established advocacy groups, (2) becoming involved at a grassroots level, and (3) conducting and publishing research in this area.

Advocacy Groups

Advocates for consumer safety play a critical role in product safety. A number of advocacy groups work to identify and publicize hazards associated with consumer products. These groups often petition the CPSC to take action to ban, recall, or draft standards for products of concern. Below is a description of three such advocacy organizations.

Consumer Federation of America

The Consumer Federation of America (CFA) is the nation's largest consumer advocacy organization, representing more than 280 state, local, and national consumer organizations. A nonprofit organization, started in 1968, the CFA works to advance pro-consumer policies on a variety of issues, including those relating to consumer products, before the Congress, White House, regulatory agencies, and courts. The CFA also researches consumer issues, publishing their findings to assist consumer advocates, policy makers, and the general public.

The CFA has been active in a number of areas relating to nursery products. In 2000, the CFA joined with other advocacy groups to petition the CPSC to ban bath rings. The following year, the CFA launched a comprehensive Web site focusing on children's safety and health. This Web site includes all recalls of products intended for children from 1990 to the present. In 2004, the CFA supported the introduction of the California Infant Crib Safety Act (California Health and Safety Code Section 24500-24506: Article 1 2010), which would make mandatory and voluntary standards applicable to the sale or use of secondhand cribs. Currently, these standards only apply to new cribs.

Keeping Babies Safe

Keeping Babies Safe is a free information resource for parents that provides crib safety and sleep environment information, product recall information, and safety tips so that parents can be vigilant about keeping their babies safe. The organization is headed by Joyce Davis, whose baby died in a portable crib. Joyce founded Keeping Babies Safe to educate parents about crib and sleep safety and to advocate for more stringent consumer safety regulations and laws.

In addition to providing education and safety guidelines to parents, Keeping Babies Safe has mounted Project Safe Crib, a nonprofit program designed to educate social workers and other health care personnel on safe crib practices, as well as help parents from economically challenged environments obtain safe cribs through health and human service organizations nationwide. Once personnel have been trained, Project Safe Crib purchases safe cribs at an industry discount and provides them to hospitals, clinics, and other health and human service organizations for distribution to the public. Since 2007, Project Safe Crib has donated more than 2000 cribs to families nationwide. Consumers can participate in Project Crib Safe. With every $100 donation, Keeping Babies Safe purchases a new crib for those in need.

Kids in Danger

Kids In Danger (KID) is a nonprofit organization dedicated to improving children's product safety. KID was founded in 1998 by the parents of 16-month-old Danny Keysar, who died at his Chicago home day care when a portable crib collapsed, entrapping him by the neck. Although the portable crib had been recalled 5 years earlier, word of its danger had not reached Danny's parents, caregiver, or a state inspector who visited the home just 8 days before Danny's death.

KID is an advocacy group that seeks to protect children from dangerous products. In 1999, KID worked with state legislators to have the Children's Product Safety Act enacted, making it illegal to sell or lease recalled or dangerous children's products or to use those products in licensed child care facilities. KID sponsors a number of outreach programs to further their objectives. For example, the Health Care Providers Outreach Program educates health care providers and parents about dangerous and recalled children's products. Also, the Teach Early Safety Testing program encourages designers and engineers to incorporate safety and testing into product development.

Grassroots Efforts

Despite the work of the Commission and advocacy groups, the safety of a nursery is not assured. Consumers must be advocates for their own children's safety. Following are some actions that can be taken:

1. Report injuries and safety concerns about products to the CPSC. The CPSC Web site (http://www.cpsc.gov) makes it easy to fill out and submit a form, or call the hotline at 1-800-638-2772 (1-800-638-CPSC).
2. Check the CPSC Web site and http://www.recalls.gov regularly for recalls. Create your own recall network among parents of young children.
3. Encourage your neighborhood schools and community groups, such as Scouting USA and Boys and Girls Clubs, to join in CPSC's Neighborhood Safety Network, a grassroots effort to distribute monthly e-mail lists with safety and recall information. See the CPSC's Web site for details.
4. Petition the CPSC to remedy a product. Anyone can petition the agency. A petition is a formal request to the agency seeking rule-making for a product, revision of an existing rule, or a product ban. The petition should identify the consumer product for which a safety rule or change is sought, along with the basis for the request. This may include personal experience or published research findings. The petition should describe the specific risk of injury, including data on severity and likelihood of injury, along with possible reasons for the injury potential (e.g., product defect, design flaw, unintentional misuse). For more information on how to file a petition, see the CPSC Web site.
5. Become a consumer member of an ASTM subcommittee and take part in the development of standards. ASTM International is one of the largest voluntary standards development organizations in the world. ASTM Committee F15 on Consumer Products has jurisdiction over and maintains more than 80 standards for a variety of consumer products, including those mentioned in this chapter. Standards are drafted by subcommittees that are composed of industry, government (usually the CPSC), and consumer representatives. Most subcommittees have openings for consumer members and in many cases will pay the expenses of consumers so they can travel to attend the meetings. (For more information on joining the ASTM as an affiliate member, go to the ASTM Web site at http://www.astm.org.)
6. Read and follow product instructions for use, paying special attention to age-grading, weight-grading, warnings, and maintenance issues.
7. Inspect nursery products for continued integrity throughout the life of the product.

Conduct Research

Practitioners and researchers can awaken the public to product safety issues when they publish their findings. Moreover, published works can prompt the development of new standards or cause industry, advocacy groups, and the CPSC to revisit and update existing standards. For example, after a study of head entrapment in side ladders of bunk beds (Pollack-Nelson, 2011), the Commission docketed a petition (CPSC 2010c) and is seeking comments in consideration of revising the mandatory standard for bunk beds. By using free and available data from the CPSC, researchers are encouraged to investigate product safety issues and publish their findings.

Conclusions

Major changes at the CPSC are leading to stronger, mandatory standards for nursery products. Although the agency is using existing voluntary standards as a starting point, the mandatory standards it develops can have additional requirements and could therefore be more comprehensive in the hazard patterns they address. It is hoped that these changes will lead to reduced injuries and deaths associated with nursery products.

Although more comprehensive federal standards for nursery products will surely make these products safer, injuries and fatalities will continue. Nursery products that meet a standard are not necessarily "safe." A product that complies with a standard will only be as good as that standard's requirements. Standards are not designed for any particular manufacturer's product. Rather, they apply to a class of products. As a result, unique characteristics of a product may present unaddressed hazards. Identifying such hazards requires an assessment of the individual product. Although some manufacturers conduct "hazard analyses" of their designs before production, others do not.

For these reasons, consumers and those who interact with them—teachers, nurses, and other health care providers—are encouraged to educate themselves about nursery product hazards and spread the word to other parents. By visiting the CPSC Web site (at http://www.cpsc.gov), consumers can learn about safety concerns, recalls, new regulations, and much more. Other Web sites (such as http://www.KidsInDanger.org) provide valuable recall information and updates on the Commission and standards' activities. A consumer can join the listservs of these sites so that information comes directly to them regularly through e-mail. On noticing a potential product hazard, consumers are advised to contact the CPSC. In these ways, every consumer can have an impact on nursery product safety.

References

American Academy of Pediatrics. 2005. The changing concept of sudden infant death syndrome: diagnostic coding shifts, controversies regarding the sleeping environment and new variables to consider in reducing risk. *Pediatrics.* 116:1245–1255.

American Society for Testing and Materials (ASTM). 1986. *F1004 Standard Consumer Safety Specification for Expansion Gates and Expandable Enclosures.* West Conshohocken, PA: ASTM International.

American Society for Testing and Materials (ASTM). 1988. F1822 Standard Consumer Safety Specification for Non-Full-Size Baby Cribs. West Conshohocken, PA: ASTM International.

American Society for Testing and Materials (ASTM). 2000. F966 Consumer Safety Specification for Full-Size and Non-Full-Size Baby Crib Corner Post Extensions. West Conshohocken, PA: ASTM International.

American Society for Testing and Materials (ASTM). 2008a. F404 Standard Consumer Safety Specification for High Chairs. West Conshohocken, PA: ASTM International.

American Society for Testing and Materials (ASTM). 2008b. F1917 Standard Consumer Safety Performance Specification for Infant Bedding and Related Accessories. West Conshohocken, PA: ASTM International.

American Society for Testing and Materials (ASTM). 2009a. F1004 Standard Consumer Safety Specification for Expansion Gates and Expandable Enclosures. West Conshohocken, PA: ASTM International.

American Society for Testing and Materials (ASTM). 2009b. F2008 Standard Consumer Safety Specification for Infant Swings. West Conshohocken, PA: ASTM International.

American Society for Testing and Materials (ASTM). 2009c. F2050 Standard Consumer Safety Specification for Hand-Held Infant Carriers. West Conshohocken, PA: ASTM International.

American Society for Testing and Materials (ASTM). 2009d. F2057 Standard Consumer Safety Specification for Chests, Door Chests, and Dressers. West Conshohocken, PA: ASTM International.

American Society for Testing and Materials (ASTM). 2009e. F2236 Standard Consumer Safety Specification for Soft Infant Carriers. West Conshohocken, PA: ASTM International.

American Society for Testing and Materials (ASTM). 2009f. F2388 Standard Consumer Safety Specification for Baby Changing Tables for Domestic Use. West Conshohocken, PA: ASTM International.

American Society for Testing and Materials (ASTM). 2010a. F406 Standard Consumer Safety Specification for Non-Full-Size Baby Cribs/Play Yards. West Conshohocken, PA: ASTM International.

American Society for Testing and Materials (ASTM). 2010b. F833 Standard Consumer Safety Performance Specification for Carriages and Strollers. West Conshohocken, PA: ASTM International.

American Society for Testing and Materials (ASTM). 2010c. *F1169 Standard Specification for Full-Size Baby Cribs.* West Conshohocken, PA: ASTM International.

American Society for Testing and Materials (ASTM). 2010d. F1967 Standard Consumer Safety Specification for Infant Bath Seats. West Conshohocken, PA: ASTM International.

American Society for Testing and Materials (ASTM). 2010e. F2085 Standard Consumer Safety Specification for Bed Rails. West Conshohocken, PA: ASTM International.

American Society for Testing and Materials (ASTM). 2010f. F2167 Standard Consumer Safety Specification for Infant Bouncer Seats. West Conshohocken, PA: ASTM International.

American Society for Testing and Materials (ASTM). 2010g. F2194 Standard Consumer Safety Specification for Bassinets and Cradles. West Conshohocken, PA: ASTM International.

Bukatko, D. and M. Daehler (1992). *Child Development: A Topical Approach.* Boston, MA: Houghton Mifflin Company: p. 214.

California Health and Safety Code Section 24500-24506: Article 1. 2010. *The Infant Crib Safety Act.* Available at: http://www.law.justa.com/California/codes/2009/hsc/24500-24506. Accessed October 1, 2010.

Chen X, Beran M, Altkorn R, et al. 2007. Frequency of caregiver supervision of young children during play. *Int J Inj Contr Saf Promot.* 14:122–124.

Chowdhury R. 2009. Nursery Product-Related Injuries and Deaths Among Children Under Age Five. Consumer Product Safety Commission.

Consumer Product Safety Commission (CPSC). 2008. *Consumer Product Safety Improvement Act of 2008,* Public Law 100-314, 110th Congress, Aug. 14.

Consumer Product Safety Commission (CPSC). 2010a. *Deaths Prompt CPSC, FDA Warning on Infant Sleep Positioners.* Available at: http://www.cpsc.gov/cpscpub/prerel/prhtm10/10358.html. Accessed October 2, 2010.

Consumer Product Safety Commission (CPSC). 2010b. *Draft Federal Register Notice: Safety Standard for Infant Bath Seats: Final Rule.* Available at: http://www.cpsc.gov/library/foia/foia10/brief/bathseatFRrev.pdf. Accessed October 2, 1010.

Consumer Product Safety Commission (CPSC). 2010c. Petition requesting standard for bunk bed cornerposts. *Federal Register.* 67:68017. Available at: http://edocket.access.gpo.gov/2010/2010-16918.htm. Accessed July 15, 2010.

Gipson K. 2009. Instability and Tipover of Appliances, Furniture and Televisions: Estimated Injuries and Reported Fatalities. Washington, DC: Consumer Product Safety Commission.

Gottesman BL, McKenzie LB, Coner K, Smith GA. 2009. Injuries from furniture tipovers among children and adolescents in the United States 1990-2007. *Clin Pediatr (Phila).* 48:851–858.

Jensen LR, Williams SC, Thurman DJ, Keller PA. 1992. Submersion injuries in children younger than five years in urban Utah. *West J Med.* 157:641–644.

Morrongiello BA, Ondejko L, Littlejohn A. 2004. Understanding toddlers' in-home injuries: I. Context, correlates, and determinants. *J Pediatr Psychol.* 29:415–431.

O'Carroll PW, Alkon E, Weiss B. 1988. Drowning mortality in Los Angeles County 1976 to 1984. *JAMA.* 260:380–383.

Pearn JH, Brown J, Wong R, Bart R. 1979. Bathtub drownings: report of seven cases. *Pediatrics.* 64:68–70.

Peterson L, Ewigman B, Kivlahan C. 1993. Judgments regarding appropriate child supervision to prevent injury: the role of environmental risk and child age. *Child Dev.* 64:934–950.

Pollack-Nelson C. 2000. Injuries associated with in-home use of infant seats and baby carriers. *Pediatr Emerg Care.* 16:77–79.

Pollack-Nelson C, Drago D. 2002. Supervision of children aged two through six years. *Inj Control Saf Promot.* 9:121–126.

Pollack-Nelson, C. (2011). Fatality in the side of a bunk bed. *Ergonomics in Design,* 19:9–11.

Rauchschwalbe R, Brenner RA, Smith GS. 1997. The role of bathtub seats and rings in infant drowning deaths. *Pediatrics.* 100e1.

Saluja G, Brenner R, Morrongiello B, et al. 2004. The role of supervision in child injury risk: definition, conceptual and measurement issues. *Inj Control Saf Promot.* 11:17–22.

CFR part 1508. 1973. Requirements for full-size baby cribs. *Federal Register.* 38:32129.

CFR part 1509. 1976. Requirements for non-full-size baby cribs. *Federal Register.* 41:6240.

CFR part 1303. 1977. Ban of lead-containing paint and certain consumer products bearing lead-containing paint. *Federal Register.* 42:44199.

CFR part 1130. 2009. Requirements for consumer registration of durable infant or toddler products, final rule. *Federal Register.* 74:68668–68679.

CFR part 1215. 2010. Safety standard for infant bath seats: final rule. *Federal Register.* 75:31691–31699.

CFR part 1218. 2010. Safety standard for bassinets and cradles; notice of proposed rulemaking, comment request. *Federal Register.* 75:22303–22318.

CFR parts 1219, 1220, 1500. 2010a. Safety standards for full-size baby cribs and non-full-size baby cribs; notice of proposed rulemaking; proposed rule. *Federal Register.* 141:43308–43327.

CFR parts 1219, 1220, 1500. 2010b. Full-size baby cribs and non-full-size baby cribs: safety standards; revocation of requirements; third party testing for certain children's products; final rules. *Federal Register.* 248:81766–81788.

CFR part 1102. 2011. Publicly available consumer product safety information database. Final rule. *Federal Register.* 75:76832–76872.

Snyder RG, Schneider LW, Owings CL, et al. 1977. *Anthropometry of Infants, Children, and Youths to Age 18 for Product Safety Design.* Washington, DC: Consumer Product Safety Commission. Report UM-HSRI-77-17.

Snyder RG, Spencer ML, Owings CL, Schneider LW. 1975. *Physical Characteristics of Children as Related to Death and Injury for Consumer Product Safety Design.* Washington, DC: Consumer Product Safety Commission: Report UM-HSRI-75-5.

Steenbekkers LP. 1993. *Child Development, Design Implications and Accident Prevention. No 1 in Physical Ergonomics Series.* The Netherlands: TU, Delft: Delft University of Technology.

Thompson KM. 2003. The role of bath seats in unintentional infant bathtub drowning deaths. *MedGenMed.* 5:36. Available at: http://www.medscape.com/viewarticle/450989. Accessed October 1, 2010.

Chapter 4

Motor Vehicle and Pedestrian Injuries Among Children and Adolescents: Risk and Prevention

Bruce G. Simons-Morton, EdD, MPH[1] *and Laura J. Caccavale, BA*[1]

HOLLYWOOD, Fla.—It was a double date like countless others: two teenage girls and their teenage boyfriends, with plans to see a movie on a summer night. But this one ended in grief. Sixteen-year-old Gerald Miller swerved his sport-utility vehicle to miss a car stalled on Interstate 95. The SUV, traveling about 78 mph, rolled five times. The boys were injured. The girls—Casey Hersch, 16, and Lauren Gorham, 15—were thrown from the SUV and died.

Jayne O'Donnell, USA Today, *March 1, 2005*

Sadly, motor vehicle crashes (MVCs) take the lives of all too many children and adolescents. The crash described above is illustrative: a teenage driver with multiple teenage passengers not wearing safety belts driving a not very safe vehicle at night. Rollover crashes tend to result in serious injuries and modern passenger vehicles are built to prevent rolling over, but the higher center of gravity of many sport utility vehicles makes them susceptible to rolling in certain types of crashes. Of course, being thrown from a vehicle is the most dangerous result of a crash, and safety belts are effective at keeping passengers in the vehicle and free from contact with cabin objects only when they are worn. Many fatalities such as these could be prevented through the combination of improved technology, strict policies, enhanced enforcement, and effective education.

The United States has a long and romantic history with vehicles and roads (Vanderbilt 2009), despite their ongoing and substantial contribution to national injury and death tolls. Because the country is geographically large and relatively wealthy, the United States has developed a greater reliance on motor vehicle transportation than any other nation, with only Australia and Canada similarly dependent on motor vehicles. Consequently, the United States leads the world in annual miles driven per driver and has one of the highest rates of injury and death due to MVCs, with more than 33,000 fatalities in 2009 (National Highway Traffic Safety Administration [NHTSA] 2010), approximately 35% of deaths for all causes.

Despite improvements in crashes per mile driven (NHTSA 2010), MVCs remain one of the leading causes of death for every age group in the United States (Centers for Disease Control, 2010a) (Figure 4.1) and the leading cause of death and disability among children and adolescents (NHTSA 2009a). Moreover, because access to motor vehicles and miles of driving are increasing in many parts of the world, notably India and China, world crash and injury rates have increased dramatically over the past decade in rapidly developing nations (World Health Organization 2009).

[1]Prevention Research Branch, Division of Epidemiology Statistics and Prevention Research, Eunice Kennedy Shriver National Institute of Child Health and Human Development, Bethesda, Maryland.

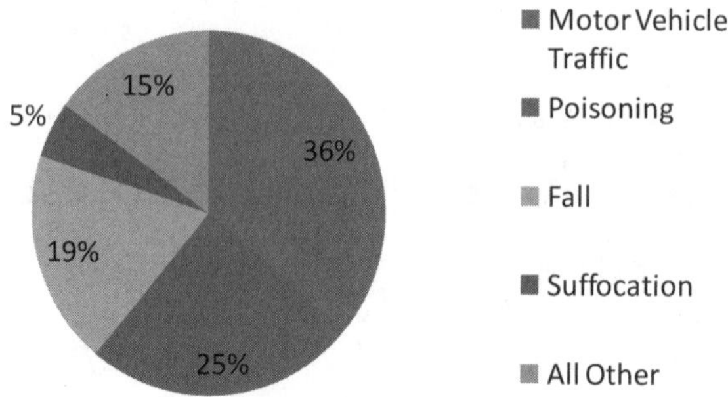

Figure 4.1. Percentage of Unintentional Injury Deaths by Category, 2007.

Source: Centers for Disease Control and Prevention, Injury Prevention and Control: Data and Statistics. 2010a. Web-based Injury Statistics Query and Reporting System (WISQARS) Leading Causes of Death Reports, 1999-2007.

To put the annual 33,000 U.S. fatalities due to MVCs into perspective, consider other statistics on fatalities that are generally perceived to have significant impacts on society and require attention. For example, 4500 Americans (and an estimated 100,000 Iraqis) were killed during the 7 years of the Iraq war (GlobalSecurity.org 2009), and 500 to 600 people die in U.S. airplane crashes annually (National Transportation Safety Board 2010). Although deaths due to any cause are unfortunate, it is surprising and disappointing that there is not greater urgency about the vast number of motor vehicle–related injuries and deaths, particularly because many of them could be prevented. Sadly, children and adolescents are overrepresented in MVC injury statistics—children because they are so vulnerable and adolescents because as drivers they are inexperienced, are easily distracted, and drive in a risky manner. As passengers, adolescents frequently ride with inexperienced adolescent drivers. Teenage drivers have the highest rate of fatal crash involvement of any age group, and adolescents and young children have high rates of passenger and pedestrian injuries and deaths (NHTSA 2009a–d).

Prevention Principles

Although there are many unique risk factors for motor vehicle and pedestrian crashes and injuries, the basic principles of injury prevention were conceptualized by Haddon and Baker (1981) according to pre-injury, injury, and post-injury events, with contributing factors that include human, vehicle, physical environment (road and driving conditions), and social environment (including driver attitudes and style) (Christoffel and Gallagher 2006). On the basis of a Haddon-type analysis of crash causes, the principles of crash causation are listed in Table 4.1 and summarized as follows: (1) Crashes are associated with mileage; the more people drive the more they crash; (2) crashes occur when vehicles get too close to other vehicles and objects, and road and traffic designs can influence crash likelihood; (3) driver error is frequently associated with crashes, (3a) inattention is the primary cause of driver error, (3b) driver inexperience, risk taking, driving complexity, and impairment increase crash likelihood; and (4) road designs, vehicle size and engineering properties, and occupant safety behavior can increase or decrease the likelihood and severity of injuries.

These contributing factors can be linked to the Haddon terminology as follows: (1) relates to the social and physical environments; (2) relates to the physical environment; (3) relates to human factors; and (4) relates to agent/vehicle factors. Actually, all contributing factors are

Table 4.1. Crash Phases, Injury Causes, and Preventive Measures

Crash Phase and Injury Causes	Prevention Objectives
Pre-Crash Phase	
Exposure causes crashes (i.e., the more people drive the more they crash, although the rate of crashing declines with experience)	Increase the use of public transportation Increase the number of passengers and reduce the number of drivers and amount of driving Provide safe walking/biking environments Reduce access to parking Increase road use fees Increase gasoline prices
Road designs are associated with crashes (i.e., some intersections and merges are more dangerous than others, roundabouts are safer than other merges, better signage improves safety, etc.)	Implement best practices in road designs Road designs Road signage Improve road laws Improve enforcement of road laws
Crashes occur when vehicles get too close to other vehicles and objects	Reduce aggressive and risky driving through enforcement of driving laws
Crashes are often due to driver error: inattention/distraction risky driving judgment, and impairment	Driver attention Driver risk behavior GDL policies Driving regulations Road designs
Phase 2. Crash Events	
Crash outcomes are affected by: road designs and vehicle size and engineering, including air bags and safety belts occupant use of safety belts and car safety seats	Improve road designs Divide roads Eliminate roadside objects Improve signage Improve merges and intersections Regulate (reduce) vehicle size and safety Engineer vehicles for safety Energy absorption Air bags Anti-lock breaks Regulate, enforce, and educate occupants regarding safety belts and car safety seats
Phase 3. Post-Crash Events	
Emergency procedures	Support road emergency services

GDL = Graduated Driver Licensing.

human in the sense that humans create these systems and conditions and only humans can fix these problems. The primary goals of crash prevention are to reduce exposure, facilitate the separation of pedestrians and vehicles from each other and from other objects, improve vehicle safety, reduce driving complexity, encourage driver attention, and discourage driver risk taking, distraction, and impairment.

Although the primary goal is to prevent *crashes*, Haddon's conceptualization reminds us that the *effects* of crashes can be mitigated by safe road designs and vehicle engineering. Therefore, it is possible to reduce the severity of injuries caused by crashes by improving roads to minimize vehicle contact with other vehicles and objects, particularly stationary objects such as trees and posts (Transportation Research Board 2004). Moreover, modern vehicles have many advanced safety features that absorb energy, protect occupants, and reduce damage to those involved in crashes (Mahmood and Fileta 2004). Efficient emergency services can save lives and reduce lasting damage from MVCs. Therefore, secondary prevention objectives call for improved vehicle safety and modern emergency services.

Although this chapter is primarily concerned with children and adolescents, many transportation safety measures are designed to benefit the entire population regardless of age. For example, modern road designs that increase the separation of vehicles from other vehicles and stationary objects have decided safety benefits (American Association of State Highway and Transportation Officials 2002; Roadway Safety Foundation 2004). Also, modern vehicles have many safety features that reduce injuries in the case of a crash, although some vehicles are much safer than others (Insurance Institute for Highway Safety [IIHS] 2010d), and lower speed limits, occupant protection laws, and vigorous enforcement of safety laws improve safety (Transport Canada 2010).

Because the causes of MVCs are complex, only a comprehensive approach to prevention and control is likely to be effective. Ultimately, the only truly substantial solution to transportation injuries is to reduce reliance on personal vehicles. On the basis of miles traveled, the most common measure of exposure, public transportation is many times safer than personal vehicles and is less polluting and increases physical activity. Although reducing exposure is a long-term goal, more immediate prevention goals can be achieved through safe road and vehicle designs, enlightened regulations and policies, vigorous enforcement of driving rules, and education to improve driver, occupant, and pedestrian behavior. To prevent or reduce crashes and injuries, both technology and safety behaviors must be improved. Concerted advocacy is needed for safe road designs, improved vehicle safety technology, creative policies, and education.

This chapter presents three separate sections focusing on young drivers, child occupant protection, and pedestrian safety. Bicycle-related injuries are covered in Chapter 9. Each section presents the prevalence, risk factors, preventive measures, and recommendations for improving policies, vehicle and road designs, enforcement, and safety behavior; and examples of effective programs that have improved safety.

The Young Driver Problem

Crash rates increase sharply in early adolescence as teenagers begin to ride with other teenage drivers, peak at age 16 to 17 years when teenagers are first licensed, and remain high relative to experienced drivers well into age 20 to 29 years (IIHS 2010b; NHTSA 2008a; Williams 2003). The dramatic increase in MVCs during adolescence and the maintenance of high crash rates through age 20 to 25 years is known as the "young driver problem."

Prevalence

In 2008, 3500 U.S. teens died and 350,000 were injured in MVCs (Centers for Disease Control and Prevention, Injury Prevention and Control 2010a; NHTSA 2009b). In every Western country studied, newly licensed teenagers have the highest crash rates of any age group, except the very old. Regardless of age, crash rates are highest immediately after licensure, decline rapidly for a period of months, and then decline slowly for a period of years before stabilizing at age 20 to 29 years (Twisk and Stacey 2007). However, the younger the age at licensure, the higher the crash rate (IIHS 2010a; Twisk and Stacey 2007), as shown in Figure 4.2. It is not surprising that preventing MVCs among adolescents is a prominent health objective in most developed and many developing countries.

In the United States, MVCs are the major cause of deaths among adolescents (Heron et al. 2009). Crash rates for U.S. adolescents are higher for 16- to 19-year-olds than for any age group younger than 70 years, and 16-year-old drivers have crash rates approximately four times that for drivers of all ages (IIHS 2010a). Fatal crash rates increase dramatically during adolescence, decline steadily during age 20 to 29 years, and stabilize at age 30 to 49 years, as shown in Figure 4.3 (NHTSA 2009a). Compared with older, more experienced drivers, young drivers are more likely to be at fault in crashes and to be involved in crashes that are speed-related and due to overcorrection errors, the types of crashes that are associated with going too fast for conditions, judgment errors, inattention, and risky driving (McKnight and McKnight 2003; Williams 2003). Fatal crash rates are somewhat higher for male teens than female teens, as shown in Figure 4.3 for fatalities and Figure 4.4 for nonfatal motor vehicle injuries. Rates are similar for White, Hispanic, and Black adolescents, but on average White adolescents get their driver's license earlier, and therefore begin to drive at younger ages, have more crashes, and suffer more injuries than Black or Hispanic adolescents (NHTSA 2009b). Approximately 40% of the MVC deaths of 16- to 19-year-olds are sustained by passengers, which increase substantially from approximately age 13 years to 20 years, presumably because of increased riding with young drivers (IIHS 2010a; Williams 2003). Fortunately, fatal crashes among 16- to 19-year-olds have declined somewhat over the past two decades, mainly because adolescents today get their driver's licenses at somewhat older ages.

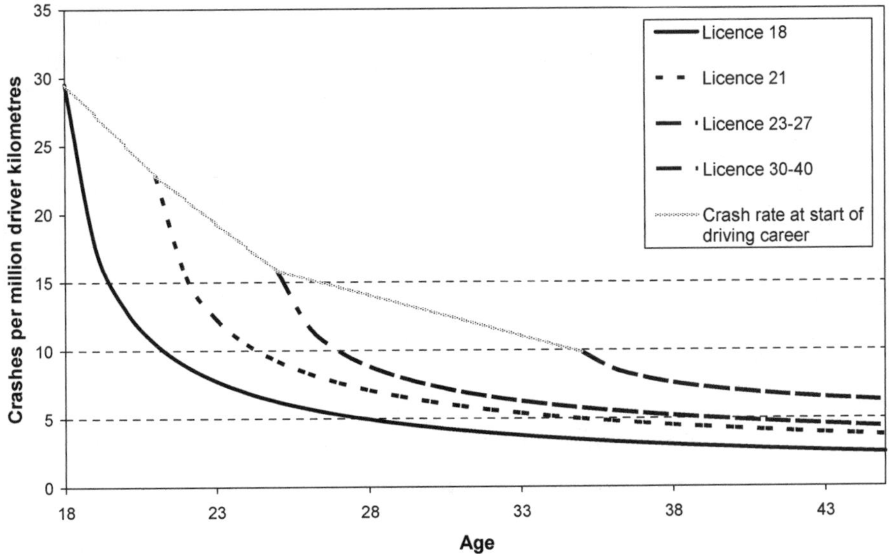

Figure 4.2. Crash Rates by Age of Licensure Among European Member Countries of the Organization of Economic Co-operation and Development.

Source: Organization for Economic Co-operation and Development 2006.

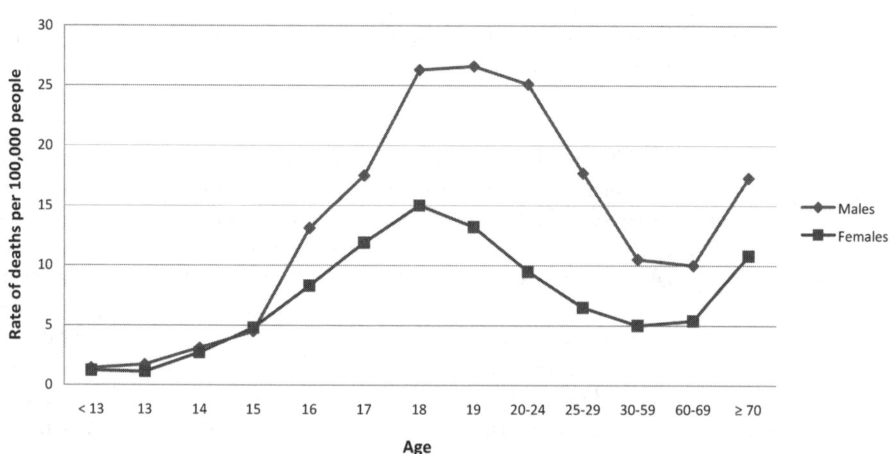

Figure 4.3. Figure 4.3. Deaths in Passenger Vehicles Per 100,000 People by Age and Gender, 2008. Source: U.S. Department of Transportation's Fatality Analysis Reporting System (FARS), 2008.

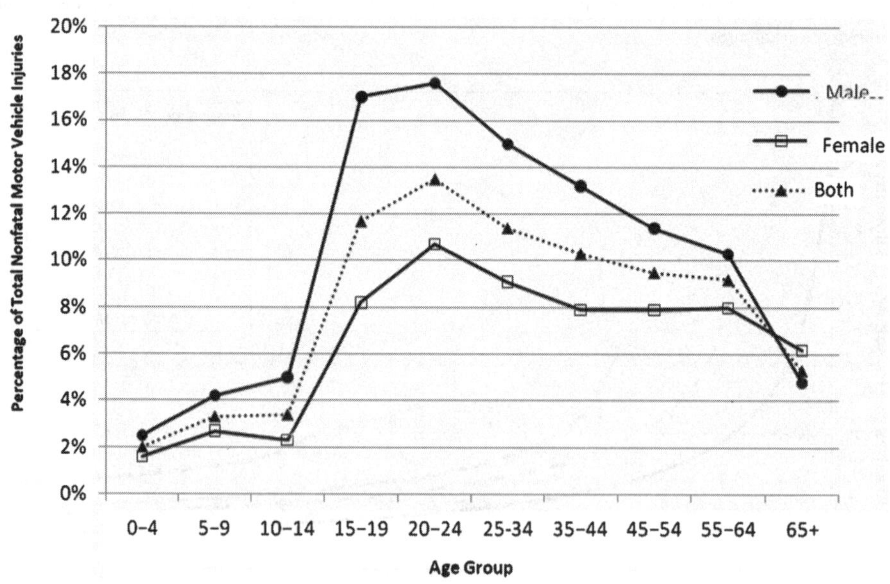

Figure 4.4. Percentage of Total Nonfatal Motor Vehicle Injuries, United States, 2008, all races, male, female, and both.

Source: Centers for Disease Control and Prevention, Injury Prevention and Control: Data and Statistics. 2010a. Web-Based Injury Statistics Query and Reporting System (WISQARS) Leading Causes of Death Reports, 1999-2007.

Risk Factors

The causes of the young driver problem are generally considered to include young age, inexperience, inattention, and risky driving. Certain driving conditions, notably night driving and teen passengers, seem to exacerbate crash risk (Williams 2003). The younger the age at licensure, the greater the crash rate (Twisk and Stacey 2007), and young age seems to interact with other factors to increase risk. For example, young age and inexperience are related. Adolescents are relatively less experienced in general and have little experience with driving. Young age also seems to be associated with risk taking in general (Steinberg 2004) and driving in particular (Williams 2003). Because males are generally higher risk takers, males tend to have higher rates of fatal crashes, although the rates of nonfatal crashes are relatively similar among males and females (Williams 2003). Although it is not entirely clear whether adolescents engage in risky driving because they prefer riskiness, do not perceive their behavior as risky, or are unable to regulate their behavior, it is certain that they drive in a manner that is highly risky.

Recent "naturalistic driving" research using sensitive instrumentation of study participants' own vehicles installed during the first 18 months of licensure shows that teenagers relative to adults on average drive faster, follow more closely, accelerate faster, brake harder, and turn more rapidly (Simons-Morton 2010). Hard braking is a good case in point. On average, novice adolescent drivers have approximately eight times the rate of hard braking events as experienced adults. Indeed, experienced drivers rarely brake so hard that passengers are made uncomfortable ($\geqslant -0.45$ g-force), but young drivers do this routinely. Mostly, hard braking is a matter of beginning to brake relatively late, either because of a failure to anticipate the need to stop or a style of driving in which late braking is acceptable or preferred. The risk associated with late braking, of course, is that it reduces the margin for error. If the lead vehicle suddenly brakes hard, the trailing vehicle is more likely to crash if the driver has waited until the last second to brake. Hard turns provide another case in point. Experienced adults rarely exceed g-forces of +0.5 or greater in turns, but young drivers do routinely (Simons-Morton et al. 2010), placing themselves at increased risk for skidding, overcorrecting, and losing control of the vehicle. Strangely, high rates of risky driving persist for at least the first 18 months of licensure, although crashes and near crashes decline rapidly, suggesting that novice teenagers adapt to risky driving, becoming better at driving in a risky manner without crashing. Curiously, when teenagers drove with their parents in the vehicle, their rate of elevated g-force events was almost identical to the rates of adults, suggesting that teens can drive in a smooth and careful manner, but they don't unless their parents are present (Simons-Morton 2010).

Survey data also indicate that on average young drivers drive in a more risky fashion than older drivers, tailgating, weaving through traffic, and speeding (Hartos, Eitel, and Simons-Morton 2001; Hatfield and Fernandes 2009). Other survey data show that on average teenagers assess their driving skill to be quite high even during the early months of licensure when they clearly are not very good (Mayhew et al. 2006). Drinking and driving is highest among college-aged youth and relatively low among novice teenage drivers, but nonetheless, drinking and driving is particularly dangerous for novices, with alcohol involved disproportionately in fatal crashes among young drivers, as shown in Figure 4.5 (Centers for Disease Control 2009; NHTSA 2009c).

Laws of Crash Causation

To understand the young driver problem, it is useful to understand the nature of crash risk in general and then apply it to young drivers. Elvik (2006) listed four laws of crash causation, to which we provide two additional laws. Each law is introduced and then applied to young drivers.

1. The universal law of learning: The ability to detect and control traffic hazards increases as the amount of travel increases.

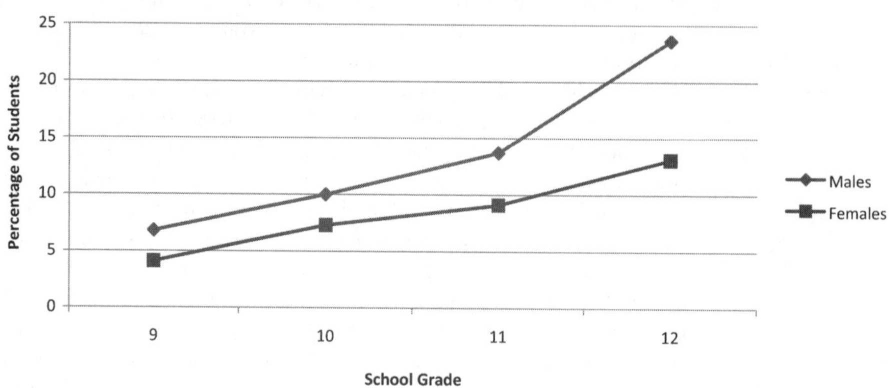

Figure 4.5. Percentage of Students Who Drove a Vehicle One or More Times in the Past 30 Days When They had Been Drinking Alcohol.

Source: Centers for Disease Control and Prevention. Youth Risk Behavior Surveillance – 2009. MMWR 2010;59(No. SS-5).

This law can best be understood in terms of the development of expertise of complex activities, which develops gradually over a long period of time with substantial experience. In contrast with novices, experts in almost any area, for example, mathematics, chess, sports, and driving, are quickly able to allocate their attention to the important elements and patterns in structured and unstructured problems and have immediate access to a huge cognitive store of memorized and automated knowledge about problems and solutions (Keating and Halpern-Felsher 2008). Likewise, driving competence can be expected to advance only through feedback from frequent experience with a wide variety of driving situations encountered over a long period of time.

Safe driving requires the ability to maneuver in a variety of complex traffic conditions, identify and react to hazards, anticipate the actions of other vehicles, manage distractions, correctly signal intended actions, and otherwise drive in a manner that keeps the vehicle well separated in space and time from other vehicles and objects. Maintaining attention to the road, extensive visual scanning, and the ability to recognize and reacting to subtle variations in the driving environment that suggest the potential for danger are more important for safety than the physical management of the vehicle. Inexperienced drivers in general are less able to recognize and anticipate potential hazards and are prone to extended inattention at inopportune times. With experience, expertise increases and errors and crash rates decline.

Driving expertise seems to advance mainly through independent driving experience. Crash rates during supervised practice driving are very low, but regardless of the amount of supervised practice novices obtain before licensure, crash rates are high early in licensure (Mayhew, Simpson, and Pak 2003; McCartt, Shabanova, and Leaf 2003). This is most likely because during supervised practice driving the adult supervisor co-drives, helping the novice to prepare for maneuvers, looking out for hazards, and controlling the vehicle environment. This is as it should be, but upon licensure, novices must learn how to perform these tasks on their own.

2. The law of rare events: The more rarely a certain factor is encountered, the larger is its effect on the likelihood of a crash. Although the most common risk factors are the most important, rare causes are responsible for crashes at disproportionate rates to their prevalence.

   For novices, nearly everything is rare and cannot quickly be understood and dealt with in a safe manner. Night is a good example. Night driving is more dangerous than day driving for drivers of all ages, but much more dangerous for young drivers, even when the nature of the trip, number of passengers, and risk taking are accounted (Williams 2003). This is probably because night driving can be disorienting, even for young eyes, and only through experience does a person learn to limit his or her driving at night because of the inherent difficulties. Likewise, it has been well demonstrated that novices are not as good as more experienced drivers at recognizing and reacting to potential road hazards (Pradhan et al. 2005). Experienced drivers are better able to identify that something in the driving scene is unusual and may be hazardous, and therefore are able to anticipate and react better than novices.

3. The law of complexity: The greater the amount of information to which a road user must attend, the greater the probability of an error.

   Complexity increases errors in all activities, and driving is no exception. This is one reason that cell phone use and other secondary tasks are associated with crashing. Making a right turn is a simple process, but it becomes more complex when there is an indefinite shoulder to the right of the road, a pedestrian crossing the street, or heavy traffic. Weather is another factor that notably increases complexity and leads to crashes. Actually, managing a vehicle is a relatively simple task that can be learned by almost anyone with a few hours of instruction, but driving safely is altogether more complex. Safety requires complex judgments about how to maneuver a vehicle in traffic where the intentions and actions of other vehicles and pedestrians must be anticipated correctly.

   Young drivers are at particular risk because the complexity of driving is greatest among the inexperienced. In addition, the driving task is more complex when the driver engages in secondary tasks, which young drivers do frequently. Also, the social environment in the vehicle, with loud music and highly active passengers, may increase the complexity of driving, particularly among young drivers. Notably, the presence of multiple passengers has no effect on crash rates for older drivers, but greatly increases crash rates among young drivers (Ouimet et al. 2010).

4. The law of cognitive capacity: The more cognitive capacity approaches its limits, the higher the error rate.

   Novices must devote a relatively greater proportion of their cognitive capacity on the driving task because it is unfamiliar to them and they have developed little expertise. Experienced drivers develop what is called automaticity, where they are able to drive with little conscious effort, often thinking about other things, but instantly aware when some untoward event occurs (Groeger 2000). However, novices must concentrate on the mechanics of driving and have little cognitive capacity available for other activities, which makes secondary task engagement among adolescent drivers so dangerous.

5. The law of space and time: The less distance in time and space between objects, the greater likelihood of a crash.

The main way to avoid crashes is to minimize the vehicle's proximity in space and time to other vehicles and hazards. Crashes occur when a vehicle hits another object—another vehicle, a stationary object, or a person. So anything that increases space and time between the vehicle and the other object provides safety effects. This principle is used successfully in road design to separate vehicles from each other, such as in divided highways, and vehicles from stationary roadside objects, such as trees and buildings. A key responsibility of drivers is to maintain safe time and distance from other objects, and this is another area where on average novices perform badly. Inattention and risky driving reduce space and time and increase crash risk.

The primary cause of crashes for drivers of all ages is inattention because it leads to reductions in time and space (Klauer et al. 2006). Drivers can react to hazards only to the extent they see them, recognize them as a hazard, and initiate avoidance maneuvers in a timely manner. When a driver takes his or her eyes off the forward roadway for any reason for a period of 2 seconds, the likelihood of a crash doubles (Klauer et al. 2006). Inattention is the dominant risk factor for crashes because it reduces the amount of time available for the driver to identify potential hazards and respond by braking or turning. Crashes are best avoided by early reaction to potential hazards because last second maneuvers are not effective and can lead to more serious problems.

Driving is a fairly routine task most of the time, and experienced drivers engage in a variety of secondary tasks, taking their eyes off the frontal roadway for brief periods of time, and are still able to maintain safety. Inattention, however brief, becomes dangerous when a driver is distracted for any reason, dialing a phone, reaching for an object, maintaining a prolonged glance away from the forward roadway, and something untoward occurs, for example, a vehicle or pedestrian enters the road ahead, altering the driving situation and demanding a reaction by the unobserving driver.

A recent study illustrates the heightened risk of inattention among novice young drivers. Sixteen newly licensed teenagers and 16 experienced adults drove with a research assistant on a test track with a lighted intersection. After a few passes, the study participants were given a cell phone and asked to complete a call and obtain certain information. As each participant engaged in the task, the intersection signal was turned amber at approximately 200 feet. All of the adults but less than 70% of the novices stopped at the light. The teens were good at the cell phone task, but many of them kept their eyes off the road for too long, whereas the experienced adults divided the task, looked up after dialing a few numbers, and were able to stop. Six months later the test was repeated with the same study participants with the identical result (Lee, Olsen, and Simons-Morton 2006). The conclusion of this research is that novices are not as good as adults at dividing their attention and are at risk for long periods of inattention, leading to driving errors, such as running a red light.

Likewise, driving is risky when it reduces time and space. Speeding, late braking, and close following are examples of risky driving that reduce space and time. Unfortunately, novices tend to stop late, turn hard, and follow closely, relative to adults, and this risky driving has the effect of reducing the amount of time to recognize and respond to potential hazards (Simons-Morton 2010).

6. The law of exposure: The more one drives, the greater the risk of crashing (although the rate per mile driven goes down with increased mileage).

   This law poses the following dilemma: Novices develop safe driving skills only with experience, but the more novices drive the more they crash. The solutions to this dilemma are to delay licensure and then to allow novices to drive for a time only under less risky driving conditions, such as during the day, without passengers, in fair weather, and on less congested, lower speed roads. Of course, ultimately, injuries due to MVCs will only be reduced substantially by reducing exposure of drivers in general. This can happen only by reducing the demand for individual modes of transportation and greater reliance on public modes of transportation.

Virtually all crash causes can be linked to one of these "laws." Crashes are more likely in inclement weather, particularly in areas where such weather is rare (NHTSA 2009d), consistent with Law 1. Crash rates are higher at night because night driving is more complex and cognitively challenging. Speeding and risky driving are causes of crashes and injury severity because they reduce the amount of space and time between vehicles or vehicles and objects (Klauer et al. 2006). Alcohol, drugs, and drowsiness are important risk factors for MVCs (Shope and Bingham 2008), because they diminish cognitive capacity, increase risk taking, and reduce attention. Secondary, nondriving tasks such as using cell phones, personal grooming, and reaching for objects result in inattention to the forward roadway, which reduces the amount of time available to react to potential road hazards (Klauer et al. 2006).

Moreover, although these universal laws apply to all drivers, they are particularly applicable to young and inexperienced drivers. The effect of teenage passengers on crash risk is a good example. Research has demonstrated an increased risk of teenage passengers on fatal crash risk among young drivers (Ouimet et al. 2010). In addition, it has been shown that in the presence of teenage passengers, teenage drivers drive faster and closer to the vehicle ahead, two good measures of risky driving (Simons-Morton, Lerner, and Singer 2005). However, it is not clear whether teenage passengers increase driving complexity, cognitive demands, or inattention, or they alter the in-vehicle social environment in such a way as to increase driver error or risk taking, thereby increasing crash risk.

Prevention Approaches

As with so many areas of prevention in general and injury prevention in particular, MVC injuries are multicausal and therefore may require comprehensive solutions. Indeed, any prevention measures that increase motor vehicle safety of the general population are likely to increase the safety of children and adolescents. Therefore, improvements in road designs, driving policies and enforcement, and vehicle safety are to be encouraged. However, because novice teenage driving is uniquely dangerous, considerable energy and resources have been devoted to programs to reduce young driver crash rates and improve safety. In this section, we describe the effectiveness and potential of the programs that have been developed specifically for adolescents. These include driver education, supervised practice driving, Graduated Driver Licensing (GDL), and parent involvement. In addition, a myriad of special prevention programs targeting safety belt use and drinking and driving have been reported, with generally negative findings (Table 4.2).

Although there are no special and efficacious programs for preventing crashes among the general population of drivers, there are such programs for novices. Effective prevention of novice teenage driving problems is based on the understanding that teenagers are not safe when first licensed and particularly at risk under more complex driving situations. Therefore, it is protective to delay licensure as long as possible and then limit driving to less risky conditions, at least for a time, while novices gain experience and develop competence. The special programs and policies directed at young drivers are shown in Table 4.2 and described next in terms of their purposes and safety effects.

Driver Education

Driver education generally achieves its primary goal of training novices in basic vehicle management skills and preparing them for licensure. Completing a driver education course certified by the state almost always leads to successful attainment of a license. These courses generally consist of a minimum of 6 hours of classroom and 4 to 8 hours of behind-the-wheel driving with an instructor. The classroom training is designed to prepare students to pass the licensing exam covering the "rules of the road." The on-road instruction is designed to prepare the student to pass the state driving test. Indeed, in many states these days the driving school instructor actually conducts the driving test and grades the student.

Although driver education does a good job at preparing novices for the licensing exam, there is no evidence that driver education provides safety effects. Indeed, recent reviews of studies in multiple countries found no evidence of safety effects of driver education programs (Clinton and Lonero 2006; Mayhew and Simpson 2002). In the United States, there is great variability in emphases by various driving schools and instructors and no evidence-based standards linking skills typically taught by driving instructors and independent driving outcomes. Meanwhile, there is evidence that hazard detection skills are important in safe driving, and training can improve hazard detection skills of novices (Pradhan et al. 2009), but these skills are seldom taught in

Table 4.2. Effectiveness of Prevention Solutions to the Young Driver Problem

Solution and Premise	Effectiveness
Driver Education: teach driving rules and vehicle management skills	No effectiveness demonstrated
Supervised Practice Driving: provide experience and improve vehicle management skills	No effectiveness demonstrated
GDL: limit driving under high-risk conditions	Significant reductions in crash outcomes demonstrated in multiple studies
Parenting: delay licensure, limit driving under high-risk conditions, set expectations for safe driving	Significant reductions in negative outcomes demonstrated in multiple studies
Safety belt use programs	Safety belt use can be increased through primary laws, vigorous enforcement, and education.
Drinking and driving prevention programs	Public information campaigns can be credited with reducing the prevalence of drinking and driving.

GDL = Graduated Driver Licensing.

driver education. "Advanced skills training" courses are now popular in many parts of the United States.

Basically, these programs teach novices how to get into and out of skids and the basics of avoiding a crash through last-second maneuvering. These programs have generally not been evaluated, but one study showed that participants actually had higher crash rates after the course than the controls (Gregersen 1996). In a subsequent trial with greater emphases on prevention, the same authors reported better results (Gregersen et al. 2000). However, to the extent these courses teach teenagers that crashes are a matter of maneuvering ability and not the prevention of the situations that require such maneuvering, they should be considered a threat to safety. In general, it is safe to conclude that driver education does an effective job of preparing novices for the licensing exam, but does not provide safety effects.

Supervised Practice Driving

In the United States, the minimum licensing requirements for parent-supervised driving have increased in recent years from a few hours to an average of 50 hours, similar to the amounts required and obtained in Australia and Canada. Many European countries require even more supervised practice driving than in the United States, and it is not uncommon for learners to complete more than 100 miles of supervised driving (Shope and Molnar 2003). The idea is that the more supervised practice driving novices get before licensure, the better they should be able to manage the vehicle, the more experience they should have under a wide range of driving conditions, and the more time parents would have to impress on their children the importance of safe driving behavior.

Although supervised practice driving is undoubtedly a good thing, there is surprisingly little evidence that the amount of parent-supervised practice driving is associated with reduced post-licensure crash rates. None of the few U.S. studies that have examined this question have shown effects. Likewise, no effect was found in a French study. A Swedish study of 18- to 20-year-old drivers found an effect on independent driving safety from a dramatic extension of the learner period and extensive supervised practice driving (Sagberg and Gregersen 2005). With respect to the United States, experts have argued for delaying training and licensure rather than moving it forward (Simons-Morton, Ouimet, and Catalano 2008). Indeed, the primary advantage of requirements for a high amount of supervised practice driving is that it delays the age at which adolescents get their driver's license and reduces driving exposure (McKnight and Peck 2002).

As shown in Figure 4.6, pre-license supervised practice driving is very safe, but as soon as adolescents get their license, their crash rates increase. No matter how much supervised practice driving teenagers obtain or the quality of instruction parents provide, there are a number of reasons that the safety benefits of supervised practice driving are likely to be limited. When supervising novice teenage drivers, instructors and parents can be expected to maintain a high priority on safety, guiding teenagers through complex driving situations, anticipating and warning of hazards, keeping the internal vehicle environment free from distraction, and otherwise co-driving. Most supervised practice is routine, exposing novices to limited variety in driving. The lack of varied practice and co-driving by parents could largely explain why parent-supervised practice driving is very safe relative to the early period of independent driving. Only with the onset of independent driving do teenagers begin to deal on their own with complex driving situations—some not encountered previously while supervised—often in the presence of teenage passengers (Simons-Morton et al. 2008).

Graduated Driver Licensing

GDL is based on the recognition that newly licensed teenagers need independent driving experience to become better, but this early experience should be gained under the least dangerous driving conditions possible (Williams and Ferguson, 2002). GDL has gradually been adopted by

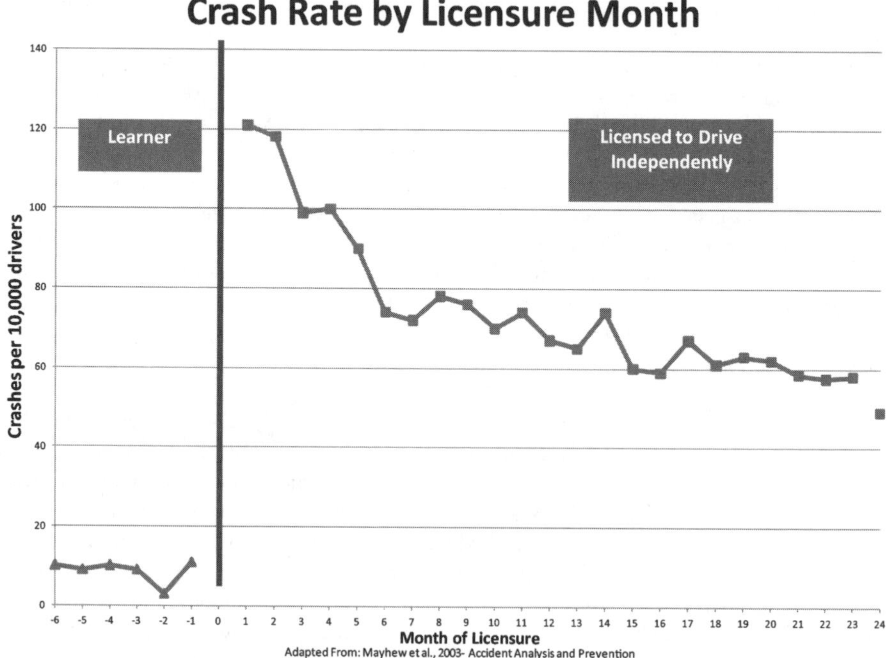

Figure 4.6. Crash Rates Based on Motor Vehicle Office Records for Nova Scotia, Canada. Source: Adapted from Mayhew, Simpson, and Pak 2003.

all Australian and Canadian provinces and each US state. GDL includes three stages: (1) the learner permit, with a long period of required adult-supervised practice driving; (2) the provisional license, with limits on late night driving, alcohol, and the number of teen passengers and the use of electronic devices while driving; and (3) the unrestricted license, usually after 12 months with a provisional license or at age 18 years and only when no violations have occurred. GDL has been evaluated frequently, and significant reductions in crashes and injuries have generally been reported. One of the effects of GDL is the requirement for approximately 50 hours of supervised practice during the learner permit, which has had the effect of delaying licensure, thereby reducing exposure.

GDL is generally enforced only when a teenager is stopped for another reason and is found by the police to also be in violation of GDL, for example, after midnight (Foss and Goodwin 2003). However, GDL does alter norms regarding the safety of novice teenage driving, delays licensure and reduces the amount of driving, and empowers parents to set limits on their newly licensed teenage children (Ferguson and Williams 2002; Simons-Morton 2007; Simons-Morton and Ouimet 2006). In any case, GDL has been demonstrated to improve safety outcomes in a range of evaluations (Chen, Baker, and Li 2006; Foss, Feaganes, and Rodgman 2001; Shope and Molnar 2003).

GDL is a developmentally appropriate approach to driving safety. It attempts to minimize the high risk of learning to drive by requiring much practice with supervising adults, presumably parents, so that teens gain experience and parents have ample opportunity to set standards and expectations. Then, adolescents are allowed to drive, but not under the most dangerous conditions, late at night, with multiple teenage passengers, or while impaired. However, GDL is not really enforced, and its main strengths are that it delays licensure and possibly the amount or nature of driving after licensure, and empowers parents to manage the first year of driving.

Parental Management of Novice Teenage Driving

Parenting practices and modeling provide important influences on adolescent behaviors of all kinds, and driving is no exception. Modest associations have been shown between parent and teenage child driving records, crash experience, and risky driving behavior. A major goal of parental management is to limit the complexity of driving conditions for some months after licensure while newly licensed teenagers develop complex driving skills. There are two promising and complementary approaches to parental management of novice teenage driving. The first is parent limit setting and the second provides electronic feedback to novice teenagers and parents about the teen's driving behavior.

Parent Limit Setting

Nearly all parents set modest limits on their newly licensed teenagers (Hartos et al. 2000). However, in general, these limits tend not to be strict, tend to focus on the details of the trip and not on safety, and quickly fade altogether in a matter of months. However, teenagers whose parents imposed more strict limits on teenage passengers and night driving reported less risky driving behavior and fewer traffic violations and crashes (Hartos, Eitel, and Simons-Morton, 2001; Simons-Morton et al. 2006a). The Checkpoints Program has been shown in several randomized trials to increase parental limit setting and improve safety outcomes by fostering the adoption of a parent–teen driving agreement that clarifies novice teenage driving limits and the requirements and timing for gaining additional driving privileges (Simons-Morton et al. 2006b, 2008).

Electronic Feedback

Teenagers may not realize their driving is risky, and there is no way for parents to know how their teenagers drive because they don't drive the same way on their own as they do when the parent is a passenger in the vehicle. Several recent studies have evaluated the effects of electronic devices installed in the vehicles of novice teenager drivers that provide visual feedback in the form of a blinking light each time the vehicle exceeds a set g-force limit (e.g., fast starts and hard braking and turning) assessed by an accelerometer. Some of these devices include cameras that record driver behavior and the forward roadway. The events are stored, downloaded, evaluated by remote staff, and made available each week for teen and parent access on a password-protected Web site.

Evaluations have shown that most teens reduce the number of triggered events within a few weeks after installation and maintain a low rate of events as long as their parents bother to review the weekly feedback (Carney et al. 2010; Farmer, Kirley, and McCartt 2009; McGehee et al. 2007). Unfortunately, only a small percentage of parents are willing to use these devices because they trust their teenager and do not want to invade teenage privacy or like the expense (Farmer, Kirley, and McCartt 2009). Moreover, in two of the studies, many participating parents quickly lost interest and stopped regularly reviewing the weekly reports.

Safety Belt Use

Safety belt use has dramatically increased in the United States since mandatory safety belt laws were instituted nationally in the 1980s. However, there remains a great deal of variability, with much higher rates in states with primary safety belt laws (where one can be ticketed for not wearing a safety belt) compared with states with secondary use laws (where one can be ticketed for not wearing a safety belt only if stopped for another reason). Moreover, use rates are lower for young drivers than for older drivers (NHTSA 2009d). Therefore, advocacy for primary safety belt laws is a public health priority. Vigorous enforcement, combined with public education, has been credited with improving safety belt use rates.

Drinking and Driving

Drinking and driving prevalence increases dramatically during adolescence and is higher among 18- to 24-year-olds than any other age group (Centers for Disease Control and Prevention, Injury Prevention and Control 2009; NHTSA 2009c). Of motor vehicle fatalities among teenagers and young adults, 22% are alcohol related (NHTSA 2009c). Drinking prevalence among adolescence is actually much lower in the United States than in Canada and many European countries (Simons-Morton et al. 2009), but the rates of drinking and driving are higher. The high rate of drinking and driving in the United States has been attributed to the strict policies against underage drinking (Grube and Nygaard 2001), which seems to lead to teenage drinking in cars (Chen et al. 2008). The risk factors for adolescent drinking and driving include early initiation and heavy drinking (Shope and Bingham 2002; Stoduto and Adlaf 2001; Zakrajsek and Shope 2006), tolerance for deviance (Bingham and Shope 2004), expectancies (Chen et al. 2008), lack of parental monitoring, and peer approval (Chen et al. 2008).

Rates of drinking and driving and alcohol-related crashes have declined in the past decade (NHTSA 2009c), and this decline is probably due to the decline in alcohol use among U.S. adolescents (Simons-Morton et al. 2009). This is in part due to more strict enforcement and public information campaigns, although it seems that the effectiveness of these campaigns depends on parental management and enforcement, and not simply on strict enforcement (Chen et al. 2008; Yu 1998). A major campaign to reduce youth drinking through coalitions was conducted in ten states from 1995 to 2004. The results for most outcomes were favorable, although not always significant (Wagenaar et al. 2006).

Recommendations

Given the importance of the problem, the clear identification of risk factors, and the known efficacy of some programs, reductions in young driver crashes can be facilitated by advances in research, dissemination of evidence-based practice, and advocacy with respect to policies and practices related to (1) safe roads, vehicles, and enforcement; (2) GDL laws; (3) parent management of novice teenage driver programs; (4) safety belt use; and (5) drinking and driving.

Child Passenger Protection

Riding in a motor vehicle is one of the most dangerous childhood activities. Children are at high risk for injuries due to MVCs because they are frequent passengers, highly vulnerable, and dependent on adults to drive safely and secure them appropriately. Also, child protective devices are complicated to use consistently and correctly.

Prevalence

MVCs are the leading cause of death for children from age 2 years (Centers for Disease Control and Prevention, Injury Prevention and Control 2010a, 2010b, 2010c; NHTSA 2008a, 2008b), an age group that is otherwise very healthy. This age group accounts for 4% of motor vehicle fatalities and 8% of injuries in 2008. When 15- to 20-year-olds are included, children and adolescents account for 21% of passenger fatalities, some 6379 deaths in 2006. Fatalities increase with age, being lowest among infants, somewhat higher among 1- to 7-year-olds, twice as high among 8- to 14-year-olds, and increasing dramatically among 15- to 20-year-olds, consistent with overall exposure and particularly to the increase in riding with young drivers.

Risk Factors

Child passengers experience the same risks as all passengers. Therefore, unsafe vehicles, unsafe roads, and unsafe driving put them at risk for crash-related injuries. Although risk increases with miles driven, the single most important risk factor is occupant restraint. Restraint use reduces fatalities by approximately half (NHTSA 2008b). Child passenger restraint use varies by child age and ethnicity. According to one NHTSA estimate (2009e), infants had relatively high restraint use, approximately 100% among White non-Hispanics, 96% among Hispanics, and 94% among Blacks. However, among children aged 1 to 3 years, restraint use was 99% among Whites, 84% among Hispanics, and 74% among Blacks. Likewise, rates were significantly lower for 4- to 12-year-olds among Hispanics and Blacks than Whites.

Prevention Approaches

Although the same principles that apply to the protection of adults from crashes and crash-related injuries apply to children, children are not adults and need special protection. The protection of occupants in MVCs requires attention to crash dynamics, the size and seat position of the occupants, and safety behavior. Engineering, education, and enforcement are required to ensure optimal protection (Bonnie, Fulco, and Liverman 1999), but engineers, educators, enforcement officers, legislators, and policy advocates speak different languages, and their efforts are not always in concert with each other or with sound evidence. As a result, some safety technology has been introduced that produced unacceptable levels of injurious side effects to children, and policy has lagged behind best practice, making education about passenger restraint complicated and relatively ineffective.

Since at least the 1950s, it has been understood that properly harnessed occupants could better survive crashes, and eventually vehicle manufacturers were required to install seat belts in new vehicles. However, there being no national seat belt law, each state created its own (under pressure from the federal government). Research regarding the unique safety requirements of child passengers came later. As with seat belts, state laws regarding childhood restraint vary by state. The development of child restraint systems has evolved gradually. Unlike new drug treatments for disease, vehicle safety technology is not evaluated by premarket clinical trials before licensure. Rather, the theoretic effectiveness of safety devices is based on laboratory studies and then introduced into the vehicle fleet. Over time, the effectiveness of the device and the unintended consequences emerge. Likewise, policy and advocacy regarding child restraint have evolved.

A range of passenger protective devices are now available, including seat belts, child car seats and booster seats, and air bags. Federal policy long emphasized passive rather than active restraints, and this resulted in some unintended consequences. Of note, for many years air bags were promoted by the NHTSA as an essential passenger protective device, particularly in light of then low rates of seat belt use. Consequently, policies and programs encouraging safety belt use lagged, and safety belt use remained generally less than 50% (Evans 2004). It is unfortunate that the expected benefits of air bags were not fully realized. Subsequent research demonstrated that safety belts alone are much more effective than air bags alone, and the safety effects of air bags are much greater in combination with safety belts than without (Evans 2004; NHTSA 2001). Moreover, as in other areas of passenger protection, the effects of air bags on the safety of children turned out to be even more complex than it was for adults.

Passenger protective devices are estimated to have saved 328,551 lives, approximately 25,000 in 2002 alone (NHTSA 2008a). However, some children are injured in crashes because restraint systems are improperly selected, positioned, or fitted (Bull and Durbin 2008). An increase in deaths due to air bag deployment among children aged less than 10 years has been noted (Braver et al. 1997). Appropriate rear seat restraint is protective in crashes with air bag deployment, whereas improper front seat restraint sharply increases injury risk (Bull and Durbin, 2008; Durbin et al. 2003).

We emphasize the objectives for preventing injuries to vehicle occupants after a crash, which include maximizing the prevalence of correct seat belts, child restraints, and air bags. As noted previously, proper road designs, signage, vehicle engineering, policies, and enforcement strategies are important for preventing crashes and injuries but are not discussed further except as they relate specifically to seat belts and child restraints. Air bags remain important to safety only when passengers are safely restrained.

Seat Belts

About the worst thing that can happen to a person in a crash is to be buffeted about the vehicle, striking the many dangerous objects within or, even worse, being thrown from the vehicle (Evans 2004). The secondary impact often causes as much damage as the initial impact in a crash. Therefore, seat belts, which secure the occupant within the vehicle, have proven to be highly effective in preventing injuries in the case of a crash (NHTSA 2008a). Seat belts dramatically improve the effectiveness of air bags; indeed, air bags are not very effective with unbelted passengers (NHTSA 2008a). Seat belts are appropriate for most children aged more than 8 years, although they could be ineffective or dangerous for 8-year-olds who are small for their age.

Despite their effectiveness, overall rates of seat belt use are approximately 82%, 79% for males (NHTSA 2008a). However, rates are lower among teenagers (77%) and Blacks (75%), and although use rates have increased approximately 5 percentage points since 2002, they have improved less among adolescents and declined somewhat among Blacks during that period (NHTSA 2008a). Occupants in fatal crashes have lower rates of restraint use than the general public, 68% among drivers and 63% among passengers. Risk factors other than male sex and Black race include riding as a passenger with a driver who is not buckled (NHTSA 2009d).

Although some educational programs have shown effects on safety belt use, many have not. However, primary enforcement laws have been shown to increase safety belt use (Calkins and Zlatoper 2001; Masten 2007; Scott 2007), and statewide media campaigns may be an important part of seat belt promotion (Decina et al. 2009), suggesting that some of the recalcitrance is simply the failure to develop the habit. However attitudes about seat belt use seem to vary by age among 8- to 15-year-olds, with information from peers and parents most valued (Kuhn and Lam 2008).

MVCs are the leading cause of injury and death during pregnancy in the United States (Weiss 2001a; Weiss, Songer, and Fabio 2001b), contributing to adverse fetal outcomes (Hyde et al. 2003). Restraint use is protective against injury in the case of a crash (Hyde et al. 2003), and women increase the frequency of restraint use once pregnant, but not always correctly, and in a crash, incorrect use can result in harm to the mother and fetus (Astarita and Feldman 1997). Many mothers do not know the correct way to wear a seat belt and do not believe that wearing a seat belt would be protective to them and to the fetus (McGwin et al. 2004). In addition, many pregnant women complain about the discomfort of wearing safety belts (McGwin et al. 2004). The shoulder belt should lay across the chest (between the breasts) and away from the neck. Move the front seat back as far as possible, while still comfortably reaching the pedals with at least 10 inches between the center of the chest and the steering wheel cover or dashboard.

The primary intervention to encourage pregnant mothers to wear seat belts is through prenatal counseling, but most pregnant women do not report being counseled about seat belt use (Siren et al. 2007).

Child Occupant Restraints

Child safety seats and booster seats have been credited with saving thousands of lives, reducing fatalities by 50% or more, and dramatically reducing injury severity (NHTSA 2008b). However, the systems are complex, installation procedures and requirements are not uniform, and some are better than others (American Academy of Pediatrics [AAP] 2002). Children should ride in a rear-facing seat to the highest weight that is allowed by the manufacturer of the seat to at least 1 year of age and at least 20 pounds (AAP 1996). When the child approaches 20 pounds, when his or her head is within 1 inch of the top of the seat, the child should be transferred to a convertible seat that is approved for rear-facing use to higher weight and height limits (AAP 2002).

Subsequently, at approximately age 4 years and weighing 40 pounds or larger, the child should be transferred to a forward-facing car seat secured in the back seat or to a booster seat, which allows the seat belt to work well with these children. Children aged less than 8 years should not be restrained simply by a seat belt, because seat belts often do not fit correctly. One study reported a 59% lower rate of injuries among 4- to 7-year-old children riding in a belt-positioning booster seat than in a seat belt alone (Durbin, Elliott, and Winston 2003). Moreover, children (and all passengers) are much safer in the rear than in the front seat of the vehicle (Bull and Durbin 2008). Using car and booster seats can be complicated because they only work well when the seat is well secured to the vehicle and the occupant to the seat. In 2002, the NHTSA required a new system, Lower Anchors and Tethers for Children (LATCH), in vehicles, greatly simplifying the task of securing the seat to the vehicle. Similarly, belt position systems have improved the security of car and booster seats (Durbin, Elliott, and Winston 2003).

Although there have been substantial improvements in the prevalence of restraint use in recent years, particularly among children aged 1 to 3 years, rates are lower among Hispanic children and still lower for Black than other children for all age groups, and rates decline with age among Blacks (Glassbrenner and Ye 2007). Glassbrenner and Ye note the findings in a national study indicating that 99% of 1- to 3-year-old White children were restrained, but only 93% of Hispanic and 89% of Black children were restrained. Among Blacks, restraint use was only 74% for 4- to 7-year-olds and 79% for 8- to 12-year-olds. Moreover, misuse of car seats remains substantial, up to 73% in a 2004 study (Decina and Lococo 2004). In a recent study, 34% of children from birth to 4 years, 40% of children aged 5- to 7-year-olds, and 52% of 8- to 12-year-olds were unrestrained (NHTSA 2009e). The transition from child to booster seat remains a challenge for many parents, with only 37% of 4- to 7-year-olds appropriately restrained in one recent study (Glassbrenner and Ye 2008). Poor and minorities are at particular disadvantage because child protective devices are expensive and more complicated to use in older vehicles.

By one recent estimate, 618,337 children aged less than 13 years rode unrestrained, more than 1 million rode in the front seat of a vehicle, and 11 million children aged 8 years or less used only adult seat belts (Greenspan, Dellinger, and Chen 2010).

Improving the Use of Child Restraints

There have been many efforts to improve the use of child restraint systems, and substantial progress has been made. However, significant minorities of infants and children are not restrained or improperly restrained. In a systematic review, Zaza and colleagues (2001) concluded that child safety seat laws and distribution programs were effective and enhanced by education. In a recent study, cost, inconvenience, child discomfort, lack of understanding of how booster seats work, and perceived risk of being ticketed have been identified as reasons why more children are not correctly restrained (Decina et al. 2009). A recent study with police officers indicated that the most effective approaches for enforcing booster seat laws included a primary booster seat law; resources to support dedicated booster seat law enforcement programs; enforcement methods, such as roadside checkpoints and dedicated roving patrols; and police officer training. Finally, a recent review of interventions to increase booster seats found that in addition to legislation, education and distribution of free booster seats (or discounts) increased the acquisition of booster seats (Ehiri et al. 2006).

Recommendations

Progress on child restraint has been made in many areas. Child safety seats are now better and easier to use. It is now well established when a child should move to a booster seat and then to an adult safety belt. Use rates have improved over time. However, use rates are lowest among adolescents and unsatisfactory among children, particularly in the transition to booster seats. Many children are improperly restrained. We know that primary enforcement and active enforcement are necessary and that once in place, well-designed education and public information campaigns are effective. However, laws in many states are deficient, enforcement is often lax, and many parents, particularly low income and racial minorities, fail to make the appropriate restraint transitions for their children. Although additional research is needed, particularly with respect to methods of facilitating the transition from child safety seats to booster seats, there is also a great need to increase the number of evidence-based programs designed to promote the use of child car safety seats. In addition, advocacy is needed to increase the compliance with child safety seat laws and to develop universal laws for booster seat use.

Child Pedestrian Safety

"When a car hits a child it is often treated as an accident, when a child hits a car it is considered vandalism" (Short and Pinet-Peralta 2010). As Short and Pinet-Peralta point out, there seems to be more societal concern about the damage to vehicles than about the damage vehicles do to children. Certainly a lot more resources are devoted to the maintenance of automobiles than to the prevention of MVCs involving children.

Prevalence

With increasing levels of obesity and heart disease, health experts are urging the population to walk and use more "active transportation;" however, it can be dangerous to be a pedestrian. Just in the last 15 years, 76,000 Americans have been killed while crossing or walking along a street. In 2008 alone, there were 69,000 pedestrian injuries and 4378 deaths in the United States (NHTSA 2008c). Although pedestrian MVC deaths have declined dramatically since 1975, they still account for 12% of crash deaths in the United States, and in some developing countries, pedestrian fatalities account for half of all crash deaths (NHTSA 2008c; Short and Pinet-Peralta 2010). To put these numbers in perspective, the number of pedestrian deaths is comparable to a jumbo jet crashing every month (Ernst and Shoup 2009). Or put another way, a pedestrian is killed approximately every 120 minutes and injured every 8 minutes (NHTSA 2008c).

Children, the elderly, and minority groups are disproportionately represented in the total number of pedestrian injuries (Ernst and Shoup 2009). Approximately 630 child pedestrian fatalities occur every year (National Safe Kids Campaign USA 2007), and 51,000 child pedestrians are injured (AAP 2009). Black children have a pedestrian injury death rate approximately twice that of White children (National Safe Kids Campaign USA 2007). Although the number of child pedestrian fatalities among children aged less than 14 years of age has decreased by 49% from 1997 to 2007, the decline is probably due to less walking and lower exposure to traffic (AAP 2009). Approximately 42% of school-aged children walked or biked to school in 1969 compared with only 16% today (AAP 2009).

Apart from the problems resulting from the various physical injuries, many preventable child pedestrian injuries result in emergency department visits. Pedestrian injuries account for 61% of all pediatric trauma admissions to U.S. hospitals and 34% of all pediatric critical care admissions (DiMaggio and Durkin 2002). Most pediatric pedestrian injuries are minor, but in the cases in which the injury is at least "moderate," traumatic brain injury is the most common pedestrian injury followed by extremity injury (Gunnels 2002). In addition to possible long-term physical complications, child pedestrian injury victims may also struggle with psychologic aftermath, such as acute stress disorder and posttraumatic stress disorder (AAP 2009). Depending on the age of the child, certain areas where children may be playing or walking pose more of a risk for injury. Younger children are more often injured in driveways when cars are backing up, children aged 4 to 6 years are injured in parking lots or mid-block while darting out into the street, and school-aged children are injured at street intersections (Agran, Winn, and Anderson 1994).

Risk Factors

Children aged 5 to 9 years have the highest population-based injury rate (Retting, Ferguson, and McCartt 2003). Although the improvements in pedestrian injury rates have been greatest among the youngest and oldest people (Figure 4.7), these groups are still at highest risk for pedestrian injury (Hotz et al. 2009; IIHS 2010c). In addition to age, sex is also a risk factor for pedestrian injuries. In 2008, 70% of pedestrians killed were male (NHTSA 2008c).

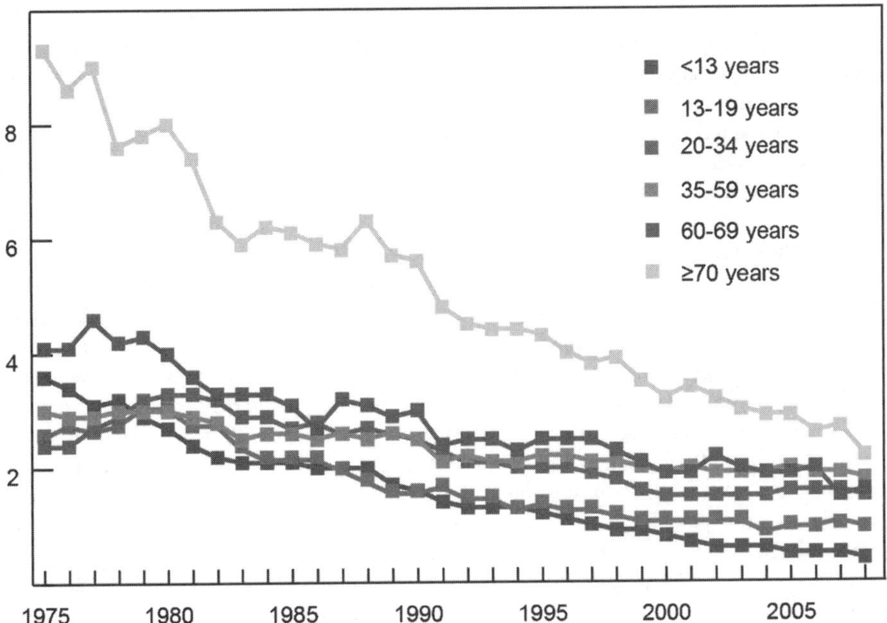

Figure 4.7. Pedestrian Deaths Per 100,000 People by Age, 1975–2008.
Source: Insurance Institute of Highway Safety 2010c.

Living in an urban area is an added risk factor for pedestrian injury. Children in urban neighborhoods cross the street more often and are exposed to more traffic and vehicles traveling at increased speeds. In addition, many urban neighborhoods have inadequate play areas that lead to children playing in the streets, often around parked cars that might obstruct a driver's view (AAP 2009; Posner et al. 2002). Seventy-two percent of pedestrian deaths in 2008 occurred in urban areas, up from 59% in 1975 (NHTSA 2008c). In urban areas, 54% of pedestrian deaths in 2008 occurred on roads with speed limits of 40 mph or less; in rural areas 24% of deaths occurred on such roads (NHTSA 2008c). In rural areas, lack of traffic-control devices and poor lighting are risk factors for pedestrians (AAP 2009). Adult pedestrians are more likely to be injured on major roads in contrast with children, who are more likely to be injured on neighborhood roads (Rothman et al. 2010). For children, 36% of pedestrian fatalities occur during the day (between 3 P.M. and 7 P.M.), and injury is more common during the spring and summer when children are playing outside.

Young children may have the motor skills to cross the roadways, but they often lack the cognitive, perceptual, and behavioral abilities to negotiate traffic (AAP 2009). The ability to identify safe and dangerous road-crossing sites and to ignore interference from irrelevant stimuli increases with age (Tabibi and Pfeffer 2003). Older children are better at identifying a safe place to cross the road, perceiving traffic and road dangers, and managing information from various parts of the traffic environment (AAP 2009; Whitebread and Neilson 2000). In general, children aged less than 10 years lack the maturity to correctly gauge the speed of vehicles and effectively use visual strategies to determine where to cross the road and how often to check for cars before crossing. The American Academy of Pediatrics policy statement on pedestrian safety states that because of developmental limitations that prevent children from being able to independently negotiate traffic, children should be supervised until at least age 10 years (AAP 2009).

Prevention Approaches

With increasing numbers of pedestrian injuries, different policy groups and organizations have recognized the importance of advocacy for child pedestrians. In the late 1980s, the World Health Organization stated that communities should adopt education, engineering, and enforcement strategies to limit child pedestrian injury through joint community and environmental interventions. Safe Kids Worldwide and other child safety organizations strongly support these recommendations (Hotz et al. 2009). In 2005, the Safe, Accountable, Flexible, Efficient Transportation Equity Act established a Safe Routes to School program with goals aimed to fix or improve sidewalks, execute traffic calming and speed reduction measures, improve pedestrian and bicycle crossings, and conduct public education campaigns to encourage walking and biking to school (National Safe Kids Campaign USA 2007). Recent state and local laws focus on trying to control and modify the environment with lower speed limits in residential areas, protecting pedestrians in crosswalks, improving pedestrian walkways, prohibiting vehicles from passing school buses while loading and unloading passengers, improving crossing guards, and requiring pedestrians to not cross streets at locations other than designated crosswalks (National Safe Kids Campaign USA 2007).

Many of the policies, such as lowering speed limits or reducing traffic in residential areas, protect adults as well as children, but the reality is that children have less developed pedestrian skills and therefore should receive effective pedestrian safety education. Despite the need, literature reviews suggest that there are few well-designed interventions that truly decrease child pedestrian injury (Hotz et al. 2009). The majority of child pedestrian safety programs take place in classrooms where educators teach children about traffic and how to use that information in real-life traffic situations, but classroom education and environmental modification alone are not effective solutions; thus, recent prevention programs have tried to focus on skills training in addition to behavioral evaluation (Hotz et al. 2009). There have been numerous educational interventions focused on child pedestrian safety, but none of the randomized clinical trials have shown a decrease in pediatric pedestrian injury rates. However, traffic skills-training programs have improved children's knowledge and observed street-crossing behaviors. From these studies,

Table 4.3. Pedestrian Injury Causes and Preventive Measures

Injury Causes	Preventive Measures
ENVIRONMENT	
Road design	Walking paths separated from traffic Wide sidewalks, fences, barriers, and raised medians/refuge islands Protected pedestrian crossings Improve signs Traffic signals exclusively for pedestriansImprove lighting Create more visibility for cars with landscaping
	No playing in driveways and alleyways Reflective clothing in low-light conditions Sidewalks near schools Safe routes for children to walk to school Well-trained crossing guards Community play areas away from traffic
	Traffic-calming measures, such as lower speed limits, rumble strips, speed bumps, and sidewalk bulbs Roundabouts Improve road laws and enforcement Improve signs
Vehicle traffic	Decrease traffic flow (especially during high-risk hours on residential streets)
VEHICLE	Automobile manufacturers develop designs that decrease injury from automobile–child pedestrian collisions
PERSON	
Driver	Driver education about pedestrians Driver manuals that teach drivers how to avoid pedestrian collisions
Child pedestrian's lack of developmental skills	Child pedestrian education programs Education interventions focused on parents, school safety personnel, school bus drivers, and community leaders Parents should be good role models. Parents should decide when a child can independently cross a street on the basis of age, maturity, volume and speed of traffic on street, and amount of on-street parking. American Academy of Pediatrics recommends that children should be supervised until age 10 years.

educators have learned that prevention strategies should be age specific (Brison, Wicklund, and Mueller 1988; Calhoun et al. 1998), and having parents or trainers as role models could increase the effectiveness of the program (Rivara et al. 1991). Table 4.3 presents pedestrian injury causes and preventive measures.

Recommendations

As with MVCs and occupant protection, a great deal is known about the nature of child pedestrian risks and how to reduce the prevalence of pedestrian injuries. Children often walk to school and around the neighborhood, which are both a good form of exercise and a risk factor for pedestrian injuries. Given the declining rates of physical activity and high rates of obesity, there are many good reasons to encourage children to walk, as noted in *Healthy People 2010* (U.S. Department of Health and Human Services 2010). However, to ensure safety, additional research is needed to develop evidence-based programs to encourage safe pedestrian behavior and parental management of child pedestrians. In addition, advocacy is needed to foster road and walkway designs that advance child pedestrian safety.

Conclusions

Motor vehicles remain the primary cause of injury and death to children, adolescents, and pregnant mothers and their fetuses. Progress has been made over the years as fatal crash rates have declined because of improvements in road designs, vehicle safety, and safety belt use. Behavior has also changed with higher rates of safety belt and car seat use in the past decade and lower prevalence of drinking and driving. However, mortality and morbidity rates remain high, particularly for population subgroups. The potential for prevention remains high, but progress is likely to occur through multiple approaches, including continued improvements in transportation safety and child safety seat and safety belt use. These improvements can only occur in an environment where safety is highly valued by the public and policymakers. There remains a great need for advocacy for improvements in road and vehicle safety, thoughtful licensing and driving policies and enforcement, public education, and targeted prevention efforts for vulnerable subgroups.

Acknowledgment

This work was supported by the Intramural Research Program of the National Institutes of Health, Eunice Kennedy Shriver National Institute of Child Health and Human Development, and the Health Resources and Services Administration.

References

Agran PF, Winn DG, Anderson CL. 1994. Differences in child pedestrian injury events by location. *Pediatrics.* 93:284–288.

American Academy of Pediatrics, Committee on Injury and Poison Prevention and Committee on Fetus and Newborn. 1996. Safe transportation of premature and low birth weight infants. *Pediatrics.* 97:758–760.

American Academy of Pediatrics, Committee on Injury and Poison Prevention. 2002. Selecting and using the most appropriate car safety seats for growing children: guidelines for counseling parents. *Pediatrics.* 109:550–553.

American Academy of Pediatrics, Committee on Injury, Violence, and Poison Prevention. 2009. Pedestrian safety. *Pediatrics.* 124:802–812.

American Association of State Highway and Transportation Officials. 2002. *AASHTO Roadside Design Guide.* 3rd ed. Available at: https://bookstore.transportation.org/item_details.aspx?ID=148. Accessed July 5, 2011.

Astarita DC, Feldman B. 1997. Seat belt placement resulting in uterine rupture. *J Trauma.* 47:738–740.

Bingham RC, Shope JT. 2004. Adolescent problem behavior and problem driving young adulthood. *J Adolesc Res.* 19:205–223.

Bonnie RJ, Fulco CE, Liverman CT. 1999. *Reducing the Burden of Injury: Advancing Prevention and Treatment.* Washington, DC: National Academy Press.

Braver ER, Ferguson SA, Greene MA, Lund AK. 1997. Reductions in deaths in frontal crashes among right front passengers in vehicles equipped with passenger airbags. *JAMA.* 278:1437–1439.

Brison RJ, Wicklund K, Mueller BA. 1988. Fatal pedestrian injuries to young children: a different pattern of injury. *Am J Public Health.* 78:793–795.

Bull MJ, Durbin DR. 2008. Rear-facing car safety seats: getting the message right. *Pediatrics.* 121:619–620.

Calhoun AD, McGwin G Jr, King WD, Rousculp MD. 1998. Pediatric pedestrian injuries: a community assessment using a hospital surveillance system. *Acad Emerg Med.* 5:685–690.

Calkins LN, Zlatoper TJ. 2001. The effects of mandatory seat belt laws on motor vehicle fatalities in the United States. *Soc Sci Q.* 82:716–732.

Carney C, McGehee DV, Lee JD. 2010. Using an event-triggered video intervention system to expand the supervised learning of newly licensed adolescent drivers. *Am J Public Health.* 100:1101–1106.

Centers for Disease Control and Prevention, Injury Prevention and Control: Data and Statistics. 2009. *Web-Based Injury Statistics Query and Reporting System (WISQARS) Leading Causes of Nonfatal Injury Reports, 2008.* Washington, DC: U.S. Department of Health and Human Services. Available at: http://webappa.cdc.gov/sasweb/ncipc/nfilead2001.html. Accessed July 5, 2011.

Centers for Disease Control and Prevention, Injury Prevention and Control: Data and Statistics. 2010a. *Web-Based Injury Statistics Query and Reporting System (WISQARS) Leading Causes of Death Reports, 1999-2007.* Washington, DC: U.S. Department of Health and Human Services. Available at: http://webappa.cdc.gov/sasweb/ncipc/leadcaus10.html. Accessed July 5, 2011.

Centers for Disease Control and Prevention, Injury Prevention and Control: Motor Vehicle Safety. 2010b. *Child Passenger Safety: Fact Sheet.* Washington, DC: U.S. Department of Health and Human Services. Available at: http://www.cdc.gov/ncipc/factsheets/childpas.html. Accessed July 5, 2011.

Centers for Disease Control and Prevention, Injury Prevention and Control: Motor Vehicle Safety. 2010c. *Teen Drivers: Fact Sheet.* Washington, DC: U.S. Department of Health and Human Services. Available at: http://www.cdc.gov/motorvehiclesafety/teen_drivers/teendrivers_factsheet.html. Accessed July 5, 2011.

Centers for Disease Control and Prevention. Youth Risk Behavior Surveillance – 2009. *MMWR* 2010;59(No. SS-5).

Chen L-H, Baker SP, Li G. 2006. Graduated driver licensing programs and fatal crashes of 16-year-old drivers: a national evaluation. *Pediatrics.* 118:56–62.

Chen M-J, Grube JW, Nygaard P, Miller BA. 2008. Identifying social mechanisms for the prevention of adolescent drinking and driving. *Accid Anal Prev.* 40:576–585.

Christoffel T, Gallagher SS. 2006. *Injury Prevention and Public Health: Practical Knowledge, Skills, and Strategies.* 2nd ed. Sudbury, MA: Jones and Bartlett Publishers.

Clinton KM, Lonero L. 2006. *Evaluating Driver Education Programs: Comprehensive Guidelines.* Washington, DC: AAA Foundation for Traffic Safety. Available at: http://www.aaafoundation.org/pdf/EvaluatingDriverEducationProgramsGuidelines.pdf. Accessed July 5, 2011.

Decina LE, Lococo KH. 2004. *Misuse of Child Restraints.* Washington, DC: National Highway Traffic Safety Administration. Available at: http://www.nhtsa.gov/people/injury/research/misuse/images/misusescreen.pdf. Accessed July 5, 2011.

Decina LE, Lococo KH, Ashburn W, Rose J. 2009. *Identifying Strategies to Reduce the Percentage of Unrestrained Young Children.* Washington, DC: National Highway Traffic Safety Administration. Available at: http://www.nhtsa.gov/DOT/NHTSA/Traffic%20Injury%20Control/Articles/Associated%20Files/811076.pdf. Accessed July 5, 2011.

DiMaggio C, Durkin M. 2002. Child pedestrian injury in an urban setting: descriptive epidemiology. *Acad Emerg Med.* 9:54–62.

Durbin DR, Elliott MR, Winston FK. 2003. Belt-positioning booster seats and reduction in risk of injury among children in vehicle crashes. *JAMA.* 289:2835–2840.

Durbin DR, Kallan M, Elliott M, et al. 2003. Risk of injury to restrained children from passenger air bags. *Traffic Inj Prev.* 4:58–63.

Ehiri J, King W, Ejere HOD, Mouzon P. 2006. *Effects of interventions to increase use of booster seats in motor vehicle for 4-8 year olds.* Washington, DC: AAA Foundation for Traffic Safety Available at: http://www.aaafoundation.org/pdf/BoosterSeatsReport.pdf. Accessed July 5, 2011.

Elvik R. 2006. Laws of accident causation. *Accid Anal Prev.* 38:742–747.

Ernst M, Shoup L. 2009. *Dangerous by Design: Solving the Epidemic of Preventable Deaths (and Making Great Neighborhoods).* Washington, DC: Transportation for America. Available at: http://t4america.org/docs/dangerousbydesign/dangerous_by_design.pdf. Accessed July 7, 2011.

Evans L. 2004. *Traffic Safety.* Bloomfield Hills, MI: Science Serving Society.

Farmer CM, Kirley BB, McCartt AT. 2009. Effects of in-vehicle monitoring and the driving behavior of teenagers. *J Safety Res.* 41:39–45.

Ferguson SA, Williams AF. 2002. Awareness of zero tolerance laws in three states. *J Safety Res.* 33:293–299.

Foss FD, Goodwin A. 2003. Enhancing the effectiveness of graduated driver licensing legislation. *J Safety Res.* 34:79–84.

Foss RD, Feaganes JR, Rodgman EA. 2001. Initial effects of graduated driver licensing on 16-year-old driver crashes in North Carolina. *JAMA.* 286:1588–1592.

Glassbrenner D, Ye TJ. 2007. *Child Restraint Use in 2006: Demographic Results.* Washington, DC: National Highway Traffic Safety Administration. Available at: http://www-nrd.nhtsa.dot.gov/Pubs/810797.PDF. Accessed July 5, 2011.

Glassbrenner D, Ye TJ. 2008. *Booster Seat Use in 2007.* Washington, DC: National Highway Traffic Safety Administration. Available at: http://www-nrd.nhtsa.dot.gov/Pubs/810894.PDF. Accessed July 5, 2011.

GlobalSecurity.org. 2009. *Military: U.S. Casualties in Iraq.* Available at: http://www.globalsecurity.org/military/ops/iraq_casualties.htm. Accessed July 5, 2011.

Greenspan AI, Dellinger AM, Chen J. 2010. Restraint use and seating position among children less than 13 years of age: is it still a problem? *J Safety Res.* 41:183–185.

Gregersen NP. 1996. Young drivers' overestimation of their own skill: an experiment on the relation between training strategy and skill. *Accid Anal Prev.* 28:243–250.

Gregersen NP, Berg H-Y, Engstrom I, et al. 2000. Sixteen years age limit for learner drivers in Sweden: an evaluation of safety effects. *Accid Anal Prev.* 32:25–35.

Groeger JA. 2000. Understanding Driving: Applying Cognitive Psychology to a Complex Everyday Task. Philadelphia, PA: Taylor & Francis.

Grube JW, Nygaard P. 2001. Adolescent drinking and alcohol policy. *Contemp Drug Probl.* 28:87–131.

Gunnels MD. 2002. Pedestrian trauma: what types of injury can we expect to see when an injured child arrives? *J Emerg Nurs.* 28:259–261.

Haddon W, Baker SP. 1981. Injury control. In: Clarke D, MacMahon B, editors. *Preventive and Community Medicine.* New York: Little, Brown. 109–140.

Hartos JL, Eitel P, Haynie DL, Simons-Morton BG. 2000. Can I take the car?: relations among parenting practices and adolescent problem driving practices. *J Adolesc Res.* 15:352–367.

Hartos JL, Eitel P, Simons-Morton BG. 2001. Do parent-imposed delayed licensure and restricted driving reduce risky driving behaviors among newly-licensed teens? *Prev Sci.* 2:111–120.

Hatfield J, Fernandes R. 2009. The role of risk-propensity in the risky driving of younger drivers. *Accid Anal Prev.* 41:25–35.

Heron M, Hoyert DL, Murphy SL, et al. 2009. Deaths: final data for 2006. *Natl Vital Stat Rep.* 57:1–135.

Hotz G, Kennedy A, Lutfi K, Cohn SM. 2009. Preventing pediatric pedestrian injuries. *J Trauma.* 66:1492–1499.

Hyde LK, Cook LJ, Olson LM, et al. 2003. Effect of motor vehicle crashes on adverse fetal outcomes. *Obstet Gynecol.* 102:279–286.

Insurance Institute for Highway Safety. 2010a. *Fatality Facts 2007: Teenagers.* Available at http://www.iihs.org/research/fatality_facts_2008/teenagers. Accessed July 7, 2011.

Insurance Institute for Highway Safety. 2010b. *Fatality Facts 2008: Children.* Available at: http://www.iihs.org/research/fatality_facts_2008/children.html. Accessed July 5, 2011.

Insurance Institute for Highway Safety. 2010c. *Fatality Facts 2008: Pedestrians.* Available at: http://www.iihs.org/research/fatality_facts_2008/pedestrians.html. Accessed July 5, 2011.

Insurance Institute for Highway Safety. 2010d. *Top Safety Picks 2010.* Available at: http://www.iihs.org/ratings/. Accessed July 5, 2011.

Keating DP, Halpern-Felsher BL. 2008. Adolescent drivers: a developmental perspective on risk, proficiency, and safety. *Am J Prev Med.* 35:S272–S277.

Klauer SG, Dingus TA, Neale VL. 2006. *The Impact of Driver Inattention on Near-Crash/Crash Risk: An Analysis Using the 100-Car Naturalistic Driving Study Data.* Washington, DC: National Highway Traffic Safety Administration. Available at: http://www.nhtsa.gov/DOT/NHTSA/NRD/Multimedia/PDFs/Crash%20Avoidance/Driver%20Distraction/810594.pdf. Accessed July 5, 2011.

Kuhn M, Lam J. 2008. *Increasing Seat Belt Use Among 8- to 15-Year-Olds: Volume I: Findings.* Washington, DC: National Highway Traffic Safety Administration. Available at: http://www.nhtsa.gov/DOT/NHTSA/Traffic%20Injury%20Control/Articles/Associated%20Files/810965.pdf. Accessed July 5, 2011.

Lee SE, Olsen ECB, Simons-Morton BG. 2006. Eyeglance behavior of novice teen and experienced adult drivers. *Transp Res Rec.* 1980:57–64.

Mahmood HF, Fileta BB. 2004. *Design of Vehicle Structures for Crash Energy Management.* Washington, DC: American Iron and Steel Institute. Available at: http://www.autosteel.org/AM/Template.cfm?Section=Safety_Book&CONTENTID=28388&TEMPLATE=/CM/ContentDisplay.cfm. Accessed July 9, 2011.

Masten SV. 2007. Do states upgrading to primary enforcement of safety belt laws experience increased daytime and nighttime belt use? *Accid Anal Prev* 39:1131–1139.

Mayhew DR, Simpson HM. 2002. The safety value of driver education and training. *Inj Prev.* 8:ii3–118.

Mayhew DR, Simpson HM, Pak A. 2003. Changes in collision rates among novice drivers during the first months of driving. *Accid Anal Prev.* 35:683–691.

Mayhew DR, Simpson HM, Singhal D, Desmond K. 2006. *Reducing the Crash Risk for Young Drivers.* Washington, DC: AAA Foundation for Traffic Safety (June). Available at: http://www.aaafoundation.org/pdf/ReducingTeenCrashes.pdf. Accessed July 5, 2011.

McCartt AT, Shabanova VI, Leaf WA. 2003. Driving experience, crashes, and traffic citations of teenage beginning drivers. *Accid Anal Prev.* 35:311–320.

McGehee DV, Raby M, Carney C, et al. 2007. Extending parental mentoring using an event-triggered video intervention in rural teen drivers. *J Safety Res.* 38:215–227.

McGwin G, Russell SR, Rux RL, et al. 2004. Knowledge, beliefs, and practices concerning seat belt use during pregnancy. *J Trauma.* 56:670–675.

McKnight AJ, McKnight AS. 2003. Young novice drivers: careless or clueless? *Accid Anal Prev.* 35:921–923.

McKnight AJ, Peck RC. 2002. Graduated driver licensing: what works? *Inj Prev.* 8:ii32–ii38.

National Highway Traffic Safety Administration. 2001. *Fifth/Sixth Report to Congress. Effectiveness of Occupant Protection Systems and Their Use.* Available at: http://www-nrd.nhtsa.dot.gov/Pubs/809-442.PDF. Accessed July 5, 2011.

National Highway Traffic Safety Administration. 2008a. *2006 Motor Vehicle Occupant Protection Facts.* Available at: http://www.nhtsa.gov/DOT/NHTSA/Traffic%20Injury%20Control/Articles/Associated%20Files/810654.pdf. Accessed July 5, 2011.

National Highway Traffic Safety Administration. 2008b. *Traffic Safety Facts, 2007 Data: Children.* Available at: http://www.dmv.ne.gov/highwaysafety/pdf/TSFChildren2007.pdf. Accessed July 5, 2011.

National Highway Traffic Safety Administration. 2008c. *Traffic Safety Facts, 2008 Data: Pedestrians.* Available at: http://www-nrd.nhtsa.dot.gov/Pubs/811163.pdf. Accessed July 5, 2011.

National Highway Traffic Safety Administration. 2009a. *Fatality Analysis Reporting System (FARS), 2008.* Available at: http://www.nhtsa.gov/FARS. Accessed July 5, 2011.

National Highway Traffic Safety Administration. 2009b. *Traffic Safety Facts, 2006 Data: Race and Ethnicity.* Available at: http://www-nrd.nhtsa.dot.gov/Pubs/810995.pdf. Accessed July 5, 2011.

National Highway Traffic Safety Administration. 2009c. *Traffic Safety Facts, 2008 Data: Alcohol-Impaired Driving.* Available at: http://www-nrd.nhtsa.dot.gov/Pubs/811155.pdf. Accessed July 5, 2011.

National Highway Traffic Safety Administration. 2009d. *Traffic Safety Facts, 2008 Data: Overview.* Available at: http://www-nrd.nhtsa.dot.gov/Pubs/811162.pdf. Accessed July 5, 2011.

National Highway Traffic Safety Administration. 2009e. *Traffic Safety Facts, 2008 Data: Young Drivers.* Available at: http://www-nrd.nhtsa.dot.gov/Pubs/811169.pdf. Accessed July 5, 2011.

National Highway Traffic Safety Administration. 2010. *Traffic Safety Facts: Early Estimates of Motor Vehicle Traffic Fatalities in 2009.* Available at: http://www-nrd.nhtsa.dot.gov/pubs/811291.pdf. Accessed July 5, 2011.

National Safe Kids Campaign USA. 2007. *Pedestrian Safety Fact Sheet.* Safe Kids Worldwide. Available at: http://www.safekids.org/our-work/research/fact-sheets/pedestrian-safety-fact-sheet.html. Accessed July 5, 2011.

National Transportation Safety Board, Aviation Accident Statistics. 2010. *Table 1. Accidents, Fatalities, and Rates, 2009 Preliminary Statistics, U.S. Aviation.* Available at: http://www.ntsb.gov/aviation/Table1.htm. Accessed July 5, 2011.

Organization for Economic Co-operation and Development. 2006. *Young Drivers: The Road to Safety.* Available at: www.oecd.org/dataoecd/17/28/37556934.pdf. Accessed July 5, 2011.

Ouimet MC, Simons-Morton BG, Zador PL, et al. 2010. Using the U.S. National Household Travel Survey to estimate the impact of passenger characteristics on young drivers' relative risk of fatal crash involvement. *Accid Anal Prev.* 42:689–694.

Posner JC, Liao E, Winston FK, et al. 2002. Exposure to traffic among urban children injured as pedestrians. *Inj Prev.* 8:231–235.

Pradhan AK, Hammel KR, DeRamus R, et al. 2005. Using eye movements to evaluate the effects of driver age on risk perception in a driving simulator. *Hum Factors.* 47:840–852.

Pradhan AK, Pollatsek A, Knodler M, Fisher DL. 2009. Can younger drivers be trained to scan for information that will reduce their risk in roadway traffic scenarios that are hard to identify as hazardous? *Ergonomics.* 52:657–673.

Retting RA, Ferguson SA, McCartt AT. 2003. A review of evidence-based traffic engineering measures designed to reduce pedestrian-motor vehicle crashes. *Am J Public Health.* 93:1456–1463.

Rivara FP, Booth CL, Bergman AB, et al. 1991. Prevention of pedestrian injuries to children: effectiveness of a school training program. *Pediatrics.* 88:770–775.

Roadway Safety Foundation. 2004. *Roadway Safety Guide.* Available at: http://www.roadwaysafety.org/wp-content/uploads/guide3.pdf. Accessed July 5, 2011.

Rothman L, Slater M, Meaney C, Howard A. 2010. Motor vehicle and pedestrian collisions: burden of severe injury on major versus neighborhood roads. *Traffic Inj Prev.* 11:43–47.

Sagberg F, Gregersen NP. 2005. Effects of lowering the age limit for driver training. In: Underwood G, editor. *Traffic and Transport Psychology: Theory and Application.* Amsterdam, The Netherlands: Elsevier Science. 171–178.

Scott M. 2007. *The Effects of Changing to Primary Enforcement on Daytime and Nighttime Seat Belt Use.* Washington, DC: National Highway Traffic Safety Administration. Available at: http://www.nhtsa.gov/DOT/NHTSA/Traffic%20Injury%20Control/Articles/Associated%20Files/810743.pdf. Accessed July 5, 2011.

Shope JT, Bingham CR. 2002. Drinking-driving as a component of problem driving and problem behavior in young adults. *J Stud Alcohol Drugs.* 63:24–33.

Shope JT, Bingham CR. 2008. Teen driving: motor-vehicle crashes and factors that contribute. *Am J Prev Med.* 35:S261–S271.

Shope JT, Molnar LJ. 2003. Graduated driver licensing in the United States: evaluation results from the early programs. *J Safety Res.* 34:63–69.

Short JR, Pinet-Peralta LM. 2010. No accident: traffic and pedestrians in the modern city. *Mobilities.* 5:41–59.

Simons-Morton BG. 2007. Parent involvement in novice teen driving: rationale, evidence of effects, and potential for enhancing graduated driver licensing effectiveness. *J Safety Res.* 38:193–202.

Simons-Morton BG. 2010. *Driving performance and risk of novice teenagers compared with parents.* Presented at: the National Meeting of the Transportation Research Board; January 13; Washington DC.

Simons-Morton BG, Farhat T, ter Bogt TFM, et al. 2009. Gender specific trends in alcohol use: cross-cultural comparisons from 1998 to 2006 in 24 countries and regions. *Int J Public Health.* 54:S199–S208.

Simons-Morton BG, Hartos JL, Leaf WA, Preusser DF. 2006a. Do recommended driving limits affect teen-reported tickets and crashes during the first year of teen independent driving? *Traffic Inj Prev.* 7:1–10.

Simons-Morton BG, Hartos JL, Leaf WA, Preusser DF. 2006b. The effect on teen driving outcomes of the checkpoints program in a state-wide trial. *Accid Anal Prev.* 38:907–912.

Simons-Morton BG, Lerner N, Singer J. 2005. The observed effects of teen passengers on the risky driving behavior among young drivers. *Accid Anal Prev.* 37:973–982.

Simons-Morton BG, Ouimet MC. 2006. Parent involvement in novice teen driving: a review of the literature. *Inj Prev.* 12:i30–i37.

Simons-Morton BG, Ouimet MC, Catalano RF. 2008. Parenting and the young driver problem. *Am J Prev Med.* 35:S294–S303.

Simons-Morton BG, Ouimet MC, Wang J, et al. 2010. Hard braking events among novice teenage drivers by passenger characteristics. Driving Assessment. In: *Procedings, Fifth International Driving Symposium on Human Factors in Driving Assessment, Training and Vehicle Design, Big Sky, Montana.* The University of Iowa, Iowa City. 236–242.

Siren H, Weiss HB, Sauber-Schatz EK, Dunning K. 2007. Seat belt use, counseling and motor-vehicle injury during pregnancy: results from a multi-state population-based survey. *Matern Child Health J.* 11:505–510.

Steinberg L. 2004. Risk taking in adolescence: what changes, and why? *Ann N Y Acad Sci.* 1021:51–58.

Stoduto G, Adlaf EM. 2001. A typology of adolescent drinking-drivers. *J Child Adolesc Subst Abuse.* 10:43–58.

Tabibi Z, Pfeffer K. 2003. Choosing a safe place to cross the road: the relationship between attention and identification of safe and dangerous road-crossing sites. *Child Care Health Dev.* 29:237–244.

Transport Canada. 2010. *Road and Motor Vehicle Safety.* Available at: http://www.tc.gc.ca/eng/roadsafety/menu.htm. Accessed July 5, 2011.

Transportation Research Board. 2004. National Cooperative Highway Research Program report 500: Guidance for Implementation of the AASHTO Strategic Highway Safety Plan. Washington, DC: American Association of State Highway and Transportation Officials.

Twisk DAM, Stacey C. 2007. Trends in young driver risk and countermeasures in European countries. *J Safety Res.* 38:245–257.

U.S. Department of Health and Human Services. 2010. *Healthy People 2010.* Washington DC: Office of Disease Prevention and Health Promotion. Available at: http://www.healthypeople.gov/. Accessed July 5, 2011.

Vanderbilt T. 2009. *Traffic: Why We Drive the Way We Do and What It Says About Us.* New York: First Vantage Books.

Wagenaar AC, Erickson DJ, Jarwood EM, O'Malley PM. 2006. Effects of state coalitions to reduce underage drinking: a national evaluation. *Am J Prev Med.* 31:307–315.

Whitebread D, Neilson K. 2000. The contribution of visual search strategies to the development of pedestrian skills by 4-11 year-old children. *Br J Educ Psychol.* 70:539–557.

Weiss HB. 2001a. The epidemiology of traumatic injury related fetal mortality in Pennsylvania, 1995-1997: the role of motor vehicle crashes. *Accid Anal Prev.* 33:449–454.

Weiss HB, Songer TJ, Fabio A. 2001b. Causes of traumatic death during the pregnancy. *JAMA.* 285:2554–2555.

Williams AF. 2003. Teenage drivers: patterns of risk. *J Safety Res.* 34:5–15.

Williams AF, Ferguson SA. 2002. Rationale for graduated licensing and the risks it should address. *Inj Prev.* 8:ii9–ii13.

World Health Organization. 2009. *Global Status Report on Road Safety: Time for Action.* Available at: http://whqlibdoc.who.int/publications/2009/9789241563840_eng.pdf. Accessed July 5, 2011.

Yu J. 1998. Perceived parental/peer attitudes and alcohol-related behaviors: an analysis of the impact of the drinking age law. *Subst Use Misuse.* 33:2687–2702.

Zakrajsek JS, Shope JT. 2006. Longitudinal examination of underage drinking and subsequent drinking and risky driving. *J Safety Res.* 37:443–451.

Zaza S, Sleet DA, Thompson RS, et al. 2001. Reviews of evidence regarding interventions to increase use of child safety seats. *Am J Prev Med.* 21(4S):31–47.

Chapter 5

Home Injuries

Eileen M. McDonald, MS,[1] *Deborah C. Girasek, PhD, MPH,*[2,3] *and Andrea Carlson Gielen, ScD, ScM, CHES*[1]

Mid pleasures and palaces though we may roam,
Be it ever so humble, there's no place like home.

—John Howard Payne

The first two lines of American poet and playwright John Howard Payne's popular 1822 song, "Home Sweet Home," belies the potential for harm that can occur in the typical American home. We like to think of our homes as a retreat; somewhere to unwind, recharge, and—most of all—be with our families. It is unsettling to realize, then, that the home is one of the most common settings in which injuries are sustained, especially for young children. Most young children spend their days in and around their homes or that of caregivers. Older children are most likely to be injured at home during after school hours. The U.S. Census Bureau reports that more than 5 million school-age children are left home alone during a typical week (Laughlin 2005). It is not surprising, then, that more than 4 million children younger than 19 years visit emergency departments for the treatment of home injuries each year (Runyan and Casteel 2004a), and more than 2500 in this same age group die as a result of injuries sustained in the home (Runyan and Casteel 2004b).

Children younger than 15 years are considered one of two high-risk age groups for unintentional injuries in the home; adults older than 70 years comprise the other high-risk group. Among children aged 0 to 14 years, the leading causes of home injury death are fire/burns, choking/suffocation, drowning/submersion, firearms, and poisonings (Table 5.1). As children approach adulthood, their risk of dying from injuries suffered at home generally declines, although the risk of unintentional poisoning increases dramatically. Males throughout their life span are at higher risk of death from home injury, compared with females (Runyan et al. 2005).

For every home injury death among children younger than 15 years, there are approximately 1500 nonfatal home injuries (Runyan and Casteel 2004a). Of injuries that result in visits to the emergency department, children aged 0 to 14 years experienced a higher rate of serious nonfatal home injury than any other age group. Falls are the leading cause of these nonfatal injuries (Table 5.2) (Casteel and Runyan 2004a).

This chapter will touch on many of the major threats that children and adolescents face at home: unintentional fire/burns, poisoning, falls, and choking/suffocation. We will also cover animal bites and stings, an often unrecognized home injury risk despite being the fifth leading cause of injury-related hospital emergency department visits among children in the United States

[1]Johns Hopkins Bloomberg School of Public Health, Department of Health, Behavior and Society, and the Johns Hopkins Center for Injury Research and Policy, Baltimore, Maryland.

[2]Uniformed Services University of the Health Sciences, Bethesda, Maryland.

[3]The views expressed are those of the author, who was not writing as a representative of any government agency.

Table 5.1. Unintentional Home Injury Deaths Involving Children: Leading Causes of Death, Ranked by Rate (per 100,000 persons): United States, 1992–1999.

Rank	<1	1–4	5–9	10–14	Total <15
1	Choking/ suffocation	Fire/burn	Fire/burn	Fire/burn	Fire/burn
2	Fire/burn	Drowning/ submersion	Drowning/ submersion	Firearm	Choking/ suffocation
3	Drowning/ submersion	Choking/ suffocation	Choking/ suffocation	Choking/ suffocation	Drowning/ submersion
4	Fall[a] Poisoning[a]	Fall	Firearm	Poisoning	Firearm
5	. . .	Struck by/ against	Fall	Drowning/ submersion	Poisoning

[a]Tied as fourth leading cause.

From Home Safety Council 2004.

(National Center for Injury Prevention and Control 2007b). We also briefly address a few new and novel household items that have been recently linked to unintentional home injury. Home-related drowning, nursery products, playground equipment, firearms, and violence will be addressed in other chapters.

Table 5.2. Nonfatal Unintentional Home Injury Resulting in Emergency Department Visits and Involving Children: Leading Causes of Injury, Ranked by Rate (per 100,000 persons): United States, 1993–2000

Rank	<1	1–4	5–9	10–14	Total <15
1	Fall	Fall	Fall	Fall	Fall
2	Struck by/ against	Struck by/ against	Struck by/ against	Struck by/ against	Struck by/ against
3	Miscellaneous	Miscellaneous	Cut/pierce	Cut/pierce	Cut/pierce
4	Fire/burn	Cut/pierce	Miscellaneous	Miscellaneous	Miscellaneous
5	Unspecified	Natural/ environmental	Natural/ environmental	Natural/ environmental	Natural/ environmental

From Home Safety Council 2004.

Each section is organized to give readers a sense of why we have included the topic: its importance, how such injuries occur, what is known about high-risk populations and circumstances, and what can be done to prevent each type of injury. There are also stories about children—*true* stories of children who were hurt or killed in their homes.

It is important to remember that the statistics in this book represent real families, like that of a 4-year-old girl who was found by her mother pinned under the garage door of an apartment building where she had been playing in the basement. The girl was resuscitated at the scene but died 70 days later of her injuries (Kriel et al. 1996).

Such tragedies evoke calls for safer products, better supervision, government regulation, and public education. Each of these remedies has a role to play in reducing child home injuries. We will share success stories as well, describing programs that have been documented as effective and advocacy efforts that have brought about important social change.

Our goal was to work from an evidence base in pulling together the material that follows, but we frequently call for more research or better data. The work by Runyan and Casteel (2004c), representing the best snapshot available of childhood injuries in the home, uses data that are now more than a decade old. More recent work by the Centers for Disease Control and Prevention (CDC) (Bornse et al. 2008) provides a more current (and slightly different) picture of childhood injuries, but it is not specific to those that occur in the home. Our desire to be evidenced-based was also challenged because a large proportion of injuries are reported to public health authorities with no information about the location of the event. Therefore, we may assume that many estimates of home injuries are underreports of the true scale of the problem. As yet, there is not even one standard definition of what constitutes a "home" for the purposes of scientific research. So, although the field of injury prevention and control continues to advocate for more systematically collected and better quality data, some progress is being made to reduce the burden of home injury, as reflected in the information in the pages that follow.

Fire and Burn Injuries

Residential fires are the most common source of burn injuries in children. Newspaper articles such as the one below (Box 5.1) are common and tell of the continuing toll wrought by fire and burns injuries. But glaring in its absence is any mention of whether working smoke alarms were in the home. The reader of such a news story also would be hard-pressed to appreciate how this house fire fits into the larger problem of residential fires in Pennsylvania or the United States. These are significant missed opportunities for enhanced advocacy for fire prevention and fire response resources and inappropriately reinforce the perception that such injury events are unavoidable, isolated, and infrequent. Nothing could be further from the truth.

According to the National Fire Protection Association, in 2009, U.S. fire departments responded to an estimated 1.3 million fires. Overall, 3010 civilians died in fires, an increase of 9.3% from the previous year; 2565 of these deaths occurred in the home, a decrease of approximately 7%. Despite the fact that many minor injuries are not reported to the fire service, 13,050 injuries occurred in residential properties. This same year, residential fires caused property damage in excess of $7.7 billion (Karter 2010).

Home fires constitute the lion's share of fatal fire and burn events. Cooking is the leading cause of home fires, but smoking materials are the cause of most home fire deaths (Ahrens 2010). Children as young as 2 years have caused home fires playing with matches and lighters (Smith, Greene, and Singh 2000), products that have been identified as a significant contributor to the fire burden both nationally and internationally (Leistikow, Martin, and Milano 2000). Other products ubiquitous to the home environment also cause fires or can produce burn injuries themselves. These common household items include wax- and oil-burning candles, stoves and microwave ovens, wood-burning stoves and fireplaces (Dunst et al. 2004), hair-curling irons

(Consumer Product Safety Commission [CPSC] 2004a), and electrical wires and sockets. One study found that kitchen-related items and household electrical appliances combined were responsible for 54% of all burn-related injuries to children aged 0 to 20 years (D'Souza, Nelson, and McKenzie 2008). Children have been burned by hot grease from cooking (Fiebiger et al. 2004) and from soup (Palmieri et al. 2008). Water and other liquids that reach temperatures above 125°F can burn a child in less than 1 minute (Feldman et al. 1978). Steam has approximately 4000 times the heat-carrying capacity of dry air (Bhoota and Kitinya 2005). A common inhalation treatment for upper respiratory tract infections in children, steam has been implicated in child burn injuries (Barrow et al. 2004) but may not be considered risky by parents, especially if they are following a physician's advice. "Shower-steamers," relatively new devices used to produce sauna-like effects in residential showers, also have been implicated in unintentional childhood injuries (Brywczynski and Arnold 2008).

Adult caretakers of children may fail to recognize the risks associated with a variety of other products used in and around the home. For example, children have experienced friction burns from treadmills (Collier et al. 2004; Maguina, Palmieri, and Greenhalgh 2004) and electrical burns from placing metal chopsticks in electric sockets (Lee, Jang, and Oh 2004). Children have been injured heating prepackaged soups in the microwave (Palmieri et al. 2008). The Consumer Product Safety Commission (CPSC) estimates that the improper use of batteries, either recharging or installing them incorrectly, was responsible for 740 children younger than 16 years being treated in hospital emergency departments for battery-related chemical burns (CPSC 2004b). Of the estimated 7000 fireworks-related injuries treated in hospital emergency departments in 2008, children and youth younger than 20 years had 58% of the estimated injuries (Greene and Granados 2010).

What Are Fire and Burn Injuries?

In general, injuries occur to the body when a threshold for absorbing some type of energy is exceeded; this is the case with fire and burn injuries. Different types of energy can be implicated in burn injuries and include thermal (heat), electrical, or chemical energy. When thermal energy is in the form of a liquid or steam and results in an injury, this is usually referred to as a scald burn. Most fire-related deaths (69%) are caused by inhaling the toxic gases produced as fires develop and spread; an additional 15% of fire-related deaths are caused by burns (Casteel and Runyan 2004b). Regardless of energy type, burn injuries can be classified by the percentage of body surface involved (e.g., 10%, 45%) or the depth of the skin involved (e.g., first- to fourth-

Box 5.1

Five Kids Die in Pittsburgh House Fire

Fire raced through a three-story row house early Tuesday, killing five children, and authorities said they were looking for a teenage baby sitter who was supposed to be watching them.... The victims, ages 2 to 7, were all found on the second floor, authorities said. One was dead on arrival at West Penn Hospital and two others died in the emergency room.... Tuesday morning, investigators were inside the gutted and blackened house skeleton of a home, examining what remained and trying to determine the cause of the fire, which officials believe started on the home's second floor. Officials said flames had been shooting from all three floors of the building in the city's East Liberty section when firefighters arrived around 1:20 A.M. The blaze also damaged a vacant building next door.

Pittsburgh, June 12, 2007.

CBSNEWS. Available at: http://www.cbsnews.com/stories/2007/06/12/national/main2918032.shtml. Accessed August 29, 2010.

degree burns). The depth of the burn depends on the temperature and duration of the heat applied and on characteristics of the skin.

Morbidity and Mortality Data

Substantial gains have been realized in protecting children from fire- and burn-related deaths. Child mortality rates from fire and burn injuries have decreased steadily for the past 20 years. For children aged 1 to 4 years, death rates per 100,000 have dipped to a low of 1.3 in 2007 compared with 5.4 in 1987 for the same age group. The death rate for older children (5–14 years) was 0.6 in 2007 (Federal Interagency Forum on Child and Family Statistics 2010). Although progress has been made, these rates translated into 457 children younger than 15 years who died of unintentional fire- and burn-related injuries in the United States in 2007 (National Center for Injury Prevention and Control 2010a).

During the same year, 97,026 children younger than 15 years suffered nonfatal, unintentional fire and burn injuries. More than half of these events occurred among children aged 1 to 4 years. For all injuries (intentional and unintentional) among infants (children aged <1 year), fire and burn injuries ranked fifth among the top ten nonfatal injury events (National Center for Injury Prevention and Control 2010b).

Child Characteristics Linked to Fire and Burn Injuries

Sociodemographic Characteristics of the Child

A variety of sociodemographic characteristics have been linked to fire deaths. According to the CDC, children younger than 5 years, poor Americans, and persons living in rural areas are at increased risk for home fire fatalities. According to a report by the National Fire Protection Association using data from 2003 to 2007, children younger than 5 years are approximately 1.5 times more likely to die in a home fire than the average person (Flynn 2010). Young children may be at increased risk because of their propensity to "play with fire" coupled with their lack of ability to "react appropriately and plan escape" (Warda, Tenenbein, and Moffatt 1999). Young children also are at increased fire-death risk because they may need to depend on others for escape. In general, younger children have faster metabolic rates and are less able to physically endure the toxic products of combustion compared with adults. Toxic gases and oxygen deprivation, collectively called "smoke inhalation," cause more fire deaths than burns (Flynn 2010). The increased risk for poor Americans and persons living in rural areas may be related to issues of housing quality, heating sources, and access by firefighters in the event of a fire.

Children's Behaviors

Istre and colleagues (2002) report that children who engage in "fireplay" (i.e., playing with any type of combustible material) are at increased risk for fire and burn injuries. Another study found that children with attention deficit/hyperactivity disorder are at increased risk for burn injuries, perhaps because of their compromised impulse control (Mangus et al. 2004).

Anatomy of the Skin

The skin is the largest organ of the body and serves as the first line of defense against trauma and infection. The skin is composed of two main layers—the epidermis and the dermis. Located under the dermis is subcutaneous tissue, such as fat and sweat glands. Muscle and bone reside below that. First-degree burns involve only the epidermis; second-degree burns affect both the epidermis and dermis. Because the epidermis varies in thickness across the body (e.g., thickest on upper back and thinnest on the eyelids), a burn of the same temperature will affect various parts of the body differently (Feldman et al. 1978; Katcher 1983). In general, children's skin is thinner than adults and therefore more susceptible to injury at lower temperatures and more serious injury at higher temperatures compared with adults.

Other Characteristics Linked to Fire and Burn Injuries

Water Temperature

A factor affecting the rate of scald burn is the temperature of the water. Water at 120°F will burn a child's skin in 3 minutes compared with 5 minutes for the skin of an adult. Water ten degrees hotter (130°F) will burn a child's skin in approximately 15 seconds, whereas water at 140°F will burn a child's skin in only 2½ seconds (Katcher 1983).

Parental Factors

In a review of the literature regarding parental factors linked to unintentional burn risk, Joseph and colleagues (2002) reported an association between child's burn risk and parent's level of education, income, employment status, and marital status, among other variables. At the same time, the authors acknowledge a variety of methodological limitations of the studies reviewed (e.g., over-reliance on self-report, single informants) that may minimize these associations and call for improved methodological approaches to better understand the link between child's burn risk and parental factors.

Alcohol Consumption

Although not associated with scald burn risk, alcohol consumption has been linked to an increased risk for fire burn injuries (Levy et al. 2004). In a meta-analysis synthesizing U.S. medical examiner studies of nontraffic fatalities, at least some of which were home fire deaths, Smith, Branas, and Miller (1999) found that unintentional injury deaths were tested for alcohol involvement in 84% of cases; among these, 31% of the accident victims were determined to be intoxicated. However, the authors could not report on the role of alcohol in child-related fatalities because of the inconsistent reporting of age across the 65 studies examined in the meta-analysis. In a review of alcohol's contribution to alcohol and fire casualties, the U.S. Fire Administration (2003) reported that 15% of children younger than 15 years "died in fires where the surviving adult was impaired by alcohol."

Housing Conditions

A variety of factors related specifically to the physical qualities of the home have been linked to injury and include the age of the house and owner occupancy, with older homes (Istre et al. 2001) and those inhabited by tenants at increased risk for fire and burn injuries (Shenassa, Stubbendick, and Brown 2004). Older homes may be less likely to be in compliance with building codes, and inadequate or deferred maintenance can be a problem with rental properties. Mobile homes, most especially single detached mobile homes, have been linked to higher fire death rates (Mullins et al. 2009).

Prevention Strategies

Smoke alarms have been established as an important, reliable, and cost-effective tool in the fight against fire-related injuries (Parmer, Corso, and Ballesteros 2006). The presence of smoke alarms is reported in 95% of homes in the United States, and recommendations call for at least one working smoke alarm on each level and in each sleeping area (Ballesteros and Kresnow 2007). Compared with homes without smoke alarms, homes with smoke alarms have approximately half as many fire-related deaths (Marshall et al. 1998). The majority of deaths due to house fires occur in the 5% of homes with no smoke alarms. The one situation in which smoke alarms seem to offer no protection from injury or death is during "fireplay" events involving children (Istre et al. 2002). On the basis of more than a decade of experience funding and evaluating community fire prevention programs, the CDC recommends the use of 10-year lithium-powered alarms with a sealed-in battery compartment and a "hush" button to temporarily deactivate the alarm during false activations (Jackson et al. 2010).

Smoke alarm manufacturers have designed products to meet the unique needs of certain segments of the population. For instance, households with people who have visual or hearing impairment are encouraged to use specially designed smoke alarms. These alarms emit audible warnings at higher than normal levels, use strobe lights, or have a mechanism that connects to a bed or pillow to create a shaking sensation to alert the person to smoke or fire (National Fire Protection Association 2010).

Having working smoke alarms in homes is necessary but not sufficient to be fully protected from house fires. Knowing what to do in the event of a residential fire is another recommended prevention strategy. However, 52% of homes report having a fire escape plan, and only 16% of them practice it every 6 months. Historically, Holmes and Jones (1996) and Hillman (1983) were successful in teaching fire escape skills to children aged 7 to 10 years, but recent research showed only modest behavioral and no significant knowledge change in children's fire safety knowledge when the intervention was directed at their parents (Duchossois, Garcia-Espana, and Durbin 2006).

Scald burn prevention skills can be taught to parents and caregivers of young children. In a pilot study that targeted residents from the zip code responsible for the majority of scald burns to a level 1 trauma and burn center, Cagle and colleagues (2006) used health educators to conduct a home-based risk assessment with parents and then discussed ways to mitigate the scald-burn risks. In addition, anti-scald devices were installed wherever the parent requested. Follow-up home visits revealed significant differences from pre- to post-intervention for parents' scald knowledge and scald risks in the home (both $P < .01$). Scald injuries among young children residing in the study area were evaluated using the burn registry and compared with a 2-year period before and after the intervention; statistically significant differences were found in scald injuries ($P < .01$). Passive prevention techniques, such as requiring water heaters to be preset by manufacturers at safe temperatures, play an important role in preventing unintentional scald burns to children (Erdmann et al. 1991). However, preset temperature settings do not completely eliminate the threat of scald burns, so interventions that combine education with passive techniques are necessary.

Recent Research Findings

The benefit of smoke alarms cannot be overstated. The CDC-sponsored Smoke Alarm Installation and Fire Safety Education program recommends the installation of lithium-battery smoke alarms with a hush feature for high-risk households (Ballesteros, Jackson, and Martin 2005). DiGuiseppi and colleagues (2002) found that families who had their smoke alarm directly installed were more likely to have a functioning alarm 6 months later compared with families who received a voucher for a free smoke alarm.

Given the increased rate of fire fatality when people are sleeping, research is being conducted to better understand the response to different types and levels of audible warnings from smoke alarms among different groups of people. For instance, Smith and colleagues (2006) compared a personalized parent recording with a traditional audible tone (both at 100 decibels) to awaken sleeping children and found that the parent recording outperformed the traditional alarm. Others have tested different auditory, visual, and tactile signals with hard-of-hearing adults, intoxicated adults, adults who are heavy sleepers, and children to find the most effective warning signal (Bruck and Ball 2007; Bruck and Thomas 2009).

Finally, despite their nascent stage, two recent developments may have considerable impact on reducing the human toll caused by fires. The adoption of "fire-safe cigarettes" in all 50 states may ultimately result in a decrease in fire deaths. Cigarettes have long been implicated as the leading cause of home-fire deaths. New York State, the first to adopt reduced ignition propensity cigarettes, is already showing positive results. They experienced a 35% reduction in fire deaths in 2006 and 2007, the first year it was illegal to buy anything other than fire-safe cigarettes (Coalition for Fire Safe Cigarettes 2010). The other development is residential fire sprinklers. Residential fire sprinklers are increasingly being advocated as another important fire prevention and injury prevention tool. A growing number of communities have adopted ordinances requiring sprinklers in new or renovated homes (U.S. Fire Administration 2010). When sprinklers are present, fatalities are reduced by one half to two thirds compared with when sprinklers are absent (Rohr and Hall 2005). Research is needed to better understand ways to facilitate adoption of residential sprinkler policies across the United States.

Advocacy Efforts

Diane Denton, a nurse at the Kosair Children's Hospital in Louisville, Kentucky, appealed to the CPSC in 1985 to require that disposable cigarette lighters be child resistant (CPSC 1998). Nurse Denton's request came after seeing numerous children suffering from burns, talking to their parents about the incidents, and identifying a common culprit—disposable cigarette lighters (Sleet and Gielen 1998). Together with members of the burn prevention community, Diane Denton compiled sufficient evidence to prompt the CPSC to further study the matter. Through their own epidemiologic study of the issue during 1986 and 1987, the CPSC estimated that such lighters could be found in 30 million households and that children younger than 5 years playing with them caused more than 5000 residential fires, approximately 150 deaths, and 1000 injuries (Smith, Greene, and Singh 2000). On July 12, 1994, a decade after being prompted by the actions of one nurse, the CPSC issued a product safety standard requiring disposable and novelty cigarette lighters to have a child-resistant mechanism that makes the lighters difficult to operate for children younger than 5 years. The passion of a few individuals, coupled with solid data, brought about policy change to keep children safer from one consumer product. This change has been effective in saving lives. Researchers compiled data from 1997 to 1999 about residential fires caused by children younger than 5 years playing with cigarette lighters and compared them with similar data from 1985 to 1987. They found a statistically significant reduction (odds ratio = 0.42, $P < .01$) that could be attributed to the child-resistant lighter standard (Smith, Greene, and Singh 2002).

Poisoning

In 2008, more than 4.3 million calls were received by the 61 regional Poison Centers that serve the United States and its territories. Of those calls, approximately 2,491,049 were confirmed human exposures, 52% of which occurred in children younger than 6 years (Bronstein et al. 2009). Most calls to poison control centers do not result in hospital or emergency department visits. In fact, 73% of calls to Poison Centers are managed at the site of the exposure.

It is fortunate that most poisonings in children are not fatal. Pediatric fatal poisonings ranged from a low of 15 in 1987 to a high of 47 in 2007 (Bronstein et al. 2009). In 2008, 39 children died of a poisoning event.

What Is a Poisoning?

A poison exposure is defined as an ingestion of or contact with a substance that can produce toxic effects (National Center for Injury Prevention and Control 2001). Despite the fact that there is no universally agreed on definition of a poisoning from either a clinical or epidemiologic perspective (Institute of Medicine 2004a), we will define a poisoning as the result of "either a brief or long-term exposure to a chemical agent" that results in physical harm (National Center for Injury Prevention and Control 2001). Physical harm can range in severity from mild to fatal, and the physical effects of nonfatal injuries caused by poisonings can be temporary in nature or can result in lifelong disability.

This section focuses primarily on acute poisonings in children and will therefore not address the issue of lead poisoning. Although foodborne illnesses are an acute condition, they are not typically considered a form of poisoning and also will not be addressed.

How Do Children Get Poisoned?

Most poisoning exposures to children younger than 12 years are unintentional and occur in either their own or someone else's home (Bronstein et al. 2009). Potentially poisonous products are ubiquitous in the typical American home. Consider these common household items found throughout various rooms in a typical home: oven cleaner in the kitchen, nail polish remover in the bathroom, adult medications in the bedroom, and bleach in the laundry room. What follows is a brief review of some of the most common poisonous products encountered by children.

Nonpharmaceutical Products

The most frequently reported poison exposures involve nonpharmaceutical products. McKenzie and colleagues (2010) used the National Electronic Injury Surveillance System (NEISS) data set to determine rates of cleaning-product poisonings treated in U.S. emergency departments between 1990 and 2006. Although they report a 46% decrease in poisoning events among children younger than 6 years over that 17-year period, an estimated 267,269 children were treated for household cleaning product-related injuries during that same time. The most common product associated with injury was bleach (37%), and the most common container type was a spray bottle (40%).

Pharmaceutical Products

In 2008, Franklin and Rodgers (2008) reported national estimates of unintentional child poisoning trends using the CPSC's NEISS. From this nationally representative sample of hospital emergency departments, they were able to estimate that 86,194 child poisonings were treated in emergency departments in 2004. Further, they estimate that 70% of these events occurred in children aged 1 to 2 years. Oral prescription drugs, oral nonprescription drugs, and supplements were implicated in approximately 60% of the poisoning events. With the use of the American Association of Poison Control Center's Toxic Exposure Surveillance System data set for a different time period, 1990 to 2000, and for children less than 2 years of age, Bar-Oz, Levichek, and Koren (2004) identified medicines that were responsible for fatal poisonings. They reviewed all available drugs in North America and identified medicinal preparations that can be fatal for a 10-kg toddler (~22 pounds) on ingestion of a one-dose unit of the drug (1–2 teaspoons). Included among their top ten fatal drug products were prescription medications for asthma, heart disease, and psychiatric problems. These drugs were responsible for 72% of fatal cases reported to the American Association of Poison Control Center's Toxic Exposure Surveillance System from 1990 to 2000. Iron was implicated in the remaining fatal cases (38%) among children younger than 2 years.

Unique differences among substances within the same class or category can yield very different clinical outcomes. For instance, although child pediatric multivitamins containing iron rarely result in fatalities because of their low toxicity, adult-use multivitamins with iron can result in serious and sometimes fatal iron poisoning in young children (McGuigan 1996).

Pesticides

The use of pesticides, insecticides, and yard chemicals are ubiquitous in the United States. The Environmental Protection Agency identifies 900 pesticides that may be used in the home, including insecticides, herbicides, rodenticides, and fungicides; 150 of these products were implicated in calls to poison control centers in a 2-year period (Spann, Blondell, and Hunting 2000). Children in urban environments may be exposed to insecticides that are used to control insects and other infestations in the housing units where they live (Landrigan et al. 1999). Children in rural areas may be exposed to chemicals that are applied in agricultural settings. The need for seasonal applications of pesticides raises concern about the cumulative nature of such exposures to children in these situations (Garry et al. 2002). Children can be exposed by the air they breathe, the food they eat, the water they drink, or through other means of contamination.

Carbon Monoxide

Carbon monoxide (CO) is a colorless, odorless gas produced from the incomplete combustion of carbon-containing substances. In addition to being present during house fires, common sources of CO include car exhaust, wood-burning or gas fire places that are improperly vented, and malfunctioning furnaces, gas space heaters, and stoves (Zimmerman and Tuxal 1981). CO is absorbed through the lungs and displaces oxygen in the body. Depending on the amount and duration of exposure to CO, symptoms can range from headache and dizziness to convulsions and loss of consciousness. Of the 14,461 cases of CO exposures reported to poison centers in the United States in 2008, 1773 involved children younger than 6 years and 2273 involved children aged 6 to 19 years. Forty-seven of these cases resulted in death (Bronstein et al. 2009).

Morbidity and Mortality Data

The death toll from unintentional poisoning among young children has decreased dramatically over the last 30 years and is identified as one of the signature successes of the field of injury prevention and control (Sleet, Schieber, and Gilchrist 2003). According to the CDC (National Center for Injury Prevention and Control 2010a), 53 children younger than 5 years died of unintentional poisoning in 2007. For children aged 10 to 14 years, unintentional poisoning is a growing threat when ranked against all types of injuries (both intentional and unintentional) over a 3-year period. In 2005, the CDC ranked unintentional poisoning as the tenth leading cause of injury-related death among 10- to 14-year-olds. In 2006 and 2007, unintentional poisoning ranked ninth and seventh, respectively (National Center for Injury Prevention and Control 2010a).

As with all injuries, deaths represent just a small proportion of the problem. Children aged 0 to 4 years have the highest rates of nonfatal poisonings (213 per 100,000) compared with children aged 5 to 9 years (32 per 100,000) and 10 to 14 years (49 per 100,000) (National Center for Injury Prevention and Control 2010b).

Child Characteristics Linked to Poisoning Exposures and Injuries

More than half of all poison exposures occur among children younger than 6 years. What is it that makes young children so susceptible to poisoning exposures and their resultant injuries?

Developmental Characteristics

Children younger than 6 years are most vulnerable to accidental poisoning because they are in growth and development stages that focus on exploration of their environment. Young children often rely on touch and taste to learn about new things, and this increases their risk of ingesting poisons.

Physical Characteristics

Size is an important factor in the risk of poisoning, not only weight but also height. Compare the ingestion of a single drug tablet in a child who weighs 20 pounds with an adult who weighs 150 pounds. Clearly the concentration of the substance in the child's body is higher than it will be for the heavier adult. Height is important in certain poisoning scenarios, particularly related to poisonous gases. Being lower to the ground may increase a child's exposure to vapor (particularly those that are heavier than air) compared with a taller adult (Garry et al. 2002).

Compared with adults, children generally have faster respiration, heartbeat, and metabolism rates. These developmental features may increase a child's exposure to certain poisons by facilitating their absorption into the child's body.

Other Risk Factors for Poisoning Injuries

Other variables come into play and must be considered when addressing the issue of poison prevention among young children.

Supervision of Child

Children need adult care and supervision until they are mature enough to navigate the world safely. Parents and caretakers of children may store dangerous products safely but fail to supervise the child adequately when the product is being used (American Association of Poison Control Centers 2004). Many children are exposed to harmful substances when those substances are in use by adults (e.g., floor cleaner). Children must rely on the assistance of an adult for administration of medications. Research suggests that less than one third of caregivers are able to accurately measure a correct dosage when dispensing over-the-counter medications to their children, which could lead to unintentional poisoning (Safe Kids 2004a). Separate from creating a safe home environment, parenting style has been shown to be protective of injuries, particularly techniques such as interactive play with children and increased frequency of praise (Schwebel et al. 2004; Soubhi 2004).

Characteristics of Product Packaging

The U.S. Poison Prevention Packaging Act of 1970 (Technical Advisory Committee 1971) requires certain household chemicals and medicines to be packaged in such a way that it will be difficult to open for children younger than 5 years. Such "child-resistant caps" do not guarantee that a child cannot access the contents; however, they do serve as a deterrent and increase the amount of time that it takes a child to open such a container.

When first adopted, the Poison Prevention Packaging Act was limited to aspirin (Walton 1982). Other prescription medicines (CPSC 2002), over-the-counter drug products (CPSC 2001a), and household chemicals (Blumenthal 1989) have been added to the list of products over the years, broadening the reach and strengthening the impact of the Poison Prevention Packaging Act.

Amount of Product Available

Once a container with a child-resistant cap is open, the child could potentially access all the contents, creating conditions for a fatal ingestion. The amount of product available in the container is a risk factor for a poisoning injury if the quantity is sufficient to cause harm.

Characteristics of the Product

Different substances have different levels of toxicity and need to be taken into consideration when brought into a home with young children. In the event of a poisoning exposure, poorer medical outcomes are associated with higher levels of toxicity (Spann, Blondell, and Hunting 2000). Likewise, products in concentrated form are more likely to cause serious harm to young children.

Other characteristics of a product, namely, appearance, taste, and smell, can be manipulated to minimize the product's "attractiveness" to a child, possibly minimizing the risk of its unintentional use or ingestion by young children. For instance, one study posited that young children being treated for rat poison ingestion could have mistaken it for a breakfast cereal because the product itself resembled corn meal (Schum and Lachman 1982). Others have noted similarities between candy and various drug products, including iron (Spann, Blondell, and Hunting 2000). In the same vein as adding a smell to improve the detection of natural gas, drug and product manufacturers should be encouraged to add bittering agents to make products less attractive to young children.

Prevention Strategies

Cabinet Locks

As with many injury areas, primary prevention is an important focus, and a variety of countermeasures are available for averting poisoning exposures and poisonings. Many countermeasures require action and vigilance on the part of adult caretakers of children. Safety advocacy groups consistently recommend, for instance, that household poisons be stored in cabinets and drawers that close with locks or latches (Safe Kids 2004a). However, a survey of homes where children younger than 6 years live or visit found that medicines were easily accessible to children; respondents reported keeping medicines out in the open (33%), in an unlocked drawer or cabinet (82%), or in their purse (43%) (Coyne-Beasley et al. 2005).

Packaging

Another important step that adults can take to minimize a child's risk of unintentional poisoning is to request the use of child-resistant containers on all their prescription medications. Numerous studies indicate that the Poison Prevention Packaging Act of 1970 and child-resistant packaging significantly reduce the morbidity and mortality of childhood poisonings (Dole, Czajka, and Rivara 1986; Walton 1982). Likewise, when adults buy any hazardous products that will be used in the home (e.g., household cleaners, over-the-counter preparations), they should carefully consider the toxicity and packaging of the product.

Packaging is an important prevention consideration. Unit-dose packaging (Hingley 1997), also known as unit-of-use packaging, encases one pill or unit of medication in a see-through plastic blister. To access the pill, the consumer simply pushes it through the paper or foil backing. Child-resistant features can be integrated into such packaging by increasing the toughness of the backing material. The potential for fatal ingestions is minimized because access to fatal amounts of the medicine is limited.

An aspect of packaging that is less clear in protecting children is warning labels that are directed to children, commonly referred to as "Mr. Yuk." First created by the National Poison Control Center in Pittsburgh, "Mr. Yuk" is a bright green picture of a scowling face with a protruding tongue designed to be placed onto containers of harmful substances. "Mr. Yuk" stickers are well known among many parents and frequently perceived as an effective countermeasure to protecting children from hazardous substances. However, one study of 2-year-olds showed no effect in reducing poisonings with the use of "Mr. Yuk" stickers (Fergusson et al. 1982). A second study of children aged 12 to 30 months showed an actual increase in the children's handling of medicines labeled with "Mr. Yuk" stickers (Vernberg, Culver-Dickinson, and Spyker 1984). Children at these young ages seem to be attracted to the colorful stickers, thus potentially increasing their risk of poisoning.

Syrup of Ipecac

Once previously recommended by pediatric and poison control groups, syrup of ipecac, a pharmaceutical agent that induces vomiting, is now contraindicated for home use (Committee on Injury, Violence, and Poison Prevention 2003). This change in policy and practice was brought about by several factors, including the dramatic decrease in childhood poisonings over the last 40 years and recent research evidence that failed to show a benefit for children who were treated with syrup of ipecac (Bond 2003). This policy change has clearly had an impact on practice. In 2008, less than 1% of all pediatric poisoning exposures involved administration of ipecac compared with 17% in 1985 (Bronstein et al. 2009).

Carbon Monoxide Detectors

Proper maintenance of potential sources of CO in the home is perhaps the best way to avoid CO poisoning. CO alarms, designed as an early warning device, offer another layer of protection by sounding a loud warning when CO surpasses a safe threshold. Two studies reviewed deaths classified as unintentional CO poisoning and estimated the number of deaths that could have been saved had a CO alarm been in use (Centers for Disease Control and Prevention 2004; Yoon, Macdonald, and Parrish 1998). Despite this evidence and that garnered via the smoke alarm experience, legislation requiring CO alarms in all residences is only slowly being adopted. In 2005, Massachusetts was the first state to pass legislation requiring CO alarms in residential properties. Since then, 24 other states have passed some type of legislation to prevent CO-related deaths by requiring CO alarms (National Conference of State Legislators 2010). However, not all of these mandate alarms in all residences. Instead they may focus only on new construction or specific types of buildings (e.g., state-owned buildings, hotels).

Poison Control Centers

In the United States, poison control center staff are available 24 hours per day on an emergency hotline to dispense information and treatment advice. In 2008 alone, poison control centers fielded more than 4.3 million such calls (Bronstein et al. 2009). Poison control centers have been identified as the "lead agencies in the pursuit of poisoning control and prevention" and are well positioned to provide specialized services to both the general public and health professionals alike (Woolf 2004). Among the other nonemergency services performed by poison control centers are public education, professional education, data collection and management, and information and referral resources. Miller and Lestina (1997) found that the average public call to a poison control center prevented $175 in other medical spending.

Until recently, access to the nation's 70 poison control centers was "hampered by a confusing array of telephone numbers and disjointed local prevention efforts" (Institute of

Medicine 2004b). Today, because of recent legislation, there is one nationwide toll-free number that routes people to their closest regional center: 1-800-222-1222.

Recent Research Findings

Although legislation streamlined some aspects of poison control centers in the United States, the Institute of Medicine (2004b) outlined significant additional steps that are needed to create a truly coordinated and comprehensive national system for poison control and prevention. Included among the 12 specific recommendations are that all poison control centers should perform a core set of functions, be better integrated into the public health system, and be supported by sufficient and stable funding to fulfill their mission. The Institute of Medicine report also identifies new realities of the 21st century, including public health preparedness needs, especially those related to bioterrorism and chemical terrorism.

Another challenge for poison control centers across the country is to provide services to non-English-speaking populations (Shepherd et al. 2004). Creating awareness of poison control centers within non-native English-speaking groups will likely be enhanced through culturally appropriate education, outreach efforts, and innovative use of technology. Kelly and colleagues (2003) created a 9-minute videotape (available in both English and Spanish) that described general information about poison control centers' hours and staff and depicts a poisoning scenario with a Hispanic family and one with an African American family. The study improved the knowledge, attitudes, behaviors, and behavioral intentions regarding the use of poison control centers among low-income and Spanish-speaking parents.

A systematic review and meta-analysis published recently by Kendrick and colleagues (2008) demonstrated that parent safety education coupled with the provision of poison prevention-related safety equipment resulted in increased safe storage of medicines and household cleaning supplies, the acquisition of syrup of ipecac, and having the poison center number readily available. Most of these interventions occurred via home-visiting programs, and therefore occurred one-on-one. An area that could benefit from additional investigation is the effectiveness of community-based models for injury prevention to complement the educational (Kendrick et al. 2008), regulatory (CPSC 2001a), and legislative (Walton 1982) efforts that have contributed greatly to the reduction in poisonings among children. Nixon and colleagues (2004) characterize community-based models as having shared ownership of the injury problem and its solution by members of the community and injury prevention experts. These researchers argue that "successful implementation of a poisoning prevention program in communities depends on embedding the countermeasures in the contextual practices of social structures and that a multi-strategy program for preventing childhood poisoning is essential." However, these authors, after conducting a comprehensive review of the literature, could find no examples of such work, and this remains the case today.

Advocacy Efforts

The role of data has been central to reducing the death toll from unintentional poisoning among young children by contributing to the identification of the problem and to the creation and dissemination of effective solutions. Few people know the name "Homer A. George," a Missouri pharmacist whose concern about the lack of pharmaceutical information in the 1950s is credited with the national public awareness campaign, Poison Prevention Week, which still exists today (Centers for Disease Control and Prevention 1986). Troubled by missing or misleading information about pharmaceutical products, George convinced his town's mayor (1958) and later his state's governor to proclaim a Poison Prevention Week to bring attention to preventable deaths and injuries caused by poisonings. By 1961, President John F. Kennedy signed legislation creating the Poison Prevention Week Council. By 1966, almost every state had some type of campaign to improve the public's understanding of childhood poisonings, which continues today to educate parents and caretakers of young children.

The establishment of the first poison control center in Chicago, Illinois, in 1953 began a chain of events that has led to the current system of regional poison control centers across the entire United States. Toward the end of the 1950s, another critical information need was beginning to be met—textbooks on emergency advice and treatment for poisoning victims became available, in part because of the experience and data being collected in poison control centers around the country (Fisher 2004). Four decades later, the passage of the 1970 Poison Prevention Packaging Act, which ultimately has resulted in numerous hazardous pharmaceutical and other household products being in child-resistant containers, has been credited with the clear declines in poisonings and the prevention of poisoning exposures (Harborview Injury Prevention and Research Center 2004).

Falls

Falls in the home can have dire consequences for children. Many serious fall injuries among young people occur on playgrounds and during sports and recreational activities, but the most common causes of fall injuries to children are in the home: stairs, furniture, and windows. Risks differ for children of different ages, but there are effective and promising prevention strategies for all of these sources of fall injuries.

In 2007, 92 deaths and 4,381,877 injuries were caused by falls among children and teens (birth to 14 years) (National Center for Injury Prevention and Control 2010a; National Center for Injury Control and Prevention 2010b). The enormous costs associated with fall injuries include those associated with the millions of emergency department visits and the additional burden of long hospital stays and rehabilitation for survivors, but, more important, the burden of human suffering must be considered, as this real-life example suggests.

Eric Clapton wrote the famous song "Tears in Heaven" after the death of his son, Conor Clapton, who died at the age of 4 years on March 20, 1991. He fell from a 53rd floor window in New York City, landing on the adjacent roof of a four-story building. Although high-rise apartments were required by a 1984 law to have window guards, condominium buildings, such as the one Conor Clapton lived in, were exempt (Tears in Heaven 2004).

What Is a Fall Injury?

A fall is an event that results in a person coming to rest inadvertently on the ground or floor or other lower level (World Health Organization 2010). Falls can occur on the same level as when a child trips or loses his balance, or falls can occur from one level to another as when a child falls from a window, down the stairs, or off furniture. When these events result in seeking medical care or are fatal, they are coded as fall injuries.

How Do Children Get Injured by Falls?

The degree to which an injury results from a fall depends on many factors. Most important to consider are the distance of the fall and the type of landing surface (Barlow et al. 1983). The shorter the distance and the greater the energy-absorbing surface, the less severe the injury is likely to be. Individual differences in anatomy also affect fall injuries. Bone structure and fat composition affect injury severity and depend in part on the individual's age. An infant's head is proportionally larger relative to his body, and his bones are still soft. These contribute to making an infant particularly susceptible to both falling over and suffering head injury as a result (American Academy of Pediatrics 2001a; Chiaviello, Christof, and Bond 1994; Wilson et al. 1991).

Morbidity and Mortality Data

Fall injuries remain the most common nonfatal unintentional injury event in 2007, ranked as number one for all age groups except 15- to 24-year-olds (ranked as number two) (National Centers for Injury Prevention and Control 2010b). During this year, 2,158,522 fall injuries occurred among children younger than 15 years. In this same year, unintentional falls ranked among the top ten causes of injury death for only two pediatric age categories, for which it ranked the tenth for both those younger than 1 year and those aged 1 to 4 years (National Center for Injury Prevention and Control 2010b). According to an analysis of data on children younger than 15 years by Ballesteros and colleagues (2003), for every child injury death due to falls, there are 19,000 nonfatal fall injuries seen in an emergency department.

Fall injuries that occur in the child's home and require medical attention are estimated to be 1.5 million annually among children younger than 15 years (Runyan et al. 2005). Of note, this number is 2.5 times larger than the next leading cause of home injury, which is being struck. According to the Safe Kids Worldwide, more than 80% of fall injuries to children younger than 4 years occur in the home environment (Safe Kids 2004b). In an analysis specifically focused on unintentional home injuries from 1993 to 2000, the Home Safety Council found that among all children the rate of falls seen in emergency departments is highest for children younger than 5 years (3756 per 100,000 for boys; 3001 per 100,000 for girls). In fact, this age group experiences nonfatal fall injuries in the home at a rate that is second only to that observed in the elderly population (Casteel and Runyan 2004a).

Risk Factors for Fall Injuries

Characteristics of both the child and the environment have been identified as risk factors for fall injuries in the home. In this section, we highlight some of the most prominent ones.

Child's Age and Development

The data presented above demonstrate the increased fall risk among children younger than 5 years. In fact, there are many developmental stages that children go through from birth to 5 years, each of which confers its own unique risks.

In the first year of life, babies go from being reflexive and unable to control their body to becoming mobile but having generally poor balance. In these early stages, infants are at risk of wiggling off a changing table or other surfaces, as well as being dropped by adults (Sethi et al. 2008). From approximately 1 to 3 years of age, children's balance and locomotion improve, and they learn to walk, run, and climb, and assert independence while at the same time being able to follow only simple directions. This combination of attributes can be particularly hazardous as children try to attempt things that are beyond their skill level, such as climbing on furniture, negotiating stairs, or running on uneven pavement, all of which pose serious fall risks.

Preschoolers and young children become increasingly independent, develop the ability to understand relationships between objects, and begin to understand danger as well as warnings. They typically can understand a specific risk but may not be able to generalize to new situations. Children at these ages are still susceptible to fall injuries from their increased independence and the amount of time at play in or around the home.

Environmental Risk Factors

The physical environment is particularly relevant for fall injuries. In an analysis of the ten leading products ranked by percentage of nonfatal home injury costs in the United States in 2000,

Zaloshnja and colleagues (2005) identified beds as the leading product for children younger than 5 years, followed closely by stairs, floors, and tables. Although these analyses focused on all causes of nonfatal injuries, the nature of the products is strongly suggestive that falls would be the cause of many of them.

Other important fall hazards in the home environment include stairways and windows above ground level. Handrails on stairs offer some protection, yet a recent national survey found that 43% of homes with young children and stairs did not have banisters or handrails (Casteel and Runyan 2004a). Stair gates are recommended for homes with infants and toddlers, yet their use does not appear to be widespread. In The Netherlands, Beirens and colleagues (2007) found that although 83% of parents of toddlers report having a stair gate, 50% of them report not using it consistently. A U.S. study of households in a low-income, urban environment found that one quarter to one third of families with young children used stair gates (Gielen et al. 2002).

Shields, Burkett, and Smith (2011) recently conducted the first-ever study of balcony-related falls using a nationally representative sample and found that over the 17-year study period, the injury rate for children significantly decreased from 3.9 in 1990 to 1.6 in 2006 ($P <$ .01; slope −0.138), whereas the rate for adults (1.6) did not change over time. By focusing exclusively on falls among children in Dallas County, Texas, Istre and colleagues (2003) studied falls from apartment balconies and windows among 98 children younger than 15 years. The two important environmental hazards identified were balcony railings more than 4 inches apart and windows that were within 2 feet of the floor. Window locks or safety guards are recommended for homes with floors above ground level, yet a national survey recently found that 73% of households in which children live or visit did not have such devices installed (Casteel and Runyan 2004a).

The placement and type of furniture in the home are also relevant for fall injuries. For example, furniture placed under a window can be an enticement to young children that allows them access to an open window. Furniture with sharp edges can increase the risk of serious injury when children fall. Beds are a type of furniture associated with injury. Bunk beds compared with conventional beds have been shown to have an increased risk of injury and more serious injury (Belechri, Petridou, and Trichopoulos 2002; Macgregor 2000). D'Souza, Smith, and McKenzie (2008) recently completed a review of the NEISS database from 1990 to 2005 for all bunk bed-related injuries among individuals aged 21 years or less and estimated that they cause 37,790 nonfatal injuries each year. Because of the increased risk of injuries from bunk beds, the CPSC (2004c) recommends they not be used with children younger than 6 years.

Products specifically made for children can also be hazards. Numerous products have been designed to hold a child and allow him to sit, recline, bounce, jump, or walk; some of these devices hang from a doorway, and others contain the child in a stationary or mobile unit. Since 1971, the CPSC had regulations that banned certain features on these products that were linked with serious injury, namely, accessible coils or openings that could cause entrapment or edges that could scissor, shear, or pinch. Redesigned products entered the market, injuries continued, and safety advocates and agencies pushed for safer designs from manufacturers through voluntary safety standards. More than 25 years later, despite these efforts, baby walkers were found to account for more injuries among young children than any other nursery product, with 14,300 emergency department visits among children younger than 15 months estimated in 1997 (CPSC 2004d).

With estimated sales of 2 million yearly, baby walkers reached their peak of popularity in the early 1990s (CPSC 2010a). Since 1995, the American Academy of Pediatrics (2001a) has had an official policy on baby walkers. Noting "no clear benefit from their use" coupled with the risk for serious injury, the Academy called for a ban on the manufacture and sale of baby walkers. The CPSC instead called for product redesign and revision to the 1986 voluntary safety standard, effective June 30, 1997, that required walker bases too wide to fit through a standard door and a "break" that prevented the walker from falling down stairs. These public education, advocacy, and engineering interventions resulted in declining sales and use of walkers and a concomitant decrease in injuries from them, down to 3000 annually (CPSC 2010a). Most recently, the CPSC "is revoking its existing regulations pertaining to baby walkers because those regulations are being replaced by a new and more comprehensive safety standard" (CPSC 2010b). Effective December 2010, any infant walker manufactured or imported into the United States is required to comply with a more stringent set of mandatory safety features, meet predefined performance and testing standards, and include specific warning notices on the products.

Prevention Strategies

There are myriad prevention strategies for fall injuries consistent with the vast array of risk factors. Mandating the use of safety guards to reduce children falling from windows is an example of how legislation can be used for prevention. Issuing regulations for safer product design, as was done by the CPSC for bunk beds (2001b) and baby walkers (2010a), is another. Making caregivers aware of the fall risks and what they can do to prevent them—using age-appropriate and safe products, using safety devices, and providing close supervision—is also an essential educational prevention strategy. It is worth noting that even when safer products have been introduced to the market, there is typically a lag time in which many of the unsafe products are still in use and available at secondhand retail outlets. Modifying the living environment could happen through manufacturing redesign (e.g., more energy-absorbing flooring in homes, counters with rounded corners), but more typically consumers must redesign their own living environment by making safety-conscious choices when furnishing their homes or by installing safety products (e.g., well-padded non-skid rugs, padded furniture corner guards).

Recent Research Findings

Research on how to protect children from fall injuries is emerging through studies that seek to understand the psychologic determinants of parental safety practices (Morrongiello and Kiriakou 2004) and intervention trial results (Lyons et al. 2004). Research by Morrongiello and Major (2002) found that risk compensation does occur, in that parents report being more permissive with risk taking (including during climbing, jumping, and running activities) when their children are in safer environments, wearing safety gear, and perceived to be more experienced. The Cochrane Library contains a systematic review of interventions that attempted to modify the home environment (Lyons et al. 2004), which included fall-related injuries among other topics. Although the majority of studies with fall-related outcomes were focused on older adults, several focused on children. Clamp and Kendrick (1998) did find significant effects for "safe practices for windows," and a study by Gielen and colleagues (2002) found significant increases in the use of stair gates as a result of interventions that included safety counseling by a pediatrician and use of a Children's Safety Center in the clinic setting where low-cost safety products are available for purchase.

Advocacy Efforts

Two particularly noteworthy advocacy efforts to reduce children's in-home fall injuries are the window guard legislation in New York City and the baby-walker ban in Canada. The role of solid data in stimulating a policy change is clear in these two examples.

Data available in 1976 demonstrated that window falls accounted for 12% of unintentional childhood injury deaths among children younger than 15 years. A pilot program that included distribution of free window guards and education about their importance resulted in a 35%

reduction in deaths due to window falls and a 50% reduction in fall incidents (Spiegel and Lindaman 1977). In response to the data on the injury problem and the effectiveness of window guards, the New York City Board of Health passed a law requiring owners of multistory buildings to provide window guards in apartments where children aged 10 years and younger lived. A reduction of up to 96% in admissions to local hospitals for window fall injury followed, making this combination of legislation, education, and free products a remarkable success in protecting children (Barlow et al. 1983). A voluntary program in Boston achieved significant reductions in fall injuries (Vinci, Freedman, and Wolski 1996), but safety advocates in Massachusetts have yet to be successful in passing legislation mandating such safe guards. To date, only New York and New Jersey require window guards.

On April 7, 2004, the Canadian Minister of Health, Pierre Pettigrew, announced that Canada would be the first in the world to ban the sale, advertisement, and importation of baby walkers. A voluntary retail industry ban on baby walkers had been in place since 1989, but children were still being injured by them years later. Safe Kids Canada estimated that as many as 1000 Canadian children were injured each year using baby walkers, and in response they launched a successful letter-writing campaign in support of a ban (Safe Kids 2004c).

Choking/Suffocation Injuries

Children experience a variety of airway injuries from events and products in their homes. Three types of airway injuries are at issue: choking on objects or foods such that the airway is internally obstructed; suffocation, in which there is an external obstruction such as an object that covers the mouth and nose; and strangulation, in which external compression, such as from strings around the neck or head entrapment, causes the injury. All three of these are included under the typically used rubric of "choking/suffocation."

Choking, suffocation, and strangulation resulting in mechanical airway obstruction have been important causes of fatal unintentional injury in children (Tarrago 2000). In 2007, among all injury deaths (both intentional and unintentional) in children younger than 15 years, suffocation ranked *first* for those younger than 1 year, *fifth* for those aged 1 to 9 years, and *eighth* for those aged 10 to 14 years (National Center for Injury Prevention and Control 2010a). Among children younger than 15 years in 2007, unintentional inhalation or suffocation events appeared among the ten leading causes of nonfatal injury events only for those younger than 1 year, in whom it ranked seventh (National Center for Injury Prevention and Control 2010b).

In August 2000, the CPSC (2004e) announced that Kentucky Fried Chicken was voluntarily recalling 425,000 Tangled Treeples toys included with their kids' meals when a 19-month-old girl nearly suffocated on the toy's container. The bottom of the plastic container was stuck over the child's nose and mouth, causing her distress. Her mother was able to remove it, but the container was recalled because it posed a suffocation hazard to children younger than 3 years.

What Is a Choking/Suffocation Injury?

In choking and suffocation injuries, breathing is partially or completely obstructed. When the airway is completely blocked, oxygen is prevented from getting to the lungs and the brain. When the brain is deprived of oxygen for more than 4 minutes, brain damage or death may occur (American Academy of Pediatrics 2001b; Tarrago 2000).

How Do Choking and Suffocation Occur in Children?

Many activities and products that are a normal part of every child's daily life can pose a hazard for airway obstruction injury. For example, 60% of infant suffocation occurs in the sleeping environment—infants can suffocate when their faces become wedged against something soft in the crib or if someone they are sleeping with rolls over on them (Safe Kids 2004d).

The most commonly cited strangulation hazards include cords on children's clothing or on window blinds that infants or toddlers have access to, as well as cribs with improperly spaced slats and toy chests with improper latching mechanisms. Product modification and caregiver vigilance can reduce these risks in the child's environment.

Foods are the most common choking hazard for young children, and include small round foods such as hot dogs, candies, nuts, grapes, carrots, raisins, and popcorn. Toys and other small objects are also commonly encountered choking hazards, and round objects such as coins and marbles or those that conform to the shape of the windpipe (e.g., balloons) are particularly hazardous.

In a national study of nonfatal choking episodes treated in emergency departments among children younger than 14 years, 59.5% were due to food products, 12.7% were due to coins, and 18.7% were due to other non–food products (Centers for Disease Control and Prevention 2002). Toy balloons were the product most frequently responsible for deaths in a 10-year study of fatal aspirations among children younger than 14 years in Cook County, Illinois (Lifschultz and Donoghue 1996).

When an object partially blocks the windpipe, the child's cough or gag reflex will usually clear it without any intervention. However, immediate action is required if the child stops breathing or crying, has a weakening cough that becomes wheezing or gasping, or starts turning blue in the face. Knowing the proper emergency response to an airway injury event is critical for caregivers of young children.

Morbidity and Mortality Data

In 2007, the CDC estimated that unintentional suffocation injuries killed 959 infants and an additional 251 children aged 1 to 14 years (National Center for Injury Prevention and Control 2010a). There were also an estimated 15,653 children younger than 14 years who were treated in emergency departments just for choking-related episodes (National Center for Injury Prevention and Control 2010b).

Airway obstruction incidents are particularly lethal. Ballesteros and colleagues (2003) found that the ratio of emergency department visits to deaths for these types of injuries was 14:1 for children aged 0 to 14 years, making airway obstruction injuries the second most lethal type of childhood injury, just behind drowning, which had a ratio of 6:1.

The Home Safety Council's analysis of injuries in the home provides the most current information on the national scope of the problem (Runyan and Casteel 2004c). When location of the airway injury death was recorded (which is true for only 40% of all such deaths), 65% occurred in the home. When location of nonfatal airway injuries that required emergency department treatment was recorded (in 43% of the cases), the majority (94%) occurred in the home. Although these data are for all age groups, children (especially those aged <5 years) tend to spend much of their time in and around their homes. More recent work by Hu and Baker (2009) (not exclusive to the home setting) revealed an increase in suffocation deaths among White children (from 301 in 1999 to 496 in 2005) younger than 1 year. The death rate is 2.6 for boys and 1.9 for girls per 100,000 population. The rate of nonfatal choking/suffocation injuries that required an emergency department visit is 100.3 among boys and 92.9 among girls per 100,000 population (Ballesteros et al 2003).

Risk Factors for Choking/Suffocation

Characteristics of both the child and his/her environment are linked to the occurrence of choking/suffocation injuries.

Child Characteristics

Infants from birth to 1 year have a large head relative to the size of their body, and they have limited ability to control their body movements. These characteristics combine to put them at risk for getting into deadly situations from which they cannot extricate themselves. For example, infants can go feet first through a small opening and strangle; this could happen in an older crib with slats that are too far apart (i.e., $>2\frac{3}{8}$ inches). Infants can also suffocate by becoming wedged into a tight space or rolling face down onto a soft surface and being unable to move.

Mouthing and teething behaviors in infancy also put children at risk for choking, and as their curiosity and mobility increase as toddlers, their exposure to choking/strangulation hazards increases. Incisors appear at approximately 6 months of age, but molars may not emerge until 18 months of age. The emotional maturity and developmental abilities needed to sit quietly and chew food thoroughly may require several years to be fully realized by some children. Despite a strong gag reflex, a child's airway is vulnerable to obstruction because of its small size and the inability to produce a strong enough cough to dislodge foreign bodies (American Academy of Pediatrics 2010). Only a few pounds of force on the blood vessels of a small child's neck can cause strangulation. Most young children cannot untwist a cord or strap or extricate themselves if they become entrapped (CPSC 2004f). Combining the increased exploratory behavior and growing independence as toddlers become preschoolers with a lack of ability to assess risk and understand danger makes the years from birth to 5 years extremely hazardous for choking/strangulation.

Older children have more independence, play with other children, and often engage in make-believe play. Yet their cognitive abilities are still limited with regard to awareness of risk and danger, and being able to generalize from one risky situation to a new one. Playtime activities can easily become dangerous because so many products that are part of the adult home environment may be attractive but hazardous for child play (e.g., coins, cords on window blinds).

In 2008, the CDC reported 82 probable deaths between 1995 and 2007 among children aged 6 to 19 years resulting from a "choking game," strangulation by self or others to achieve a feeling of euphoria from temporary lack of oxygen (Toblin et al. 2008). Most of the deaths were among males aged 11 to 16 years. Ramowski and colleagues (2010) surveyed eighth-grade students in Oregon to better understand their familiarity with and participation in this activity. Survey results indicated that 38% of eighth-grade students had heard of it, 30% heard of someone participating in it, and 6% had tried it themselves. Factors associated with an increased likelihood of participation included rural area residence (7%), presence of a mental health risk factor only (4%), substance use only (8%), or both a mental health risk factor and substance use (16%).

Environmental Risk Factors

As the above discussion suggests, the characteristics of a child's environment are critical determinants of choking and strangulation risk. Foods that are served, household products and toys that are accessible, and availability of adult supervision are all elements of the environment that influence risk. Some of the most commonly cited hazards are described in this section.

Foods

The size, consistency, and shape of food influence its likelihood of being a choking hazard. A landmark 1984 study published in the *Journal of the American Medical Association* (Harris et al. 1984) reported on an analysis of national data on child choking deaths during a 3-year period and identified the hazards of round foods, including hot dogs, candy, nuts, and grapes. Morley and colleagues (2004) analyzed data from 51 children younger than 3 years who were treated for a foreign body aspiration and found that nuts, raw carrots, and popcorn accounted for 64% of the aspirations.

Toys and Other Household Products

Myriad products in the home environment can be choking/suffocation hazards to children. To assess which are particularly risky, Rimell and colleagues (1995) conducted a review of 165 children who underwent endoscopy for foreign body aspiration or ingestion and 449 deaths due to choking. Among those children who died, balloons caused 29% of the deaths overall; 33% of the deaths were among children younger than 3 years, but 60% of the deaths were among children older than 3 years. Lifschultz and Donoghue (1996) analyzed 10 years of cases at the Cook County Medical Examiner's Office in which deaths in children aged 0 to 14 years were due to aspiration of foreign objects. Toy balloons were responsible for more fatal aspirations than any other product. Data from autopsy examination of a series of five children who died from aspirating a balloon indicated that the common scenario is the child playing with an uninflated balloon, sucking or mouthing it (Abdel-Rahman 2000). Other products identified as choking hazards include marbles and small balls, toys with small parts or toys that can compress to fit entirely into a child's mouth, pen and marker caps, small batteries, and medicine syringes (American Academy of Pediatrics 2001b).

Cribs, Beds, and Bedding

According to the CPSC (2010c), more than 600 models of cribs are sold in the United States and approximately 2.4 million cribs are sold each year. Through a pilot project known as the "Early Warning System," the CPSC became aware of 3584 crib-related incidents between November 2007 and April 2010, including 153 fatalities and 1703 nonfatalities. The CPSC is in the process of adopting crib standards for all cribs manufactured or sold in the United States; these enhanced safety standards cover issues related to hardware systems, mattress fit and supports, assembly instructions, and slat integrity and spacing, among other things. Since 2005, the CPSC has used a dedicated product code to track injuries from toddler beds and has recorded 4 deaths and 81 injuries since that time (CPSC 2010d). Again, the CPSC is in the process of enhancing the voluntary standards currently in place for such products and making them mandatory if the product is to be manufactured or sold in the United States. Since 1992, the CPSC has banned infant cushions (soft, loosely fitted with a granular material that conforms to the face or body of an infant) that were involved in 36 infant suffocations. Safety advocates continue to warn caregivers about the potential dangers related to (1) soft bedding, pillows, and water beds; (2) overlaying or rolling on top of or against an infant while sleeping; (3) wedging or entrapment of the child between two surfaces; and (4) strangulation, as when the child's head and neck become trapped between slats or around a window blind cord.

Strings and Cords

The CPSC estimates that in 2009, 17,035 children aged 0 to 4 years and 35,372 children aged 5 to 14 years were injured by clothing (CPSC 2010e). Common injuries include strangulations by strings, cords, ribbons, or necklaces around their necks. Despite a ban on the use of drawstrings or cords on children's clothing by the CPSC, such products still find their way into the U.S. market and the CPSC is forced to use its limited resources to produce product recalls (*Child Health Alert* 2007). From 1991 to 2000, the CPSC received reports of 160 strangulations involving cords on window blinds, of which 140 involved the outer pull cords and 20 involved the inner cords that run through the blind slats.

Prevention Strategies

Small, round, or hard foods are to be avoided. For example, hot dogs can be difficult to chew, and they are the perfect shape to form a plug in the child's throat. Soft, smooth-textured foods that are easy to chew are best for young children. The American Academy of Pediatrics recommends cutting foods for infants and young children into pieces no larger than one-half inch. Round foods like hot dogs and grapes should be cut lengthwise to reduce their plug-like qualities. Food items generally agreed to be dangerous for young children are grapes, nuts, chunks of meat or cheese, hard or gooey candy, chewing gum, popcorn, and raw vegetables. Although the recommended age for serving these items varies from 4 to 6 years depending on the group, there is wide agreement that when these items are served, they should be prepared in a way to reduce the choking risk by cutting or chopping to change the item's shape or by cooking to soften the item.

Warning labels on toys and household products should be read and treated seriously. Toys labeled as choking hazards for children younger than 3 years should be kept away from infants and toddlers. As older siblings begin to understand directions, they should be taught to participate in keeping the environment safe for their younger brothers and sisters. Warnings and instructions on other household products (e.g., cribs, bunk beds, toy chests) should be inspected and followed as well. Older models of dangerous products (e.g., toy chests with self-closing lids, infant cushions) should be removed and destroyed. Purchases made at secondhand shops or yard sales need to be carefully inspected to make sure that the product has not been recalled or identified as dangerous (e.g., jackets with drawstrings). The CPSC Web site (at http://www.cpsc.gov) or help line (800-638-2772 [TTY 800-638-8270]) can be helpful in determining the safety of children's products; the CPSC is also using various social media (e.g., YouTube, Twitter, Flickr) to reach out to consumers.

Because of the immediacy of the risk when a child is choking, prompt intervention can be lifesaving. Therefore, adult caregivers should be trained in infant/child cardiopulmonary resuscitation (CPR). The American Heart Association recently revised their CPR guidelines from airway, breathing, chest compressions (ABC) to chest compressions, airway, breathing (CAB) (Field et al. 2010).

Beyond what individuals can do to protect their children, everyone can be encouraged to become involved in promoting safer products. If there is an incident (a death or near miss) or a concern about a dangerous product, it should be reported to the CPSC. Local community groups can organize events to collect and destroy old unsafe products. Groups that have access to parents of young children (e.g., childbirth classes, parenting groups, pediatric care providers) should take whatever steps available to them to alert families to the dangers of choking/strangulation in young children and instruct them in ways to avoid the risks. Increased access to CPR training could also help reduce the risk to children.

Recent Research Findings

Childhood suffocation/choking is a complex topic because of the myriad ways in which these injuries occur and the variation in underlying causes as children age. Although improving, research available in the standard medical/public health databases such as Medline seems to be limited. Two issues stand out in the recent research. First, new hazards are continually being identified. Second, there remains controversy over safety issues in the sleep environment for infants.

Button batteries, an increasingly common household item, seem to be involved in increasing numbers of childhood ingestions, frequently with serious, even fatal results. Litovitz, et al. (2010)

reviewed data from three sources: the national poison data system from 1985 to 2009, the national battery ingestion hotline from 1990 to 2008, and the medical literature. In all, they found an approximately seven-fold increase in button battery ingestions. In 92% of fatal cases, no one witnessed the ingestion, making diagnosis and appropriate clinical response difficult. Another analysis of battery ingestion revealed that the batteries were obtained from the product in 62% of cases, suggesting that manufacturers should redesign products to better secure the batteries (Litovitz, Whitaker, and Clark 2010).

Despite an increase in infant suffocations and more than a decade of recommendations to place children to sleep on their backs, the safe sleep controversy continues. The debate centers on whether safe co-sleeping can exist to promote bonding and breastfeeding or whether all co-sleeping is unsafe. Risk factors for unsafe co-sleeping include sleeping with an adult smoker or one who is intoxicated; sleeping in a bed with soft, fluffy bedding or in a water bed; and "wedging" hazards (e.g., a mattress up against a wall). Overlying is also a concern when an adult and infant share the same bed (O'Hara et al. 2000). Two recent qualitative studies shed light on the different motivations that drive caregivers' decisions about how and where a child sleeps. By using focus groups to explore various motivators, Chianese et al. (2009) found that perceptions of better sleep for parent and child, convenience, tradition, and emotional needs outweigh concerns about safety among African American women in Pittsburgh. However, in a qualitative study of African American women in the Washington, DC area, other researchers found that sleep decisions are often based on whether there is space for or availability of a crib (Joyner et al. 2010).

Although research will likely continue, the CPSC, the American Academy of Pediatrics, and others will continue to promote safe sleep practices and environments for infants (CPSC 2000).

Advocacy Efforts

The Consumer Product Safety Improvement Act (CPSIA) of 2008 was signed into law by President George W. Bush on August 14, 2008. The law not only increased the CPSC budget but also set new testing and documentation requirements for the manufacture or sale of consumer products in the United States. Section 104 of the CPSIA covers the safety of various infant and toddler products, such as cribs, toddler beds, high chairs, and bath seats, among others. Current CPSC Chairman Inez M. Tenenbaum credits the CPSIA with making it easier for "CPSC to create an appropriate and effective mandatory standard" for a variety of durable nursery products (CPSC 2010f). By strengthening the CPSC, the CPSIA should have an important impact on reducing the number of dangerous consumer products available in the United States.

Animal Bites

The dog is the biting animal that children are mostly likely to encounter at home. Forty-six percent of U.S. households own dogs (American Pet Products Manufacturers Association 2010). They are associated with approximately 80% of the bite-related injuries inflicted by vertebrate animals (Patronek and Slavinski 2009). Cats are next, but because of their smaller size, cat bites are less likely to cause severe injuries. Much of the focus in this section is on dog bites.

Dog bites occur most often in the home setting and are more likely to involve dogs that are familiar to the victim (Patronek and Slavinski 2009), which may surprise parents who have cautioned young children about the dangers of "stranger dogs." This problem is complex, because unlike other home hazards (i.e., unsafe products), dogs do not sit by passively in reaction to children's exploration. They can initiate contact on their own and change their behaviors on the basis of both internal and external stimuli. However, there is considerable epidemiologic data available about how dog bites occur. These will be reviewed for their relevance to prevention. Because the primary focus of this volume is prevention, how animal bites should be treated is not discussed.

Half of the 800,000 Americans who seek medical attention for dog bites each year are children (National Center for Injury Prevention and Control 2004). One retrospective study of children aged 4 to 18 years indicated that 45% had been bitten by dogs in their lifetimes (Beck and Jones 1985). Most such incidents are minor and self-treated, but the serious dog bites that do occur can be devastating.

Domestic pets, most notably dogs, are responsible for most animal bites (Patronek and Slavinski 2009). Children, boys in particular, are their most frequent victims. Approximately two thirds of the injuries suffered by children younger than 5 years are to the head or neck (Beck and Jones 1985), which may explain why 80% of the people killed by dog attacks in the United States from 1995 to 1996 were children (National Center for Injury Prevention and Control 1997).

This public health problem also produces considerable financial loss. It is estimated that one third of all liability claims associated with homeowners are dog-bite related, and that U.S. insurance companies pay out more than one billion dollars per year on claims related to dog bite injuries (Overall and Love 2001).

What Are Animal Bites?

A bite has been defined as "any break in the skin caused by an animal's teeth, regardless of the intention" (Beck and Jones 1985). Our discussion will focus primarily on dog bites, because they cause the majority of such injuries among American children. During a 3-year period in Philadelphia, for example, 86% of animal "attacks" reported to authorities involved dogs, followed by cats (10%), rats, and squirrels (<1% each) (Stull and Hodge 2000). This is not surprising because so many U.S. families "include" a canine member. Most households with children also have pets, and dogs make up more than half of the animals in those homes (Villar et al. 1998).

How Do Children Get Bitten?

Eighty percent of dog bites inflicted on people aged 18 years or less are attributed to the family's own pet or a neighbor's dog (Beck and Jones 1985). Children are more likely to be bitten during the spring or summer (Daniels et al. 2009; Sinclair and Zhou 1995; Stull and Hodge 2000) in the late afternoon or early evening (Bernardo et al. 2000). One study of dogs that were referred to a veterinary behavior clinic for human-directed aggression found that children were bitten most often when dogs were guarding their food, a bone or toy, or territory (Reisner, Shofer, and Nance 2007).

Although children are most likely to be bitten by dogs, female adults are overrepresented among cat bite victims. One Texas study that compared biting dogs and cats found that implicated felines were more likely to be less than 3 months of age, unrestrained, off their owner's property, and unvaccinated for rabies (American Pet Products Manufacturers Association 2010). A Spanish study of aggressive cats found that most of the offending animals were female and owned by the victim's family (Palacio et al. 2007). Although dog bites tend to be distributed all over the body, most cat bites are inflicted to the hands or arms. In particular, dog bites are three to four times more likely to affect the head, neck, or face than cat bites (Moore et al. 2000). In addition, cat bites are much less likely than dog bites to be characterized as "unprovoked."

Morbidity and Mortality Data

Accurate incidence data for animal bites are not available, in part because they are grossly underreported. For example, one study found that the actual dog bite rate among children aged 4 to 18 years was 36 times the reported rate (Beck and Jones 1985). This is likely because most bites are perceived as minor and not called to the attention of a medical professional. Reporting bias favors more vicious attacks, those brought on by large or wild animals, and those that occur in nonrural locations (Sinclair and Zhou 1995).

In an average year, 19 people die in the United States as a result of being attacked by a dog. Victims younger than 10 years account for the majority of those deaths, with infants experiencing the highest risk (Langley 2009). In a series describing 18 babies killed by dogs, 17 involved unrestrained animals that were on their owner's property. In 11 instances, the infants were sleeping at the time of the attack (Sacks et al. 1996). There have also been multiple reports of newborns who were killed by dogs after having been left in a mobile infant swing (Chu et al. 2006). Three quarters of fatal dog bites overall are inflicted on household members of the attacking canine or guests on the family's property (Sacks et al. 2000). The rate of dog bite fatalities in the United States appears to be increasing by approximately 2% per year (Langley 2009).

For every fatality attributed to dog bites, it is estimated that there are 670 hospitalizations and 16,000 emergency department visits (Weiss, Friedman, Coben 1998). In 1994, it is estimated that approximately 2% of all Americans (4.7 million people) sustained a dog bite. It is estimated that 585,000 Americans a year receive dog bites that require medical attention or result in restricted activity. This makes dog bites the 12th leading cause of nonfatal injury in the United States (Overall and Love 2001). Children who have multiple or deep dog bites may be at increased risk for posttraumatic stress disorder (Peters et al. 2004).

It is estimated that 11,476 children younger than 18 years are treated in emergency departments for cat bites each year (O'Neill, Mack, and Gilchrist 2007). Although cats are less likely to bite than dogs, cat bites are more likely to cause infection. This is because cat bites cause puncture wounds, which are more difficult to clean. Also, cats tend to bite hands, which are more prone to infection (Stefanopoulos and Tarantzopoulou 2005). It has been reported that 20% to 50% of cat bites become infected. Stray cats are more likely than pet cats to be involved in biting incidents.

Because cats are less likely to be vaccinated against rabies, and more likely to be exposed to nocturnal animals that carry disease, they are more likely than dogs to be reported as rabid in the United States (Centers for Disease Control and Prevention 2008). It is not surprising that cat victims are therefore more likely than dog victims to be subjected to prophylaxis treatment for rabies, an expensive and potentially unpleasant ordeal (Moore et al. 2000). Although bites from nonimmunized domestic animals do carry a risk of rabies in the United States, bites from wild animals are more likely to transmit the disease. For the past few decades, the majority of human rabies cases acquired in the United States have come from bats. Raccoons, skunks, and foxes are the carnivores most likely to carry this life-threatening infection (Centers for Disease Control and Prevention 2008).

For boys, snakebites are the third most common type of animal bite treated in hospital emergency departments (O'Neill, Mack, and Gilchrist 2007). Fatal snakebites are rare in the United States. Children are at lower risk for snakebites than adults, and more than 80% of snakebites are from nonpoisonous snakes. When children are bitten by venomous snakes, however, they are more likely to experience a serious reaction (Seifert et al. 2009). More than half of all people treated for venomous snakebites in U.S. emergency departments each year require hospital admission. Sixty-eight percent of such injuries are inflicted by rattlesnakes (O'Neil, Mack, and Gilchrist 2007). Snakebites occur more frequently during warmer months and in warmer states (Seifert et al. 2009).

Florida has been experiencing problems from pythons. In July 2009, a Florida toddler was strangled by her mother's boyfriend's pet python that escaped its cage in the middle of the night and wrapped itself around the girl, killing her (Msnbc.com 2010). Pythons, native to Africa and Asia, have no known predators in Florida. Irresponsible pet owners who release them into the wild when they get too large to handle are blamed for the reported 10,000 pythons that live in the Everglades area. Concerned about the growing problem, Florida's governor recently authorized ten python hunters to trap the animals (Clark 2010).

Risk Factors for Dog Bites

Risk factors for dog bites include characteristics of the animal, the child, and the environmental factors, as reviewed in this section. We should mention, however, that there is a need for improved surveillance of such injuries and the circumstances that surround them.

Animal Factors

Breed of Dog

Listing "breed of dog" as a risk factor is controversial, in part because previous studies have been criticized for lacking accurate denominator data. Also, dog owners do not always know their dog's breed, and most household pets are a product of cross-breeding. There are also many confounding factors that make researching this question a challenge (Overall and Love 2001). Keeping those caveats in mind, we can report that between 1989 and 1994, Rottweilers and "pit bull-type" dogs were responsible for half of all dog bite–related fatalities in the United States (Sacks et al. 1996). Other studies of dog bites have also implicated these breeds along with German Shepherds, Dobermans, and Chow Chows (Cornelissen and Hopster 2010; Gershman, Sacks, and Wright 1994; Kaye, Belz, and Kirschner 2007; Schalamon et al. 2006; Stull and Hodge 2000). Nevertheless, parents need to remember that all dogs can bite.

Other Animal Characteristics

The most reliable indicator of a dog's ability to inflict serious injury to a child is probably its size. Despite this, a survey of Arizona parents found that 20% of families with children aged 0 to 1 years had large dogs in their homes (Villar et al. 1998). Male and unneutered dogs are more likely to bite (Sacks et al. 2000). We also know that animals with a history of biting or exhibiting aggressive behavior are at higher risk for inflicting future bites. Anxious dogs and those with painful medical conditions may also pose greater risk (Reisner, Shofer, and Nance 2007).

Child Factors

Age

Children are at least three times more likely to receive an injury-producing dog bite than adults (Overall and Love 2001). The incidence of dog bites peaks among 5- to 9-year-olds (National Center for Injury Prevention and Control 2004; Sinclair and Zhou 1995). One- to 4-year-olds, however, may be at higher risk for incurring a dog bite that requires hospitalization (Ozanne-Smith, Ashby, Stathakis 2001).

In the United States, 70% to 80% of fatal dog bite victims are children (National Center for Injury Prevention and Control 2010a). Infants younger than 3 months seem to experience the highest rate of fatal dog bites, with those younger than 1 month experiencing a risk that was once calculated to be 370 times that of adults aged 30 to 49 years (Sacks, Sattin, and Bonzo 1989).

Children's increased vulnerability stems, undoubtedly, from cognitive and physical limitations imposed by their phase of development. For example, although most adult victims are bitten on the extremities, greater than 70% of child victims receive an injury to the head, neck, or face (Overall and Love 2001). In one study, younger children's bites were more likely to be inflicted when dogs are resource-guarding or responding to potentially painful interaction (e.g., child fell on dog) (Reisner, Shofer, and Nance 2007).

Gender

Studies have shown that boys are more likely than girls to be bitten by dogs (Overall and Love 2001). There is some suggestion that this disparity is related to different play patterns, because it seems to be more common among dogs other than the family pet (Daniels et al. 2009) and is more true of older boys who may be permitted to play farther from home (Overall and Love 2001). Males are also overrepresented among fatal dog bite victims (Langley 2009).

Personality

Cruelty to animals is a symptom of certain types of personality disorders, which may provoke an animal to bite (Sinclair and Zhou 1995). It should be noted, however, that many behaviors common to healthy children (e.g., yelling, grabbing, making darting movements) can trigger dog bites (American Veterinary Medical Association 2001).

Adult Supervision

For minor bites, the relationship between adult presence and dog bite occurrence are mixed. Observers point out, however, that being present and monitoring are not necessarily the same behavior. With regard to fatal dog bites, it has been reported that most child victims are alone with a dog at the time of the attack (Overall and Love 2001).

Other Environmental Factors

Because of issues of exposure, it is not surprising that dog ownership by household has emerged repeatedly as a risk factor for dog bites. Most children are bitten by dogs at home, rather than in public places (Ozanne-Smith, Ashby, and Stathakis 2001). Exposure is probably at play again, when we observe that younger children are more likely to be bitten at home than older children (Beck and Jones 1985). It has been reported that poor children are at higher risk of dog bite than children of higher socioeconomic status (Overall and Love 2001). Urban dwellers also seem to be at higher risk than rural or small town residents for experiencing an animal bite (Sinclair and Zhou 1995). Animal bites have been shown to increase in the aftermath of hurricanes (Centers for Disease Control and Prevention 2009; Warner 2010). The southern United States has the highest death rate for fatal dog attacks, and the Northeast has the lowest (Sacks et al. 1996).

Between 1989 and 1994, 27% of fatal dog attacks involved more than one dog. Fifty-nine percent of deaths involved an unrestrained dog on the owner's property, and 22% involved unrestrained dogs off the owner's property (Sacks et al. 1996). Despite these findings, a number of studies have reported that chained dogs are overrepresented in biting incidents (Gershman, Sacks, and Wright 1994).

Prevention Strategies

Before acquiring a pet, parents should speak to a veterinarian about which types are most suitable for households with children. The American Veterinary Medical Association (2010) advises parents to put off getting a dog in their home until their children are more than 4 years of age. Adults should socialize family pets and seek immediate professional help if their dog exhibits aggressive behaviors. Finally, they should understand that young children should not be left alone with any dog (National Center for Injury Prevention and Control 2004). The Arizona study cited earlier (Villar et al. 1998) found that 63% of dog owners with children aged 0 to 5 years believed that a 4-year-old would be safe if left unsupervised with their dog(s). A survey of Australian parents found that 70% "always" allowed their child to play unsupervised with the family dog, and that most believed their dog would never bite their child regardless of its circumstances (e.g., eating, sleeping) (Wilson, Dwyer, Bennett 2003).

The CDC (National Center for Injury Prevention and Control 2004) also recommends that children be taught some basic safety tips, such as not to approach unfamiliar dogs, how to approach dogs they know, and how to react if they are knocked over or bitten by a dog. Canines should also be spayed or neutered. By taking these measures, families can enjoy the benefits of dog ownership while minimizing the likelihood that their child will be harmed in the process.

The acquisition of wildlife/wild animal hybrids as pets should be discouraged (Centers for Disease Control and Prevention 2008; Sinclair and Zhou 1995). This is particularly true of raccoons, which represent an important reservoir for human and domestic pet exposure to rabies (Moore et al. 2000). Ferrets can also carry rabies, and pet ferrets have been implicated in vicious attacks on young children (Applegate and Walhout 1998).

At present, most pediatricians do not seem to discuss pet-related injuries with parents, despite the fact that they believe such counseling to be worthwhile (Villar et al. 1998). One simple message that clinicians might want to communicate is that female dogs seem to be a safer choice than male dogs (Reisner, Shofer, and Nance 2007). Additional outreach channels could include pet stores, veterinarian offices, local dog clubs and trainers, and the media (American Veterinary Medical Association 2010; Villar et al. 1998). It has been recommended that such counseling begin before a dog is acquired and evolve in response to the behavior of individual animals and the developmental stage of the children in the home. A number of resources have been developed to guide providers through such sessions (Hart 1997; Love and Overall 2001).

The importance of maintaining rabies vaccination is another message that should be stressed to parents. Educational resources geared toward adults, as well as children, can be accessed via the American Veterinary Medical Association Web site (at http://www.avma.org/animal_health/brochures/dog_bite/dog_bite_brochure.asp). Schools should clearly be involved in dissemination campaigns, because children in grades K to 4 are at highest risk of dog bites.

At the community level, animal control programs should be supported, along with strict regulation of vicious dogs (National Center for Injury Prevention and Control 1997). The literature contains mixed reports on the effects of breed-specific legislation. The Netherlands abolished breed-specific legislation after evaluating its impact (Cornelissen and Hopster 2010). In Spain, declines in hospitalizations due to dog bites were seen after the enactment of regulations that imposed a multitude of requirements on the owners of dogs that were deemed potentially dangerous (i.e., because of their breed, physical traits, or behavioral history) (Villalbi et al. 2010). In the United States, a local ordinance that focused on restricting dogs that had exhibited "dangerous" behavior in the past also achieved positive results (Oswald 1991). Feral cat populations should also be controlled, and owners should be discouraged from allowing their cats to roam freely (American Pet Products Manufacturers Association 2010). Better surveillance of animal bites, and the circumstances under which they occurred, would also facilitate preventive efforts. Finally, to prevent medical treatment and morbidity secondary to animal bites, municipalities should consider linking the ability to obtain a pet license with the requirement for documenting that the pet has a current rabies vaccination (Moore et al. 2000).

Recent Research Findings

Most recommendations for reducing dog bite incidence are not evidence-based. In updating this review, we were encouraged to find multiple peer-reviewed reports of prevention programs that had been evaluated. Most used brief educational interventions targeting young children. This body of work demonstrates that such programs can increase participants' awareness and recognition of risky situations and concluded that parental involvement enhanced children's learning (Meints and de Keuster 2009; Wilson, Dwyer, and Bennett 2003). We were most impressed by a randomized controlled trial of "Prevent-a-Bite," a program conducted in Australia. That intervention was designed to instill precautionary behaviors in children when they are around dogs. Its authors showed that 7- to 8-year-old students who were exposed to a half-hour instructional program were significantly less likely to pet a "strange" dog on the playground 10 days after the intervention (Chapman et al. 2000). We did not identify any evaluations that measured injury outcomes. Noting this gap in the literature, a Cochrane review concluded that education of children should not be the only public health strategy advanced for reducing dog bites (Duperrex et al. 2009).

Advocacy Efforts

The American Veterinary Medical Association (2010) Task Force on Canine Aggression and Human-Canine Interactions has developed a comprehensive set of recommendations that could guide community-based prevention efforts while a more solid scientific foundation is being built. They advise advocates to promote this issue in collaboration with public officials and other community leaders, veterinarians and allied personnel, animal behaviorists, responsible dog breeders and trainers, physicians and nurses, animal control personnel, members of the judicial and educational systems, public health professionals, law enforcement representatives, business leaders (e.g., pet stores, insurance companies), groups with occupational safety interests (e.g., meter readers and postal workers), voluntary/nonprofit organizations (e.g., Safe Kids Worldwide, 4-H clubs), members of the animal welfare community (i.e., the Humane Society, animal shelter/rescue personnel), recreational groups, and the media.

Conclusions

Home injuries remain all too common. This is especially true during the earliest years of children's lives, before they venture out into the world on their own. Parents who are informed of potential sources of risk within the home environment can remove or modify them. Even when such steps have been taken, however, children's levels of physical and cognitive development pose inherent dangers. That is why vigilance is required of those responsible for protecting young children. Such advice can be hard to follow, however, in a household where siblings need attention, phones are ringing, and chores must be completed. Up to now, our field has not helped parents determine what constitutes "adequate supervision." Recently, however, important research has been undertaken to define and measure supervision (Morrongiello and House 2004). These efforts will enable us to understand which styles of caretaking are associated with injury risk, providing a basis for parental advice that is more specific and useful. In many cases, safety products already exist, such as smoke alarms and cabinet locks, and the challenge is finding effective ways to promote their use. Evaluation studies of programs designed to prevent specific types of home injuries are still needed.

Improved surveillance is also a critical need. As noted in this chapter, we do not even know how many U.S. children are killed or injured in their homes each year. Surveillance data on home injuries per se are not routinely collected. However, since 1971 a nationally representative sample of hospital emergency departments have provided the CPSC with data on consumer product-related injuries, many of which affect children (CPSC 2004g). This system is known as the NEISS. In 2000, the CPSC and the National Center for Injury Prevention and Control at the CDC began jointly funding the NEISS All Injury Program, meaning that data are now provided routinely on all injuries, not just those that are product related. This more comprehensive data source has substantially strengthened our ability to document the burden of injury, and new reports from this data set have appeared in the published literature. Improved data-collection processes should be put in place, and organizations that carry out related work (e.g., the CPSC, poison control centers) should be provided with adequate and secure funding.

An important new resource in the efforts to prevent home injury is the CPSIA, legislation passed in 2008 that strengthens the CPSC's efforts to keep unsafe products from the marketplace. The Act also increased the CPSC's budget, which is critical to provide the necessary resources to address consumer product safety in a comprehensive manner. From surveillance of injury events, to consumer education and product recalls, to continuous advocacy with product manufactures to design the safest products possible, the CSPC's activities mirror what should be done by all sectors of society to keep our children safe, especially in their own homes.

References

Abdel-Rahman HA. 2000. Fatal suffocation by rubber balloons in children: mechanism and prevention. *Forensic Sci Int.* 108:97–105.

Ahrens M. 2010. *Home Structure Fires.* Quincy, MA: National Fire Protection Association.

American Academy of Pediatrics. 2001a. Injuries associated with infant walkers. *Pediatrics.* 108:790–792.

American Academy of Pediatrics. 2001b. *Choking: Common Dangers for Children, Information Sheet.* Elk Grove, IL: American Academy of Pediatrics.

American Academy of Pediatrics. 2010. Prevention of choking among children. *Pediatrics.* 125:601–607.

American Association of Poison Control Centers. 2004. *Poison Prevention Tips to Keep Our Children Safe.* Available at: http://www.aapcc.org/children.htm. Accessed August 29, 2004.

American Pet Products Association (APPA). 2010. *2009/2010 National Pet Owners Survey.* Greenwich, CT: APPA. Available at: http://americanpetproducts.org/press_industrytrends.asp. Accessed July 30, 2010.

American Veterinary Medical Association. 2001. A community approach to dog bite prevention. *J Am Vet Med Assoc.* 218:1732–1746.

American Veterinary Medical Association (AVMA). 2010. *Dog Bite Prevention, revised 3/10.* Schaumburg, IL: AVMA. Available at: http://www.avma.org/animal_health/brochure/public_health.asp. Accessed May 20, 2010.

Applegate JA, Walhout MF. 1998. Childhood risks from the ferret. *J Emerg Med.* 16:425–427.

Ballesteros M, Jackson M, Martin MW. 2005. Working towards the elimination of residential fire deaths: CDC's smoke alarm and fire safety education. *J Burn Care Res.* 26:434–439.

Ballesteros MF, Kresnow MJ. 2007. Prevalence of residential smoke alarms and fire escape plans in the U.S.: results from the Second Injury Control and Risk Survey (ICARIS-2). *Public Health Rep.* 122:224–231.

Ballesteros MF, Schieber RA, Gilchrist J, et al. 2003. Differential ranking of causes of fatal versus non-fatal injuries among US children. *Inj Prev.* 9:173–176.

Barlow B, Niemirska N, Gandhi RP, Leblanc W. 1983. Ten years experience with falls from a height in children. *J Pediatr Surg.* 18:509–511.

Bar-Oz B, Levichek Z, Koren G. 2004. Medications that can be fatal for a toddler with one tablet or teaspoon: a 2004 update. *Paediatr Drugs.* 6:123–126.

Barrow RE, Spies M, Barrow LN, Herndon DN. 2004. Influence of demographics and inhalation injury on burn mortality in children. *Burns* 30:72–77.

Beck AM, Jones B. 1985. Unreported dog bites in children. *Public Health Rep.* 100:315–321.

Beirens TMJ, Brug J, van Beeck EF, et al. 2007. Presence and use of stair gates in homes with toddlers (11-18 months old). *Accid Anal Prev.* 39:964–968.

Belechri M, Petridou E, Trichopoulos D. 2002. Bunk versus conventional beds: a comparative assessment of fall injury risk. *J Epidemiol Community Health.* 56:413–417.

Bernardo LM, Gardner MJ, O'Connor JO, Amon N. 2000. Dog bites in children treated in a pediatric emergency department. *J Soc Pediatr Nurses.* 5:87.

Bhoota BL, Kitinya J. 2005. Deaths from accidental steam inhalation during traditional therapy. *J Clin Forensic Med.* 12:214–217.

Blumenthal D. 1989. Artificial nail remover poses poisoning risk. *FDA Consumer.* 23:26–33.

Bond GR. 2003. Home syrup of ipecac use does not reduce emergency department use or improve outcome. *Pediatrics* 112:1061–1064.

Bornse NN, Gilchrist J, Dellinger AM, et al. 2008. *The CDC Childhood Injury Report: Patterns of Unintentional Injuries Among 0-19 Year Olds in the United States, 2000–2006.* Atlanta, GA: Centers for Disease Control and Prevention, National Center for Injury Prevention and Control.

Bronstein AC, Spyker DA, Cantilena LR, et al. 2009. 2008 Annual Report of the American Association of Poison Control Centers' National Poison Data System (NPDS): 26th Annual Report. *Clin Toxicology.* 47:911–1084.

Bruck D, Ball M. 2007. Optimizing emergency awakening to audible smoke alarms: an update. *Human Factors.* 49:585–601.

Bruck D, Thomas IS. 2009. Smoke alarms for sleeping adults who are hard-of-hearing: comparison of auditory, visual and tactile signals. *Ear Hear* 30:73–80.

Brywczynski J, Arnold DH. 2008. Shower steamer burns in a toddler: care report and brief review of steam burns in children. *Pediatr Emerg Care.* 24:782–784.

Cagle KM, Davis JW, Dominic W, Gonzales W. 2006. Results of a focused scald-prevention program. *J Burn Care Res.* 27:859–863.

Casteel C, Runyan CW. 2004a. Leading causes of unintentional home injury in high-risk groups. In: Runyan CW, Casteel C, editors. *The State of Home Safety in America: Facts About Unintentional Injuries in the Home,* 2nd ed. Washington, DC: Home Safety Council:61–68.

Casteel C, Runyan CW. 2004b. Leading causes of unintentional home injury death. In: Runyan CW, Casteel C, editors. *The State of Home Safety in America: Facts About Unintentional Injuries in the Home,* 2nd ed. Washington, DC: Home Safety Council:33–60.

Centers for Disease Control and Prevention. 1986. Perspectives in disease prevention and health promotion National Poison Prevention Week: 25th anniversary observance. *MMWR.* 35:149–152.

Centers for Disease Control and Prevention. 2002. Nonfatal choking-related episodes among children—United States, 2001. *MMWR.* 51:945–948.

Centers for Disease Control and Prevention. 2004. Use of carbon monoxide alarms to prevent poisonings during a power outage—North Carolina, December 2002. *MMWR.* 53:189–192.

Centers for Disease Control and Prevention. 2008. Human rabies prevention—United States, 2008. *MMWR.* 57;RR03:1–26, 28.

Centers for Disease Control and Prevention. 2009. Morbidity and mortality associated with hurricane Floyd-North Carolina, September-October 1999. *MMWR.* 49:369–372.

Chapman S, Cornwall J, Righetti J, Sung L. 2000. Preventing dog bites in children: randomized controlled trial of an educational intervention. *BMJ.* 320:1512.

Chianese K, Plof D, Trovato C, Change JC. 2009. Inner-city caregivers' perspectives on bed sharing with their infants. *Acad Pediatr.* 9:26–32.

Chiaviello CT, Christof RA, Bond GR. 1994. Infant walker-related injuries: a prospective study of severity and incidence. *Pediatrics.* 93:974–976.

Child Health Alert. 2007. Recall: children's hooded sweatshirts with drawstrings ... and Kids II teethers. 25:6.

Chu AY, Ripple MG, Allan CH, et al. 2006. Fatal dog maulings associated with infant swings. *J Forensic Sci.* 51:403–406.

Clamp M, Kendrick D. 1998. A randomized controlled trial of general practitioner safety advice for families with children under 5 years. *BMJ.* 316:1575–1579.

Clark A. 2009. "Snakes on the Glades"—Florida launches mass python hunt. Guardian.co.uk. Available at: http://www.guardian.co.uk/world/2009/jul/19/florida-santions-mass-python-hunt. Accessed November 5, 2010.

Coalition for Fire Safe Cigarettes. 2010. *The New York Experience.* Quincy, MA: National Fire Protection Association. Available at: http://www.firesafecigarettes.org. Accessed September 1, 2010.

Collier ML, Ward S, Saffle JR, et al. 2004. Home treadmill friction injuries: a five year review. *J Burn Care Rehab.* 25:441–444.

Committee on Injury, Violence, and Poison Prevention. 2003. Poison treatment in the home. *Pediatrics.* 112:1182–1185.

Consumer Product Safety Commission (CPSC). 1998. CPSC initiates rulemaking for cigarette lighters. Press release #880001. Washington, DC: CPSC.

Consumer Product Safety Commission (CPSC). 2000. Babies in adult beds. *Consumer Product Safety Rev.* 4:5.

Consumer Product Safety Commission (CPSC). 2001a. Child-resistant packaging for certain over-the-counter drug products, final rule. *Federal Register.* 6:40111–40116.

Consumer Product Safety Commission (CPSC). 2001b. Requirements for Bunk Beds, 16 C.F.R. Part 1213, 1500, and 1513. Washington, DC: CPSC.

Consumer Product Safety Commission (CPSC). 2002. Poison prevention packaging requirements: exemption of hormone replacement therapy products. *Federal Register.* 67:66550–66552.

Consumer Product Safety Commission (CPSC). 2004a. *Consumer Product Safety Alert: Young Children and Teens Burned by Hair Curling Irons.* Washington, DC: CPSC. Available at: http://www.cpsc.gov. Accessed August 15, 2004.

Consumer Product Safety Commission (CPSC). 2004b. *Consumer Product Safety Alert: Household Batteries can Cause Chemical Burns.* Washington, DC: CPSC. Available at: http://www.cpsc.gov. Accessed August 15, 2004.

Consumer Product Safety Commission (CPSC). 2004c. *Just the Facts: Bunk Beds.* Washington, DC: CPSC. Available at: http://www.cpsc.gov/CPSCPUB/PUBS/071.html. Accessed September 15, 2004.

Consumer Product Safety Commission (CPSC). 2004d. *CPSC Gets New, Safer Baby Walkers on the Market (2001).* Washington, DC: CPSC. Available at: http://www.cpsc.gov/CPSCPUB/PUBS/5086.pdf. Accessed September 15, 2004.

Consumer Product Safety Commission (CPSC). 2004e. *CPSC, KFC Corporation Announce Recall of Toy Included with KFC Kids Meal.* Washington, DC: CPSC. Available at: http://www.recall-warnings.com/cpsc-content-00-00162.html. Accessed September 15, 2004.

Consumer Product Safety Commission (CPSC). 2004f. *Strings and Straps on Toys can Strangle Young Children.* Washington, DC: CPSC. Available at: http://www.cpsc.gov/cpscpub/pubs/5100.html. Accessed September 15, 2004.

Consumer Product Safety Commission (CPSC). 2004g. *The National Electronic Injury Surveillance System: A Tool for Researchers.* Washington, DC: CPSC. Available at: http://www.cpsc.gov/Neiss/2000d015.pdf. Accessed September 15, 2004.

Consumer Product Safety Commission (CPSC). 2010a. Safety standard for infant walkers. *Federal Register.* 75:35266–35278.

Consumer Product Safety Commission (CPSC). 2010b. Revocation of regulations banning certain baby walkers. *Federal Register.* 75:35279–35280.

Consumer Product Safety Commission (CPSC). 2010c. Safety standards for full-size baby cribs and non-full-size baby cribs: notice of proposed rulemaking. *Federal Register.* 75:43308–43327.

Consumer Product Safety Commission (CPSC). 2010d. Safety standard for toddler beds. *Federal Register.* 75:2291–2303.

Consumer Product Safety Commission (CPSC). 2010e. *National Electronic Injury Surveillance System (NEISS) Data Highlights—2009.* Washington, DC: CPSC. Available at: http://www.cpsc.gov/neiss/2009highlights.pdf. Accessed November 5, 2010.

Consumer Product Safety Commission (CPSC). 2010f. Minutes of the Commission Meeting: Statement of Chairman Inez M. Tenenbaum on the Commission Decision Regarding the Final Rule on the Mandatory Safety Standard for Infant Walkers. Washington, DC: CPSC. Available at: http://www.cpsc.gov/LIBRARY/FOIA/ballot/ballot10/cm05262010.pdf. Accessed November 5, 2010.

Cornelissen JMR, Hopster H. 2010. Dog bites in The Netherlands: a study of victims, injuries, circumstances and aggressors to support evaluation of breed specific legislation. *Vet J.* 186:292–298. Epub 2009 Oct 29.

Coyne-Beasley T, Runyan CW, Baccaglini L, et al. 2005. Storage of poisonous substances and firearms in homes with young children visitors and older adults. *Am J Prev Med.* 28:109–115.

Daniels DM, Ritzi RBS, O'Neil J, Scherer LRT. 2009. Analysis of nonfatal dog bites in children. *J Trauma.* 66:S17–S22.

DiGuiseppi C, Roberts I, Wade A, et al. 2002. Incidence of fires and related injuries after giving out free smoke alarms: cluster randomized controlled trial. *BMJ.* 325:995–997.

Dole EJ, Czajka PA, Rivara FP. 1986. Evaluation of pharmacists' compliance with the Poison Prevention Packaging Act. *Am J Public Health.* 76:1335–1336.

Duchossois HV, Garcia-Espana JF, Durbin DR. 2006. Impact of a community based fire prevention intervention of fire safety knowledge and behavior in elementary school children. *Inj Prev.* 12:344–346.

Dunst CM, Scott EC, Kraatz JJ, et al. 2004. Contact palm burns in toddlers from glass enclosed fireplaces. *J Burn Care Rehabil* 25:67–70.

Duperrex O, Blackhall K, Burri M, Jeannot E. 2009. Education of children and adolescents for the prevention of dog bite injuries. *Cochrane Database Syst Rev.* (2):CD004726. Review.

D'Souza AL, Nelson NG, McKenzie LB. 2008. Pediatric burn injuries treated in US emergency departments between 1990-2006. *Pediatrics.* 124:1424–1430.

D'Souza AL, Smith GA, McKenzie LB. 2008. Bunk bed-related injuries among children and adolescents treated in emergency departments in the United States, 1990-2005. *Pediatrics.* 121:e1696–702.

Erdmann TC, Feldman KW, Rivara FP, et al. 1991. Tap water burn prevention: the effect of legislation. *Pediatrics.* 88:572–577.

Federal Interagency Forum on Child and Family Statistics. [n.d.] *Child Injury and Mortality: Death Rates Among Children Ages 1-14 by Gender, Race, and Hispanic Origin, and All Causes and All Injury Causes of Death, 1980-2007.* Washington, DC: U.S. Department of Education, National Center for Education Statistics. Available at: http://www.childstats.gov/americaschildren/tables/phy6b.asp. Accessed September 10, 2010.

Feldman KW, Schaller RT, Feldman JA, McMillon M. 1978. Tap water scald burns in children. *Pediatrics.* 62:1–7.

Fergusson DM, Horwood LJ, Beautrais AL, Shannon FT. 1982. A controlled field trial of a poisoning prevention method. *Pediatrics.* 69:515–520.

Fiebiger B, Whitmire F, Law E, Still JM. 2004. Causes and treatment of burns from grease. *J Burn Care Rehabil.* 25:374–376.

Field JM, Hazinski MF, Sayre MR, et al. 2010. Part 1: Executive summary: 2010 American Heart Association guidelines for cardiopulmonary resuscitation and emergency cardiovascular care. *Circulation.* 122(18 Suppl 3): S640–656.

Flynn J. 2010. *Characteristics of Home Fire Victims.* Quincy, MA: National Fire Protection Association.

Franklin RL, Rodgers GB. 2008. Unintentional child poisonings treated in United States hospital emergency departments: national estimates of incident cases, population-based poisoning rates, and product involvement. *Pediatrics.* 122:1244–1251.

Garry VF, Harkins ME, Erickson LL, et al. 2002. Birth defects, season of conception, and sex of children born to pesticide applicators living in the Red River Valley of Minnesota, USA. *Environ Health Perspect.* 110(Suppl 3):441–449.

Gershman KA, Sacks JJ, Wright JC. 1994. Which dogs bite? A case-control study of risk factors. *Pediatrics.* 93:913–917.

Gielen AC, McDonald EM, Wilson MEH, et al. 2002. Effects of improved access to safety counseling, products, and home visits on parents' safety practices. *Arch Pediatr Adolesc Med.* 156:33–40.

Greene MA, Granados DV. 2010. *2008 Fireworks Annual Report: Fireworks Related Deaths, Emergency Department Treated Injuries, and Enforcement Activities During 2008.* Available at: http://www.cpsc.gov/LIBRARY/2008fwreport.pdf. Accessed August 29, 2010.

Harborview Injury Prevention and Research Center. 2004. *Poisoning Interventions: Child Resistant Packaging and the Poison Prevention Packaging Act.* Available at: http://depts.washington.edu/hiprc/practices/topic/poisoning/packaging.html. Accessed September 15, 2004.

Harris CD, Baker SP, Smith GA, Harris RM.1984. Childhood asphyxiation by food: a national analysis and overview. *JAMA.* 251:2231–2235.

Hart BL. 1997. Selecting, raising and caring for dogs to avoid problem aggression. *J Am Vet Med Assoc.* 210:1129–1134.

Hillman HS. 1983. Memory Processing and Overlearning in the Acquisition and Maintenance of Fire-Safety Skills. Pittsburgh, PA: University of Pittsburgh.

Holmes GA, Jones RT. 1996. Fire evacuation skills: cognitive behavior versus computer-mediated instruction. *Fire Technology.* First Quarter:51–64.

Hingley AT. 1997. Preventing childhood poisoning. *FDA Consumer Magazine* 30:1–7.

Hu G, Baker SP. 2009. Trends in unintentional injury deaths, U.S., 1999–2005: age, gender, and racial/ethnic differences. *Am J Prev Med.* 37:188–194.

Institute of Medicine. 2004a. *Forging a Poison Prevention and Control System.* New York: The National Academy of Sciences.

Institute of Medicine. 2004b. *The Future of Poison Prevention and Control Services.* New York: The National Academy of Sciences.

Istre GR, McCoy MA, Osborn L, et al. 2001. Deaths and injuries from house fires. *N Engl J Med.* 344:1911–1916.

Istre GR, McCoy MA, Carlin DK, McClain J. 2002. Residential fire related deaths and injuries among children: fireplay, smoke alarms, and prevention. *Inj Prev.* 8:128–132.

Istre GR, McCoy MA, Stowe M, et al. 2003. Childhood injuries due to falls from apartment balconies and windows. *Inj Prev.* 9:349–352.

Jackson M, Wilson JM, Akoto J, et al. 2010. Evaluation of fire-safety programs that use 10-year smoke alarms. *J Community Health.* 35:543–548.

Joseph KE, Adams CD, Goldfarb IW, Slater H. 2002. Parental correlates of unintentional burn injuries in infancy and early childhood. *Burns.* 28:455–463.

Joyner BL, Oden RP, Ajao TI, Moon RY. 2010. Where should my baby sleep: a qualitative study of African American infant sleep location decisions. *J Natl Med Assoc.* 102:881–889.

Karter MJ. 2010. *Fire Loss in the United States During 2009.* Quincy, MA: National Fire Protection Association.

Katcher ML. 1983. Scald burns from hot tap water. *Pediatrics.* 71:145–146.

Kaye AE, Belz JM, Kirschner RE. 2007. Pediatric dog bite injuries: a 5-year review of the experience at The Children's Hospital of Philadelphia. *Plast Reconstr Surg.* 124:551–558.

Kelly NR, Huffman LC, Mendoza FS, Robinson TN. 2003. Effects of a videotape to increase use of poison control centers by low-income and Spanish-speaking families: a randomized, controlled trial. *Pediatrics.* 111:21–26.

Kendrick D, Smith S, Sutton A, et al. 2008. Effect of education and safety equipment on poisoning-prevention practices and poisoning: systematic review, meta-analysis and meta-regression. *Arch Dis Child.* 2008;93:599–608.

Kriel RL, Gormley ME, Krach LE, Luxemberg MG, Bartsh SM, Bertrand JR. 1996. Automatic garage door openers: hazard for children. *Pediatrics.* 98:770-773.

Landrigan PJ, Claudio L, Markowitz SB, et al. 1999. Pesticides and inner city children: exposures, risks, and prevention. *Environ Health Perspect.* 117(Suppl 3):431–437.

Langley RL. 2009. Human fatalities resulting from dog attacks in the United States, 1979–2005. *Wilderness Environ Med.* 20:19–25.

Laughlin L. 2005. Who's minding the kids? Child care arrangements: Spring 2005 and Summer 2006. *Curr Popul Rep.* 70121.

Lee JW, Jang YC, Oh SJ. 2004. Pediatric electrical burn: outlet injury caused by steel chopstick misuse. *Burn.* 30:244–247.

Leistikow BN, Martin DC, Milano CE. 2000. Fire injuries, disasters, and costs from cigarettes and cigarette lights: a global overview. *Prev Med.* 31:91–99.

Levy DT, Mallonnee S, Miller TR, et al. 2004. Alcohol involvement in burn, submersion, spinal cord, and brain injuries. *Med Sci Monit.* 10:CR17–24.

Lifschultz BD, Donoghue ER. 1996. Deaths due to foreign body aspiration in children: the continuing hazard of toy balloons. *J Forensic Sci.* 41:247–251.

Litovitz T, Whitaker N, Clark L, et al. 2010. Emerging battery-ingestion hazard: clinical implications. *Pediatrics.* 125:1168–1177.

Litovitz T, Whitaker N, Clark L. 2010. Preventing battery ingestions: an analysis of 8648 cases. *Pediatrics.* 125:1178–1183.

Love M, Overall KL. 2001. How anticipating relationships between dogs and children can prevent disasters. *J Am Vet Med Assoc.* 219:446–453.

Lyons RA, John A, Brophy S, et al. *Modification of the home environment for the reduction of injuries.* Cochrane Database of Systematic Reviews 2006, Issue 4, Art. No.: CD003600. DOI: 10.1002/14651858. CD003600.pub2.

Macgregor DM. 2000. Injuries associated with falls from beds. *Inj Prev.* 6:291–292.

Maguina P, Palmieri TL, Greenhalgh DG. 2004. Treadmills: a preventable source of pediatric friction burn injuries. *J Burn Care Rehabil.* 25:201–204.

Mangus RS, Bergman D, Zieger M, Coleman JJ. 2004. Burn injuries in children with attention-deficit/hyperactivity disorder. *Burns.* 30:148–150.

Marshall S, Runyan CW, Bangdiwala SI, et al. 1998. Fatal residential fires: who dies and who survives. *JAMA.* 279:1633–1637.

McGuigan MA. 1996. Acute iron poisoning. *Pediatr Ann.* 25:33–38.

McKenzie LB, Ahir N, Stolz U, Nelson NG. 2010. Household cleaning product-related injuries treated in US emergency departments in 1990-2006. *Pediatrics.* 126:108–116.

Meints K, de Keuster T. 2009. Brief reports: don't kiss a sleeping dog: the first assessment of "The Blue Dog" Bite Prevention program. *J Pediatr Psychol.* 334:1084–1090.

Miller TR, Lestina DC. 1997. Costs of poisoning in the United States and savings from poison control centers: a benefit-cost analysis. *Ann Emerg Med.* 29:246–247.

Moore DA, Sischo WM, Hunter A, Miles T. 2000. Animal bite epidemiology and surveillance for rabies postexposure prophylaxis. *J Am Vet Med Assoc.* 217:190–194.

Morley RE, Ludemann JP, Moxham JP, et al. 2004. Foreign body aspiration in infants and toddlers: recent trends in British Columbia. *J Otolaryngol.* 33:37–41.

Morrongiello BA, House K. 2004. Measuring parent attributes and supervision behaviors relevant to child injury risk: examining the usefulness of questionnaire measures. *Inj Prev.* 10:114–118.

Morrongeillo BA, Major K. 2002. Influence of safety gear on parental perceptions of injury risk and tolerance for children's risk taking. *Inj Prev.* 8:27–31.

Morrongiello BA, Kiriakou S. 2004. Mothers' home safety practices for preventing six types of childhood injuries: what do they do and why? *J Pediatr Psychol.* 29:285–297.

Msnbc.com. 2009. Girl, 2, strangled by pet python, police say. Available at: http://www.msnbc.msn.com/id/31684161/ns/us_news-life. Accessed November 5, 2010.

Mullins RF, Alarm B, Huq Mian MA, et al. 2009. Burns in mobile home fires—descriptive study at a regional burn center. *J Burn Care Res.* 30:694–699.

National Center for Injury Prevention and Control. 1997. Dog-bite-related fatalities—United States, 1995-6. *MMWR.* 46:463–467.

National Center for Injury Prevention and Control. 2001. *Injury Fact Book 2001–2002.* Atlanta, GA: Centers for Disease Control and Prevention.

National Center for Injury Prevention and Control. 2004. *Dog Bite Prevention.* Atlanta, GA: Centers for Disease Control and Prevention. Available at: http://www.cdc.gov/HomeandRecreationalSafety/index.html. Accessed August 2, 2004.

National Center for Injury Prevention and Control. 2010a. *Fatal Injury Data 2007.* Atlanta, GA: Centers for Disease Control and Prevention. Available at: http://www.cdc.gov/injury/wisqars/index.html. Accessed October 10, 2010.

National Center for Injury Prevention and Control. 2010b. *10 Leading Causes of Nonfatal Injury, United States, 0–14 Age Group, 2007, All Races, Both Sexes, Disposition: Treated and Released.*

Atlanta, GA. Centers for Disease Control and Prevention. Available at: http://www.cdc.gov/injury/wisqars/index.html. Accessed October 10, 2010.

National Conference of State Legislators (NCSL). 2010. *Carbon Monoxide Detectors-State Statutes.* Washington, DC: NCSL. Available at: http://www.ncsl.org/Default.aspx?TabId=13238. Accessed October 15, 2010.

National Fire Protection Association. 2010. *Smoke Alarms for People Who Are Deaf or Hard of Hearing.* Quincy, MA: National Fire Protection Association. Available at: http://www.nfpa.org/assets/files/pdf/public%20education/alarmguidedeaf.pdf. Accessed September 1, 2010.

Nixon J, Spinks A, Turner C, McClure R. 2004. Community based programs to prevent poisoning in children 0-15 years. *Inj Prev.* 10:43–46.

O'Hara M, Harruff R, Smialek JE, Fowler DR. 2000. Sleep location and suffocation: how good is the evidence. *Pediatrics.* 105; 915–920.

O'Neil ME, Mack KA, Gilchrist J. 2007. Epidemiology of non-canine bite and sting injuries treated in the U.S. emergency departments, 2001–2004. *Public Health Rep.* 122:764–775.

Oswald M. 1991. Report on the potentially dangerous dog program: Multonomah County, Oregon. *Anthrozoos.* IV:247–254.

Overall KL, Love M. 2001. Dog bites to humans—demography, epidemiology, injury and risk. *J Am Vet Med Assoc.* 218:1923–1934.

Ozanne-Smith J, Ashby K, Stathakis VZ. 2001. Dog bite and injury prevention—analysis, critical review and research agenda. *Inj Prev.* 7:321–326.

Palacio J, León-Artozqui M, Pastor-Villalba E, et al. 2007. Incidence of and risk factors for cat bites: a first step in prevention and treatment of feline aggression. *J Feline Med Surg.* 9:891–895.

Palmieri TL, Alderson TS, Ison D, et al. 2008. Pediatric soup scald burn injury: etiology and prevention. *J Burn Care Res.* 29:114–118.

Parmer JE, Corso PS, Ballesteros MF. 2006. A cost analysis of a smoke alarm installation and fire safety education program. *J Safety Res.* 37:367–373.

Patronek GJ, Slavinski SA. 2009. Animal bites. *J Am Vet Med Assoc.* 234:336–345.

Peters V, Sottiaux M, Appelboom J, Kahn A. 2004. Posttraumatic stress disorder after dog bites in children. *J Pediatrics.* 121–122.

Ramowski SK, Nystrom RJ, Chaumeton NR, Rosenberg KD. 2010. "Choking game" awareness and participation among 8th graders—Oregon, 2008. *MMWR* 59:1–5.

Reisner IR, Shofer FS, Nance ML. 2007. Behavioral assessment of child-directed canine aggression. *Inj Prev.* 13:348–351.

Rimell FL, Thome A, Stool S, et al. 1995. Characteristics of objects that cause choking in children. *JAMA.* 13;274:1763–1766.

Rohr KD, Hall JR. 2005. *U.S Experience With Sprinklers and Other Fire Extinguishing Equipment.* Quincy, MA: National Fire Protection Association.

Runyan CW, Casteel C. 2004a. Nonfatal home injuries. In: Runyan CW, Casteel C, editors. *The State of Home Safety in America: Facts about Unintentional Injuries in the Home.* 2nd ed. Washington, DC: Home Safety Council:25–32.

Runyan CW, Casteel C. 2004b. Unintentional home injury deaths. In: Runyan CW, Casteel C, editors. *The State of Home Safety in America: Facts About Unintentional Injuries in the Home.* 2nd ed. Washington, DC: Home Safety Council; 2004:21–24.

Runyan CW, Casteel C, editors. 2004c. *The State of Home Safety in America: Facts About Unintentional Injuries in the Home.* 2nd ed. Washington, DC: Home Safety Council.

Runyan CW, Casteel C, Perkis D, et al. 2005. Unintentional injuries in the home in the United States; Part I-Mortality. *Am J Prev Med.* 28:73–79.

Sacks JJ, Lockwood R, Hornreich J, Sattin RW. 1996. Fatal dog attacks, 1989-1994. *Pediatrics.* 97:891–895.

Sacks JJ, Sattin RW, Bonzo SE. 1989. Dog bite-related fatalities from 1979 to 1988. *JAMA.* 262:1489–1492.

Sacks JJ, Sinclair L, Gilchrist J, et al. 2000. Breeds of dogs involved in fatal human attacks in the United States between 1979 and 1998. *J Am Vet Med Assoc.* 217:836–840.

Safe Kids USA. 2004a. *Injury Facts: Poisoning.* Washington, DC: Safe Kids USA. Available at: http://www.safekids.org/tier3_printable.cfm?content_item_id=1152&folder_id+540. Accessed September 2, 2004.

Safe Kids USA. 2004b. *Injury Facts: Falls.* Washington, DC: Safe Kids USA. Available at: http://www.safekids.org/tier3_cd.cfm?folder_id=540&content_item_id=1050. Accessed September 15, 2004.

Safe Kids USA. 2004c. *Safe Kids Thrilled by Government's Ban on Baby Walkers: Asks Parents to Take Action and Wipe Out Walkers.* Washington, DC: Safe Kids USA. Available at: http://www.safekidscanada.ca/ENGLISH/Media/Media_babywalkersbanned.html. Accessed September 15, 2004.

Safe Kids USA. 2004d. *Injury Facts: Airway Obstruction.* Washington, DC: Safe Kids USA. Available at: http://www.safekids.org/tier3_cd.cfm?folder_id=540&content_item_id=991. Accessed September 15, 2004.

Schalamon J, Ainoedhofer H, Singer G, et al. 2006. Analysis of dog bites in children who are younger than 17 years. *Pediatrics.* 17:e374–379.

Schum TR, Lachman BS. 1982. Effect of packaging and appearance on childhood poisoning: Vacor Rat Poison. *Clin Pediatr.* 21:282–285.

Schwebel DC, Brezausek CM, Ramey SL, Ramey CT. 2004. Interactions between child behavior patterns and parenting: implications for children's unintentional injury risk. *J Pediatr Psychol.* 29:93–104.

Seifert SA, Boyer LV, Benson BE, Rogers JJ. 2009. AAPCC database characterization of native U.S. venomous snake exposures, 2001–5. *Clin Toxicol.* 47:327–335.

Sethi D, Towner E, Vincenten J, et al. 2008. *European Report on Child Injury Prevention.* Copenhagen, Denmark: World Health Organization.

Shenassa ED, Stubbendick A, Brown MJ. 2004. Social disparities in housing and related pediatric injury: a multilevel study. *Am J Public Health.* 94:633–639.

Shepherd G, Larkin GL, Velez LI, Huddleston L. 2004. Language preferences among callers to a regional Poison Center. *Vet Hum Toxicol.* 46:100–101.

Shields BJ, Burkett E, Smith GA. 2011. Epidemiology of balcony fall-related injuries, United States, 1990-2006. *Am J Emerg Med.* 29:174–180. Epub 2010 Mar 25.

Sinclair CL, Zhou C. 1995. Descriptive epidemiology of animal bites in Indiana, 1990-92—a rationale for intervention. *Public Health Rep.* 110:64–67.

Sleet DA, Gielen AC. 1998. Injury prevention. In: Gorin SS, Arnold A, editors. *Health Promotion Handbook.* St. Louis, Mosby:247–275.

Sleet DA, Schieber RA, Gilchrist J. 2003. Health promotion policy and politics: lessons from childhood injury prevention. *Health Promot Pract.* 4:103–108.

Smith GA, Splaingard M, Hayes JR, Xiang H. 2006. Comparison of a personalize parent voice smoke alarm with a conventional residential tone smoke alarm for awakening children. *Pediatrics.* 118:1623–1632.

Smith GS, Branas CC, Miller TR. 1999. Fatal non-traffic injuries involving alcohol: a metaanalysis. *Ann Emerg Med.* 33:659–668.

Smith LE, Greene MA, Singh HA. 2000. Fires caused by children playing with lighters: an evaluation of the Consumer Product Safety Commission (CPSC) safety standard for cigarette lighters. Washington, DC: CPSC.

Smith LE, Greene MA, Singh HA. 2002. Study of the effectiveness of the US safety standard for child resistant cigarette lighters. *Inj Prev.* 8:192–196.

Soubhi H. 2004. The social context of childhood injury in Canada: integration of the NLSCY findings. *Am J Health Behav.* 28(Suppl 1):S38–S50.

Spann MF, Blondell JM, Hunting KL. 2000. Acute hazards to young children from residential pesticide exposures. *Am J Public Health.* 90:971–973.

Spiegel CN, Lindaman FC. 1977. Children can't fly: a program to prevent childhood morbidity and mortality from window falls. *Am J Public Health.* 67:1143–1147.

Stefanopoulos PK, Tarantzopoulou AD. 2005. Facial bite wounds: management update. *Internat J Oral Maxillofacial Surg.* 34:464–472.

Stull JW, Hodge RR. 2000. An analysis of reported dog bites: reporting issues and the impact of unowned dogs. *J Environ Health.* 62:17.

Tarrago SB. 2000. Prevention of choking, suffocation and strangulation in childhood. *WMJ.* 99:43–46.

Mikkelson B. *Tears in Heaven.* 2007. Snopes.com. Available at: http://www.snopes.com/music/songs/tears.htm. Accessed September 15, 2004.

Technical Advisory Committee. 1971. Poison prevention packaging act of 1970. *Bull Natl Clgh Poison Control Cent.* May–June:1–2.

Toblin RL, Paulozzi LJ, Gilchrist J, Russell PJ. 2008. Unintentional strangulation deaths from the "Choking Game" among youths aged 6–19 years—United States, 1995–2007. *J Safety Res.* 39:445–448.

United States Fire Administration. 2003. *Establishing a Relationship Between Alcohol and Casualties of Fire.* Emmitsburg, MD: U.S. Fire Administration.

United States Fire Administration. 2010. *Residential Sprinkler Systems.* Emmitsburg, MD: U.S. Fire Administration. Available at: http://www.usfa.fema.gov/citizens/home_fire_prev/sprinklers/. Accessed September 6, 2010.

Vernberg K, Culver-Dickinson P, Spyker DA. 1984. The deterrent effect of poison-warning stickers. *Am J Dis Children.* 138:1018–1020.

Villar RG, Connick M, Barton LL, et al. 1998. Parent and pediatrician knowledge, attitudes, and practices regarding pet-associated hazards. *Arch Pediatr Adolesc Med.* 152:1035–1037.

Villalbi JR, Cleries M, Bouis S, et al. 2010. Decline in hospitalizations due to dog bit injuries in Catalonia, 1997–2008: an effort of government regulation? *Inj Prev.* 16:408–410.

Vinci RJ, Freedman E, Wolski K. 1996. Preventing falls from windows: the efficacy of the Boston window fall prevention program. *Arch Pediatr Adolesc Med.* 150:32.

Walton WW. 1982 An evaluation of the Poison Prevention Packaging Act. *Pediatrics.* 69:363–370.

Warda L, Tenenbein M, Moffatt MEK. 1999. House fire injury prevention update. Part I. A review of risk factors for fatal and non-fatal house fire injury. *Inj Prev.* 5:145–150.

Warner G. 2010. Increased incidence of domestic animal bites following disaster due to natural hazards. *Prehosp Disaster Med.* 25:188–190.

Weiss HB, Friedman DI, Coben JH. 1998. Incidence of dog bite injuries treated in emergency departments. *JAMA.* 279:51–53.

Wilson F, Dwyer F, Bennett PC. 2003. Prevention of dog bites: evaluation of a brief educational intervention program for preschool children. *J Comm Psychol.* 31:75–86.

Wilson MEH, Baker SP, Teret SP, et al. 1991. Falls. In: *Saving Children: A Guide to Injury Prevention.* New York, NY: Oxford University. 127–139.

Woolfe A. 2004. Challenge and promise: the future of poison control centers. *Toxicology.* 198:285–289.

World Health Organization (WHO). 2010. *Injuries and Violence Prevention.* Geneva, Switzerland: WHO. Available at: http://www.who.int/violence_injury_prevention/unintentional_injuries/falls/ falls1/en. Accessed October 22, 2010.

Yoon SS, Macdonald SC, Parrish RG. 1998. Deaths from unintentional carbon monoxide poisoning and potential for prevention with carbon monoxide detectors. *JAMA.* 279:685–687.

Zaloshnja E, Miller TR, Lawrence BA, Romano E. 2005. The costs of unintentional home injuries. *Am J Prev Med.* 28:88–94.

Zimmerman SS, Tuxal B. 1981. Carbon monoxide poisoning. *Pediatrics.* 68:215–233.

Chapter 6

Adolescent Employment and Injury in the United States

Carol W. Runyan, PhD, MPH,[1,2,3,4,5] *Michael D. Schulman, PhD,*[1,3,6,7] *and Lawrence E. Scholl, MPH*[1,3]

Working for pay, either after school or during the summer, is a usual part of teenage life in the United States, starting as early as age 12 years. Although most teens work in the retail or service sectors, others are employed in manufacturing, construction, and agriculture. Informal sector employment, although usually seen as a characteristic of teen employment in less developed nations, also occurs in the United States. Despite the presence of child labor laws (CLLs), many employers violate these laws. Even jobs in conformance with the laws may be dangerous, exposing teens to a variety of hazards, including operating dangerous tools, machinery, or vehicles, and handling cash in situations prone to robbery. Training is sometimes minimal, and supervision is limited.

Work can be an important component of adolescent development, helping teens develop skills, exercise autonomy, and achieve a greater degree of competence and control. But, in their quest to demonstrate that they are good workers with adult-like skills, teens may not question the safety of their working conditions as often or as forcefully as they should. Likewise, employers may not fully understand the laws or be motivated to comply with them. Employers may not realize that these young workers need special training and supervision because of their inexperience. Parents may assume that teen jobs are safe and may not question their child about work until a major incident occurs, especially if the child's job is obtained through family or friend networks. Parental knowledge and understanding of the relevant CLLs is limited. Enforcement agencies may have insufficient support and resources, in part because of lack of public awareness of worker safety issues.

The vignettes below reveal some of the important hidden aspects of teen work and injury. They are followed by a discussion on what is known about the risks and benefits of teen work, the epidemiology of injuries among young workers, and strategies for preventing injuries. Because there is another chapter on agricultural injury, this chapter will focus primarily on the nonagricultural settings where teens work. Also, because there is a chapter on child injury in global perspective, this chapter primarily deals with the U.S. environment with some information related to Canada.

[1]The University of North Carolina Injury Prevention Research Center, Chapel Hill.
[2]Department of Epidemiology, Colorado School of Public Health, Aurora, Colorado.
[3]Department of Health Behavior and Health Education, University of North Carolina Gillings School of Global Public Health, Chapel Hill.
[4]Department of Pediatrics, The University of North Carolina at Chapel Hill.
[5]Department of Epidemiology, University of North Carolina Gillings School of Global Public Health, Chapel Hill.
[6]Department of Sociology and Anthropology, North Carolina State University, Raleigh.
[7]Department of 4-H Youth Development and Family & Consumer Sciences, North Carolina State University, Raleigh.

Putting a Face on Injury

The December 17, 2004, broadcast of the Montel Williams daytime television show featured four working teenagers who were injured on the job. These are their stories (Montel Williams Talk Show 2005).

- On his first day of work at a metal stamping plant, Brad lost half of his right arm and his left hand when the press stamped down while he was trying to make sure that the metal part was situated correctly in the machine.
- Mallory, aged 14 years, had her hands caught in the auger of an ice-packing machine while trying to retrieve a bag that was caught in the machinery.
- John, aged 16 years, was operating a forklift without a license. When he tried to move the forklift without being seated in the driver's seat (something he had seen older workers do), he slipped on some oil on the floor and the forklift ran over him crushing his back.
- Jennifer lost three fingers while operating a dough machine at a pizza restaurant.

Videos produced by government health and safety departments, labor education programs, and teens themselves provide additional vignettes of the real conditions faced by working teens at jobs (Washington State Department of Labor and Industries 2003, 2005). Newspaper accounts provide further documentation of illegal and hazardous work. For example, in 2008 federal immigration agents raided a meatpacking plant in Postville, Iowa. They found 20 underage workers, some as young as 13 years. A 16-year-old Guatemalan male talked to reporters about his job in the kill room and the 17-hour shifts he worked six days a week (Preston 2008). A 17-year-old Guatemala native was killed at a plant in North Carolina in 2008 while operating a pallet shredding machine (Alexander and Ordonex 2008). Other stories of teen injuries and workplace death are readily available. The National Institute for Occupational Safety and Health (NIOSH)—part of the Centers for Disease Control and Prevention (CDC)—hosts the Fatality Assessment and Control Evaluation (FACE) Program Web site, which lists state-based and in-house reports of worker fatalities archived since 2002, including many instances involving workers aged less than 18 years (NIOSH 2008). For example, in March 2004, a 16-year-old Hispanic construction laborer on a framing crew died of head injuries after falling 10 feet from a scaffold onto a concrete slab. The teen was working with his father and four uncles for a subcontractor who employed a crew leader responsible for finding and paying (in cash) Hispanic workers. The fatality investigation (NIOSH 2004a) revealed that the teen had been working on the framing crew for approximately two weeks. He and the other Hispanic workers spoke little or no English, and there was no documentation of training for any of the workers. Another NIOSH FACE Report details a 17-year-old female worker who fell from a roof to a stone patio while unloading shingles from a box raised by a forklift (NIOSH 2009). Yet, youth aged less than 18 years are prohibited by state and federal regulations from roofing occupations.

Teen Work Experience in the United States

In July 2009, the labor force participation rate for youth aged 16 to 24 years was 63.0%, the lowest since 1955 (Bureau of Labor Statistics [BLS] 2009a). However, many teens begin working before their 16th birthdays. Once adolescents enter the labor market, they usually continue working, although they change jobs frequently (National Research Council and Institute of Medicine 1998). Most working adolescents are employed during both the school year and the summer, with the proportions working during both periods increasing from 60% among 16-year-olds to 68% of 17-year-olds and 77% of 18-year-olds (BLS 2001; Herman 2000). By the time they graduate from high school, approximately 80% of teens have had job experience.

However, summer employment rates are decreasing in response to increased labor market competition, the lack of funding for special employment programs, and preferences for summer school, internships, and summer enrichment programs (Morisi 2010).

Most research has focused on teens aged 14 to 17 years, the ages covered by CLLs. However, a Wisconsin study reported that 58% of teens aged 10 to 14 years (in a study group of >5000 youth surveyed in school) reported working, with approximately 16% of working youth indicating they were "self-employed" (e.g., babysitting, lawn mowing) (Zierold, Garman, and Anderson 2004). A study using school-based surveys of working teens in two Canadian provinces found that 42% to 53% of students aged 12 to 14 years reported working during the school year (Breslin, Koehoor, and Cole 2009).

The largest proportion (~60%) of working adolescents are employed in retail establishments, of which half are restaurants. The second largest number work in the service sector (Herman 2000). Work roles vary by sex, with the most common occupations for 16-year-old males being cooks, stock handlers, baggers, cashiers, and food counter operators, whereas females most often work in service occupations and as cashiers, food counter operators, sales workers, wait persons, and supervisors of food preparation (BLS 2001; Herman 2000).

Teens also work long hours. One study showed that 39% work 20 or more hours per week in a typical week during the school year (Runyan et al. 2007). Among the teens in the 10- to 14-year age group surveyed by Zierold, Garman, and Anderson (2004), 54% reported having more than one job and 30% reported working more than 10 hours per week. Although estimates of illegal child labor are difficult to find because of the lack of high-quality data, there is some evidence. By using the 1980s Current Population Survey datasets and the 1979 and 1997 National Longitudinal Survey datasets, Kruse and Mahony (2000) estimate that 153,600 U.S. children aged less than 18 years worked illegally in an average week, with illegal employment affecting all demographic and geographic segments of the population. A more recent national study of U.S. teens aged 14 to 18 years working in retail and service jobs found that 37% of survey respondents reported violations of the hazardous work order, 15% reported working off the clock, and 11% reported working past the latest hour allowed by CLLs (Rauscher et al. 2008).

Social Context of Teen Work

Labor sociologists study the way work is actually done within different organizational contexts, for example, the tools, technology, division of labor and organization of work, and the extent to which workers control the way work is done versus the way managers control workers to increase productivity and efficiency. Scholars argue that work in the 20th century has been "deskilled," that is, broken down into component parts. In addition, workers in this environment have lost control over the pace of their work (Braverman, Sweezy, and Foster 1974). Many of the jobs in food service that teens occupy have been subject to "Fordist"-type rationalization, where the production process has been broken down into minute and specific processes and steps. Although jobs in workplaces that are highly specified and that incorporate detailed risk assessment and control may be less hazardous for teen workers than jobs in disorganized workplaces, the growth in part-time jobs without benefits through outsourcing, downsizing, and temporary work is associated with declines in occupational health (Mayhew and Quinlan 2002; Quinlan, Mayhew, and Bohle 2001).

Although jobs may be broken down into a series of tasks with formal safety procedures, workers may have a variety of reasons for not adhering to safety rules. In situations where speed and efficiency are at a premium, or if wages are determined by piece rate, following safety procedures may slow down production and be a disincentive. Experienced workers may teach younger workers ways to facilitate getting the jobs done quickly, but not necessarily safely.

Furthermore, in this environment, inexperienced workers, such as teenagers, can do jobs that used to require expertise based on careful training. Rather, job tasks are organized so that managers and machines control their timing and execution. Mechanization and automation are assumed to make tasks easier and safer, but this may be a false assumption—especially given workplace demands for speed that may encourage workers to rush, a factor that has been documented to be related to injury (Evensen et al. 2000). In addition, teen workers may realize that they are easily replaceable and fear loss of employment if they complain or do not keep pace (Zakocs et al. 1998). As a result, concerns about injury prevention may take a backseat to keeping their jobs (Dwyer 1991). Adolescents are capable of making rational decisions, but the social context of their workplaces and their perceptions of coworkers and supervisors influence their risk-taking decisions (Reyna and Farley 2006; Westaby and Lowe 2005).

In addition, safety equipment may be too uncomfortable (e.g., too hot) or too cumbersome. In many industries, teens start working at low-level jobs and may attempt to "earn" respect by demonstrating their ability to do dirty, hard, and dangerous work, especially because older teens or adult coworkers started in the same positions. In some large and complex workplaces (e.g., a construction site), adolescent workers may not have the opportunity to learn how their particular job is linked or connected with others at the work site. In smaller firms where work group cohesion exists, coworkers keep each other's safety in mind, and they share in knowledge of both safe and unsafe practices (Dwyer 1991). Because of efforts to curb costs, employers have increased the use of lesser qualified and more inexperienced workers (Dwyer 1991). Poorly trained workers often will not have the necessary knowledge to deal with problematic workplace hazards. Frequent and low-severity injuries may be perceived as a "normal part of the job," and teens may not complain to supervisors about working conditions so they can appear mature and competent among their adult coworkers (Breslin, Polzer et al. 2007).

According to Scharf and colleagues (2001), constant change is a core feature of the most hazardous work environments, such as agriculture, construction, and transport. Related to this is the observation that workplace hazards vary by the degree of control the worker has over the labor process and the predictability, visibility, movement, speed, and force of the tools, equipment, and exposures that are specific to the work environment (Schulman and Slesinger 2004). Agriculture, transportation, and construction are inherently dangerous work environments because of the complex interactions of environment, job tasks, tools, and other workers. These sites may be hot, cold, wet, or sandy; workers are alone, in small groups, or with many other crews; machinery is large and complex; and raw materials, from lumber to soil, are not uniform. The combination of inexperienced workers looking to demonstrate competence and the constantly changing hazards in dangerous environments creates high-risk situations for young workers in these settings.

Teen Work and Employment as a Stage in the Life Course

The life course perspective emphasizes stages and transitions that individuals experience in the social context of normal development and aging. This perspective reflects the interaction of social and historical factors with personal biography. Transitions (changes in status that are discrete and bounded in duration) and trajectories (long-term patterns of stability and change) are key parts of the life course perspective (George 1993). A life course perspective views work and employment for pay outside of the home as a key stage in adolescent development.

Whether work has a positive or negative impact on adolescent life course development is a topic of debate (Call and Mortimer 2001). For example, there is literature suggesting that work is beneficial in reducing violent behaviors with working teens, developing improved job skills (e.g., time management), and improving self-esteem, future time perspective, and social consciousness (National Research Council and Institute of Medicine 1998; Phillips and Sandstrom 1990). Call and Mortimer (2001) emphasize the benefits of work, arguing that work is an "arena of comfort" that can provide a safe haven for adolescents who experience stress from family, school, or peers. By using survey data from the Youth Development Study conducted in Minnesota, Finch, Mortimer, and Ryu (1997) argued that the majority of teens find work to be satisfying and low stress and that positive support from supervisors can buffer family-based distress for working teens. They also found few significant differences between working and nonworking teens except for an association between working long hours and alcohol abuse. Another study using these same data found that employment increased self-efficacy for teens in multiple realms, including family, community, and personal health (Cunnien, MartinRogers, and Mortimer 2009).

Studies addressing the impact of work on teen violence emphasize the impact of work intensity (Heimer 1995; Miller and Matthews 2001; Ploeger 1997; Safron, Schulenberg, and Bachman 2001; Wofford and Elliot 1997; Wright, Cullen, and Williams 1997). Traditionally, working more than 20 hours per week during the school year was considered to have negative impacts on a variety of teen outcomes. However, contemporary work shows that working long hours does not necessarily result in students dropping out of high school (Lee and Staff 2007; Staff and Mortimer 2008). Studies also have found that the relationships between work hours and adolescent problem behaviors may be spurious because of problems involved in measuring the differences between working and nonworking teens (Apel et al. 2006, 2008). Some researchers argue for the importance of considering aspects of the work other than intensity (Wright, Cullen, and Williams 1997). A study of affluent teens working at coffee franchises found that their jobs provided feelings of empowerment and individuality (Besen 2006). Staff and Uggen (2003) have reported that adolescents with more autonomy at work, with jobs that raise their status among peer groups, and with high-paying jobs are more likely to engage in substance use. However, adolescents with jobs that are compatible with their schoolwork or that provide opportunities for useful learning are less likely to engage in substance use. Work settings provide opportunities for teens to learn and model behaviors, either positive or negative, from coworkers and supervisors.

Descriptive Epidemiology of Injuries to Teen Workers in the United States

Fatal Injuries

Despite its potential benefits, employment can be dangerous for many adolescents. Several studies in the last two decades have documented the magnitude of fatal injuries to young workers (American Academy of Pediatrics 1995; Castillo, Landen, and Layne 1994; Castillo and Malit 1997; Centers for Disease Control and Prevention [CDC] 2010; Cooper and Rothstein 1995; Derstine 1996; Dunn and Runyan 1993; Rivara 1997; Schenker, Lopez, and Wintemute 1995; Suruda and Halperin 1991; Windau, Sygnatur, and Toscano 1999). Statistics on work-related fatalities among youth aged 17 years or less are compiled by the U.S. Department of Labor, Bureau of Labor Statistics (BLS) Census of Fatal Occupational Injuries (CFOI)—an annual census covering all sectors of the U.S. economy. According to CFOI data for 2003 to 2008, an average of 42 workplace deaths occurred annually among youth aged less than 18 years (BLS 2004–2009). This contrasts with the average of 67 workplace deaths that occurred annually between 1992 and 1998 among youth aged less than 18 years (Herman 2000). Between 1998 and 2007, 374 workers aged 15 to 17 years and 5719 workers aged 15 to 24 years died of occupational injuries (CDC 2010). A review of pooled CFOI data for the 6-year period (2003–2008) conducted by the BLS is shown in Table 6.1. Table 6.1 shows an overall decline in fatal occupational injuries for employed workers aged 16 to 17 years, with fatality rates declining from 1.2 (per 100,000 workers) in 2003 to 0.9 (per 100,000 workers) in 2007 (BLS 2004–2009). For workers aged 18 to 19 years, the fatality rates (per 100,000 workers) changed little, from 2.3 in 2003 to 2.6 in 2007 (BLS 2004–2009). Fatality rates for both age groups were calculated per

Table 6.1. Numbers and Rates of Fatal Occupational Injuries Among Workers Aged 16-17 and 18-19 Years, 2003-2008

	No.		Rate[a]	
Year	Age 16-17 y	Age 18-19 y	Age 16-17 y	Age 18-19 y
2003	28	84	1.2	2.3
2004	25	103	1.1	2.7
2005	31	111	1.4	2.9
2006	21	106	0.9	2.8
2007	20	97	0.9	2.6
2008[b]	23	66	2.5	2.4

[a]Rates are per 100,000 workers for years 2003-2007.

[b]In 2008, the CFOI began using hours worked for fatal work injury rate calculations rather than employment. These rates are expressed per 100,000 FTE workers.

Source: Bureau of Labor Statistics. *Census of Fatal Occupational Injuries.* 2004-2009 [cited June 8, 2010]. Available at: http://www.bls.gov/iif/oshcfoiarchive.htm#rates. Accessed July 6, 2011.

100,000 full-time equivalent (FTE) workers beginning in 2008 and are not directly comparable with those reported through 2007 (BLS 2004–2009). However, a separate analysis calculated fatality rates per 100,000 FTE workers for prior years. This analysis found that fatality rates between 1998 and 2007 were 2.9 per 100,000 FTE workers for 15- to 17-year-olds and 3.6 per 100,000 FTE workers for 15- to 24-year-olds—both of which were below the rate of 4.4 per 100,000 FTE workers for those aged 25 years or more (CDC 2010).

According to the 1998–2007 CFOI data, 90% of fatally injured youth aged 15 to 17 years were male; 65% were White, non-Hispanic; 5% were Black, non-Hispanic; and 27% were Hispanic. These percentages were similar for those aged 15 to 24 years (CDC 2010). The fatality rate for young Hispanic workers (5.6 per 100,000 FTE workers) between 1998 and 2007 was greater than the rates for White, non-Hispanic youth workers (3.3 per 100,000 FTE workers) and Black, non-Hispanic youth workers (2.3 per 100,000 FTE workers) (CDC 2010).

In sharp contrast with the industry distribution of fatalities for older workers, approximately 80% of the deaths of youth workers aged less than 18 years were concentrated in two industries: 1) natural resources and mining (primarily agriculture, forestry, fishing, and hunting) and 2) construction (Table 6.2) (BLS 2010a). Separate analyses by the BLS revealed that the burden of youth fatalities in agriculture is disproportionately borne by the youngest workers, approximately three quarters of all deaths to workers aged less than 15 years, and commonly involves farm machinery (Herman 2000), usually tractors (Cimini 1999). Data reported by the Department of Labor (Herman 2000) suggest that the risk of a fatality, per hour worked, in an agriculture wage and salary job was more than four times greater than the average risk for all working youth. (See Chapter 8 for detailed information about farm injuries.) For this same time period, the Department of Labor's *Report on the Youth Labor Force* (Herman 2000) identified youth working in family businesses as having an especially high fatality risk, irrespective of whether these jobs were inside or outside of agriculture. The majority (54.5%) of events or exposures commonly responsible for the reported fatal occupational injuries during the 2003–2008 period involved

Table 6.2. Distribution and Number of Fatal Occupational Injuries Among Workers Aged ≤17 Years, by Industry: 2003–2008

	Year						2003–2008	
Private industry[a]	2003	2004	2005	2006	2007	2008	No.	Percent
Construction	5	5	7	5	9	7	38	19.8
Leisure and hospitality (e.g., food services)	. . .	. . .	4	. . .	. . .	5	9	4.7
Natural resources and mining (e.g., agriculture, forestry, fishing, and hunting)	24	17	29	13	20	13	116	60.4
Professional and business services	8	. . .	. . .	. . .	. . .	. . .	8	4.2
Trade, transportation, and utilities (e.g., retail trade)	7	4	4	. . .	. . .	. . .	15	7.8
Other services, except public administration	. . .	3	. . .	3	. . .	. . .	6	3.1
Total	44	29	44	21	29	25	192	

Note: Dashes (. . .) indicate no data reported or data do not meet BLS publication criteria. Data may not add to totals because of BLS confidentiality suppression (i.e., data for categories and subcategories with one or two cases are removed to reduce the possibility of identifying specific cases) (BLS, personal communication, August 2, 2010).

[a]Based on the North American Industry Classification System, 2002.

Source: Bureau of Labor Statistics. 2010a. Youth worker fatal injury data received on July 22, 2010.

Table 6.3. Distribution and Number of Fatal Occupational Injuries Among Workers Aged ≤17 Years, 2003–2008

Event or Exposure	No.	%
Transportation incidents	120	54.5
Highway	41	
Nonhighway (farm, industrial premises)	40	
Pedestrian struck by vehicle, mobile equipment	8	
Assaults and violent acts	14	6.4
Contact with objects and equipment	58	26.4
Falls	8	3.6
Exposure to harmful environments	20	9.1
Total	220	

Note: Data may not add to totals because of BLS confidentiality suppression (i.e., data for categories and subcategories with one or two cases are removed to reduce the possibility of identifying specific cases) (BLS, personal communication, August 2, 2010).

Source: Bureau of Labor Statistics. 2010a. Youth worker fatal injury data received on July 22, 2010.

transportation incidents (Table 6.3), with 68% of the transportation incident fatalities occurring on highways, farms, or industrial premises (BLS 2010a). Contact with objects and equipment (26.4%) was followed by exposure to harmful environments (9.1%), and 6% were fatally assaulted (BLS 2010a).

Comparisons of Fatal Injury Patterns With Adult Workers

It is hard to compare fatal injury risks for teen and adult workers because teens typically work part-time, and comparable FTE data have only recently been compiled (BLS 2010a; CDC 2010). In a study of fatal teen injuries in the U.S. construction industry, Suruda and colleagues (2003) noted that adolescent rates are greater than for adults on an hour-worked basis. This research also indicated that teenage workers killed while doing construction work were more likely than their adult counterparts to be working in nonunion firms and smaller firms, and to be employed by employers with more safety citations from the U.S. Department of Labor Occupational Safety and Health Administration. In fact, approximately half the teen workers killed were in apparent violation of child labor regulations (Suruda et al. 2003).

Nonfatal Injuries Among Working Youth

Although teens have a rate per population of fatal work injury slightly less than that of adults (Castillo and Malit 1997), the number of injuries per hour worked may be greater for youth. Layne and colleagues (1994) estimated that 64,100 youth aged 14 to 17 years were treated in emergency departments for occupational injuries in 1992, whereas NIOSH estimates that approximately 200,000 adolescents are injured at work every year (NIOSH 1995). Several studies have examined workers' compensation data to determine the incidence of nonfatal injuries to teen workers (Banco, Lapidus, and Braddock 1992; Belville et al. 1993; Brooks and Davis 1996; Cooper et al. 1999; Cooper and Rothstein 1995; Heyer et al. 1992; Miller and Kaufman 1998; Schober et al. 1988). Other studies have examined first reports of injury records (Parker et al. 1994a) or used surveys of adolescents (Bowling et al. 1998; Cohen et al. 1996; Dunn et al. 1998; Knight, Castillo, and Layne 1995; Parker et al. 1994a, 1994b; Schulman et al. 1997). For example, a Washington State study using 4 years of workers' compensation data estimated the injury rate among 16- to 17-year-olds to be more than three times that for adult workers (Miller and Kaufman 1998). This is particularly troubling because CLLs prohibit teens from working in occupations of highest risk, such as mining and manufacturing. More recent evidence from Canada suggests that lost time claims for workers of all ages in their first month on the job are as much as five to seven times greater than those in the second or subsequent months (Chapeskie and Breslin 2003). Given that young workers change jobs frequently, the overall impact of this factor puts young workers at increased risk. An analysis of workplace injury claims involving British Columbia workers aged 14 to 24 years found that 10% of young worker injuries occurred in the first week and 20% in the first month of employment (Holizki et al. 2008).

Annual national data on nonfatal injuries and illnesses come from the BLS Survey of Occupational Injuries and Illnesses (SOII), which provides annual numbers of workplace injuries and illnesses in private industries and the frequency of these incidents. These data are not without limitations with respect to measurement of work injuries to youth. The exclusion of agriculture and family businesses omits an important source of jobs for youth, whereas the threshold for case inclusion (not being able to return to work on the "next regular workday") may underemphasize the incidence for younger workers because they tend to work part-time compared with the majority of the labor force. Thus, the estimates derived from these data are more likely to undercount the magnitude of nonfatal injuries to working youth.

Trend analyses of SOII data from 2003 to 2008 (Table 6.4) show nonfatal injuries and illnesses involving days away from work to be low for workers aged 14 to 15 years. There were a total of 1200 reported cases of nonfatal occupational injury and illness involving days away from work for 14- to 15-year-olds between 2003 and 2008, ranging from a low of 90 in 2005 to a high of 400 in 2007 (BLS 2010b). The number of reported cases for this age group decreased to 130

Table 6.4. Number of Nonfatal Occupational Injuries and Illnesses Involving Days Away From Work Among Young Workers in Private Industry, 2003–2008

	No.		
Year	14–15 y	16–19 y	20–24 y
2003	210	42,210	143,800
2004	200	38,230	141,730
2005	90	41,530	133,760
2006	170	39,330	132,120
2007	400	35,250	124,550
2008	130	31,010	107,880

Source: Bureau of Labor Statistics. 2010b. Youth worker nonfatal injury data received on July 22, 2010.

in 2008 (BLS 2010b). Workers in the age group 16 to 19 years also experienced overall decreases in injuries for the same time period, ranging from a high of 42,210 in 2003 to a low of 31,010 in 2008 (BLS 2010b). Although the rates are declining, and may be small relative to all workers, the number of young workers injured is substantial.

The national perspective on nonfatal injuries also can be illustrated by examining the number of nonfatal injuries treated in hospital emergency departments using the National Electronic Injury Surveillance System (NEISS). According to NEISS data between 1998 and 2007, 598,000 youth workers aged 15 to 17 years sustained nonfatal injuries while working (CDC 2010). Sixty-three percent of these were male workers; 65% were White, non-Hispanic; 8% were Black, non-Hispanic; and 5% were Hispanic (CDC 2010). These data also indicate that 7,946,000 youth workers aged 15 to 24 years sustained nonfatal injuries during the same time period with sex and ethnicity patterns similar to those of the younger group (CDC 2010).

It is important to note that the NEISS data do not reflect rates of worker injuries by employment status, so these data may give the impression that minorities experience lower rates (Breslin, Day et al. 2007). Other research suggests Hispanic and Black teens may be more likely to report having a serious injury at work compared with their White counterparts, even though their overall jobs were similar (Zierold and Anderson 2006a). A study of a New England high school found that students of lower socioeconomic status (as measured by mother's education) had more work-related injuries (Rauscher and Myers 2008). Other analyses, although finding no racial differences in reporting occupational injuries, note that race and ethnicity may influence the duration of absence from work (Strong and Zimmerman 2005).

There are noteworthy gender differences with respect to frequency and type of nonfatal injury. Male workers represent two thirds (62.5%) of adolescent injuries tracked in Massachusetts (NIOSH 2004b). For 1997, sprains, strains, and tears occurred more often during the work time of female youth (37%) than of male youth (22%), whereas cuts and lacerations were more common among male youth (NIOSH 2004b). Analysis of Oregon workman's compensation data from 16- to 19-year-old claimants found that males had more than twice the rate of females (McCall, Horwitz, and Carr 2007). Data from Canada showed that even after adjusting for job characteristics, adolescent and young male workers had an elevated risk status (Breslin and Smith 2005). Teen workers also encounter a variety of forms of violence at work. One third of the respondents in a national study of working teens reported some form of workplace violence, including physical attacks and verbal threats from customers and sexual harassment from coworkers (Rauscher 2008). Fifty-two percent of females in a New England private high school reported that they had been sexually harassed at work during the past year and that half of the perpetrators were coworkers (Fineran and Gruber 2009). More information is needed to fully understand how gender, ethnicity, and socioeconomic status are related to teen worker injury.

Severity of Nonfatal Injuries

A commonly used measure for injury severity involves the median number of workdays away from work. The most current available information on lost workdays reported by the BLS (Table 6.5) is based on 2008 data and supports the observation that work loss experienced by young workers tends to be moderate. In 2008, workers in both the 14- to 15-year and 16- to 19-year age groups experienced a median of 4 lost workdays as the result of nonfatal injury (BLS 2010b). This relatively small number of days of lost work for adolescent workers is compared with 5 days for workers aged 20 to 24 years, 6 days for workers aged 25 to 34 years, and 9 days for workers aged 35 to 44 years (BLS 2010b). Although approximately 31% of workers aged 14 to 15 years lost 6 to 10 days of work, approximately 39% were out of work for 2 days as a result of occupational injuries (BLS 2009b). The distribution of days lost from work for 16- to 19-year-olds, which parallels that for 20- to 24-year-old workers, reflects that 38% of workers aged 16 to

Table 6.5. Percentage Distribution of Occupational Injuries and Illnesses Involving Days Away From Work Among Workers Aged 14–24 Years in Private Industry, by Number of Days Away From Work, 2008

Age Group	Days Away From Work 1	2	3–5	6–10	11–20	21–30	≥31
14–15 y	. . .	38.5%	. . .	30.8%	15.4%	. . .	. . .
16–19 y	20.1%	17.9%	21.1%	12.5%	11.2%	4.8%	12.4%
20–24 y	20.3%	13.2%	20.7%	12.3%	11.7%	5.5%	16.2%

Note: Dashes (. . .) indicate no data reported or data do not meet BLS publication criteria. Because of rounding, data for a given age range may not sum to 100%.

Source: Bureau of Labor Statistics. 2009b. Lost-Worktime Cases–Characteristics, Worker Demographics, and Resulting Lost Time, 2008. Washington, DC: U.S. Department of Labor, 2008 News Release USDL-09-1454.

19 years lost 1 to 2 days of work, whereas approximately 21% were out of work for 3 to 5 days, 12.5% were out of work 6 to 10 days, and 16% were out of work 11 to 30 days as the result of injuries sustained at work (BLS 2009b).

Older data revealed that lost work time injuries to youth aged 16 to 17 years are distributed across the six industries where youth employment is most concentrated: eating and drinking establishments, food stores, general merchandise stores, health services, amusement and recreation, and business services (Herman 2000). Analyses conducted by the U.S. Department of Labor indicate that the risk of an injury resulting in lost work time in health services was greater than the risk in eating and drinking establishments, food stores, or general merchandise industries (Herman 2000). A review of data from 2008 for 16- to 19-year-old workers noted that the majority of cases of days lost from work because of injury or illness resulted from work performed in several industries: goods producing and manufacturing, construction, service providing, trade transportation and utilities, retail trade, leisure and hospitality, and accommodation and food service (BLS 2010b). As an important note, data regarding lost workdays do not take into account the numbers of days typically worked by adolescents in these different settings, so they must be interpreted with caution.

Other measures of severity are limited, although several studies have examined disabilities subsequent to injury. For example, a New York State study found that 44% of teens injured at work who filed workers' compensation claims suffered a permanent disability (Belville et al. 1993). An analysis of 1990–1997 Oregon workers' compensation data from 16- to 19-year-olds noted that occupational injuries are a major source of trauma for adolescent workers, evidenced by an average of 22.3 days of indemnity per insurance claim (McCall, Horwitz, and Carr 2007).

Comparisons of Nonfatal Injury Patterns With Adult Workers

Between 1998 and 2007, rates of nonfatal injury were significantly higher for younger workers than for their adult counterparts. During this time period, workers aged 15 to 17 years had a nonfatal injury rate of 4.6 per 100 FTE workers, and 15- to 24-year-old workers had a nonfatal injury rate of 5.0 per 100 FTE workers (CDC 2010). In contrast, workers 25 years of age and older had a nonfatal injury rate of 2.4 per 100 FTE workers (CDC 2010).

Comparisons of the distribution of lost workdays between adults and youth suggest that injured adult workers lose more workdays than injured youth. For example, in 1997 approximately 25% of all workers with lost workdays were away from work for more than 20 days (⩾4 weeks on a full-time schedule), whereas only approximately 10% of employed youth experienced this same amount of lost workdays. A 2004 study by Ehrlich and colleagues (2004) examined workers' compensation data for West Virginia and noted that the rate of injuries requiring surgical intervention among workers aged less than 19 years (9.3% per year) was slightly higher than that for adults (8.9% per year). Of particular note was the nearly four times higher incidence of amputations among teen versus adult workers (Ehrlich et al. 2004).

It is important to note that the use of lost workdays as an indicator of injury severity may overemphasize the relative severity of adult work injuries because youth are more likely to hold short-term jobs or work intermittent schedules than adults. Twenty or more lost workdays reflect a longer recuperation period for workers on intermittent schedules. Likewise, workers with short-term jobs often do not have the opportunity to work additional days. It is conceivable that recuperation time for youth includes nonscheduled work time, which would not be included in counts of days away from work, thereby underestimating the severity of youth injuries.

Industry and Job-Related Characteristics

Some industries and their associated job-related conditions present high injury risk settings for teen workers (NIOSH 1996; Runyan et al. 1997; Stueland et al. 1996; Zakocs et al. 1998). Absence of safety devices and being rushed also constitute potential risk factors. Certain industries are more dangerous simply because of the types of jobs they offer. For example, the majority of young worker fatalities occur in agricultural settings (Castillo, Landen, and Layne 1994; Derstine 1996), mostly associated with operating tractors and other machinery (CDC 1998; Rivara 1997; Schenker, Lopez, and Wintemute 1995; Stueland et al. 1996; Swanson et al. 1987). Retail establishments involve exchange of cash, a known risk factor for robbery and worker assaults (Loomis et al. 2001; Loomis et al. 2002; Moracco et al. 2000; Peek-Asa, Erickson, and Kraus 1999; Runyan, Schulman, and Hoffman 2003) and for which potentially modifiable cash handling practices appear to be influential in the level of risk experienced (Loomis et al. 2001, 2002). Hendricks et al. (1999) identified the specific safety practices of fast food restaurants that are associated with teens' increased risks of burns and falls in those settings, including the floor surfacing and how fryers are operated and maintained. Likewise, there is evidence that the types of cutting instruments provided in grocery stores influence the incidence of cut injuries among teen workers (Banco, Lapidus, and Braddock 1992). Similarly, youth working in construction are exposed to various types of hazardous equipment (e.g., electrical equipment, machinery) and working conditions (e.g., heights, extreme weather) that are associated with injury (Lipscomb and Li 2001; O'Connor et al. 2005; Suruda et al. 2003). Youth working in jobs involving transportation are subjected to other hazards associated with operating, riding in, or working near motor vehicles (Dunn and Runyan 1993).

A recent review of NEISS data found that contact with objects and equipment accounted for approximately half of nonfatal occupational injuries for workers aged 15 to 17 years (52%) and 15 to 24 years (49%) between 1998 and 2007 (CDC 2010). These injuries included events such as being struck by or against equipment and being caught in or crushed by various tools, equipment, machinery, parts, or materials (CDC 2010). During this same 10-year period, workers aged 15 to 17 years suffered additional nonfatal injuries due to falls (13%), bodily reaction and exertion (14%), exposure to harmful substances (14%), and assaults and violent acts (3%) (CDC 2010). For workers aged 15 to 24 years, additional nonfatal injuries between 1998 and 2007 were due to falls (11%), bodily reaction and exertion (22%), exposure to harmful substances (9%), transportation incidents (2%), fires and explosions (1%), and assaults and violent acts (4%) (CDC 2010). A separate review of NEISS data found that young workers aged 15 to 19 years had a higher rate of nonfatal motor vehicle injuries than workers in other age ranges between 1998 and 2002 (Chen 2009).

Additional studies have identified specific tasks that were responsible for a large or increased number of the occupational injuries sustained by youth, despite the fact that many tasks included are not prohibited by the Fair Labor Standards Act (FLSA). These tasks include handling hot liquids and grease (Hayes-Lundy et al. 1991; Mardis and Pratt 2003; Parker et al. 1994a), using cutting and other nonpowered hand tools (Banco, Lapidus, and Braddock 1992; Brooks, Davis, and Gallagher 1993; Mardis and Pratt 2003; Munshi et al. 2002; National Center for Health Statistics 1994; Schober et al. 1988; Zierold, Garman, and Anderson 2004), using power machinery (Knight, Castillo, and Layne 1995; Mardis and Pratt 2003), lifting or moving heavy objects (Knight, Castillo, and Layne 1995; Munshi et al. 2002; Parker et al. 1994a), operating tractors and other farm vehicles (e.g., all-terrain vehicles) (Children's Safety Network 1992; Kerr and Fowler 1988; Munshi et al. 2002; Rivara 1985), and working late at night or alone (Knight, Castillo, and Layne 1995; National Consumers League Child Labor Coalition 1993; Strong and Zimmerman 2005).

Preventing Teen Worker Injury in the United States

A huge gap exists in understanding the prevention of teen worker injury and in evaluating the effectiveness of specific interventions. As with most types of injuries, the prevention of injuries at work requires broad thinking and multiple types of strategies. However, unlike some other areas of injury control, there is limited evidence about successful approaches to prevention of teen worker injuries or other negative outcomes that may be associated with teen work.

Training

Although data on the effects of worker training are scant, the lack of training seems to place workers at increased risk (Dong et al. 2004; Goldenhar and Schulte 1994; National Research Council and Institute of Medicine 1998; NIOSH 1996, 1997; Office of Technology Assessment 1985). There is little information on training and its effects on teen worker safety, although one recent study (Dong et al. 2004) suggests that trained teens working in construction experienced a 42% reduction in workers' compensation claims compared with untrained teens. Several studies (Bush and Baker 1994; Knight, Castillo, and Layne 1995; Layne et al. 1994; Lewko et al. 2010; Runyan et al. 2007) have documented that youth receive very limited training on workplace safety. In a survey in the mid-1990s of teen workers in Massachusetts, California, Pennsylvania, and North Carolina, few teens reported having been trained about safety procedures related to their specific job tasks (Bowling et al. 1998; Runyan et al. 1997; Runyan, Schulman, and Hoffman 2003; Runyan et al. 2005). Knight and colleagues (1995) also reported 54% of the injured adolescent workers had not received safety training. Focus group discussions with teen workers have surfaced their concerns about the quality of the training they have received (Zakocs et al. 1998). Other studies have noted that training is very often not offered at all or on a limited basis (Delp et al. 2002; Miara et al. 2003; O'Connor et al. 2005; Runyan et al. 2007; Zierold, Garman, and Anderson 2004), and training may not be in a language appropriate to the workers (O'Connor et al. 2005).

In a national study of U.S. teens working in retail and service jobs, about the training they had received to do their jobs, approximately two thirds reported having received some sort of training, mostly by demonstration at the workplace (Runyan et al. 2007). Few respondents reported that they received worker safety training at school (Runyan et al. 2007). Despite the fact many teens report having received training at work, the content of their training is widely variable and may or may not be well matched to their job duties or inexperience. For example, less than half of respondents reported that they had been taught what to do in case of a robbery—one of the main causes of fatal injury in the retail sector (Runyan et al. 2007).

Among teens in the retail and service trades, most reported that they had been taught about safe use of equipment or generally how to avoid getting hurt while working (Runyan et al. 2007). Fewer had received training related to workplace violence (e.g., what to do in the event of a robbery or when dealing with angry customers and threats) (Runyan et al. 2007). In a companion study of 14- to 19-year-olds in Ontario, Canada, in 2008, almost all the young workers reported having received some training, although only approximately half received training on workplace violence issues ranging from sexual harassment to angry customers (Lewko et al. 2010). Of note, in the Canadian sample, females were more likely to report having been trained than males (Lewko et al. 2010).

Supervision

Given this lack of training, the fact that many teens work alone, without adult supervision, or after dark is particularly troublesome (Runyan and Zakocs 2000; Runyan et al. 2007). This lack of adequate supervision has been linked to injury risks (National Research Council and Institute of Medicine 1998; NIOSH 1997). For example, approximately one fourth of the teens interviewed by Knight and colleagues (1995) had been alone at the time of their injury event, and 80% had no supervisor present. Several studies indicate teens routinely work without supervision and alone. One study found the average young worker spent only 12% of his or her time in the presence of a supervisor (Greenberger and Steinberg 1986).

In a study of construction workers in North Carolina, 20% of teens aged less than 18 years reported that they had worked in situations where no one was within hearing or visual range (Runyan et al. 2006). Likewise, approximately 10% of 14- to 17-year-olds working in retail and service sector jobs in the United States and 14% of those working in Ontario (aged 14–19 years) reported that they had worked completely alone for at least 1 day during the past year during daylight hours (Lewko et al. 2010; Runyan et al. 2007). Similar numbers had worked alone for at least half an hour after dark once a week or more (9% in the United States and 17% in Ontario) (Lewko et al. 2010; Runyan et al. 2007). Furthermore, 15% of these teen workers reported having worked alone in one or both of these circumstances (daytime or night hours) at least one time each week (Lewko et al. 2010; Runyan et al. 2007).

Aside from working totally alone, working with inexperienced supervisors is a potential problem. In response to a question about working without adult (age ≥ 21 years) supervisors present, 22% of the females and 30% of the males working in retail and service sector jobs in the United States reported that in a typical week they worked without adult supervision at least 1 day (Runyan et al. 2007). Another form of supervision is checking workers to ensure they are performing tasks appropriately. Among service and retail workers, only 60% of the teens in the U.S. study (Runyan et al. 2007) reported that someone checked at least daily to make sure they were doing their work correctly.

Regulatory Approaches

In 1938, the federal government included child labor provisions in the FLSA. These laws were most recently updated in July 2010 (U.S. Department of Labor 2010). Most states have since passed laws to supplement the FLSA. These federal and state laws, commonly known as CLLs, are designed to protect youth aged less than 18 years from hazardous work conditions. CLLs specify minimum ages for general and specific types of employment, prohibit work during night hours ("night work restrictions"), prohibit certain kinds of employment ("hazardous orders"), and dictate maximum daily and weekly hours of work. The Occupational Safety and Health Administration, which establishes and enforces mandatory safety and health standards for workers of all ages, also protects teen workers.

Forty-one states have laws that require young workers (aged 14–17 years) to obtain a work permit, with the intent that these procedures will ensure greater compliance with worker safety standards and teen labor laws. However, the effectiveness of the work permit system is unclear. There is some suggestion that work permits appear to be effective in limiting performance of certain types of hazardous tasks (Dal Santo, Bowling, and Harris 2010; Delp et al. 2002), although teens with permits may not be any less likely to experience injuries (Zierold and Anderson 2006b). It also seems there are major gaps in enforcing permit laws (Dal Santo and Bowling 2009).

Enforcement of other CLLs is also uneven. For example, several studies report that large proportions of teens killed at work had been employed in situations in, or appearing to be in, violation of the FLSA or involving youth working in unregulated settings (Dunn and Runyan 1993; Suruda and Halperin 1991). Nationally, it has been estimated that 19% of teens treated in emergency departments for work-related injuries had been hurt while doing jobs prohibited by CLLs (Knight, Castillo, and Layne 1995). The Department of Labor found 1475 serious injuries of illegally employed children between 1983 and 1990, 85% of which were associated with "hazardous order" violations (U.S. General Accounting Office 1998). More recent research examined youth employed in construction, noting that more than 80% were working in violation of at least one restriction (Runyan et al. 2006) and that there were apparent violations in nearly half of the deaths of teen workers (Suruda et al. 2003).

To be effective, regulations must be enforced. Federal documents have called for employers to "strive to implement available prevention strategies for hazards that are not covered by existing standards" (Wegman and Davis 1999). A school-based Wisconsin survey found that the percentage with and without work permits varied by gender and job, but that teens with permits were not any more likely to be injured than those without permits (Zierold and Anderson 2006b). Similar data from North Carolina found that 44% of working teens lacked a state-required work permit (Dal Santo and Bowling 2009; Dal Santo, Bowling, and Harris 2010). Having a work permit appeared to be protective in terms of teens doing illegal tasks, but not in terms of self-reported working hour violations (Dal Santo and Bowling 2009; Dal Santo, Bowling, and Harris 2010).

A national study of U.S. teens and their parents found significant gaps in enforcement of labor laws, with 40% to 50% of teen workers reporting engaging in practices that were violations—most of which involved exposures to hazardous tasks or equipment (Rauscher et al. 2008; Runyan et al. 2007). Also, this same study discovered that although most working adolescents are aware of the presence of laws, they know little about the specifics of the restrictions. However, teens appear to be more knowledgeable than their parents (Rauscher, Runyan, and Schulman 2010).

Worker Safety Programs

There is little published evidence about the implementation or effectiveness of specific intervention strategies to improve teen worker safety in the United States or Canada despite the implementation of multiple curricula to enhance young worker understanding of labor laws, workers' rights, and safety (Hendricks and Layne 1999; Miara et al. 2003). Only one controlled study (Banco et al. 1997) assessed the implementation of a worker safety program designed to reduce risks for teen workers—a randomized trial that examined the effects of worker safety training and changes in the types of box cutters used by grocery store workers. Their results indicate that the greatest decrease in case-cutting injuries were in stores that introduced both new safety cutters and worker safety education, although stores with just an education program also had decreases in case-cutting injuries (Banco et al. 1997). However, the study was small and may not be generalizable to other settings or risks.

Parental Perspectives

Parents of teen workers often express approval and pride when their adolescents enter the workforce (Lescohier and Gallagher 1996; Phillips and Sandstrom 1990), and both teens and parents evaluate their own early work experiences as favorable (Aronson et al. 1996; Runyan et al. 2009). Parents can play a vital role in helping teens to develop a better understanding of the world of work and to use their personal and social resources to find desirable jobs (Runyan et al. 2011; Schneider and Stevenson 1999). However, little is known about parental roles in assisting teens in learning about CLLs and developing workplace safety behaviors and attitudes, although one study reported how parents engaged with their teen children around work issues (Runyan et al. under review). Most parents reported helping their adolescents find jobs and consider work hours, but were less involved in helping teens address safety issues. When confronted with hypothetic situations involving workplace dangers encountered by their teens, most parents indicated they would be very likely to actively engage in dealing with the situation. However, when parents were actually told by their teens about safety issues, fewer had reported doing what they indicated hypothetically that they would do (Runyan et al. 2011).

These findings are consistent with the low level of concern parents express about worker safety, indicating a need for efforts to increase their awareness of workplace safety hazards and protective strategies, including CLLs in their respective states (Runyan et al. 2009).

Although parents have not been a frequent target of teen occupational injury prevention efforts, a few resources targeting parents do exist. The National Consumers League Web site (National Consumers League Child Labor Coalition 2010) has a detailed "Parent's Primer" about teen work that recommends that parents set limits, talk frequently with their son/daughter about work, visit their teenager's workplace, meet the boss, and check on the employer's history of labor law violations. Likewise, NIOSH's publication (NIOSH 2005) "Promoting Safe Work for Young Workers: A Community Based Approach" encourages young worker safety projects to partner with parents in the effort to promote safety.

Conclusions

Employment of teens, although highly variable in nature, is a common and important element of this phase of development, as teens learn independence and develop new skills. Teens work for a variety of reasons and derive varied benefits from their employment. At the same time, work experiences vary widely with respect to type of work, hours worked, duration of employment, and quality of the experience. As a result, the positive and negative effects of adolescent employment differ.

Measuring and quantifying the effects of teen labor is difficult. Furthermore, making assessments of the risks and benefits are complex, and comparisons with adult workers are especially challenging. Unlike adults, most teen workers work part-time, change jobs frequently, and in a given position may perform a wide variety of tasks. For example, those working in service and retail settings do such diverse tasks as cleaning, lifting, handling cash, working at heights, using knives and ovens, and operating fryers. Even where data on young workers exist, there are variations in how information is recorded and which age groups are included.

Despite the difficulties in understanding the work patterns and experiences of teens, a fair amount is known. In the United States, the majority of young workers are employed in the retail and service industries, with smaller proportions working in agriculture, construction, and manufacturing. Within these work environments they are exposed to an array of hazards, including working alone or late at night, handling cash, dealing with potentially angry customers, and working with dangerous equipment and chemicals or in other dangerous conditions (e.g., heights)—despite legal requirements designed to protect young workers. Employers often provide very limited training and supervision to these young employees.

Although both child labor and general worker safety laws are designed to protect these young workers from many hazards, they are not fully enforced and gaps exist. In addition, many teens are not aware of the laws or their rights as workers, so they may not always raise questions when they are asked to perform dangerous tasks. Likewise, parents may not be familiar with CLLs or the safety issues in the places their adolescents work.

A common tendency in the social sciences and public health is to examine a problem in terms of a limited set of organizing categories (e.g., Black vs. White; rural vs. urban). These categories are useful for discovering and analyzing disparities in health, but they can also lead to divisions among scholars and health professionals. The state of research and intervention on health consequences of adolescent employment is indicative of this type of division. The work is good versus work is bad debate is only one part of the division. Different groups of scholars and health professionals deal with violence and delinquency, school achievement and occupational attainment, and occupational injury and fatality outcomes. There is a great need to understand more fully the interactions among teens, parents, employers, and the work environment and to develop intervention strategies that address the complexity of the contexts in which teens work and how adolescent development and workplace competence occur in the transition to adulthood. In taking this approach, there needs to be close involvement of professionals involved in youth development, such as teachers, pediatricians, and school counselors, as well as parents, employers, and the adolescents themselves. Integrating across perspectives is one way to advance understanding and progress.

Implications for Future Research and Prevention Efforts

Little evidence exists about successful interventions to protect young workers from injury on the job. Although increasing attention has been paid to development of worker safety training programs for youth, no one knows what elements of these programs are successful and how to deliver them in the most effective manner. Furthermore, to focus the majority of interventions on education directed at teen employees has only limited potential effect and runs the risk of communicating that adolescents are responsible for the safety of their workplaces. New efforts are needed that bring together diverse expertise to design interventions that address not only the knowledge, attitudes, skills, and behaviors of the teen workers but also the need for changes in the social and physical environments where work takes place. The Haddon Matrix is a useful model for generating ideas about multiple approaches to interventions (Haddon Jr. 1980a, 1980b; Runyan 1998). Using the matrix in a multidisciplinary group has great benefit in identifying options that derive from varied areas of expertise and that speak to the pros and cons of teen employment experiences.

Once interventions of any type are developed, they need to be carefully designed to allow for sound evaluations. This will enable good decision-making about continuing strategies that work and abandoning interventions that have no effect or that may, in fact, be harmful. These evaluations must be done rigorously, and efforts should be made to disseminate the findings of their work, both positive and negative. Others must be able to learn from these evaluations to replicate the high-quality interventions in new locales and either modify or avoid interventions that have proven to be unsuccessful.

Careful research needs to examine the nature, implementation, and enforcement of policies that are designed to protect young workers and those that may have unintended effects (positive or negative) on the employment prospects and experiences of teen workers.

Although further scientific evidence about the problem and the interventions is being developed, we suggest that efforts be made to continue to engage parents, teens, employers, and teachers in developing and implementing strategies to improve awareness of workplace safety issues. Efforts should incorporate education, regulation, legislation, and, as necessary, litigation.

Youth advocacy and workers' rights organizations should take advantage of their abilities to advance teen worker safety as they advocate with decisionmakers in schools, health care settings, and government bodies. Every working teen and his/her parents should receive clear, understandable information about the policies that affect teen work in their locale, as well as information about workers' rights and safety measures, whether covered by existing law or not. They should have guidance with regard to hazards in specific types of workplaces and suggestions for how to assess the safety of a particular job, questions to ask employers, and where to get help if safety is in question. Much of this information can be obtained from the sources listed in Figure 6.1. Advocacy should also focus on ensuring that worker safety policies, whether general or specific to teens, are properly disseminated to employers with clear expectations and assistance for achieving compliance. Advocacy groups should also monitor the regulatory process and promote clear and complete enforcement of measures designed to protect young workers.

Educators should incorporate basic information about worker safety into standard school-based health and safety curricula to help raise teen awareness of the issues and encourage a culture of safety. Curricula should target all teens, not just those in work-based learning programs. New social media, from the Internet to the smart phone, should be explored as means to deliver safety messages.

Parents should engage with advocacy groups and support their efforts to monitor and enhance regulatory measures and their enforcement. They should also discuss workplace safety with their teen workers and help them assess the safety of jobs they are considering and monitor safety conditions and exercise their rights as workers once employed.

Health care professionals who care for adolescents should become familiar with worker safety issues, regulations, and strategies for providing guidance to their teen patients. They should become advocates for worker safety regulatory measures and assist parents in providing guidance to teens (Runyan 2007).

Employers need to assume the major burden for ensuring a safe workplace for teens by developing their own and their managers' knowledge and awareness of safety issues, including ensuring full compliance with workplace safety and youth labor regulations. They should implement carefully considered training and supervision practices based on sound evidence and should monitor safety regularly, inform young workers of their rights, and encourage and reward safety consciousness among teen workers and their supervisors.

Legislative bodies should ensure that regulatory organizations are adequately funded and that they are ensuring high standards for businesses and enforcing existing laws to the full extent, while providing employers with assistance in finding ways to increase safety for teen workers. They should collect surveillance data and use them to monitor teen worker safety issues so as to make appropriate adjustments in policies, enforcement, educational, and assistive efforts and use scarce resources wisely. In addition, the federal government should ensure sufficient funding for research on teen labor safety and support mechanisms for periodic exchange of information both within the United States and with international colleagues to enhance dissemination of evidence-based and best practices for reducing teen worker injury.

The media should continue to give coverage of the issue of occupational health and safety through both news and feature stories, helping to reinforce that injury at work is aberrant and should not be considered just "the cost of doing business" and noting that teen workers are a group requiring special attention. It is hoped this will help establish a social norm that reinforces the importance of a culture of safety at work.

CDC National Center for Injury Prevention and Control

http://www.cdc.gov/injury/

Children's Safety Network

http://www.childrenssafetynetwork.org/

National Injury and Violence Prevention Resource Center

http://www.edc.org/projects/childrens_safety_network_national_injury_and_violence_prevention_resource_center

National Children's Center for Rural and Agricultural Health and Safety

http://www.marshfieldclinic.org/nccrahs/

Economics and Data Analysis Resource Center

http://www.edarc.org/

National Injury Data Technical Assistance Center

http://www.injuryprevention.org/info/data.htm

These are four national resource centers that provide information, training, and technical assistance for injury and violence prevention programs for state and local health departments, as well as publications and resource guides for professionals to assist with injury control and violence prevention programs for adolescents.

Federal Network for Young Workers Safety and Health (FedNet)

http://www.cdc.gov/niosh/fednet/

Web site gateway to nine federal agencies.

Labor Occupational Health Program, UC Berkeley, Young Workers' Health and Safety Web site

http://www.youngworkers.org/

Information for teens, parents, employers, and teachers.

National Consumer's League: Child Labor Coalition

http://www.stopchildlabor.org/

A private nonprofit organization that is a major advocate for youth safety at work, both for teens working in traditional jobs and especially for teens working in traveling sales crews.

The National Council for Occupational Safety and Health (National COSH)

http://www.coshnetwork.org/

Network of nonprofit organizations working on workers' rights, health, and safety.

New York Committee for Occupational Safety and Health (NYCOSH)

http://www.nycosh.org

Nonprofit provider of occupational safety and information training and information to workers and unions in the New York metropolitan area.

Occupational Health Surveillance Program, Massachusetts Department of Public Health, Teens at Work Surveillance and Prevention Project

http://www.mass.gov/dph/teensatwork

Collects information on work-related injuries to teens aged less than 18 years in Massachusetts and recommendations for targeted interventions and prevention activities.

U.S. Department of Labor, BLS, Injuries, Illnesses, and Fatalities Home Page

http://www.bls.gov/iif

Provides data on illnesses and injuries on the job and data on worker fatalities.

U.S. Department of Labor, FLSA Child Labor Rules Advisor

http://www.dol.gov/elaws/esa/flsa/cl/default.htm

U.S. Department of Labor, Occupational Safety and Health Administration, Teen Workers Safety and Health Page

http://www.osha.gov/SLTC/teenworkers/

Designed to educate teen workers, parents, employers, and educators about workplace safety. Provides fact sheets on job hazards, rights and responsibilities, ways to prevent injuries, CLLs, and links to state resources.

WorkSafeBC Young Workers Health and Safety Centre

http://www2.worksafebc.com/Topics/YoungWorker/Home.asp

Workman's Compensation Board of British Columbia with online resources for workers, employers, parents, and educators.

Young Worker Safety and Health Network

http://www.osha.gov/SLTC/teenworkers/networkmembers.html

Network of researchers, educators, physicians, and other professionals working to ensure the safety of youth in the workplace.

Figure 6.1. Selected resources for further information.

Finally, all the various groups and activities identified will work best if there is clear communication and networking among them and commonality in the message. Advocacy groups and health professionals should take a leadership role in developing community-based programs for teenage occupational injury. This approach would engage parents, teens, and employers in developing and disseminating a package of health promotion and information tools to reduce the risks of teen occupational injury in their community. Ultimately, through these various means, we may be able to find the "tipping point" (Gladwell 2002) by which safety of young workers is highly valued and considered normative as something that is not left to a few safety professionals to advocate.

References

Alexander A, Ordonex F. 2008. Danger Stalks Teens on the Job. *The News & Observer.* November 10.

American Academy of Pediatrics, Committee on Environmental Health. 1995. The hazards of child labor. *Pediatrics.* 95:311–313.

Apel R, Bushway SD, Paternoster R, et al. 2008. Using state child labor laws to identify the causal effect of youth employment on deviant behavior and academic achievement. *J Quant Criminol.* 24:337–362.

Apel R, Paternoster R, Bushway SD, Brame R. 2006. A job isn't just a job: the differential impact of formal versus informal work on adolescent problem behavior. *Crime Delinq.* 52:333–369.

Aronson PJ, Mortimer JT, Zierman C, Hacker M. 1996. Generational differences in early work experiences and evaluations. In: Mortimer J, Finch M, editors. *Adolescents, Work, and Family: An Intergenerational Developmental Analysis.* Thousand Oaks, CA: Sage Publications. 25–62.

Banco L, Lapidus G, Braddock M. 1992. Work-related injury among Connecticut minors. *Pediatrics.* 89 (5 Pt 1):957–690.

Banco L, Lapidus G, Monopoli J, Zavoski R. 1997. The Safe Teen Work Project: a study to reduce cutting injuries among young and inexperienced workers. *Am J Ind Med.* 31:619–622.

Belville R, Pollack SH, Godbold JH, Landrigan PJ. 1993. Occupational injuries among working adolescents in New York State. *JAMA.* 269:2754–2759.

Besen Y. 2006. Exploitation or fun?: the lived experience of teenage employment in suburban America. *J Contemp Ethnogr.* 35:319–340.

Bowling MJ, Runyan C, Miara C, et al. 1998. Teenage workers' occupational safety: results of a four-school study. Paper read at The Fourth World Conference on Injury Prevention and Control; Amsterdam, The Netherlands; May.

Braverman H, Sweezy PM, Foster JB. 1974. Labor and Monopoly Capital: The Degradation of Work in the Twentieth Century. New York: Monthly Review Press.

Breslin FC, Day D, Tompa E, et al. 2007. Non-agricultural work injuries among youth: a systematic review. *Am J Prev Med.* 32:151–162.

Breslin FC, Koehoor M, Cole DC. 2009. Employment patterns and work injury experience among Canadian 12 to 14 year olds. *Can J Public Health.* 99:201–205.

Breslin FC, Polzer J, MacEachen E, et al. 2007. Workplace injury or 'part of the job'?: towards a gendered understanding of injuries and complaints among young workers. *Soc Sci Med.* 64:782–793.

Breslin FC, Smith P. 2005. Age-related differences in work injuries: a multivariate population-based study. *Am J Ind Med.* 28:50–56.

Brooks DR, Davis LK. 1996. Work-related injuries to Massachusetts teens, 1987–1990. *Am J Indust Med.* 29:153–160.

Brooks DR, Davis LK, Gallagher SS. 1993. Work-related injuries among Massachusetts children: a study based on emergency department data. *Am J Indust Med.* 24:313–324.

Bureau of Labor Statistics. 2001. *Youth Employment, Unemployment Both Rise in the Summer* [cited August 9, 2010]. Available at: http://stats.bls.gov/opub/ted/2001/aug/wk3/art03.htm. Accessed July 6, 2011.

Bureau of Labor Statistics. *Census of Fatal Occupational Injuries.* 2004–2009 [cited June 8, 2010]. Available at: http://www.bls.gov/iif/oshcfoiarchive.htm#rates. Accessed July 6, 2011.

Bureau of Labor Statistics. 2009a. *News: Employment and Unemployment Among Youth-Summer 2009.* Available at: http://www.bls.gov/news.release/pdf/youth.pdf. Accessed July 5, 2011.

Bureau of Labor Statistics. 2009b. Lost-Worktime Cases—Characteristics, Worker Demographics, and Resulting Lost Time, 2008. Washington, DC: U.S. Department of Labor, 2008 News Release USDL-09-1454.

Bureau of Labor Statistics. 2010a. Youth worker fatal injury data received on July 22, 2010.

Bureau of Labor Statistics. 2010b. Youth worker nonfatal injury data received on July 22, 2010.

Bush D, Baker R. 1994. *Young Workers at Risk: Health and Safety Education and the Schools.* Berkeley, CA: Labor Occupational Health Program, University of California.

Call KT, Mortimer JT. 2001. *Arenas of Comfort in Adolescence: A Study of Adjustment in Context.* Mahwah, NJ: Lawrence Erlbaum Associates.

Castillo DN, Landen DD, Layne LA. 1994. Occupational injury deaths of 16-and 17-year-olds in the United States. *Am J Public Health.* 84:646–649.

Castillo DN, Malit BD. 1997. Occupational injury deaths of 16 and 17 year olds in the US: trends and comparisons with older workers. *Inj Prev.* 3:277–281.

Centers for Disease Control and Prevention. 1998. Youth agricultural work-related injuries treated in emergency departments: United States, October 1995-September 1997. *MMWR Morb Mortal Wkly Rep.* 47:733–739.

Centers for Disease Control and Prevention. 2010. Occupational injuries and deaths among younger workers—United States, 1998-2007. *MMWR Morb Mortal Wkly Rep.* 59:449–455.

Chapeskie K, Breslin FC. 2003. Securing a safe and healthy future: the road to injury prevention for Ontario's young workers. *Infocus: Current Workplace Research—A Supplement to at Work.* Fall 2003(34a).

Chen GX. 2009. Nonfatal work-related motor vehicle injuries treated in emergency departments in the United States, 1998–2002. *Am J Ind Med.* 52:698–706.

Children's Safety Network. 1992. Injury Prevention Outlook: An Assessment of Injury Prevention in State MCH Agencies. Newton, MA: Education Development Center, Inc.

Cimini MH. 1999. Research summary: fatal injuries and young workers. *Compensation and Working Conditions.* 27–29.

Cohen LR, Runyan CW, Dunn KA, Schulman MD. 1996. Work patterns and occupational hazard exposures of North Carolina adolescents in 4-H clubs. *Inj Prev.* 2:274–277.

Cooper SP, Burau KD, Robison TB, et al. 1999. Adolescent occupational injuries: Texas, 1990-1996. *Am J Ind Med.* 35:43–50.

Cooper SP, Rothstein MA. 1995. Health hazards among working children in Texas. *South Med J.* 88:550–554.

Cunnien KA, MartinRogers N, Mortimer JT. 2009. Adolescent work experience and self-efficacy. *Int J Sociol Soc Policy.* 29:164–175.

Dal Santo JA, Bowling JM. 2009. Characteristics of teens with and without work permits. *Am J Ind Med.* 52:841–849.

Dal Santo JA, Bowling JM, Harris TA. 2010. Effects of work permits on illegal employment among youth workers: findings of a school-based survey on child labor violations. *Am J Public Health.* 100:635–637.

Delp L, Runyan CW, Brown M, et al. 2002. Role of work permits in teen workers' experiences. *Am J Ind Med.* 41:477–482.

Derstine B. 1996. Job-related fatalities involving youths, 1992-1995. *Compensation and Working Conditions.* 1:40–42.

Dong X, Entzel P, Men Y, et al. 2004. Effects of safety and health training on work-related injury among construction laborers. *J Occup Environ Med.* 46:1222–1228.

Dunn KA, Runyan CW. 1993. Deaths at work among children and adolescents. *Am J Dis Child.* 147:1044–1047.

Dunn KA, Runyan CW, Cohen LR, Schulman MD. 1998. Teens at work: a statewide study of jobs, hazards, and injuries. *J Adolesc Health.* 22:19–25.

Dwyer T. 1991. Life and Death at Work: Industrial Accidents as a Case of Socially Produced Error. New York, NY: Plenum Publishing Corporation.

Ehrlich PF, McClellan WT, Hemkamp JC, et al. 2004. Understanding work-related injuries in children: a perspective in West Virginia using the state-managed workers' compensation system. *J Pediatr Surg.* 39:768–772.

Evensen CT, Schulman MD, Runyan CW, et al. 2000. The downside of adolescent employment: hazards and injuries among working teens in North Carolina. *J Adolesc.* 23:545–560.

Finch MD, Mortimer JT, Ryu S. 1997. Transitions into part-time work: health risks and opportunities. In: Schulenberg J, Maggs J, Hurrelmann K, editors. *Health Risks and Developmental Transitions During Adolescence.* New York, NY: Cambridge University Press. 321–344.

Fineran S, Gruber JE. 2009. Youth at work: adolescent employment and sexual harassment. *Child Abuse Negl.* 33:550–559.

George LK. 1993. Sociological perspectives on life transitions. *Ann Rev Sociol.* 19:353–373.

Gladwell M. 2002. The Tipping Point: How Little Things Can Make a Big Difference. Boston, MA: Little Brown and Company.

Goldenhar LM, Schulte PA. 1994. Intervention research in occupational health and safety. *J Occup Environ Med.* 36:763–775.

Greenberger E, Steinberg L. 1986. When Teenagers Work: The Psychological and Social Costs of Adolescent Employment. New York, NY: Basic Books Inc. Publishers.

Haddon W Jr. 1980a. Advances in the epidemiology of injuries as a basis for public policy. *Public Health Rep.* 95:411–421.

Haddon W Jr. 1980b. Options for the prevention of motor vehicle crash injury. *Isr J Med Sci.* 16:45–65.

Hayes-Lundy C, Ward RS, Saffle JR, et al. 1991. Grease burns at fast-food restaurants: adolescents at risk. *J Burn Care Res.* 12:203–208.

Heimer K. 1995. Gender, race, and the pathways to delinquency: an interactionist explanation. In: Hagan J, Peterson R, editors. *Crime and Inequality.* Stanford, CA: Stanford University Press. 140–173.

Hendricks KJ, Layne LA. 1999. Adolescent occupational injuries in fast food restaurants: an examination of the problem from a national perspective. *J Occup Environ Med.* 41:1146–1153.

Herman AM. 2000. *Report on the Youth Labor Force.* Washington, DC: Office of Publications and Special Studies, U.S. Department of Labor, Bureau of Labor Statistics.

Heyer NJ, Franklin G, Rivara FP, et al. 1992. Occupational injuries among minors doing farm work in Washington State: 1986 to 1989. *Am J Public Health.* 82:557–560.

Holizki T, McDonald R, Foster V, Guzmicky M. 2008. Causes of work-related injuries among young workers in British Columbia. *Am J Ind Med.* 51:357–363.

Kerr G, Fowler B. 1988. The relationship between psychological factors and sports injuries. *Sports Med.* 6:127–134.

Knight EB, Castillo DN, Layne LA. 1995. A detailed analysis of work-related injury among youth treated in emergency departments. *Am J Ind Med.* 27:793–805.

Kruse DL, Mahony D. 2000. Illegal child labor in the United States: prevalence and characteristics. *Ind Labor Relat Rev.* 54:17–40.

Layne LA, Castillo DN, Stout N, Cutlip P. 1994. Adolescent occupational injuries requiring hospital emergency department treatment: a nationally representative sample. *Am J Public Health.* 84:657–660.

Lee JC, Staff J. 2007. When work matters: the varying impact of work intensity on high school dropout. *Sociol Educ.* 80:158–178.

Lescohier I, Gallagher GS. 1996. Unintentional injury. In: DiClemente R, Hansen W, Ponton L, editors. *Handbook of Adolescent Health Risk Behavior.* New York, NY: Plenum Publishing Corp. 225–258.

Lewko JH, Runyan C, Tremblay CL, et al. 2010. Workplace experiences of young workers in Ontario. *Can J Public Health.* 101:380–384.

Lipscomb HJ, Li L. 2001. Injuries among teens employed in the homebuilding industry in North Carolina. *Inj Prev.* 7:205–209.

Loomis D, Marshall SW, Wolf SH, et al. 2002. Effectiveness of safety measures recommended for prevention of workplace homicide. *JAMA.* 287:1011–1017.

Loomis D, Wolf SH, Runyan CW, et al. 2001. Homicide on the job: workplace and community determinants. *Am J Epidemiol.* 154:410–417.

Mardis AL, Pratt SG. 2003. Nonfatal injuries to young workers in the retail trades and services industries in 1998. *J Occup Environ Med.* 45:316–323.

Mayhew C, Quinlan M. 2002. Fordism in the fast food industry: pervasive management control and occupational health and safety risks for young temporary workers. *Sociol Health Illn.* 24:261–284.

McCall BP, Horwitz IB, Carr BS. 2007. Adolescent occupational injuries and workplace risks: an analysis of Oregon workers' compensation data 1990–1997. *J Adolesc Health.* 41:248–255.

Miara C, Gallagher S, Bush D, Dewer R. 2003. Developing an effective tool for teaching teens about workplace safety. *Am J Health Educ.* 35(5 Suppl):30–34.

Miller ME, Kaufman JD. 1998. Occupational injuries among adolescents in Washington State, 1988–1991. *Am J Ind Med.* 34:121–132.

Miller WJ, Matthews RA. 2001. Youth employment, differential association, and juvenile delinquency. *Sociol Focus.* 34:251–268.

Montel Williams Talk Show. 2005. *Working Teens: Dangerous Jobs 2004* [cited January 13, 2005]. Available at: www.montelshow.com/show/past_detail_11_17_2004.htm. Accessed July 6, 2011.

Moracco KE, Runyan CW, Loomis DP, et al. 2000. Killed on the clock: a population-based study of workplace homicide, 1977–1991. *Am J Ind Med.* 37:629–636.

Morisi TL. 2010. The early 2000s: a period of declining summer employment rates. *Monthly Labor Review.* 133:23–35.

Munshi, K, Parker DL, Bannerman-Thompson H, Merchant D. 2002. Causes, nature, and outcomes of work-related injuries to adolescents working at farm and non-farm jobs in rural Minnesota. *Am J Ind Med.* 42:142–149.

National Center for Health Statistics. 1994. *Healthy People 2000 Review, 1993.* Hyattsville, MD: U.S. Public Health Service.

National Consumers League Child Labor Coalition. 1993. Late night hours can be killers. *Child Labor Monitor.* 3:1–2, 8.

National Consumers League Child Labor Coalition. 2010. *Working the Smart Shift: Helping Parents Help Their Teens Avoid Dangerous Jobs* [cited August 9, 2010]. Available at: http://www.stopchildlabor.org/USchildlabor/kidprime.htm. Accessed July 6, 2011.

National Institute for Occupational Safety and Health (NIOSH). 1995. *NIOSH Alert: Request for Assistance in Preventing Deaths and Injuries of Adolescent Workers.* Washington DC: U.S. Department of Health and Human Services, Publication 95–125.

National Institute for Occupational Safety and Health (NIOSH). 1996. *Violence in the Workplace: Risk Factors and Prevention Strategies.* Cincinnati, OH: Publications Dissemination, EID. Publication 96–100.

National Institute for Occupational Safety and Health (NIOSH). 1997. *NIOSH Special Hazard Review-Child Labor Research Needs: Recommendations from the NIOSH Child Labor Working Team.* Washington DC: U.S. Department of Health and Human Services. Publication 97–143.

National Institute for Occupational Safety and Health (NIOSH). 2004a. *Sixteen-Year-Old Hispanic Youth Dies After Falling From a Job-Made Elevated Platform During Construction—South Carolina.* Cincinnati, OH: NIOSH In-house FACE Report 2004-06.

National Institute for Occupational Safety and Health (NIOSH). 2004b. *Worker Health Chartbook, 2004.* Cincinnati, OH: NIOSH Publications, Publication 2004-146. Available at: http://www.cdc.gov/niosh/docs/2004-146/. Accessed June 2010.

National Institute for Occupational Safety and Health (NIOSH). 2005. *Promoting Safe Work for Young Workers: A Community Based Approach* [cited January 25, 2005]. Available at: http://www.cdc.gov/niosh/99-141.html. Accessed June 2010.

National Institute for Occupational Safety and Health (NIOSH). *Youth Fatality Investigation Reports.* 2008 [cited August 9, 2010]. Available at: http://www.cdc.gov/niosh/face. Accessed January 9, 2008.

National Institute for Occupational Safety and Health (NIOSH). 2009. *Seventeen Year Old Female Laborer Falls From Residential Roof and Dies Nine Days Later—Connecticut.* Cincinnati, OH: NIOSH In-house FACE Report 2007-10.

National Research Council and Institute of Medicine. 1998. *Protecting Youth at Work: Health, Safety, and Development of Working Children and Adolescents in the United States.* Washington DC: National Academy Press.

O'Connor T, Loomis D, Runyan C, et al. 2005. Adequacy of health and safety training among young Latino construction workers. *J Occup Environ Med.* 47:272–277.

Office of Technology Assessment. 1985. *Preventing Illness and Injury in the Workplace.* Washington DC: U.S. Government Printing Office. Publication OTA-H-256.

Parker DL, Carl WR, French LR, Martin FB. 1994a. Characteristics of adolescent work injuries reported to the Minnesota Department of Labor and Industry. *Am J Public Health.* 84:606–611.

Parker DL, Carl WR, French LR, Martin FB. 1994b. Nature and incidence of self-reported adolescent work injury in Minnesota. *Am J Ind Med.* 26:529–541.

Peek-Asa C, Erickson R, Kraus JF. 1999. Traumatic occupational fatalities in the retail industry, United States 1992-1996. *Am J Ind Med.* 35:186–191.

Phillips S, Sandstrom KL. 1990. Parental attitudes toward youth work. *Youth Soc.* 22:160–183.

Ploeger M. 1997. Youth employment and delinquency: reconsidering a problematic relationship. *Criminology.* 35:659–676.

Preston J. 2008. After Iowa Raid, Immigrants Fuel Labor Inquiries. *New York Times.* July 7, 2008.

Quinlan M, Mayhew C, Bohle P. 2001. The global expansion of precarious employment, work disorganization, and consequences for occupational health: a review of recent research. *Int J Health Serv.* 31:335–414.

Rauscher KJ. 2008. Workplace violence against adolescent workers in the US. *Am J Ind Med.* 51:539–544.

Rauscher KJ, Myers DJ. 2008. Socioeconomic disparities in the prevalence of work-related injuries among adolescents in the United States. *J Adolesc Health.* 42:50–57.

Rauscher KJ, Runyan C, Schulman M. 2010. Awareness and knowledge of the U.S. child labor laws among a national sample of working adolescents and their parents. *J Adolesc Health.* 47:414-417.

Rauscher KJ, Runyan CW, Schulman MD, Bowling JM. 2008. US child labor violations in the retail and service industries: findings from a national survey of working adolescents. *Am J Public Health.* 98:1693–1699.

Reyna VF, Farley F. 2006. Risk and rationality in adolescent decision making. *Psychol Sci Public Interest.* 7:1–44.

Rivara FP. 1985. Fatal and nonfatal farm injuries to children and adolescents in the United States. *Pediatrics* 76:567–573.

Rivara FP. 1997. Fatal and non-fatal farm injuries to children and adolescents in the United States, 1990-3. *Inj Prev.* 3:190–194.

Runyan CW, Vladutiu CJ, Schulman MD, Rauscher KJ. 2011. Parental involvement with their working teens. *J Adolesc Health.* 49:84–86.

Runyan C, Zakocs RC, Dunn KA, et al. 1997. Teen workers' training and concerns about safety. Presented at the 125th Annual Meeting of the American Public Health Association, Indianapolis, IN, November 9–12, 1997.

Runyan CW. 1998. Using the Haddon matrix: introducing the third dimension. *Inj Prev.* 4:302–307.

Runyan CW. 2007. Advocating the inclusion of adolescent work experience as part of routine preventive care. *J Adolesc Health.* 41:221–223.

Runyan CW, Bowling JM, Schulman M, Gallagher SS. 2005. Potential for violence against teenage retail workers in the United States. *J Adolesc Health.* 36:267.e1–267.e5.

Runyan CW, Dal Santo J, Schulman M, et al. 2006. Work hazards and workplace safety violations experienced by adolescent construction workers. *Arch Pediatr Adolesc Med.* 160:721–727.

Runyan CW, Schulman M, Dal Santo J, et al. 2007. Work-related hazards and workplace safety of US adolescents employed in the retail and service sectors. *Pediatrics.* 119:526–534.

Runyan CW, Schulman M, Dal Santo J, et al. 2009. Attitudes and beliefs about adolescent work and workplace safety among parents of working adolescents. *J Adolesc Health.* 44:349–355.

Runyan CW, Schulman M, Hoffman CD. 2003. Understanding and preventing violence against adolescent workers: what is known and what is missing? *Clin Occup Environ Med.* 3:711–720.

Runyan CW, Zakocs RC. 2000. Epidemiology and prevention of injuries among adolescent workers in the United States. *Ann Rev Public Health.* 21:247–269.

Safron DJ, Schulenberg JE, Bachman JG. 2001. Part-time work and hurried adolescence: the links among work intensity, social activities, health behaviors, and substance use. *J Health Soc Behav.* 42:425–449.

Scharf T, Vaught C, Kidd P, et al. 2001. Toward a typology of dynamic and hazardous work environments. *Hum Ecol Risk Assess Int J.* 7:1827–1841.

Schenker MB, Lopez R, Wintemute G. 1995. Farm-related fatalities among children in California, 1980 to 1989. *Am J Public Health.* 85:89–92.

Schneider B, Stevenson D. 1999. *The Ambitious Generation: America's Teenagers.* New Haven, CT: Yale University Press.

Schober SE, Handke JL, Halperin WE, et al. 1988. Work-related injuries in minors. *Am J Ind Med.* 14:585–595.

Schulman MD, Evensen CT, Runyan CW, et al. 1997. Farm work is dangerous for teens: agricultural hazards and injuries among North Carolina teens. *J Rural Health.* 13:295–305.

Schulman MD, Slesinger DP. 2004. Health hazards of rural extractive industries and occupations. In: Glasgow N, Morton L, Johnson N, editors. *Critical Issues in Rural Health.* Ames, IA: Wiley-Blackwell. 49–60.

Staff J, Mortimer JT. 2008. Social class background and the school-to-work transition. *New Dir Child Adolesc Dev.* 2008:55–69.

Staff J, Uggen C. 2003. The fruits of good work: early work experiences and adolescent deviance. *J Res Crime Delinq.* 40:263–290.

Strong LL, Zimmerman FJ. 2005. Occupational injury and absence from work among African American, Hispanic, and non-Hispanic White workers in the National Longitudinal Survey of Youth. *Am J Public Health.* 95:1226–1232.

Stueland DT, Lee BC, Nordstrom DL, et al. 1996. A population based case-control study of agricultural injuries in children. *Inj Prev.* 2:192–196.

Suruda A, Halperin W. 1991. Work-related deaths in children. *Am J Ind Med.* 19:739–745.

Suruda A, Philips P, Lillquist D, Sesek R. 2003. Fatal injuries to teenage construction workers in the US. *Am J Ind Med.* 44:510–514.

Swanson JA, Sachs MI, Dahlgren KA, Tinguely SJ. 1987. Accidental farm injuries in children. *Arch Pediatr Adolesc Med.* 141:1276–1279.

U.S. Department of Labor. 2010. Child Labor Regulations, Orders and Statements of Interpretation. *Federal Register.* 75.

U.S. General Accounting Office. 1998. *Child Labor: Characteristics of Working Children.* Washington DC: U.S. General Accounting Office. Report No. GAO/HRD-91-83BR.

Washington State Department of Labor and Industries. Lost Youth [Video] 2003. Available at: http://www.lni.wa.gov/Safety/TrainTools/Videos/Library/catalog.asp?VID=V1117. Accessed July 5, 2011.

Washington State Department of Labor and Industries. Teen Works: Real Jobs Real Risks [Video] 2005. Available at: http://www.lni.wa.gov/Safety/TrainTools/Videos/Library/catalog.asp?VID=V1145. Accessed July 5, 2011.

Wegman DH, Davis LK. 1999. Protecting youth at work. *Am J Ind Med.* 36:579–583.

Westaby JD, Lowe JK. 2005. Risk-taking orientation and injury among youth workers: examining the social influence of supervisors, coworkers, and parents. *J Appl Psychol.* 90:1027–1035.

Windau J, Sygnatur E, Toscano G. 1999. Profile of work injuries incurred by young workers. *Monthly Labor Review.* 122:3–10.

Wofford MD, Elliot D. 1997. Short and long term consequences of adolescent work. *Youth Soc.* 28:464–498.

Wright JP, Cullen FT, Williams N. 1997. Working while in school and delinquent involvement: Implications for social policy. *Crime Delinq.* 43:203–221.

Zakocs RC, Runyan CW, Schulman MD, et al. 1998. Improving safety for teens working in the retail trade sector: opportunities and obstacles. *Am J Ind Med.* 34:342–350.

Zierold KM, Anderson HA. 2006a. Racial and ethnic disparities in work-related injuries among teenagers. *J Adolesc Health.* 39:422–426.

Zierold KM, Anderson HA. 2006b. The relationship between work permits, injury, and safety training among working teenagers. *Am J Ind Med.* 49:360–366.

Zierold KM, Garman S, Anderson H. 2004. Summer work and injury among middle school students, aged 10-14 years. *Occup Environ Med.* 61:518–522.

Chapter 7

Partnering With Schools To Prevent Injuries and Violence

Ellen R. Schmidt, MS, OT[1] and Susan Frelick Goekler, PhD, MCHES[2]

In the United States, an estimated 55 million students are enrolled in prekindergarten through 12th grade. Another 15 million students attend colleges and universities across the country. Schools are safer places than homes for children and youth during the day. However, serious injuries do occur in schools. Just as important, schools are places for learning the lessons young people will need for the rest of their lives. Because injuries are the leading cause of death and disability for children, youth, and adults up to the age of 44, it is critical that schools impart lessons about injury and violence prevention, and provide a violence-free, physically and psychosocially safe environment.

Children spend 7 to 9 waking hours 5 days per week, 8 months per year, in school or on school property. These facts demonstrate that schools are a good venue to address injuries and violence. Schools are also settings where students and staff establish safe and healthy behaviors, become role models, and create an environment of safety. Finally, they can receive education on safety that affects their lives outside of school.

Injury and violence prevention decrease risk factors and promote protective factors in many different ways. Using a social ecological model, prevention efforts influence the individual, family, peers, and social structure. An environmental modification approach involves making changes in the physical and social environments using methods including advocacy, policy (organizational protocols, regulations, and legislation), education, and training. Regardless of the approach, it should be adjusted to the needs of the particular school and/or community and evaluated to assess efficacy.

This chapter will focus on injuries and violence occurring in school and on school grounds, from preschool through high school. It will review prevalence and incidence data for injuries common on school grounds and at school events, and will offer recommendations on how schools and child care programs can develop and implement coordinated injury and violence prevention programs. The issues covered and recommendations include those relevant to child care programs located on school premises as well as those for elementary, middle, or junior high and high schools, but will not specifically address independent child care or preschool settings. This chapter will address school-based curricula and integrated programming for general injury and violence prevention, and offer recommendations on how public health and safety professionals can work with schools and education professionals to make injury and violence prevention an institutional priority and part of the student's education.

Almost all of the precautions and prevention messages addressed in this chapter apply to preschool programs and child care settings within schools. The issues for elementary school children are similar to those for younger children as are many of the training issues for providers and staff.

[1]Assistant Director, Children's Safety Network National Injury and Violence Prevention Resource Center, Education Development Center, Washington, DC.
[2]Executive Director, Directors of Health Promotion and Education, Washington, DC.

Caring for Our Children: National Health and Safety Performance Standards; Guidelines for Out-of-Home Child Care Programs (National Resource Center for Health and Safety in Child Care 2011) addresses additional safety issues that apply to child care settings but not school settings. Issues covered in *Caring for Our Children* include the following:

- Safe sleep—including crib safety and putting babies on their back to sleep
- Safe travel—installation and use of child passenger safety seats, booster seats, safety belts, and fit and use of bicycle helmets when riding bicycles; never leaving a child in a car alone
- Safe play—following U.S. Consumer Product Safety Commission (CPSC) playground safety guidelines
- Safe physical environment—product safety (CPSC recalls), poison prevention, stairway safety, fire drills, disaster planning, first aid, cardiopulmonary resuscitation (CPR), choking hazards, toy safety, sun exposure, water temperature safety, entrapment hazards, baby walkers, supervision, covered electrical outlets
- Safe social environment—sharing, respect, bully-free, acceptance of differences

Both schools and child care centers should keep complete records regarding student/child injuries. Child care providers also have opportunities to teach and demonstrate safety practices to parents and caregivers.

The actual stories that follow highlight what can happen when schools fail to provide adequate protection for students.

Chanel

Chanel was stabbed to death in 2003 by her former boyfriend, Tyrone. Both Chanel, age 15, and Tyrone, age 16, were students at the same high school, where the murder occurred. Chanel had broken up with Tyrone the day before her murder. Chanel told teachers that Tyrone was "becoming increasingly violent with her and that she was worried about her safety." Later that day, Tyrone stabbed her six times in the school hallway. After Chanel's death, Tyrone was sentenced to 40 years in prison. Chanel's mother also brought a wrongful death lawsuit against the school. The suit claimed that school officials violated Chanel's rights by failing to protect her.

Jarod

On December 19, 2003, 6-year-old Jarod Bennett was killed in school by a mobile, folding cafeteria table. He was one of over a dozen children who have been killed by tables at school. A 290-pound table (like the one that killed Jarod) can tip over with only 27 pounds of tip-over pressure. It falls with a force of over 8 tons. Although many of the tables have decals on them warning of their danger (the table that killed Jarod had two warning decals placed on the surface of the table), schools still purchase and use them. Jarod's death prompted a state law that requires annual inspections of every school in the state by the State Board of Health and reminds school staff to follow important guidelines when dealing with mobile, folding cafeteria tables (*The Plain Dealer* 2005).

Injury Risk in the School Environment

In the United States, 74% of all deaths among youth and young adults aged 10–24 years result from four causes: motor vehicle crashes (30%), other unintentional injuries (16%), homicide (16%), and suicide (12%) (Centers for Disease Control and Prevention 2007a). From 2004 to 2007, an average of 33.5 million injuries were reported each year. For females, 54% of injuries occurred inside or outside of the home, compared with 42% of injuries among males. Injuries among males were more likely to occur in recreation areas (17%) and commercial areas (13%) than injuries among females. Less than 10% of these injuries occur at school (Chen et al. 2009).

Based on the 2009 Youth Risk Behavior Survey (YRBS), approximately 20% of high school students reported being bullied at school, and over 30% reported being in a physical fight (Centers for Disease Control and Prevention 2010g). More than 656,000 young people, ages 10–24 years, were treated in emergency departments for injuries sustained from violence in 2009 (Centers for Disease Control and Prevention 2010f). In 2007, homicide was the second leading cause of death of young people, with an average of 16 youth murdered every day (Centers for Disease Control and Prevention 2010b). Fortunately, a strong and growing research base and community involvement demonstrate that there are multiple strategies that work to prevent youth violence.

In 2007, the frequency of injuries in schools, child care centers, and preschools was 2,243,000. The number of injuries among students while attending school was 760,000 (Chen et al. 2009, p. 19). Approximately one third of these injuries resulted in time lost from school; 22% resulted in 1 to 5 days lost (Chen et al. 2009). Most of the injuries that occur on school property are unintentional and minor. Serious injuries occur more frequently at home or in the community, thus the need for broad safety education for students and staff.

Highly associated with these injuries are adolescent behaviors such as physical fights, carrying weapons, making a suicide plan, and not using seat belts. The 2009 Centers for Disease Control and Prevention (CDC) YRBS provides data about high school student behavior the 2 years prior to the survey. Results show that nationally 5.5% of students reported missing school because they felt unsafe. About 8% of students had been threatened or injured with a weapon (e.g., gun, knife, club) on school property one or more times during the 12 months before the survey. The percentage of students who reported carrying a weapon on school property on at least one day and those who reported being "threatened or injured with a weapon on school property one or more times" has decreased from 1993 to 2009. However, 32% of high school students had been in a physical fight, 18% had carried a weapon in the past 30 days (not necessarily at school), and 11% had made a plan about how they would attempt suicide in the past 12 months (Centers for Disease Control and Prevention 2010g).

A safe school environment includes both the physical and psychosocial environments. Ensuring that the school building and grounds are in proper condition is as important as ensuring social climate, which includes positive and healthy relationships between students, faculty, and staff. The psychosocial environment encompasses the formal and informal policies, norms, climate, and mechanisms through which students, faculty, and staff members interact daily. A psychosocial environment can promote safety or increase risk for unintentional injuries, violence, and suicide.

Environmental Factors

The Physical Environment

Unintentional injuries can occur anywhere in a school's physical environment—walkways and grounds, playgrounds, sports fields, parking lots, school vehicles, gymnasiums, classrooms, shop and vocational education classrooms, cafeterias, hallways, and bathrooms.

Injuries due to the physical environment are most often the result of inadequate maintenance, nonuse of protective equipment such as goggles, use of equipment for purposes for which it was not intended, or equipment that is not developmentally appropriate for the user. Sometimes the problem is with the manufacturing itself. Standards exist for certain types of equipment but not all items meet standards; for other equipment no standards exist. Ensuring that flooring surfaces are slip-resistant and free of hazards and stairwells are in good repair and have sturdy handrails are important steps in reducing falls. Regular safety and hazard assessments coupled with routine maintenance of school structures, window openings, fencing, and equipment can prevent many injuries in schools and in child care settings.

According to CPSC, an estimated 156,000 injuries on public playgrounds require emergency room treatment each year (U.S. Consumer Product Safety Commission 2008). Because the types and causes of these injuries differ, schools and child care facilities need to keep records about each incident. Aggregating incidence data and developing a prevention plan can help determine areas that need repair and/or modification. The chapter on Sports and Recreation in this book includes information on sports injuries in schools and on playgrounds.

Sample strategies for reducing injuries in the school physical environment include the following:

- Install and maintain playgrounds that meet CPSC guidelines
- Ensure that materials and equipment used in schools, child care facilities, or on school grounds have not been subject to a product recall (http://www.clickcheckandprotect.org is a searchable Web site that lists recalled products [Consumers Union 2010])
- Inspect playground equipment and athletic fields regularly
- Make safety-related repairs promptly and prohibit use of or access to anything in need of repair
- Install break resistant glass in doors.
- Use slip-resistant flooring materials and keep hallways and stairways clean, dry, and clear of obstructions
- Provide adequate lighting in hallways and stairways
- Install and maintain working smoking alarms, fire extinguishers and sprinklers
- Lock roof doors and limit access to unsafe maintenance areas
- Require the use of protective equipment and safety guards in chemistry labs and shop classes
- Provide storage for student backpacks
- Install and maintain railings along stairwells
- Select materials and equipment that are developmentally appropriate for the student's abilities

To and From School

Between 2000 and 2009, of the reported 371,104 motor vehicle-related fatalities, 0.34 % (1245) were classified as school transportation-related. In that same time frame, 1386 people died in school transportation-related crashes—an average of 139 fatalities per year. Most people killed in those crashes (72%) were in other vehicles. Nonoccupants (e.g., pedestrians, bicyclists) accounted for 20% of the deaths, and occupants of school transportation vehicles accounted for 8% (National Highway Traffic Safety Administration 2009).

Between 2000 and 2009, 96 crashes occurred in which at least one occupant of a school transportation vehicle died. More than half of those crashes (59%) involved at least one other vehicle. Also during this time, 130 school-age pedestrians (younger than 19) died in school transportation-related crashes. Over two thirds (67%) were killed by school buses, 6% by vehicles functioning as school buses, and 27% by other vehicles involved in the crashes (National Highway Traffic Safety Administration 2009). About one half (43%) of the school-age pedestrians killed in school transportation-related crashes were between 5 and 7 years old. On average, ten school-age pedestrians are killed by school transportation vehicles (school buses and nonschool bus vehicles used as school buses) each year, and four are killed by other vehicles involved in school bus-related crashes. More school-age pedestrians have been killed between the hours of 3:00 P.M. and 4:00 P.M. than any other time of day (National Highway Traffic Safety Administration 2009).

Transportation-related information from YRBS indicates that 10% of high school students never or rarely wore a seat belt while riding in a car (Centers for Disease Control and Prevention 2010g). These data indicate the need for providing safety education that includes messages about the use of safety belts and bicycle helmets, and the risk of driving under the influence and at night. Although transportation to and from school is relatively safe compared to outside of school, it is important to establish safety habits in students as early as possible.

There was a time when walking and bicycling to school was part of everyday life. In 1969, about half of all students walked or bicycled to school (Federal Highway Administration 1972). Today, however, fewer than 15% of all school trips involve walking or bicycling, 25% are on a school bus, and over half of all students arrive at school in private automobiles (Centers for Disease Control and Prevention 2004).

This decline in walking and bicycling has had an adverse effect on traffic congestion and air quality around schools, as well as pedestrian and bicycle safety. In addition, a growing body of evidence has shown that children who lead sedentary lifestyles are at risk for a variety of health problems such as obesity, diabetes, and cardiovascular disease (Centers for Disease Control and Prevention 2004). Safety issues are a big concern for parents, who consistently cite traffic danger as a reason why their children do not bicycle or walk to school (Centers for Disease Control and Prevention 2005).

Overall, in 2007, 114 (down from 130 in 2006) bicyclists aged 4–19 years were killed and an additional 44,000 were injured in traffic crashes (Chen et al. 2009). Of these deaths, 94 were males. In 2009, there were 267,265 bicycle-related injuries among children and youth ages 4–19 years (Centers for Disease Control and Prevention 2010f), and among the high school students who had ridden a bicycle during the previous 12 months, 85% had rarely or never worn a bicycle helmet (Centers for Disease Control and Prevention 2010g). Considering that many states have bicycle helmet laws, this nonhelmet use seems like a very high number, indicating once again the need for education about helmet use and enforcement of existing laws.

The Safe Routes to School (SRTS) programs enable community leaders, schools, and parents across the United States to improve safety and encourage more children, including those with disabilities, to safely walk and bicycle to school. In the process, programs are working to reduce traffic congestion and improve health and the environment, making communities more livable for everyone. SRTS programs examine conditions around schools and conduct projects and activities that work to improve safety and accessibility, and reduce traffic and air pollution in the vicinity of schools. As a result, these programs help make bicycling and walking to school safer and more appealing transportation choices, thus encouraging a healthy and active lifestyle from an early age (National Center for Safe Routes to School 2010). As of June 2010, the National Center for Safe Routes to School indicates there are more than 7622 programs across the United States (National Center for Safe Routes to School 2010). These programs offer public health and education another opportunity for collaboration around a very important topic for children and youth.

Although schools have the ability to address some factors that contribute to safety of students going to and from school, other factors require policies or legislation at the municipal, county, or state levels. There are many strategies in the Motor Vehicle-Related Injury Prevention chapter of this book that provide examples of where public health and education could partner to decrease the toll of these injuries.

Environmental strategies for reducing injuries to students traveling to and from school include the following:

- Create safe pedestrian crossing areas protected from bus and auto traffic.
- Safely separate students who are riding school buses, those being dropped off by cars, and those walking or biking to school.
- Require occupants of moving cars on school property to wear safety belts and motorcycle and bicycle riders to wear helmets.

- Install and maintain adequate lighting and low shrubbery to reduce the chance of injury.
- Work with the local governmental authority to have painted crosswalks and traffic signals on the major pedestrian and bicycle routes to schools.
- Work with the local governmental authority to require sidewalks and bicycle lanes and their maintenance and snow removal on the major pedestrian and bicycle routes to schools.
- Adjust school start times as students get older to reduce crashes due to drowsy drivers.
- Enforce safety policies and regulations.
- Support passage and enforcement of graduated driver licensing (GDL) policies. These laws allow new teen drivers to get experience on the road in lower-risk situations. Strong GDL laws have been associated with up to a 40% decrease in crashes among 16-year-old drivers (Centers for Disease Control and Prevention 2010d).

The Psychosocial Environment

A safe school environment includes both physical and psychosocial environments. Ensuring that the school building and grounds are in proper condition is as important as ensuring positive and healthy relationships among students, faculty, and staff. The psychosocial environment encompasses the formal and informal policies, norms, climate, and mechanisms through which students, faculty, and staff members interact daily. A psychosocial environment can promote safety or increase risk for unintentional injuries, violence, and suicide. According to YRBS, 5% of students did not go to school because they felt they would be unsafe at school or on their way to or from school at least once a day during the 30 days before the survey (Centers for Disease Control and Prevention 2010g).

School connectedness, defined as "the degree to which a student experiences a sense of caring and closeness to teachers and the overall school environment" (Wilson 2004, p. 298), helps predict the likelihood of victimization and aggression among secondary school students (Wilson 2004). In a study of fourth graders, school connectedness was positively associated with behavior control and negatively associated with openly expressing anger and with stress (Rice et al. 2008). The 2007 National Survey of Children's Health shows that school engagement among children aged 6–17 years was overall about 80.5%; engagement of children with special health care needs was 69.5% compared to 84% of children without special health care needs (Health Resources Services Administration 2009). Students who feel connected to school believe that adults and peers in the school care about their learning as well as about them as individuals. When students feel connected to school, they are less likely to engage in a variety of risk behaviors, including violence and gang involvement. Connected students are also more likely to have higher grades and test scores, better school attendance, and stay in school longer.

In the report, *Student Victimization in U.S. Schools: Results From the 2007 School Crime Supplement to the National Crime Victimization Survey*, published by the National Center for Education Statistics at the U.S. Department of Education's Institute of Education Sciences, about 4% of students aged 12–18 years reported they were victims of crime at school in the 2006–2007 school year. The percentage of students who avoided specific places at school because of fear of attack or harm was higher for students reporting any crime (13%) versus students who were nonvictims (5%) (DeVoe and Bauer 2010). Based on her work with juveniles in trouble with the law, Juvenile Court Judge Marilyn Moores concluded that what society labels deviance or disruption is often a response to pain. Most adjudicated youth have experienced four to five significant losses in their lives, which leads them to fear others and rationalizes acting in anger, which appears less threatening than being vulnerable or rejected. If a teen keeps others at bay, or does not try to succeed, then he or she can't fail or be hurt. Acting out is better than powerlessness. In the brain, physical pain and social pain are not distinguishable. People who can verbalize their pain are better able to overcome adversity (Moores 2006). Young people who do not have the emotional support they need at home have an even greater need to benefit from feeling connected to school and to adults in the school or community.

Social ecological factors associated with improved school connectedness are critical topics for teacher and staff training. These include organizational, functional, structural, and interpersonal factors. The organizational factors associated with connectedness are a small school size and less departmentalization, which improves teacher collegiality. In the built environment (structural), well-maintained facilities that create a pleasant environment and interesting architecture of which students and staff are proud contribute to school connectedness. Although neither public health professionals nor school staff might have control over these factors, they can make changes in the functional and interpersonal realms.

Factors in the functional realm associated with school connectedness include the following (1) clear and fairly applied discipline expectations, (2) student involvement in decisionmaking, (3) high expectations for learning, (4) developmentally appropriate and student-centered teaching practices, (5) parental involvement, (6) extracurricular activities that allow student and teacher interactions, and (7) pastoral systems. Contributing interpersonal factors are positive relationships among students, between staff and students, and among staff (Waters, Cross, and Runions 2009). Strategies for enhancing students' connectedness to school include treating students fairly (Samdal et al. 1998); creating school norms for positive, prosocial, helping behaviors and discouraging bullying, discrimination, intimidation, violence, or aggression; utilizing classroom management techniques that enforce clear expectations for attendance and behaviors, rewarding students for involvement and cooperation with one another, and for attempts to comply with behavioral expectations; and during counseling and school nurse visits assessing students for school connectedness, behavioral control, angry outbursts, social confidence, and stress (Rice et al. 2008).

Sample strategies for reducing injuries and violence involving the school psychosocial environment include the following:

- Establish and enforce school-wide policies for mutual respect
- Implement an ongoing, anonymous student reporting system
- Implement a comprehensive bullying prevention program
- Implement a conflict resolution program
- Involve students in planning and implementing programs
- Provide adult supervision on playgrounds and in hallways; express disapproval of pushing, shoving, or sexual harassment; and intervene if witnessed (Centers for Disease Control and Prevention 2001a)

Sample strategies for enhancing school connectedness include the following:

- Create decisionmaking processes that facilitate student, family, and community engagement, academic achievement, and staff empowerment
- Provide education and opportunities that enable families to participate actively in their children's academic and school life
- Provide students with the academic, emotional, and social skills necessary to engage actively in school activities
- Use effective classroom management and teaching methods that foster a positive learning environment
- Provide professional development and support for teachers and other school staff that enable them to meet the diverse cognitive, emotional, and social needs of children and adolescents
- Create trusting and caring relationships that promote open communication among administrators, teachers, staff, students, families, and communities (Centers for Disease Control and Prevention 2009)
- Provide increased support to young people who experience significant losses in their lives (Moores 2006)

Developmental and Behavioral Factors

Brain Development

The ability of children and youth to perceive and assess risks, as well as their fine and gross motor skills, change as they mature. Because of inexperience and a poor understanding of cause and effect, children and youth often do not perceive that a situation or action presents a risk. Setting and enforcing safety rules is one way adults can protect children.

Although the brain of a 6 year old is 95% the size of an adult's, it continues to develop till well into early adulthood. Until puberty, the brain increases the number of neural connections. Nutritional deficiencies between conception and puberty can result in fewer brain cells and neural connections. In adolescence, the rate of creating neural connections slows and the brain begins a pruning process, eliminating unused connections. One of the last places in the brain to develop fully is the prefrontal cortex, which is not fully developed until age 25 or so. This prefrontal cortex is the area responsible for impulse control and decisionmaking (Giedd 2006).

The neural pruning that occurs in adolescence explains why some mental health problems manifest in the teen years. Autistic children have larger than normal brains—they have too many connections and do not prune the branches well. Schizophrenics' brains show fourfold the normal rate of pruning (Giedd 2006). Adolescents who are chronically exposed to violence or become dependent on alcohol or other substances often do not develop good impulse control, coping mechanisms, or decisionmaking skills. Because of the pruning process in adolescence, skills not learned during the formative years are often much harder to learn later (Giedd 2006).

Drug use and lack of sleep can affect the brain's development during the teen years in ways that have lifelong consequences. Only 31% of students have 8 or more hours of sleep on an average school night (Centers for Disease Control and Prevention 2010g). The long-term consequences of sleep deprivation are less well known, but short-term consequences include loss of coordination and poorer decisionmaking ability. The normal sleep cycle shifts during adolescence, with a later normal sleep and wake time. Unfortunately, high schools often start earlier than elementary schools, thus almost guaranteeing that large numbers of adolescents are sleep deprived much of the time. In one study that examined the effects of delaying high school start times, the average crash rates for teen drivers in the county during the 2 years after the change in school start time dropped 16.5%, compared with the 2 years prior to the change, whereas teen crash rates for the rest of the state increased 7.8% over the same time period (Danner and Phillips 2008).

Physical/Developmental Immaturity

Implications of youth development include a need to provide graduated structure and guidance for young people as they mature, while remembering that even physically mature adolescents lack the impulse control and decisionmaking ability of adults. An understanding of youth development can also inform educators as they prepare safety-related curricula so they match the curriculum sequence with the maturation sequence. The human brain is programmed for modeling, listening, flexibility, and so on, but not for reading, thus interactive activities are important components of safety instruction. Interactive, relevant safety instruction activities that appeal to students' emotions could build on an understanding that adolescent brains and hormones are limbic-driven and respond powerfully when emotionally motivated.

Effective instructional programs model learning; provide opportunities for problem-solving; engage students through teaching models, concept mapping, scaffolding; provide constant feedback to help prune the brain; and help students learn executive functions such as goal setting, setting tactics, and monitoring learning (Rose 2006).

Sample strategies for reducing injuries due to physical/developmental immaturity include the following:

- Advocate for schools to participate in school breakfast, lunch, and weekend snack programs
- Advocate for the importance of addressing extreme poverty and hunger issues that can diminish normal brain development
- Establish and enforce safety rules that take into account students' development
- Select materials and equipment that take into account students' motor abilities
- Provide leadership education for adolescents to develop executive functions for decisionmaking consistent with demonstrated abilities
- Support positive youth development programs that help reduce dependence on alcohol or other mind-altering substance use
- Explore later school start times as students get older
- Continue to provide adult guidance during adolescence
- Develop and implement sequential safety curricula that are consistent with students' development of motor skills and cognitive functioning, and that are consistent with findings from adolescent brain development research

Violence at School

While schools remain relatively safe, any amount of violence is unacceptable. Parents, teachers, and administrators expect schools to be safe havens of learning. Acts of violence can disrupt the learning process and have a negative effect on students, the school itself, and the broader community (Centers for Disease Control and Prevention 2010a).

Violence at school is a subset of youth violence, a broader public health problem. Youth violence refers to harmful behaviors that often start early and continue into young adulthood. It includes bullying, slapping, punching, weapon use, self-inflicted injury and rape. Victims can suffer serious injury, significant social and emotional damage, or even death. The young person can be a victim, an offender, or a witness to the violence-or a combination of these (Centers for Disease Control and Prevention 2010a).

The 2007 Task Force on Community Preventive Services recommends universal, school-based violence prevention programs based on strong evidence of effectiveness in preventing or reducing violent behavior. Universal school-based programs to reduce violence include instructing all students in a given school or grade about the problem of violence and its prevention, or about one or more of the following topics or skills intended to reduce aggressive or violent behavior: emotional self-awareness, emotional control, self-esteem, positive social skills, social problem-solving, conflict resolution, or teamwork. In this review, violence refers to both victimization and perpetration.

The Task Force conducted a study of school-wide interventions intended to reduce youth violence. The criteria for inclusion in the study were that the programs were implemented in prekindergarten, kindergarten, elementary, middle school, and/or high school classrooms and all children in a given grade or school, regardless of prior violence or risk for violent behavior received the programs. Some programs targeted schools in high-risk areas, including those with low socioeconomic status, high crime rates, or both. Elementary school and middle school programs usually sought to reduce disruptive and antisocial behavior using approaches that focused on modifying behavior by changing the associated cognitive and affective mechanisms. In middle and high schools, the focus of programs shifted to general violence and to specific forms of violence, including bullying and dating violence. The interventions used approaches that made greater use of social skills training and emphasized the development of behavioral skills rather than changes in cognition, consequential thinking, or affective processes. The Task Force review found the following:

- For all grades combined, the median effect was a 15.0% relative reduction in violent behavior among students who received the program (high school students: median relative reduction of 29.2%; middle school students: 7.3%; elementary school students: 18.0%; prekindergarten and kindergarten students: 32.4%)
- All intervention strategies (e.g., informational, cognitive/affective, social skills building) were associated with a reduction in violent behavior
- Programs appeared to be effective in reducing violent behavior among students in all school environments, regardless of socioeconomic status or crime rate and among all school populations, regardless of the predominant ethnicity of students (Task Force on Community Preventive Services 2007)

Bullying

Bullying is aggressive behavior that is intentional (not accidental or done in fun) and that involves an imbalance of power or strength. Often, bullying is repeated over time. Bullying can take many forms such as hitting or punching, teasing or name-calling, intimidation through gestures, social exclusion, and sending insulting messages or pictures by mobile phone or using the Internet (also known as cyber bullying). Bullying is far too often seen as an inevitable part of schoolyard culture, but the consequences of bullying can be serious (Health Resources Services Administration 2010). The 2009 YRBS indicated that 20% of students had been bullied on school property during the 12 months before the survey (Centers for Disease Control and Prevention 2010g). A 2007 survey conducted by the Gay, Lesbian, and Straight Education Network (GLSEN) indicated that 50% of principals (75% of junior and senior high schools and less than 50% of elementary school principals) believe that bullying, name calling, and/or harassment of students is a serious problem at their respective schools (Gay, Lesbian, and Straight Education Network and Harris Interactive 2008).

Bullies tend to be physically larger than their peers. They are aggressive, quick to anger, impulsive, lack empathy, and have lower self-esteem. Victims of bullying lean toward social isolation, lack of social skills, and smaller stature than their peers (Health Resources Services Administration 2010). Students who are repeatedly bullied are at increased risk for mental health problems and suicidal ideation. Sometimes bullied youth resort to violence to stop the torment.

Cyber bullying is an emerging bullying issue. The number of young people who reported being victims of electronic aggression increased 50% between 2000 and 2005. Various studies found that 35% to 50% of youths reported being targeted by cyber bullying at least once, and that 27% of youths who had been targets of cyber bullying had also carried a weapon to school at least once (Ybarra, Diener-West, and Leaf 2007; David-Ferdon and Hertz 2007). According to Kowalski and Limber, instant messaging appears to be the most common form of electronic aggression; 67% through instant messaging, 25% via e-mail, and 16% via text messages. (Kowalski and Limber 2007).

According to researchers, cyber bullying has characteristics that differ from traditional bullying. These include anonymity, disinhibition, accessibility, lack of victim reporting due to punitive fears, and ambiguous bystander roles. Research has found that both the cyber bully and the victim have higher rates of anxiety and depression and high school absenteeism than other students. In some rare cases, young people have committed suicide as an apparent result of cyber bullying (Kowalski, Limber, and Agatston, 2008).

Bullying not only involves the person who bullies and the person being bullied, but the students who witness the bullying. Bystanders are those who watch bullying happen or hear about it. They can either contribute to the problem or the solution. Most people who witness bullying are passive bystanders. There are many different reasons they do not intervene. Many fear becoming a victim themselves, think it is none of their business, feel powerless against the bully, or do not know what to do (Storey et al. 2008).

Teachers and school staff may also not know how to properly address the problem. It is important to involve everyone in bullying prevention programs.

Strategies to Prevent Bullying

Although the issue of bullying is mostly discussed in terms of tweens and older adolescents, it is also an issue for younger children. Thus lessons and activities that address respect, equity, feelings, and compassion are relevant at all levels, including child care settings. The adults in schools must embody these traits and serve as role models.

According to the *Eyes on Bullying Project*, there are two types of bystanders. Hurtful bystanders are those who may instigate the bullying, laugh at the victim or cheer for the bully, or join in on the bullying once it has begun. Hurtful bystanders also include those people who passively watch the bullying and do nothing about it. Passive bystanders provide the audience a bully wants and the silent acceptance that allows bullies to continue their behavior (Storey et al. 2008). Helpful bystanders are those who directly intervene while the bullying is happening by defending the victim or discouraging the bully. Helpful bystanders also include those who get help or gather support from other peers for the victim (Storey et al. 2008).

The *Stop Bullying Now!* (SBN) Campaign, launched in 2004 by the U.S. Department of Health and Human Services, Health Resources Services Administration (HRSA), provides free, research-based resources in multimedia formats for youth ages 9–13 years and the adults who work with them. Youth and adults can find topic-specific, tailored evidence-informed tip sheets that facilitate prevention and that suggest interventions for both bullies and victims (available at http://www.stopbullying.gov). These tip sheets provide guidance on how to respond to bullying situations as well as how to prevent bullying in schools and communities. Among the most popular resources on the Web site are 12 animated webisodes that help youth understand the power of bystanders and the importance in telling an adult about ending bullying behavior. Youth can also access games, public service announcements, and profiles of relatable characters that collectively promote discussion among youth and adults about appropriate action.

A review of bullying prevention programs and feedback from educators in the field led HRSA SBN Campaign to suggest strategies that represent "best practice" in bullying prevention and intervention. These include the following:

(1) Focus on the social environment of the school. In order to reduce bullying, it is important to change the social climate of the school and the social norms regarding bullying. This requires the efforts of everyone in the school environment: teachers, administrators, counselors, school nurses, school librarians, other nonteaching staff (e.g., bus drivers, custodians, cafeteria workers), parents, and students.

(2) Assess bullying at your school. Adults are not always very good at estimating the nature and prevalence of bullying at their school. As a result, it can be quite useful to administer an anonymous questionnaire to students about bullying.

(3) Obtain staff and parent buy-in and support for bullying prevention. Bullying prevention should not be the sole responsibility of any single individual at a school. To be most effective, bullying prevention efforts require buy-in from the majority of the staff and from parents. However, bullying prevention efforts should still begin even if immediate buy-in from all isn't achievable. Usually, more and more supporters will join the effort once they see what it's accomplishing.

(4) Form a group to coordinate the school's bullying prevention activities. Bullying prevention efforts seem to work best if they are coordinated by a representative group from the school. This coordinating team might include the following:

- An administrator
- A teacher from each grade
- A member of the nonteaching staff
- A school counselor or other school-based mental health professional
- A parent

The team should meet regularly to review findings from the school's survey; plan specific bullying prevention activities; motivate staff, students, and parents; and ensure that the efforts continue over time.

(5) Provide training for school staff in bullying prevention. All school administrators, faculty, and staff should be trained in bullying prevention and intervention. In-service training can help staff members to better understand the nature of bullying and its effects, how to respond if they observe bullying, and how to work with others at the school to help prevent bullying.

(6) Establish and enforce school rules and policies related to bullying. Developing simple, clear rules about bullying can help to ensure that students are aware of adults' expectations that they not bully others and that they help students who are bullied. School rules and policies should be posted and discussed with students and parents. Appropriate positive and negative consequences should be developed.

(7) Increase adult supervision in "hot spots" for bullying. Bullying tends to thrive in locations where adults are not present or are not watchful. Adults should look for creative ways to increase adult presence in locations that students identify as "hot spots."

(8) Intervene consistently and appropriately when you see bullying. Observed or suspected bullying should never be ignored by adults. All school staff should learn effective strategies to intervene on-the-spot to stop bullying. Staff members also should be designated to hold sensitive follow-up meetings with students who are bullied and (separately) with students who bully. Staff members should involve parents whenever possible.

(9) Devote some class time to bullying prevention. Students can benefit if teachers set aside a regular period of time (e.g., 20–30 minutes each week or every other week) to discuss bullying and improving peer relations. These meetings can help teachers to keep their fingers on the pulse of students' concerns, allow time for discussions about bullying and the harms that it can cause, and provide tools for students to address bullying problems. Anti-bullying messages can also be incorporated throughout the school curriculum.

(10) Continue these efforts. There should be no "nd date" for bullying prevention activities. Bullying prevention should be continued over time and woven into the fabric of the school environment (Health Resources Services Administration 2010).

HRSA has partnered with the U.S. Department of Education's Office of Safe and Drug-Free Schools on a program that recognizes the value and power of student leaders. A Student Leaders Tool Kit was created and is seen as critical in raising awareness about bullying and as a powerful tool in creating a successful school safety initiative.

Principals often report that their schools have an anti-harassment or anti-bullying policy (Gay, Lesbian, and Straight Education Network 2010). As of this writing, 22 states have adopted cyber bullying statutes and 45 states have laws regarding bullying. The National Conference on State Legislatures (NCSL) is tracking bullying prevention laws. NCSL's tracking also shows the variance among the laws (National Conference on State Legislatures 2010). Very few of the anti-bullying laws identified by NCSL specifically address creating a safe environment for lesbian, gay, bisexual, and transgender students (Gay, Lesbian, and Straight Education Network and Harris Interactive 2008). In an effort to begin to address this need, the Human Rights Campaign Foundation (HRCF) created "Welcoming Schools Guidelines," a comprehensive guide with tools, lessons, and resources on family diversity, gender stereotyping, and name-calling (Human Rights Campaign Foundation 2010).

Bullying prevention researchers, Hinduja and Patchin, suggest the following six components that schools should include in anti-bullying and harassment policies and practices: (1) specific definitions of harassment, intimidation, and bullying (including electronic variants); (2) graduated consequences and remedial actions; (3) procedures for reporting; (4) procedures for investigating; (5) language specifying that if a student's off-campus speech or behavior results in "substantial disruption of the learning environment," the student can be disciplined by the school; and (6) procedures for cyber bullying (Hinduja and Patchin 2009).

Evaluation is an important component of any program. The CDC's National Center for Injury Prevention and Control has released a new publication, *Measuring Bullying Victimization, Perpetration, and Bystander Experiences: A Compendium of Assessment Tools* (Centers for Disease Control and Prevention 2011b). The resources and time to do evaluation are often not provided with the mandate or need to implement a program. However, it is also a waste of resources and time if we implement a program that does not work.

Homicide and Suicide

Although a student who dies by violence in school is a rare occurrence, it is always a tragedy that attracts a great deal of attention. It is a rare but an emotionally charged event. Violent deaths at schools accounted for less than 1% of the homicides and suicides among children ages 5–18 years (Kachur et al. 1996). During the past 7 years, 116 students were killed in 109 separate incidents—an average of 16.5 student homicides each year. Most school-associated homicides included gunshot wounds (65%), stabbings or cuttings (27%), and beatings (12%) (Centers for Disease Control and Prevention 2010b). Rates of school-associated student homicides decreased between 1992 and 2006. However, they have remained relatively stable in recent years. Rates were significantly higher for males, students in secondary schools, and students in central cities. From 1991 to 2009, there has been a 50% decrease in students who report seriously considering suicide and those who made a plan for how they would commit suicide. Still, 11% to 14% of students still report considering suicide, and 6% had attempted suicide one or more times in the previous year (Centers for Disease Control and Prevention 2010g).

Strategies to Reduce Student Suicide

With the significant risk of suicide among adolescents, one of the prevention efforts includes an increase in the amount of training provided to school teachers and staff. According to the 2006 CDC School Health Policy and Programs Study (SHPPS): (1) the percentage of states that required elementary schools to teach about suicide prevention increased from 26% in 2000 to 44% in 2006; (2) the percentage of high schools in which teachers in at least one required health education course taught about suicide prevention increased from 66% in 2000 to 80% in 2006; and (3) among courses in which suicide prevention was taught, the median number of hours of required instruction teachers provided on suicide prevention was 0.4 hours among middle school courses and 1.4 hours among high school courses (Kann, Telljohann, and Wooley 2007). The chapter on Youth Suicide in this book focuses in-depth on the problem and strategies for the prevention of suicide.

Dating and Sexual Violence

Teen dating violence is a significant component of violence. Annually, one of four adolescents experience verbal, physical, emotional, or sexual abuse from a dating partner. Both middle school and high school students are exposed to dating and sexual violence. Twenty percent of tweens report that they know friends who have been struck in anger by a boyfriend or girlfriend (Liz Claiborne 2011). In a study of seventh grade students who were 44.5% Hispanic, 27% non-Hispanic African American, 24% White, and 4.5% other, 35% of boys and 24% of girls reported physical dating violence victimization in the past 12 months (Swahn et al. 2008). A nationally representative survey shows that 60% of female and 69% of male victims were first raped before age 18 (Basile et al. 2007).

Some individuals think that dating violence happens in private where no one can see. However, in one study conducted with 13- to 18-year-olds, 42% of boys and 43% of girls who reported abuse related that the violence happened on school grounds (Novas 2010). In addition, a study in three cities (Boston, Chicago, and San Antonio) showed that early involvement with antisocial peers at ages 10–15 years was linked to dating violence perpetration for Hispanic and African American students (Schnurr and Lohman 2008). A cross-sectional survey of a small sample of middle school Latino youth (316 students) between the ages of 11 and 13 years found that carrying a gun or another weapon was associated with physical dating violence victimization among boys (Yan et al. 2010).

Many of the incidents go unreported because teens are afraid to tell friends and family (Centers for Disease Control and Prevention 2010e.) Although these incidents may not occur on school grounds, it is important for school personnel and other people important in the lives of children and youth to be aware of the problem and methods for prevention. Dating violence can have a negative effect on health throughout life. Teens who are victims are more likely to be depressed and do poorly in school (Banyard and Cross 2008). They may engage in unhealthy behaviors such as using drugs and alcohol (Banyard and Cross 2008), and are more likely to have eating disorders (Ackard and Neumark-Sztainer 2002).

Strategies for Preventing Dating Violence

Dating violence is not only dangerous for the couple involved, but also puts other students at risk of violence. Comprehensive strategies to reduce dating and sexual violence should address factors at each of the levels that influence violence: the individual, relationship, community, and society. States have begun implementing policies that address dating violence. To date, 34 states have laws, or proposed legislation on dating violence (Women's Defense and Legal Education Fund 2010).

This is a positive first step. However, school staff have to take a more proactive role in preventing dating violence and intervening when they see violence. School districts need to implement teen dating violence programs, train teachers and school staff on how to intervene in situations, and support students who are victims. The most common prevention strategies currently focus on the victim, the perpetrator, or bystanders. Strategies that aim to equip the victim with knowledge, awareness, or self-defense skills are referred to as risk reduction techniques. Strategies targeting the perpetrator attempt to change risk and protective factors for sexual violence in order to reduce the likelihood that an individual will engage in sexually violent behavior. The goal of bystander prevention strategies is to change social norms supporting sexual violence and empower boys and girls to intervene with peers to prevent an assault from occurring. Other prevention strategies may target social norms, policies, or laws in communities to reduce the perpetration of sexual violence across the population (Centers for Disease Control and Prevention 2011c).

Choose Respect is a program developed by the CDC. The following suggestions for schools described below are taken from the Choose Respect CDC Web site:

> Educators_including teachers, counselors, administrators, school personnel, coaches, mentors, and other trusted adults_can take an active and important role in helping their students

understand the characteristics of healthy and unhealthy relationships, and the connection between respect and healthy relationships.

Many teens are more comfortable talking with a peer, teacher, or another trusted adult than they are with their parents. The most important thing is having someone [to] turn to for advice and that the person is a source of good information.

If a student approaches you and wants to talk about dating, they are likely to feel more comfortable if you create an open environment. Here are some ways educators can help create a climate of respect and openness that can encourage students to feel comfortable talking about difficult issues:

- Keep an open environment. Be available to listen to your students. Give them opportunities to start talking and do not to [sic] criticize them for having questions.
- Give your student your undivided attention. Listening is an important skill in healthy relationships. If a student has chosen to confide in you, focus your attention on the conversation and your student. Do not let other things distract you or divide your concentration. If it is really a bad time to talk, schedule and keep another appointment where you can talk, but first make sure that waiting is okay with the teen.
- Connect frequently. Following up with your students on a regular basis is a great way to communicate and let your students know you are interested in their lives. This is particularly important if a student has already confided in you about something.
- Understand the questions and respond genuinely. If you are not sure what the student is asking, say so. Once you understand the question, respond genuinely and assure him or her that you take his or her concerns seriously.
- Keep in mind that it is not the teacher's responsibility to "fix" the problem. Rather, as a trusted adult in the students' lives, the teacher can connect students with other resources they can access for help.

In addition to teaching students about healthy relationship behaviors, you can model these skills in their schools. Teens watch how adults handle and react to various situations, emotions, and conflict. If you do not "practice what you preach," your students may tune you out and ignore the lessons given.

It is also important that educators look for a pattern of behaviors. These patterns can potentially serve as warning signs of elevated risk for dating violence. (Centers for Disease Control and Prevention 2011a).

Educational Factors

Student Education and Training

Schools and preschool and child care settings are critical venues where students can develop the understanding, awareness, knowledge, and skills they need to navigate the world safely and become productive, successful adults. Establishing healthy behaviors during childhood and maintaining them is easier and more effective than trying to change unhealthy behaviors during adulthood (Centers for Disease Control and Prevention 2010c).

The percentage of elementary schools and middle schools required by their districts to teach injury prevention and safety has increased from 66% to 77% and 67% to 80%, respectively, from 2000 to 2006 (Kann et al. 2007). However, among classes and courses in which violence prevention was taught, the median number of hours of required instruction decreased from 4.9 in

2000 to 2.6 in 2006 among elementary school classes, and from 4.1 to 2.5 among high school classes (Kann et al. 2007).

Safety education courses for students address injury and violence prevention on school property as well as general skills for injury prevention outside the classroom. Many schools include safety lessons within the context of health education, physical education, technical/vocational education, home economics, and sciences classes. Formal safety education should include the following topics chosen based on students' ages and the school's physical and psychosocial environment:

Although many schools provide safety education, few address all categories and levels. Not noted in Table 7.1 are important categories such as bullying prevention (including cyber bullying), suicide prevention, conflict resolution, or dating violence. Strategies to address these issues can be found at several national resource centers and on government-sponsored Web sites. Those resources include but are not limited to the following:

- http://www.ChildrensSafetyNetwork.org
- http://www.SPRC.org
- http://www.childrensnational.org/emsc/
- http://www.stopbullying.gov

Table 7.1. Percentage of Schools in Which Teachers Taught* Injury Prevention Topics as Part of Required Instruction, by School Level, 2004 data

Topic	Elementary	Middle	High
Cardiopulmonary resuscitation (CPR)	15.2	37.1	48.6
Emergency preparedness	63.6	56.4	56.7
Fire safety	72.4	52.2	39.9
First aid	49.8	56.2	55.8
Motor vehicle occupant safety (e.g., seat belt use)	68.5	54.3	56.3
Pedestrian safety	68.6	35.0	29.5
Playground safety	79.9	NA	NA
Poisoning prevention	47.0	39.8	49.8
Use of protective equipment for biking, skating, or other sports	69.2	55.4	50.0
Water safety	54.6	42.8	38.0

*In at least one elementary school class or in at least one required health education course in middle schools or high schools.

NA = not asked at this level.

Adapted from Kann L et al. 2007. Health education: results from the School Health Policies and Programs Study 2006. Table 10. Percentage of All Schools in Which Teachers Taught Injury Prevention Topics as Part of Required Instruction, by School Level, SHPPS 2006.

- http://www.cdc.gov.healthyyouth
- http://www.CPSC.gov
- http://www.cdc.gov/injury
- http://www.endabuse.org
- http://www.BullyingInfo.org

Many educational programs that address reducing injuries and violence among school-aged children and youth exist. Both the *American Journal of Health Education* and the *Journal of School Health* have published descriptions of injury prevention activities as teaching ideas or techniques. Although a few have undergone evaluation, most have not. What is not known is exactly what is taught, time provided to translate the information to the students, how much they follow the training themselves, and/or whether it has resulted in improvements in school policy and physical or social environments.

A factor often omitted from safety education is youth engagement in planning, program implementation, evaluation, and policy. When students are involved in the planning and have a real voice, not just token participation, they have opportunities to develop executive functions through curricula and opportunities for decisionmaking. These opportunities can decrease the influence of negative peer pressure and the likelihood of engaging in high-risk behaviors.

Staff Education and Training

A coordinated school injury and violence prevention program requires trained school personnel who can identify and remedy hazards, prevent unintentional injury, and intervene to stop bullying and violence as well as assist and educate students while they serve as positive role models.

Quality supervision is a key element to ensuring safety in the classroom, cafeteria, hallways, stairways, gymnasium, shop, athletic field, and playgrounds. Both students and school staff, including faculty, need safety education. For example, staff members responsible for playground and recreational supervision need training in first aid and CPR (Centers for Disease Control and Prevention 2001a); and those in cafeterias need to know how to relieve obstructed airways.

Teachers and other school staff also need education about preventing injuries, bullying, and violence. All school staff and contracted personnel including bus drivers, security personnel, grounds and custodial staff members, and food service staff need training that might include the basics of recognizing risks and hazards in their areas of responsibility, child development and child supervision, first aid and CPR, and identifying at-risk students including those with autism and special needs. Training for teachers might include methods for teaching injury and violence prevention skills and for developing and maintaining a safe learning environment such as proactive classroom management, cooperative learning methods, social skills training, promoting interactive learning, and environmental modifications (Centers for Disease Control and Prevention 2001a).

The SHPPS conducted by the CDC included items about staff training. During the two years preceding the 2006 CDC SHPPS,

- The percentage of elementary schools and middle schools that participated in a program to prevent bullying increased from 63% in 2000 to 77% in 2006
- The percentage of states that provided funding for staff development or offered staff development on suicide prevention to those who teach health education increased from 50% in 2000 to 67% in 2006
- The percentage of health education classes or courses with a teacher who received staff development on injury prevention and safety increased from 25% in 2000 to 41% in 2006 (Kann et al. 2007)

At the beginning of each school year, all school staff should be trained on the school policies and identify best practices for actions. Newly hired staff may require more in-depth training. Our goal of staff training is to improve communication among school personnel (Virginia Department of Criminal Justice Services 2002). Each school community should assess the training needs of its teachers and staff. Possible training areas for school staff include the following:

- Identification and remediation of common safety hazards such as poisons and trip hazards
- Completion of injury incident report forms
- Training coaches to enforce safe play guidelines and to identify warning signs of injuries such as concussion
- Educating parents on recognition of the risks and signs of injury, violence, and suicide threat
- Bullying prevention
- Peer mediation and conflict resolution (not appropriate for bullying prevention)
- Recognizing and making referrals for signs of depression or abuse
- Gatekeeper methods to recognize risk factors for suicide

Public Health and Education as Partners

Because injuries are the leading cause of death and disability for preschool and school-aged children and youth, protecting children and youth requires that public health and safety professionals collaborate with school personnel. At first glance, the education system, responsible for the social cognitive development and academic achievement of students, and the public health system, responsible for protecting the health and safety of the population, might appear to have different goals and objectives. However, on the issue of injuries and violence in the school environment, neither system can succeed in meeting its responsibilities without the other. Strong policy development, implementation, and enforcement; comprehensive and sequential health and safety education programs; appropriate supervision; routine maintenance of buildings, grounds, and equipment; and environmental changes can prevent many injuries that occur on school grounds or during school-sponsored activities, including child care centers.

Schools can teach students essential public health skills—to assess risks, promote safety, prevent injury, and/or treat an injury using first aid and CPR skills. Other skills might include problem-solving, communication, decisionmaking, impulse control, conflict resolution, stress management, and anger management. Likewise, the community, including local universities, emergency medical services (EMS) and fire departments, police departments, and health care professionals, can partner with the school to help develop or implement safety precautions or real-world experiences as part of a safety or violence education curriculum.

The Education Perspective

Schools are asked to take on more and more responsibilities with no additional resources. School administrators are often in crisis mode—responding to the latest issue from falling test scores to labor disputes and declining revenues. Injury prevention often does not even surface as an issue, let alone a priority, until someone gets hurt. When school administrators become aware of the potential for litigation, high costs, and lost time associated with injuries, they often become motivated to take preventive actions.

According to research published by the CDC, a wide range of injuries are litigated, and such lawsuits often require schools and school districts to pay costly awards to injured parties. In two thirds of the cases, schools or school districts paid an award to plaintiffs (mean = \$562,915, median = \$50,000) (Barrios, Jones, and Gallagher 2007).

School and pre- and after-school personnel have a legal and ethical responsibility to prevent injuries from occurring on school property and at school-sponsored events to promote safety. Policies that prohibit running in the hallways, require fire drills, and helmet and mouth guard use requirements for sports are examples of safety policies.

The Public Health Perspective

Healthy People 2020 is a U.S. Department of Health and Human Services, Office of Disease Prevention and Health Promotion (ODPHP) document that outlines an agenda for health promotion, injury prevention, and disease prevention (Office of Disease Prevention and Health Promotion 2010). *Healthy People 2020* recognizes injury, violence, and mental health among the ten leading public health concerns for the nation and outlines a comprehensive set of objectives. Some of those objectives relevant to school injuries and violence include the following:

- Increase the proportion of schools that provide school health education to prevent injury, violence, and suicide
- Increase the proportion of schools that require use of appropriate head, face, eye, and mouth protection for students participating in school-sponsored physical activities
- Reduce physical fighting among adolescents
- Reduce bullying among children and youth
- Reduce weapon carrying by children and youth on school property
- Increase the proportion of infants who are put to sleep on their backs (child care settings)
- Reduce physical assaults and physical fighting among adolescents and reduce weapon carrying by adolescents on school property
- Increase the proportion of students in grades nine through twelve who get sufficient sleep
- Reduce the proportion of adolescents who report that they rode, during the previous 30 days, with a driver who had been drinking alcohol

Some of the safety education objectives for students and staff include the following:

- Reduce nonfatal unintentional injuries
- Increase the use of safety belts
- Increase age-appropriate vehicle restraint system use in children
- Reduce pedestrian deaths and injuries
- Increase the number of states and the District of Columbia with "good" GDL licensing laws
- Reduce unintentional suffocation deaths
- Reduce violence by current or former intimate partners
- Reduce children's exposure to violence
- Reduce nonfatal, intentional self-harm injuries
- Reduce suicide attempts made by adolescents
- Increase depression screening by primary care providers

An additional *Healthy People 2020* objective is to increase high school completion to 90% (Office of Disease Prevention and Health Promotion 2010). Those who drop out of school are more likely than those who complete high school to exhibit multiple social and health problems, including substance abuse, delinquency, intentional and unintentional injury, and unintended pregnancy. The Healthy People objective is consistent with President Obama's goal for the Department of Education of America again having the highest proportion of college graduates in the world (quotation from a speech delivered by President Barack Obama on 2/24/09. Available at: http://www.whitehouse.gov/issues/education/higher-education). Students who are unable to attend school because of poor health, fear of violence, or injuries will have a difficult time achieving academic success and reaching their potential.

Although *Healthy People 2020* objectives provide a guide for the public health community, education systems often have their own goals and objectives. Public health professionals who want to collaborate with schools need to compare the various sets of objectives and find strategies that address both health and educational objectives. Any successful partnership requires an understanding of the needs, goals, and objectives of the school district and the school.

Navigating the Education System

State and local public health systems and education systems have areas of commonality as well as differences. The United States does not have a national education system; constitutionally, state governments are responsible for public education and thus school districts and schools are technically agents of the state. The governance structure varies for each state, often described in the state's constitution or in its education code adopted by the legislature. The public health system, on the other hand, exists at the federal, state, and local levels. Unlike public health funding which comes from federal and state budgets, the majority of funds for kindergarten through 12th grade in public schools are from local property taxes. State funds account for less than half and federal funds account for only about 7% of the money spent for schools nationwide.

The governor, the legislature, and the state board of education (SBE) share responsibility for education. In most states, SBE establishes education goals and standards, setting graduation requirements, and establishing teacher certification requirements. In some states, SBE approves textbooks.

Just as the state health department provides guidance to local health departments, the state education agency (SEA) provides guidance to school districts. The head of SEA might be the State School Superintendent, Chief State School Officer, or State Secretary of Education. These state officials, with their employees at the state level, establish academic standards, provide financial resources to school districts, manage information and reporting systems, develop the public education infrastructure, and hold districts accountable for student performance and achievement. Many states have delegated considerable authority to local education agencies (LEAs), also called school districts.

Each LEA has a school board that establishes district-wide standards and policies, consistent with required state mandates. The head of LEA is the superintendent who, with LEA staff, monitors and reports on school performance, provides leadership, engages parents and community members, and creates partnerships with local organizations.

At the school level, the principal is the leader and key decisionmaker. The principal is responsible for academic programs, teachers, staff, students, and budget and resource allocation, and is expected to enforce federal, state, and district rules, policies, and laws. The principal is often the school's primary representative to the parents and the community. The authority and responsibility of the principals and superintendent vary from state to state and district to district.

Some schools and districts have a designated person responsible for coordinating school health and safety services, instruction, and programming. That person might be a full-time administrator such as a school health coordinator, a health services supervisor, a safe and drug-free schools coordinator, or an assistant superintendent or assistant principal. Sometimes it is a faculty or staff member who also has teaching or student services responsibilities, such as a physical educator, health educator, school nurse, or school counselor. Some schools or school districts establish a school health and safety council or committee that includes community members as well as representatives of school staff, administration, students, and their families. Such groups can assist in the oversight, management, planning, and evaluation of school health and safety programs. They might advise the school board, superintendent, principal, or coordinator about needs, available resources, and policy additions or revisions. Key stakeholders within the school who might serve as a point of entry for public health and safety professionals include school nurses or school health center staff, teachers, school resource officers, guidance counselors, school psychologists, and/or social workers.

Individual schools often have more autonomy and the ability to make independent policy and program decisions than do local health departments. While federal policy can prompt change in the education system, the state and local levels are generally more productive partners for those seeking to implement changes in safety and violence prevention programming. One common fallacy of public health personnel wishing to implement something in a school is an assumption that the schools are doing nothing about that issue. Before approaching a school official about a relationship, it is important to check the school/school district's Web site and talk to students and staff to find out what the school is already doing. In addition, one should find out what relationships already exist between the public health agency and school.

The Role of Public Health in Preventing Injuries in Schools

The public health model serves as a road map for many public health programs including injury and violence prevention. Using this model, the first step is to collect information and data about the issue to be addressed. Once the various factors have been taken into consideration, the strategies for prevention are examined and prioritized for implementation. Many factors influence program implementation including funding, staffing, acceptance of the practice, timing, and others. Plans for evaluation need to be developed and implemented simultaneously with program implementation as well as after the program or policy is in place. As the public health model unfolds, the school/education and public health (at the state and local level) agencies need to assess what each brings to the achievement of mutual goals and objectives.

Data Collection, Analysis, and Dissemination

An understanding of trends and prevalence of injury and violence can guide policymakers, school administrators, and public health professionals in setting priorities and allocating always scarce resources of money, time, and staff. In addition, data can help them determine the effectiveness and cost-effectiveness of injury or violence prevention programs. Many schools lack a comprehensive, coordinated approach to injury and violence prevention that is integrated with other aspects of school health and the academic curricula. There is still no federal guidance for collecting and recording data, thus there is little consistency of what data are recorded, their reliability, or who has access to the information. Although the vast majority of schools collect incidence data on injuries, a very limited number collect data that enumerate the cause of the injury, the location, and the outcome of that injury. Often the person responsible for collecting and recording information about injuries sustained at school receives little or no training to ensure that the data entered are accurate and consistent. Where schools have full-time nurses, they are usually in the best position to collect incident information, but they need cooperation from students and staff to obtain all the relevant information. In schools that do not have a full-time nurse, a school secretary or administrative assistant often maintains incident report records.

To gather meaningful data at the district, state, or national levels requires consistent databases across schools. The lack of comprehensive national or state data collection systems for injuries sustained in schools denies practitioners and decisionmakers with the information they need to make informed decisions at the national/federal level, and in providing information on injuries in the school environment that can help state and LEAs and health agencies provide resources, technical assistance, and policy guidance that schools could use. This information is critical to developing appropriate injury and violence prevention programs that can address a problem specific to a school, a school district, or the state system overall. In an era of increased accountability and emphasis on data gathering in both the education sector and under health care reform, more states are setting up state-level data collection systems.

Utah's Student Injury Reporting System has become a model for school surveillance systems both nationally and abroad. This is a voluntary system and therefore injuries might be underreported; however, the state has collected and reported the data back to the schools through fact sheets that can help schools learn about their injury problem and methods to implement prevention. A survey of principals revealed that about 25% of the responding schools made changes to reduce injuries as a result of receiving the feedback. Utah has a student injury rate of 11.4 injuries per 1000 students. Student injuries resulted in more than 4900 missed school days during the 2006–2007 school year. This absenteeism can interfere with student academic success (Utah Department of Health 2010).

During a sight visit to Taiwan, the lead author observed one elementary school that collects data about the incidents in their school by involving the students in the process. In a true epidemiological fashion, the school nurse placed a map of the school outside of her office. The students are sent to the school nurse for any injury-causing incident. After the student is examined and treated, the child places a dot on the map where the incident occurred. The collection of dots provides information regarding locations that might present safety hazards.

Creating new data collection systems, plans, educational interventions for students and staff, and evaluations for each factor that places students at risk for injury, illness, or academic failure is wasteful, inefficient, and ultimately unaffordable. Adopting an all-hazards approach creates the systems that can respond to many situations, and new hazards identified in the future. In this approach, a data collection system would collect information not only on injuries, but also on illnesses, absenteeism, tardiness, and academic performance. It supports a robust health education curriculum that builds skills such as decisionmaking, goal setting, negotiating, and refusing unwanted suggestions that students can use in many situations (Joint Committee on National Health Education Standards, 2007).

Because data are the fundamental building blocks of all public health programs and policies, including school-based interventions, public health and safety personnel have much to offer schools. Public health and safety professionals could contribute to preventing injuries and violence by helping schools establish data collection systems that track all incidents of injury and violence. The type of data might include the nature, extent, location, and cause of the incident as well as the victim's age, grade, and sex (Centers for Disease Control and Prevention 2001b). Additionally, they could analyze and interpret data, making recommendations to school officials and policymakers for implementing, modifying, revising, or eliminating programs, policies, educational interventions, or environmental conditions. They could conduct surveys to determine students' concerns and priorities; and could contribute epidemiological expertise and interpretation of evidence with respect to causes, consequences, and prevention of injuries and violence.

Program Selection, Prioritization, Implementation, and Evaluation

Data collection has utility only when the information gathered drives decisions and interventions. A comprehensive school-focused injury and violence prevention program includes policies and procedures; environmental changes; education for students that addresses behaviors that place students at risk for injury; and training for all school staff about ways to prevent and mitigate injuries, bullying, and violence that includes proper supervision techniques during student activities (Kaldahl and Blair 2005). These interventions fall into one of three categories, often referred to as the three Es: Environmental Modifications, Educational Programs, and Enforcement of Policies.

Public health professionals could assist educators in developing a school health council/ committee or an injury and violence prevention subcommittee associated with a school health council. They could collaborate in creating a coordinated safety plan; or assessing, identifying and implementing environmental changes that increase safety on playgrounds, school grounds, and in transportation areas (i.e., bus stops and student drop-off areas).

A school health council/committee includes representatives of students and their families, business and community leaders, and school staff, with the goal of supporting and guiding school health and safety practices, programs, and policies (Shirer and Miller 2003). For injury and violence prevention, schools need strong relationships with public safety departments (fire, EMS, and police), local health departments, mental health counselors, environmental designers, and transportation officials and planners. A council, which might advise the school board, the superintendent, the school health and safety coordinator, or the school principal, could offer assistance in program planning, curriculum review, advocacy, fiscal planning, evaluation, accountability, and identifying resources (Brener et al. 2004).

A considered approach for selecting interventions might begin by asking the following questions: (1) Do the data indicate a need? (2) Is the timing right for this program? (3) Is there political support for the program? (4) Are there resources for the program? (5) Is the program effective in similar settings? Answering these questions requires the input of multiple partners and is often the task of the school health council. After selecting one or more program(s), the next step is for the school health council or a team of school staff members to develop a plan of action with timed and measurable goals and objectives, specific strategies, responsibility assigned for each task, and an evaluation plan.

The CDC created the Health Education Curriculum Analysis Tool (HECAT) to help school districts, schools, and others conduct an analysis of health education curricula based on the National Education Standards and the CDC's Characteristics of Effective Health Education Curricula. HECAT results can help schools select or develop appropriate and effective health education curricula and improve the delivery of health education to address safety, violence prevention, and other health education topics (Centers for Disease Control and Prevention 2007b).

Emergency Preparedness/Disaster Planning

The 2006 SHPPS found that about 90% of states (60% of districts) provided funding for staff development or offered staff development on emergency preparedness to school nurses (Brener et al. 2007a). Almost 95% of schools provided counseling when needed after a natural disaster or other emergency or crisis situation (Brener et al. 2007b). Slightly fewer (92%) states required districts or schools (84% of districts) to have a comprehensive plan for crisis preparedness, response, and recovery for natural disaster or other emergency or crisis situation (Jones et al. 2007). These results are among the highest for injury- and violence-related issues and are aimed at protecting students during and after an event.

For a plan to work, public safety and health department personnel should work collaboratively on a school/district's plan. Public safety officers need to be familiar with key places in schools before there is a crisis. School officials need to know and trust public safety officers. Lines of authority and communication need to be clearly delineated so during an emergency all systems work together and not at cross-purposes.

Advocacy, Policy, and Enforcement

Because most school safety policies are developed and implemented at state and local levels, public health and professionals at the state and local levels are often effective advocates for policies, regulations, and laws that address the safety of students and school staff. Policies that public health and safety professionals might support include incorporating injury and violence prevention into curricula and school-based programs, safer playground standards, and mandating dating violence prevention programs at the high school level.

In a perfect world, policy is data-driven; however, policy is often created through anecdote. As a result, public health and school officials need to know what is happening throughout the community. People do not live or work in isolation, so what happens in one arena often affects others and can influence the creation and implementation of policies, regulations, and laws. Timing can be everything; thus advocates need to have established networks and partnerships that they can activate when an opportunity presents itself.

Those in the public health community concerned with injury prevention can share with school administrators the data on the impact of injuries and violence on the academic success of students and the associated litigation costs of injuries. Nonfatal school-related injuries result in an estimated $10 billion in lost future work and $34 billion in lessened quality of life (Danseco, Miller, and Spicer 2000).

Schools have made some policy efforts to address violence occurring on school grounds. Below are several findings from the CDC 2006 SHPPS:

- The percentage of districts that required schools to conduct routine locker searches increased from 35% in 2000 to 57% in 2006 for middle schools, and from 44% to 63% for high schools
- The percentage of schools that used security or surveillance cameras increased from 17% in 2000 to 43% in 200, and the percentage that used communication devices increased from 80% in 2000 to 92% in 2006
- Seventy-six percent of states and 95% of districts required students to wear appropriate protective gear when engaged in classes such as wood shop or metal shop, and among the 33% of schools with these classes, 95% required students to wear appropriate protective gear when engaged in those classes
- The percentage of districts that had adopted a policy on the inspection or maintenance of smoke alarms increased from 72% in 2000 to 90% in 2006, and the percentage of schools that inspected smoke alarms during the 12 months preceding the study increased from 85% to 97%
- The percentage of districts that required elementary schools to use the safety checklist and equipment guidelines published in the *Handbook for Public Playground Safety* by CPSC increased from 30% in 2000 to 47% in 2006 (Jones et al. 2007)

Two sets of nationally developed guidelines suggest ways public health and safety professionals can work with school personnel to reduce injuries and violence in schools. These are as follows:

School Health Guidelines to Prevent Unintentional Injuries and Violence. Developed by the CDC in 2001, these guidelines are still considered best practice. Recommendations address the following:

- A social environment that promotes safety
- A safe physical environment
- Health education curricula and instruction
- Safe physical education, sports, and recreational activities
- Health, counseling, psychological, and social services for students
- Appropriate crisis and emergency response
- Involvement of families and communities
- Staff development to promote safety and prevent unintentional injuries, violence, and suicide (Centers for Disease Control and Prevention 2001a)

Health, Mental Health, and Safety Guidelines for Schools. In this resource, the American Academy of Pediatrics, the National Association of School Nurses, the American School Health Association (ASHA), and the Health Resource Services Administration's Maternal and Child

Health Bureau brought together guidance from a variety of sources in order to help school administrators, school personnel, and those working with schools address important health, mental health, and safety issues (Taras et al. 2004).

National guidance is a good place to start, but effective school policies also must consider the needs of students, staff, and community members. When those potentially affected by the policies, as well as those responsible for implementing the policies, are active participants in policy development, the policies are more likely to be workable, realistic, and enforceable. In order to be effective, school policies must be clear, implemented consistently and fairly, and evaluated for effectiveness.

Conclusions and Recommendations

Implementing school-based injury and violence prevention programs is good policy and practice not only because schools are where children and adolescents spend most of their time, but because health, safety, and academic success are reciprocal. Sometimes the association between safety and achievement is obvious (e.g., an injury that causes absence from school). At other times the association between student achievement and health and safety is not easily observed (e.g., when a student's anxiety about a real or perceived threat of violence affects his/her attention to class work, such as in bullying situations). Many groups want to partner with schools to reach students. Any group that wishes to partner with schools needs to consider what they bring to schools to make it worthwhile. Because there are so many schools and usually so few public health professionals who address safety, it may be most beneficial to work through systems rather than school by school. There are many entry points including the school board, the PTA, the principals, LEA and SEA, preschool programs, and school counselors, nurses, and/or psychologists.

In conclusion, the following suggestions shared at a 2001 ASHA conference by school superintendents for strengthening the working relationships between school administrators and health and safety professionals still hold true. By working together public health professionals and educators can develop those interventions and strategies that will strategically and effectively decrease injuries among children and adolescents.

- Link health and safety education and programs to academic performance, attendance, litigation prevention, holistic education, and budget.
- Approach school administrators with an offer of what you can do for the school, rather than asking the school to do something for you. Clearly identify the benefit to the school, students, and school personnel when you propose a project or policy.
- Be aware that words often have different meanings. For example, the term "surveillance" commonly used by public health professionals to mean data collection and trend analysis might mean the use of security cameras for school personnel.
- Use a team approach that involves school personnel, students and their families, and community members.
- Make presentations at school administrator conferences and invite administrators to present at school health and safety conferences. Joint presentations are often especially effective.

References

Ackard DM, Neumark-Sztainer D. 2002. Date violence and date rape among adolescents: associations with disordered eating behaviors and psychological health. *Child Abuse Negl.* 26:445–473.

Banyard VL, Cross C. 2008. Consequences of teen dating violence: understanding intervening variables in ecological context. *Violence Against Women.* 14:998–1013.

Barrios LC, Jones SE, Gallagher SS. 2007. Legal liability: the consequences of school injury. *J Sch Health.* 77:273–279.

Basile KC, Chen J, Black MC, Saltzman LE. 2007. Prevalence and characteristics of sexual violence victimization among U.S. adults, 2001–2003. *Violence Vict.* 22:437–448.

Brener ND, Kann L, McManus T, et al. 2004. The relationship between school health councils and school health policies and programs in US schools. *J Sch Health.* 74:130–135.

Brener ND, Weist M, Adelman H, et al. 2007, Mental health and social services: results from the School Health Policies and Programs Study 2006. *J Sch Health.* 77:486–499.

Brener ND, Wheeler L, Wolfe LC, et al. 2007. Health services: results from the School Health Policies and Programs Study 2006. *J Sch Health.* 77:464–485.

Centers for Disease Control and Prevention, 2001a. School health guidelines to prevent unintentional injuries and violence. *MMWR Morb Mortal Wkly Rep.* 50:1–84.

Centers for Disease Control and Prevention. 2001b. Temporal variations in school-associated student homicide and suicide events–United States, 1992–1999. *MMWR Morb Mortal Wkly Rep.* 50:657–660.

Centers for Disease Control and Prevention. 2004. *Healthy Youth! Physical Activity and the Health of Young People.* Atlanta, GA: National Center for Chronic Disease Prevention and Health Promotion. Available at: http://www.cdc.gov/healthyyouth/physicalactivity/facts.htm. Accessed August 14, 2011.

Centers for Disease Control and Prevention. 2007a. The effectiveness of universal school-based programs for the prevention of violent and aggressive behavior: a report on recommendations of the Task Force on Community Preventive Services. *MMWR Morb Mortal Wkly Rep.* 56:1–16.

Centers for Disease Control and Prevention. 2007b. *Health Education Curriculum Analysis Tool (HECAT).* Atlanta, GA: Centers for Disease Control and Prevention, National Center for Chronic Disease Prevention and Health Promotion. Available at: http://www.cdc.gov/healthyyouth/hecat/index.htm. Accessed August 14, 2011.

Centers for Disease Control and Prevention. 2009. *School Connectedness: Strategies for Increasing Protective Factors Among Youth.* Atlanta, GA: Centers for Disease Control and Prevention, National Center for Chronic Disease Prevention and Health Promotion. Available at: http://www.cdc.gov/HealthyYouth/AdolescentHealth/pdf/connectedness.pdf. Accessed August 14, 2011.

Centers for Disease Control and Prevention. 2010a. *Electronic Aggression.* Atlanta, GA: Centers for Disease Control and Prevention, National Center for Injury Prevention and Control. Available at: http://www.cdc.gov/ViolencePrevention/youthviolence/electronicaggression/index.html. Accessed August 14, 2011.

Centers for Disease Control and Prevention. 2010b. *National Vital Statistics System.* Hyattsville, MD: Division of Vital Statistics, National Center for Health Statistics. Available at: http://www.cdc.gov/nchs/deaths.htm. Accessed August 14, 2011.

Centers for Disease Control and Prevention, National Center for Chronic Disease Prevention and Health Promotion. 2010c. *School Health Programs: Improving the Health of Our Nation's Youth.* Atlanta, GA: Centers for Disease Control and Prevention, National Center for Chronic Disease Prevention and Health Promotion. Available at: http://www.cdc.gov/chronicdisease/resources/publications/aag/pdf/2010/dash-2010.pdf. Accessed August 14, 2011.

Centers for Disease Control and Prevention. 2010d. *Teens Behind the Wheel: Graduated Driver Licensing.* Atlanta, GA: Centers for Disease Control and Prevention, National Center for Injury Prevention and Control. Available at: http://www.cdc.gov/MotorVehicleSafety/Teen_Drivers/GDL/Teens_Behind_Wheel.html. Accessed August 14, 2011.

Centers for Disease Control and Prevention. 2010e. *Understanding Teen Dating Violence: Fact Sheet.* Atlanta, GA: Centers for Disease Control and Prevention, National Center for Injury Prevention and

Control. Available at: http://www.cdc.gov/violenceprevention/pdf/TeenDatingViolence_2010-a.pdf. Accessed August 14, 2011.

Centers for Disease Control and Prevention. 2010f. *Web-Based Injury Statistics Query and Reporting System (WISQARS)*. Atlanta, GA: Centers for Disease Control and Prevention, National Center for Injury Prevention and Control, Office of Statistics and Programming. Available at: http://www.cdc.gov/injury/wisqars/index.html. Accessed August 14, 2011.

Centers for Disease Control and Prevention. 2010g. Youth risk behavior surveillance–United States, 2009. *MMWR Morb Mortal Wkly Rep*. 59:1–142.

Centers for Disease Control and Prevention. 2011a. *Choose Respect*. Atlanta, GA: Centers for Disease Control and Prevention, National Center for Injury Prevention and Control. Available at: http://www.cdc.gov/chooserespect/at_school/index.html. Accessed August 14, 2011.

Centers for Disease Control and Prevention. 2011b. *Measuring Bullying Victimization, Perpetration, and Bystander Experiences: A Compendium of Assessment Tools*. Atlanta, GA: Centers for Disease Control and Prevention, National Center for Injury Prevention and Control. Available at: http://www.cdc.gov/ViolencePrevention/pub/measuring_bullying.html. Accessed August 14, 2011.

Centers for Disease Control and Prevention. 2011c. *Training Professionals in the Primary Prevention of Sexual and Intimate Partner Violence: A Planning Guide*. Atlanta, GA: Centers for Disease Control and Prevention, National Center for Injury Prevention and Control.

Chen LH, Warner M, Fingerhut L, Makuc D. 2009. Injury episodes and circumstances: National Health Interview Survey, 1997–2007. *Vital Health Stat*. no. 10: 1– 64, . Available at: http://www.cdc.gov/nchs/data/series/sr_10/sr10_241.pdf. Accessed August 14, 2011.

Consumers Union. 2010. *Safety Alert: Click, Check, Protect*. Yonkers, NY: Consumers Union. Available at: http://www.clickcheckprotect.org. Accessed March 3, 2011.

Danner F, Phillips B. 2008. Adolescent sleep, school start times, and teen motor vehicle crashes. *J Clin Sleep Med*. 4:533–535.

Danseco ER, Miller TR, Spicer RS. 2000. Incidence and costs of 1987–1994 childhood injuries: demographic breakdowns. *Pediatrics*. 105:E27. Available at: http://www.pediatrics.aappublications.org/content/105/2/e27.full.pdf. Accessed August 14, 2011.

David-Ferdon C, Hertz MF. 2007. Electronic media, violence, and adolescents: an emerging public health problem. *J Adolesc Health*. 41(6 Suppl 1): S1–S5.

DeVoe JF, Bauer L. 2010. *Student Victimization in U.S. Schools: Results From the 2007 School Crime Supplement to the National Crime Victimization Survey*. U.S. Department of Education, National Center for Education Statistics. Washington, DC: U.S. Government Printing Office. Available at: http://www.nces.ed.gov/pubs2010/2010319.pdf. Accessed August 14, 2011.

Federal Highway Administration. 1972. Transportation characteristics of school children. Report No. 4, *Nationwide Personal Transportation Study*. Washington, DC: Federal Highway Administration.

The Gay, Lesbian and Straight Education Network (GLSEN) and Harris Interactive. 2008. *The Principal's Perspective: School Safety, Bullying and Harassment, A Survey of Public School Principals*. New York: GLSEN. Available at: http://www.glsen.org. Accessed August 14, 2011.

The Gay, Lesbian and Straight Education Network. 2010. Welcoming Schools. Available at: http://www.welcomingschools.org. Accessed August 14, 2011.

Giedd, JN.2006. The teen brain. Presented at: Ninth Annual Meeting of the National Coordinating Committee on School Health and Safety on Emerging Scientific Findings in Adolescent Brain Development and Their Implications for Student Learning, Behavior, and Well-Being; May 17; Arlington, VA.

Health Resources Services Administration. 2009. *The National Survey of Children's Health 2007: The Health and Well-Being of Children: A Portrait of States and the Nation*. Rockville, MD: U.S. Department of Health and Human Services, Health Resources Services Administration.

Health Resources Services Administration. 2010. *Stop Bullying Now! Campaign*. Rockville, MD: U.S. Department of Health and Human Services, Health Resources Services Administration. Available

at: http://www.stopbullyingnow.
hrsa.gov. Accessed August 14, 2011.

Hinduja S, Patchin JW. 2009. Bullying Beyond the Schoolyard: Preventing and Responding to Cyberbullying. Thousand Oaks, CA: Corwin Press.

Human Rights Campaign Foundation. 2010. Welcoming Schools. Washington, DC: Human Rights Campaign Foundation. Available at: http://www.welcomingschools.
org. Accessed March 3, 2011.

Joint Committee on National Health Education Standards. 2007. *National Health Education Standards: Achieving Excellence.* 2nd ed. Atlanta, GA: American Cancer Society.

Jones SE, Fisher CJ, Greene BZ, et al. 2007. Healthy and safe school environment, part I: results from the School Health Policies and Programs Study 2006. *J Sch Health.* 77:522–543.

Kachur SP, Stennies GM, Powell KE, et al. 1996. School-associated violent deaths in the United States, 1992 to 1994. *JAMA.* 275:1729–1733.

Kaldahl MA, Blair EH. 2005. Student injury rates in public schools. *J Sch Health.* 75:38–40.

Kann L, Telljohann SK, Wooley SF. 2007. Health education: results from the School Health Policies and Programs Study 2006. *J Sch Health.* 77:408–434.

Kowalski RM, Limber SP. 2007. Electronic bullying among middle school students. *J Adolesc Health.* 41(6 Suppl 1): S22–S30.

Kowalski RM, Limber SP, Agatston PW. 2008. *Cyber Bullying: Bullying in the Digital Age.* Malden MA: Blackwell Publishing.

Liz Claiborne Inc. 2011. *Love Is Not Abuse.* New York: Liz Claiborne. Available at: http://www.loveisnotabuse.com. Accessed March 3, 2011.

Moores MA. 2006. Implications for juvenile justice. Presented at: Ninth Annual Meeting of the National Coordinating Committee on School Health and Safety on Emerging Scientific Findings in Adolescent Brain Development and Their Implications for Student Learning, Behavior, and Well-Being; May 17; Arlington, VA.

National Center for Safe Routes to School. Safe Routes. 2010. Chapel Hill, NC: National Center for Safe Routes to School. Available at: http://www.saferoutesinfo.
org. Accessed August 14, 2011.

National Conference of State Legislatures (NCSL). 2010. *Cyberbullying and the States.* Washington, DC: NCSL. Available at: http://www.ncsl.org/default.aspx?tabid=20753. Accessed March 3, 2011.

National Highway Traffic Safety Administration (NHTSA). 2009. *Traffic Safety Facts, 2009 Data: School Transportation-Related Crashes.* Washington, DC: NHTSA. DOT HS 811 396. Available at: http://www-nrd.nhtsa.dot.gov/Pubs/811396.pdf. Accessed March 2, 2011.

National Resource Center for Health and Safety in Child Care. 2011. *Caring for Our Children: National Health and Safety Performance Standards; Guidelines for Early Care and Education Programs.* 3rd ed. Elk Grove Village, IL: American Academy of Pediatrics; Washington, DC: American Public Health Association.

Novas C. 2010. *Dating Violence: A Two Way Street, But Girls Are Hurt Most.* Washington, DC: National Research Center for Women and Families. Available at: http://www.center4research.-org/2010/05/dating-violence-a-two-way-street-but-girls-are-hurt-most. Accessed March 3, 2011.

Office of Disease Prevention and Health Promotion. 2010. *Healthy People 2020.* Washington, DC: U.S. Department of Health and Human Services, Office of Disease Prevention and Health Promotion. Available at: http://www.healthypeople.
gov/2020/default.aspx. Accessed August 14, 2011.

The Plain Dealer. Ohio School-Safety Law That Takes Effect Today Is Legacy of 6-Year-Old. *The Plain Dealer.* December 19, 2005. Available at: http://www.cleveland.
com. Accessed February 20, 2011.

Rice M, Kang DH, Weaver M, Howell CC. 2008. Relationship of anger, stress, and coping with school connectedness in fourth-grade children. *J Sch Health.* 78:149–156.

Rose DH. 2006. Implications for education. Presented at: Ninth Annual Meeting of the National Coordinating Committee on School Health and Safety on Emerging Scientific Findings in Adolescent Brain Development and Their Implications for Student Learning, Behavior, and Well-Being; May 17; Arlington, VA.

Samdal O, Nutbeam D, Wold B, Kannas L. 1998. Achieving health and educational goals through schools. *Health Educ Res.* 13:383–397.

Schnurr MP, Lohman BJ. 2008. How much does school matter? An examination of adolescent dating violence perpetration. *J Youth Adolesc* 37:266–283.

Shirer K, Miller PP. 2003. *Promoting Healthy Youth, Schools, and Communities: A Guide to Community-School Health Councils.* Atlanta, GA: American Cancer Society. Available at: http://www.schoolwellnesspolicies.org/resources/AGuideToCommunitySchoolHealthCouncils.pdf. Accessed August 14, 2011.

Storey K, Slaby R, Adler M, et al. 2008. *Eyes on Bullying: What Can You Do: A Toolkit to Prevent Bullying In Children's Lives.* Newton, MA: Education Development Center.

Swahn MH, Simon TR, Arias I, Bossarte RM. 2008. Measuring sex differences in violence victimization and perpetration within date and same-sex peer relationships. *J Interpers Violence.* 23:1120–1138.

Taras H, Duncan P, Luckenbill D, et al. 2004. *Health, Mental Health and Safety Guidelines for Schools.* Chicago, IL: American Academy of Pediatrics. Available at: http://www.nationalguidelines.org. Accessed August 14, 2011.

Task Force on Community Preventive Services. 2007. A recommendation to reduce rates of violence among school-aged children and youth by means of universal school-based violence prevention programs. *Am J Prev Med.* 33:S112–113.

U.S. Consumer Product Safety Commission. 2008. *Public Playground Safety Handbook.* Bethesda, MD: U.S. Consumer Product Safety Commission.

Utah Department of Health, Violence and Injury Prevention Program. 2010. Utah Student Injury Reporting System Database. Salt Lake City: Utah Department of Health. Available at: http://www.health.utah.gov/vipp/schoolInjuries/overview.html. Accessed August 14, 2011.

Virginia Department of Criminal Justice Services. 2002. *School Safety Training Needs Assessment: Report on Findings.* Richmond: Virginia Department of Criminal Justice Services. Available at: http://www.dcjs.virginia.gov/research/documents/vcss/trainingNeedsAssessment.pdf. Accessed August 14, 2011.

Waters SK, Cross DS, Runions K. 2009. Social and ecological structures supporting adolescent connectedness to school: a theoretical model. *J Sch Health.* 79:516–524.

Wilson D. 2004. The interface of school climate and school connectedness and relationships with aggression and victimization. *J Sch Health.* 74:293–299.

Women's Defense and Legal Education Fund, New York Civil Liberties Union. 2010. *State Law Guide: Teen Dating Abuse Education and School Policies.* New York: New York Civil Liberties Union. Available at: http://www.legalmomentum.org/assets/pdfs/teen-dating-abuse-education.pdf. Accessed March 3, 2011.

Yan FA, Howard DE, Beck KH, et al. 2010. Psychosocial correlates of physical dating violence victimization among Latino early adolescents. *J Interpers Violence.* 25:808–831.

Ybarra M, Diener-West M, Leaf PJ. 2007. Examining the overlap in internet harassment and school bullying: implications for school intervention. *J Adolesc Health.* 41:S42–S50.

Chapter 8

Childhood Agricultural Injuries

Barbara C. Lee, PhD[1] *and Barbara Marlenga, PhD*[1]

When newspapers report tragic childhood deaths or disabling injuries on farms, a casual reader might interpret these events as "freak accidents" or merely the consequence of traditional agricultural practices. These same readers often admire North American farmers for their family values and their work ethic. Yet, these very factors are frequently associated with conditions that put children at increased risk for injury or death on farms. The complex factors behind each news clipping reveal predictable and preventable circumstances that can guide interventions, research, and advocacy intended to protect young people who live on, work on, or visit farms and ranches. Consider the following actual stories.

August 12, 2009, Teen Killed in Grain Accident Was Member of Sonoma Farm Family

A 13-year-old boy who was killed in a grain loading incident was being remembered by friends as an avid Boy Scout with a wry sense of humor. David Yenni died Tuesday when he was trapped in his father's grain hauler at a Petaluma, CA mill. He was a nice kid according to his scout leader and will be sorely missed. David, a member of a Sonoma Valley farming family, was working alongside his father as he delivered a load of wheat to a local granary. David apparently climbed on top of an open trailer just as the father was emptying it into underground storage. David became trapped in the funneling material. The father heard the boy cry for help and three mill workers rushed to dig him out, grabbing a hold of his arm. He was rushed unconscious to the Petaluma Valley Hospital where he was pronounced dead about an hour later. (Payne 2009)

September 6, 2007, Boy, 12, Dies in Farm Accident

An Athens, WI boy has died of injuries suffered when he was pinned by a piece of machinery on his family's dairy farm. Joshua Root, 12, was filling the bucket of a skid steer loader (small engine-powered, four wheel or tracked machine with lift arms and front bucket) with feed Tuesday when his body became trapped between the arm of the machinery and the bucket. His brother found Joshua and alerted his father who was milking cows in the barn. Emergency crews arrived and airlifted him to the local hospital but he died about five hours later. They suspected Joshua leaned forward out of the cab and accidentally lowered the loader's bucket. It was a chore the boy had performed countless times, the brother said. (Hutton 2007)

July 23, 2009, Six-Year-Old Richland County Boy Killed in Farm Accident

Richland County Sheriff's Department dispatcher received a call for an ambulance at 5:37 p.m. reporting a skid steer loader accident. An ambulance and medical helicopter were dispatched to

[1]National Farm Medicine Center, Marshfield, WI.

> the scene. According to the report, Tristen Cornell, 6, was struck by a skid steer loader as it was backing up. The equipment operator did not notice the child who had moved behind the vehicle. When the operator backed up the child was struck. (Hillsboro Sentry-Enterprise 2009)

September 24, 2010, Child Killed in Combine Accident

> A local farming family is grieving the loss of child tragically killed in an accident. Three-year-old Reid Crosby was riding in the cab of a combine with his father, when the large front windshield broke out. The child, who had been leaning on the window, fell forward and was run over by the harvesting machine that cuts, threshes, and cleans grain. The boy was pronounced dead at the scene. Police ruled the death accidental. (Joles 2010)

October 7, 2009, 2-Year-Old Girl Dies in Gate Mishap

> In Cherryvale, KS a 2-year-old girl died as a result of injuries sustained after being crushed by a heavy farm gate. The Sheriff said Shaylee Collins sustained severe internal injuries after a heavy 16-foot farm gate fell on top of her on Sunday afternoon. When emergency personnel responded to the scene the girl was in severe medical distress. She was flown by helicopter to Wesley Medical Center where she died shortly after arrival. (Montgomery County Chronicle 2009)

Grief over a preventable death of a child often follows. In a tragic sequel to an 11-year-old's death, just 2 months later, a November 5, 2002, newspaper headline reported "Man Shoots, Kills Self in Hospital":

> Officers were called to Sacred Heart Hospital after a shooting on a mental health ward. Police haven't determined how a handgun got into a patient's room. A 43-year-old man had been under treatment for mental strain and took his own life. His 11-year-old son had died two months earlier when a tractor flipped over and pinned him beneath. (Olson 2002)

These actual cases, all reported in public newspapers, are just a sampling of the tragedies that occur on the 2.2 million farms and ranches across the United States (National Agricultural Statistics Service 2008). The fatalities have striking similarities, such as siblings working together, inadequate adult supervision, and farm machinery designed for adults who willingly choose to work in one of our nation's most dangerous occupations (National Safety Council 2004b). Beyond the news clippings is the unreported psychologic, social, and financial toll that often reaps a devastating impact on survivors, especially parents. This toll affects children living, visiting, or hired to work on farms. On some farms, children begin actively working at an early age or they may merely be bystanders to the work. Statistics regarding the ethnic or cultural characteristics of children injured on farms are limited; however, from the newspaper clippings, it is clear that no population is immune to fatal and nonfatal events.

This chapter provides an overview of the epidemiology of childhood agricultural fatal and nonfatal injuries (work-related and non-work-related), including data sources and limitations of data. We then describe common injury risk factors among children involved in agricultural work and children who are not working, but are victims of agricultural injuries. This is followed by a description of injury prevention strategies for both working and nonworking children. Advocacy efforts for children on farms were formally introduced two decades ago, trailing behind those of other child safety concerns. The major advocacy initiatives are described, followed by recommendations for action.

Epidemiology of Injuries

Population at Risk

In 2006, there were approximately 1.1 million children living on farms in the United States (National Institute for Occupational Safety and Health [NIOSH] 2010a). More than half of these children worked on the farm, with the highest proportion of youth workers aged 10 to 15 years (Hendricks 2008). In addition, 307,000 youth were hired to work on these farms in 2001 (NIOSH 2010a).

Childhood Agricultural Injury Surveillance

The National Institute for Occupational Safety and Health (NIOSH) is the primary source for U.S. surveillance data on fatal and nonfatal childhood agricultural injuries. For fatal injuries, NIOSH (a) collects death certificates from the 50 state vital statistics registrars for all traumatic deaths that occur on farms to youth aged less than 20 years and (b) works with the Bureau of Labor Statistics to report work-related fatalities of youth workers in agriculture from the Census of Fatal Occupational Injuries (CFOI) (NIOSH 2010b). For nonfatal injuries, NIOSH in partnership with the National Agricultural Statistics Service conducts periodic surveys of farm operators to collect information on farm-related youth injuries (NIOSH 2010b).

Fatal Injuries

A review of death certificate data for the 6 years from 1995 to 2000 identified 695 farm-related youth fatalities with an average annual rate of 9.3 fatalities per 100,000 youth (Goldcamp et al. 2004). The highest annual fatality rate by age was for 16- to 19-year-olds (10.4 per 100,000 youth), closely followed by youth aged less than 10 years (10.1 per 100,000 youth) (Goldcamp et al. 2004). Males accounted for 80% of the fatalities. The major sources of fatal injury were machinery (25%), motor vehicles (17%), and drowning (16%). Only 13% (94 cases) were identified as work-related on the death certificate (Goldcamp et al. 2004).

An analysis of the CFOI for the years 1992 to 2002 identified 310 work-related deaths to youth aged less than 20 years in the agriculture production sector (crops and livestock) (Hard and Myers 2006). The fatal work-related injury rate for young workers in the agriculture production sector was 3.6 times higher than that for young workers in all industries (13.7/100,000 full-time equivalents [FTEs] vs. 3.8/100,000 FTEs) and 2.9 times higher than that of adult workers in all industries combined (4.7/100,000 FTEs) (Hard and Myers 2006). On examination of trends in fatality rates from 1992 to 1996 and 1997 to 2002, rates for young workers in all industries decreased during the 1997 to 2002 period, whereas fatality rates for young workers in agriculture increased. Fatality rates increased by 81% during the period 1997 to 2002 for 15-year-olds, 45% for 16-year-olds, and 24% for 19-year-olds (Hard and Myers 2006).

Caucasian males accounted for nearly all of the fatalities per the CFOI data set. Vehicles (50.3%) and machinery (21.6%) were the leading sources of fatal injury, with tractors accounting for more than half the vehicle deaths and 27.1% of all the young worker fatalities in agriculture production (Hard and Myers 2006). The Midwest region of the United States (48%) had the highest proportion of worker fatalities, followed by the West (19%). Wisconsin, Pennsylvania, New York, Ohio, and Montana were the five states with the highest numbers of young worker fatalities (Hard and Myers 2006).

Nonfatal Injuries

NIOSH developed the Childhood Agricultural Injury Survey to collect data about injuries that occurred on the farm operation and resulted in at least 4 hours of restricted activity (NIOSH

2010b). Childhood Agricultural Injury Survey data for all youth aged less than 20 years have been collected for the years 1998, 2001, 2004, and 2006 (NIOSH 2010b).

In 2006, an estimated 22,894 injuries occurred on farms, a decline of 30% since the 1998 survey (Hendricks and Goldcamp 2010; Myers and Hendricks 2001). Males accounted for 66% of the injuries. Youth aged 10 to 15 years had the highest proportion of injuries (44%). Youth living on farms sustained the most injuries (51%), followed by visitors to the farm (40%) and hired youth workers (6%) (Hendricks and Goldcamp 2010). Approximately 25% of the injuries occurred while the youth was working. The leading sources of injury were structures and surfaces, animals (primarily horses), and vehicles (primarily all-terrain vehicles) (Hendricks and Goldcamp 2010). The South and Midwestern regions of the United States accounted for 78% of the injuries.

The past two decades have witnessed a demographic shift in agricultural workers that NIOSH attempted to capture in injury surveillance data. Data were extracted from a sampling frame of 49,270 farms, or 2% of all U.S. farms that were owned and operated by minority populations. There were an estimated 307 nonfatal injuries among the estimated 21,631 youth living on Hispanic-operated U.S. farms in 2000. Males accounted for 73% of injuries and had a rate of 20.2 compared with 8.2 per 1000 females (Layne et al. 2009).

In 2010, NIOSH released preliminary data from their 2009 surveillance. Data reveal the rate of total injuries (includes household youth, hired youth, and visitors) per 1000 farms has declined by 59% from 1998 to 2009, whereas the rate of injuries among youth who live on farms declined by 47.3% from 1998 to 2009 (NIOSH 2010c). Further breakdown of this most recent dataset will be forthcoming (Figure 8.1).

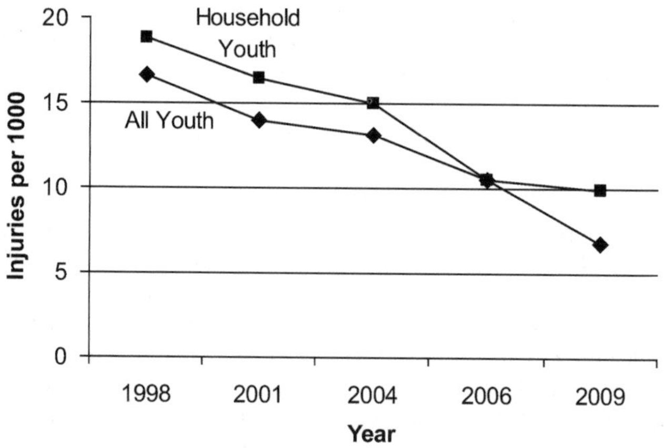

Figure 8.1. Legend: NIOSH. 2010. Trends in Childhood Agricultural Nonfatal Injury Rates, 1998 through 2009. Internal Analysis of the Childhood Agricultural Injury Survey (CAIS) Surveillance System. Morgantown, WV: National Institute for Occupational Safety and Health.

Risk Factors for Childhood Agricultural Injuries

The classic Haddon matrix of agent, host, and environment (Haddon 1972), and modifications of its use as proposed by Runyan (1998) and Rivara (2002) depict risk factors and their underlying cause in the pre-event, event, and post-event phase of any injury. Studying injury events from this public health framework offers insights that can guide injury prevention interventions. In this chapter's first agricultural case report, the agent of injury was the energy from the force of a large volume of grain rapidly moving downward via a funnel through the bottom of a hauling wagon. The host was a 13-year-old boy, unaware of the physics of grain transfer, and the environment was a semi-supervised, dangerous work site.

Stallones and Gunderson (1994) were the first to apply the Haddon theoretic framework to childhood agricultural injuries when they pieced together available data sources and demonstrated how the matrix of agent, host, and environment could identify prevention strategies. Yet, applicability of this matrix for proposing agricultural injury prevention strategies is limited for two primary reasons. First, there is a wide spectrum of agricultural conditions, many of which have no control mechanisms (e.g., weather). Second, a parent or other adult bears accountability for a minor's presence in a hazardous work setting; thus, the principle intervention is to modify underlying adult decisions rather than address modification of the agent, host, or environment. A brief description of those risk factors most amenable to interventions for preventing childhood agricultural injuries are described in the context of children involved in agricultural work, followed by children exposed to agricultural work hazards while not actively engaged in work.

Working Children and Adolescents

Worldwide, agriculture is the occupation most likely to involve children (Forastieri 2002). Unlike most occupational settings, it can be difficult to separate bona fide work from nonwork activities. A traditional farmstead in the United States includes the home contiguous with the work site where children have open access to both. To make matters more complex, there can be problems distinguishing when and where labor regulations and safety standards apply. These factors complicate injury data collection and the design and implementation of injury prevention strategies.

Mechanisms of Injury Among Working Youth

Data from several sources consistently depict the most common vehicles of injuries and fatalities on farms. Farm machinery, including tractor rollovers (victim is on the tractor when it tips over) and runovers (victim is stationary on the ground or falls off a moving tractor, and then is crushed underneath a tractor wheel), account for more than one third of deaths to youth aged less than 20 years (Adekoya and Pratt 2001). Many engineering designs for improving tractor and machinery safety on farms have been introduced by manufacturers over the past 50 years. Rollover protective structures combined with seat belts are recommended for all tractors but are mandatory in only a few situations in the United States (Swenson 2004). Likewise, safety guards for rotating machinery parts are provided by manufacturers and recommended for safety, but unlike industry settings, there are few mandates to enforce these standard safety features.

Since 1968 when the Hazardous Occupations Order for Agriculture specified restrictions to children's work, the U.S. Department of Agriculture has been authorized to address youth farm safety education and certification (National Safety Council 2004a). Local programs have been coordinated by state Cooperative Extension Service or high school agriculture instructors (National Safety Council 2004a).

Tractor and machinery training and certification programs, consisting of approximately 20 hours of lecture and driving experience, are intended to improve the safety of youth at risk of tractor-related injuries. However, these training and certification programs have not been consistently implemented. Furthermore, program evaluations have shown mixed results (Carrabba et al. 2000; Heaney et al. 2006; Schuler et al. 1994). Although engineering improvements and labor laws might be effective interventions, a more basic issue is the adult decision (i.e., work assignment to youth) that preceded the child/adolescent being on or near farm machinery and the effectiveness of training and supervision when such work is assigned.

Nonfatal work injuries among children often include livestock and horses (Hendricks and Adekoya 2001; Hendricks et al. 2004). Risk factors leading to animal injuries include inadequate fencing or other barriers, inappropriate access of children to animals, and the unpredictable and unmanageable nature of the animals themselves. Addressing these risk factors requires modification of the work setting by the farm owner in addition to training and supervision of the young worker.

Host Characteristics

In reviewing risk factors associated with the injury host (i.e., the child on the farm), data sources highlight basic demographic characteristics of age, gender, farm residency status, geographic location, and agricultural commodity. Research has demonstrated that children working on their family farm are at notably greater risk of injury than hired youth. Indeed, of all injuries to all youth on farms, only 6% occur to youth hired to work on nonfamily farms (Hendricks and Goldcamp 2010). There are often different expectations of youth working on family farms versus those hired on nonresident farms. Farm parents sometimes perceive that growing up on a farm lends itself to being more cognizant of inherent dangers and more capable of handling risky tasks at an earlier age (Neufeld et al. 2002). In addition, children strive to please their parents and willingly perform tasks that exceed their abilities (Darraugh et al. 1998; Kidd et al. 1997).

Hours of work, fatigue, training, and supervision are other host factors that put a child at risk of agricultural injury (Gerberich et al. 2001; Stueland et al. 1996). Interventions for addressing these host characteristics include parent and work supervisor training regarding child and youth development, as well as revised regulations that would mandate limited work hours, certified training, and apprenticeships.

Host risk factors also include culture, ethnicity, and assimilation into the "culture of agriculture." As the industry of agriculture opens new opportunities for niche products, minority populations have become increasingly involved in agriculture, including Hispanic/Latino immigrants, Hmong, and Anabaptist (e.g., Amish, Mennonite). Children of this new workforce are engaging in work on family and nonfamily farms. Issues such as language barriers, basic safety and hygiene principles, housing, and transportation introduce new challenges for professionals dealing with agricultural health and safety. Behind the reported demographic risk factors specific to agriculture are a myriad of general factors related to child development, including physical strength and psychologic state, which prevail in any child safety situation.

Environmental Factors

A variety of factors associated with the physical and social environment of an agricultural site have been associated with childhood agricultural injuries (Kidd et al. 1997; Myers and Hendricks 2001; Stueland et al. 1996). Environmental factors include the agricultural commodity, geographic features such as terrain or climate, economic conditions, and training and supervision standards for workers. Awareness of the inherent risks of childhood injuries associated with different agricultural enterprises can be helpful. For example, crop production accounts for more than half of all work-related fatalities to children, including hired youth (Castillo et al. 1999; National Agricultural Statistics Service 2008). When looking solely at youth residing on farms, livestock operations are slightly more hazardous than other enterprises (Myers and Hendricks 2001).

Training and supervision of youth working in agriculture differ from those of occupations such as quick service restaurants. Many industries have safety standards and compliance expectations for all employees, including young workers. This is not the case in agriculture. A recent survey of agricultural employers found that approximately half do not currently hire teen workers because of concern over labor regulations and requirements for monitoring and supervision (Lee et al. 2007).

Among those employers who do hire teen workers, the majority were interested in improving their practices related to training and supervision (Lee et al. 2007). For the many youth working on family farms, supervision and training are strictly the prerogative of the parent or farm owner.

In an ideal situation, adolescents would be hired to conduct safe, appropriate agricultural work. Training programs modeled on effective programs in other industries should be considered for agricultural settings where youth are legally hired, including seasonal jobs that fill employment needs of young workers (Vela Acosta and Lee 2001).

Labor Policy

The 2008 Census of Agriculture identified 2.2 million farms in the United States (National Agricultural Statistics Service 2008), and an estimated 90% of these are exempt from enforcement of Occupational Safety and Health Administration (OSHA) standards, because they employ fewer than 11 employees (Murphy 1992; U.S. Department of Labor 1975). It is important to note that the Department of Labor's Fair Labor Standards Act with Child Labor regulations has two primary distinctions: agricultural work and all other work (U.S. Department of Labor 1991, 2004a). Furthermore, the Hazardous Occupations Order for Agriculture that attempts to protect youth by limiting their employment activities to nonhazardous agricultural work has many exemptions applicable to family farms (U.S. Department of Labor 1991, 2004a; U.S. General Accounting Office 1998). Thus, unlike conditions for youth employed in nonagricultural jobs, regulations and safety standards are primarily voluntary, except where youth are hired to work on nonfamily farms.

Nonworking Children

Tractors and machinery are often involved in deaths and injuries of nonworking children, similar to the conditions of youth who are working. Young children are likely to fall from or be run over by tractors or farm equipment. Safety specialists strongly promote the "No Extra Rider" rule to keep young children off of tractors; however, the practice of children riding on tractors or playing near tractor pathways remains common on many farms.

Following machinery and vehicles, drowning is a major cause of childhood agricultural fatalities (Forastieri 2002), and on minority farm operations, drowning is the leading cause of death to children (Castillo et al. 1999). Unlike urban drownings, the agricultural water source can be an irrigation ditch, a farm pond for animals and wildlife, or a livestock-watering trough. Prevention strategies to minimize on-farm drownings include secure fencing or other barriers, as well as close supervision around water hazards.

Falls occur frequently among children on farms, and these events are associated with high structures, tall machinery, climate, and slippery surfaces. Interventions should first address removal of children from these work settings and then address safety hazards for adults and children. A recent case illustrates the need for a two-step intervention. A 12-year-old girl suffered a severe head injury after falling from a hayloft. The girl was playing basketball with her siblings in a makeshift upper hayloft court. A hay shoot floor latch broke open, resulting in her fall through the hole, crashing to a concrete floor 13 feet below. To prevent similar injuries, the strategy is first to prohibit children from playing in the loft and then to repair the dysfunctional shoot latch to protect adults working in the area.

Supervision

Safety professionals state that young children injured in agricultural settings are in the "wrong place…all of the time" (Esser 2001). Research has shown that parents justify children's presence in hazardous work settings on the basis of specific attitudes and subjective norms (Lee, Jenkins, and Westaby 1997). A study of Wisconsin farm fathers revealed that they allow children in the work site so they can spend time together, supervise a child while getting work done, help a child gain a strong work ethic, and provide an opportunity for fun (Lee, Jenkins, and Westaby 1997). The same study reported that the people most likely to influence parents' decisions are grandparents and spouse, whereas health professionals have little influence on such decisions. Another study, which specifically analyzed the effect of supervision on childhood agricultural injuries, noted that approximately half of all injured children were being "supervised" by an adult who was actively conducting farm work at the same time (Pryor et al. 2002).

The availability or absence of affordable, high-quality childcare services is a key determinant affecting the presence of young children in agricultural work sites. Previously, farm enterprises were generational in nature, increasing the likelihood that children could be cared for by nonworking family members or neighbors. Contemporary farms typically have one or both parents employed off the farm to augment income. Thus, dependable childcare services are needed in farming communities to the same extent as their urban counterparts, yet few options exist.

Interventions and Their Effectiveness

Concern over children being injured while living, working, or visiting farms has always been present, but a targeted effort to address these concerns was not undertaken as a national public health initiative until recently. In 1991, a Surgeon General's Conference on Agricultural Safety and Health was held in Des Moines, Iowa. During this conference, a session entitled "Intervention—Safe Behaviors Among Adults and Children" highlighted the risks faced by youth and adults involved with production agriculture (Armbruster 1991).

This was followed in 1992 by a Childhood Agricultural Injury Prevention Symposium held in Marshfield, Wisconsin. The symposium was sponsored by the National Farm Medicine Center and sought to understand key issues from the different perspectives of farm parents, pediatricians, researchers, educators, engineers, and the media. Participants formulated discussion points, identified areas for further consideration, and published their proceedings (Lee and Gunderson 1992).

As a follow-up to the 1992 Symposium, a core of 42 individuals formed the National Committee for Childhood Agricultural Injury Prevention (1996). Over a 16-month period, members of the committee finalized a National Action Plan that was released in 1996 for addressing the childhood agricultural injury problem (National Committee for Childhood Agricultural Injury Prevention 1996). The National Action Plan, endorsed by more than 80 professional organizations and agricultural groups, recommended leadership, surveillance, research, education, and public policy. Committee members advocated for formal adoption of the plan, and in October 1996 the U.S. Congress endorsed the plan and targeted funding for its implementation.

The 1996 National Action Plan recommended that the NIOSH serve as the lead federal agency in preventing childhood agricultural injury. In late 1996, NIOSH rolled out its National Childhood Agricultural Injury Prevention Initiative with goals to fill critical data needs, establish an infrastructure that facilitates the use of data to develop and improve on prevention efforts, and encourage the use of effective prevention strategies by the private and public sectors (Castillo et al. 1998). To date, NIOSH has undertaken a number of activities to address the recommendations in the National Action Plan (Centers for Disease Control and Prevention 2005). It is through this NIOSH-led initiative that the majority of intervention research and injury surveillance has been funded.

In 2004 a team of Canadian scientists published a systematic review of interventions for preventing childhood agricultural injuries (Hartling et al. 2004). Their findings, based on a comprehensive assessment of controlled research trials and observational studies, provide valuable insights into strengths and weaknesses of some of the most prominent interventions currently in place. For example, they found that school-based programs seem to be effective at increasing short-term knowledge gain among children, especially when interactive learning methods are used; and the popular 1-day farm safety day camps demonstrate children's ability to retain selected safety messages. There were mixed results from evaluations of tractor safety training and general farm safety community-based initiatives (Hartling et al. 2004).

Interventions to Prevent Agricultural Work-Related Injuries

In 1999, the North American Guidelines for Children's Agricultural Tasks (NAGCAT) were released as a new resource to help adults match a child's physical, mental, and psychosocial abilities with the requirements of agricultural jobs (Lee and Marlenga 1999). The NAGCAT enable children aged 7 to 16 years to have safe, meaningful work experiences in agriculture. It is important to note that the NAGCAT were developed for use in family farm settings, so they do not match up with child labor regulations or conditions where youth are employed in nonfamily settings (Cohen 2002). By using the job hazard analysis framework, detailed information for 62 agricultural jobs commonly performed by children is provided in a professional resource manual along with illustrated posters for parent use. These resources can be downloaded from a dedicated Web site: www.nagcat.org.

NIOSH-funded evaluation studies have demonstrated that parents' use of NAGCAT improves if dissemination is accompanied by a farm visit from a safety specialist or if child development principles are provided and promoted along with the print guidelines (Gadomski et al. 2003; Marlenga et al. 2002). A review of injury cases highlighted that if NAGCAT recommendations had been applied, 70% to 80% of the most serious work-related injuries could have been prevented (Marlenga et al. 2004). The NAGCAT resources and modifications have been used in the United States, Canada, Scandinavia, Australia, and the Philippines (Lee 2010). In some situations within the United States, the NAGCAT have been tested with underserved populations, including Hispanic and Asian farmworker families (Liller et al. 2002; Rasmussen et al. 2003).

In 2001, under the direction of the U.S. Department of Agriculture, a multifaceted program was implemented to improve tractor and machinery safety training and certification for youth. The Hazardous Occupations Safety Training in Agriculture attempted to refine a formal training program (including low-literacy resources) with a national tracking and recording system for use where employers need verification of training by minor employees (National Safety Council 2004a). (See http://hosta.nsc.org for more information.)

Other interventions for youth working in agriculture include information dissemination from the state Cooperative Extension Service, nongovernment agencies, or the Department of Labor. For example, the Department of Labor works with OSHA to regularly update the Youth Rules! Web site (at http://www.youthrules.dol.gov), providing guidance to teens, parents, educators, and employers (U.S. Department of Labor 2004b). The site includes specific information for youth working in agriculture, including OSHA safety standards, pertinent labor laws, and safety tips for jobs such as tractor operations and working in confined spaces (U.S. Department of Labor 2005).

Non-Work-Related Research and Interventions

The strategy of relying on educational interventions to protect nonworking children on farms is not universally endorsed. Because the farm is a hazardous occupational work site, children who are not actively participating in chores would ideally be separated from the work setting. Thus, there would be no need to educate children regarding injury prevention. Indeed, parents or responsible adults should be knowledgeable about the rationale for separating nonworking children from farm work sites. Although many current interventions focus on education for young children, most safety professionals promote removing young children from the work site altogether. However, this perspective (i.e., it is inappropriate for children to be in the work site) directly conflicts with populations who practice traditional agriculture.

Off-site childcare for nonworking children of farm owners and farmworkers is an ideal injury prevention option. Attempts have been made to implement rural childcare cooperative programs for farm families with mixed results. Childcare services for farm families must have flexible hours to match farmers' variable, often unscheduled, work activities. In addition, childcare services for an agricultural population must accommodate cultural values and economic limitations of parents and guardians who depend on these services. The Redlands Christian Migrant Association (RCMA) of Immokalee, Florida, is a successful cooperative venture among growers, migrant farmworker women, and churches that provides graduated levels of programming and services for children of various ages (http://www.rcma.org/). After three decades of trial and error, the RCMA now serves approximately 8000 individuals from programs in 21 Florida counties and 75 child care centers that incorporate Migrant Head Start services. Migrant, seasonal, and full-time agricultural workers use these centers for high-quality, value-added child care. The RCMA program is endorsed by major farm organizations, such as the American Farm Bureau.

When off-site childcare is not an option for nonworking children, designated safe play areas on farms are recommended (Lee et al. 2002). A safe play area on a farm is a carefully planned, designated location with limited exposure to hazards such as traffic, agricultural production, and environmental concerns. In 2003, Australia adopted a national child farm safety plan that included "safe play areas on farms" as a major national theme, promoting fencing and supervision in a manner consistent with their national swimming pool safety campaign (Farmsafe Australia 2003). In 2003, a U.S. team of agricultural safety and playground safety specialists generated a detailed guide based on playground safety and child development principles, to be used by farm owners (Esser et al. 2004). Creating Safe Play Areas on Farms serves as a guidance document to facilitate action by farm owners when off-site childcare is not a viable option (Esser et al. 2004). (The document can be downloaded at http://www.marshfieldclinic.org/proxy/mcrf-centers-nfmc-nccrahs-resources-creatingsafeplayareasbooklet.1.pdf.)

Community-based interventions, including programs developed by nonprofit organizations such as Farm Safety 4 Just Kids (FS4JK), where rural mothers introduce safety education for children, have been popular in many areas of the United States and Canada (Farm Safety 4 Just Kids 2010). Another popular approach is Farm Safety Days, with more than 400 events each year sponsored by the Progressive Agriculture Foundation (http://www.progressiveag.org/). Although these programs are presumed to have benefits for parents and children, and some have demonstrated short-term knowledge gain, there is no definitive research to demonstrate that they reduce the toll of childhood agricultural injuries (DeRoo and Rautianen 2000; Hartling et al. 2004; Reed and Claunch 2000).

Advocacy

In the early 1990s, the primary advocacy efforts toward child safety on farms involved the development, endorsement, and then implementation of the National Action Plan for Childhood Agricultural Injury Prevention (Castillo et al. 1998; National Committee for Childhood Agricultural Injury Prevention 1996). To assess the extent to which progress was being made on the National Action Plan, an in-depth assessment of activities was facilitated by the National

Children's Center for Rural and Agricultural Health and Safety (http://www.marshfieldclinic.org/NCCRAHS/).

Assessment summaries were discussed at length among 100 individuals participating in the 2001 Summit on Childhood Agricultural Injury Prevention, with proceedings published 1 year later (Lee et al. 2002). The initial 1996 plan, combined with the 2001 follow-up report, served as the primary communication tools for advocacy. NIOSH uses these reports to solicit research proposals, and individuals use the reports to justify grant requests to private foundations.

Advocacy efforts have also occurred within professional organizations and nonprofit groups. For example, the American Academy of Pediatrics developed and disseminated its policy statement on Childhood Agricultural Injuries (Committee on Injury and Poison Prevention and Committee on Community Health Services 2001). The American Academy of Pediatrics also published guidelines for the care of migrant farmworkers' children (McLaurin 2000). International Society for Agricultural Safety and Health (ISASH) is the professional organization of agricultural safety practitioners, including Cooperative Extension safety specialists and insurance company safety representatives. The ISASH convenes annual conferences and publishes technical articles that include research and practical applications for child safety on farms. The ISASH does not have formal lobbying efforts, but endorses position papers and action plans. The American Society of Agricultural Engineers has a primary focus on engineering solutions to agricultural hazards. The American Society of Agricultural Engineers also develops and endorses position articles on issues such as "buddy seats" in tractors, but does not have an official advocacy arm to the organization. The American Public Health Association indirectly addresses childhood agricultural injury prevention through two special interest groups sections: Injury Control and Emergency Health Services, and the Occupational Health and Safety group. The American Public Health Association also supports a Young Worker Network that, if called on, would propose and endorse policy changes to protect youth working on farms.

In the private sector, nongovernment organizations such as FS4JK have raised the profile of the injury problem by gaining regional and national coverage in the general media and farm press. In 2004, Marilyn Adams, the Founder and President of FS4JK, was named one of the 25 outstanding "Faces of Public Health" for her grassroots efforts to bring national attention to the problem of children being injured and killed on farms across the United States (Pfizer Global Pharmaceuticals, Pfizer Inc. 2004). Advocacy groups and coalitions can learn much from FS4JK and similar organizations regarding methods to unite professionals and laypersons in raising awareness and promoting strategies to minimize childhood agricultural injuries and deaths.

Future Directions

Although progress has been made on preventing childhood agricultural injuries in the past two decades, more can be done. Action plans for general and child-specific agricultural safety have been developed through consensus methods involving agricultural stakeholders. The various plans include general and detailed recommendations for minimizing injuries to children on farms.

National agricultural health and safety recommendations that address child and adolescent safety are as follows:

- A Report to the Nation: Agricultural Occupational and Environmental Health: Policy Strategies for the Future (Merchant et al. 1989)
- Children and Agriculture: Opportunities for Safety and Health (National Committee for Childhood Agricultural Injury Prevention 1996)
- Migrant and Seasonal Hired Adolescent Farmworkers: A Plan to Improve Working Conditions (Vela Acosta and Lee 2001)

- Childhood Agricultural Injury Prevention: Progress Report and Updated National Action Plan from the 2001 Summit (Lee et al. 2002)
- National Agenda for Action: National Land Grant Research and Extension Agenda for Agricultural Safety and Health (Committee NCR-197 2003)
- Using History and Accomplishments to Plan for the Future: A Summary of 15 Years in Agricultural Safety and Health and Action Steps for Future Directions (Petrea 2003)
- Looking Beneath the Surface of Agricultural Safety and Health: Chapter 7, Challenges, Opportunities and Ideas for the Future (Murphy 2003, pp. 81–83)
- National Agricultural Tractor and Safety Initiative: A Plan of the NIOSH Agricultural Safety and Health Centers (Swenson 2004)

There is no shortage of suggestions for improving the safety of children and adults on our nation's farms and ranches. Where we fall short is in leadership and ability to enact recommendations. For myriad reasons, individuals and organizations find it difficult to implement desired strategies for childhood agricultural injury prevention. Factors such as economic farm policy, the independent nature of farming and farmers, resistance to change, and limitations in rural services prevail. For example, farm policies in the United States have primarily focused on global trade, product safety, and environmental preservation, not on worker health and safety. In those cases where worker safety policy is addressed, it rarely incorporates issues of children living and working on family farms where the majority of childhood injuries occur.

Resistance to safety interventions can be compared with other areas of injury prevention, such as motorcycle helmet use, where the irony is that resistance is greatest among the population with the most at stake. Another limiting factor is the obvious dissonance between safety professionals and the general farm community regarding an acceptable degree of risk in agricultural work settings. Indeed, farm owners seem to have lower expectations for occupational safety than do the public health and agricultural safety professionals serving them.

Initial Action

In the near future, attention should be given to the young, nonworking children at risk of injuries. Having affordable, accessible childcare options available and used by farm owners and parents would remove the most vulnerable children from the immediate risk of injury. Government or private-sector incentives for increasing the number and quality of rural childcare programs should be encouraged (Children's Defense Fund 2001). Parents and farm owners should be held accountable for child protection, consistent with urban parents. Finally, insurance companies should offer incentives to farm owners that physically separate children from the occupational work site.

Long-Term Action

In the long run, organizational policy, public policy, and regulatory changes are warranted on several fronts. Some of these policy changes include the following:

- National, state, and organizational policies should provide financial incentives to farm owners for improving the safety environment and practices in their agricultural enterprise, especially as they affect children. Farm subsidies should be contingent on safe working conditions. Such policies could mimic other government programs that reward agricultural producers for environmental practices, or they could be filtered through property insurers.
- Policy recommendations of the 1996 National Action Plan should be addressed. These include mandating the restriction of youth aged less than 18 years from operating tractors without seat

belts and rollover protective structures, and restricting tractor operations on public roads to youth aged 16 years or older who have a valid driver's license (National Committee for Childhood Agricultural Injury Prevention 1996).

- The Hazardous Occupations Order for Agriculture that affects youth working on farms should be updated and enforced (Miller and Bush 2004). Particular attention should be given to agricultural work that is highly associated with childhood morbidity and mortality.
- OSHA's regulation of farm safety equipment should be strengthened to increase the likelihood that working conditions for adults and youth meet minimum safety standards.

Although we have focused heavily on the adverse outcomes of children's presence in agricultural work sites, it is important to maintain a balanced perspective. Agriculture offers many positive benefits for children. The largest youth-serving organization in the United States, the National FFA Organization, was chartered by the U.S. Congress on the principle that agriculture provides unique opportunities for young people to develop "premier leadership, personal growth, and career success" (https://www.ffa.org/Pages/default.aspx#). Future research should enhance our knowledge regarding the benefits and risks of living and working on farms so that injury prevention strategies, such as stricter child labor regulations, are based on scientific findings that will stand the test of time.

References

Adekoya N, Pratt SG. 2001. *Fatal Unintentional Farm Injuries Among Persons Less Than 20 Years of Age in the United States: Geographic Profiles.* Publication No. 2001-131. Cincinnati, OH: Department of Health and Human Services/National Institute for Occupational Safety and Health.

Armbruster WJ. 1991. Intervention—safe behaviors among adults and children. In: Myers ML, Herrick RF, Olenchock SA, Myers JR, Parker JE, Hard DL, Wilson K, editors. *Papers and Proceedings of the Surgeon General's Conference on Agricultural Safety and Health.* Washington DC: U.S. Department of Health and Human Services. 462–465.

Carrabba JJ, Field WE, Tormoehlen RL, Talbert BA. 2000. Effectiveness of the Indiana 4-H tractor program at instilling safe tractor operating behaviors and attitudes in youth. *J Agric Saf Health.* 6:179–189.

Castillo D, Hard D, Myers J, et al. 1998. A national childhood agricultural injury prevention initiative. *J Agric Saf Health.* [Special issue] (1):183–191.

Castillo DN, Adekoya N, Myers JR. 1999. Fatal work-related injuries in the agricultural production and services sectors among youth in the United States, 1992-96. *J Agromedicine.* 6:27–41.

Centers for Disease Control and Prevention. 2005. NIOSH Safety and Health Topic: Childhood Agricultural Injury Prevention Initiative. Available at: http://www.cdc.gov/niosh/childag. Accessed February 9, 2005.

Children's Defense Fund. 2001. *A Fragile Foundation: State Childcare Assistance Policies.* Washington DC: Children's Defense Fund.

Cohen A. 2002. *North American Guidelines for Children's Agricultural Tasks and Child Labor Regulations.* NIOSH report.

Committee NCR-197. 2003. *National Agenda for Action: National Land Grant Research and Extension Agenda for Agricultural Safety and Health.* Washington DC: U.S. Department of Agriculture.

Committee on Injury and Poison Prevention and Committee on Community Health Services. 2001. American Academy of Pediatrics: prevention of agricultural injuries among children and adolescents. *Pediatrics.* 108:1016–1019.

Darraugh AR, Stallones L, Sample PL, Sweitzer K. 1998. Perceptions of farm hazards and personal safety behavior among adolescent farmers. *J Agric Saf Health.* 1:159–169.

DeRoo LA, Rautianen R. 2000. A systematic review of farm safety interventions. *Am J Prev Med.* 18:51–62.

Esser N. In the Wrong Place—All of the Time. *Dairy Today.* 2001:44.

Esser N, Heiberger S, Lee B, 2004. *Creating Safe Play Areas on Farms.* 2nd ed. Marshfield, WI: Marshfield Clinic. Available at: http://www.marshfieldclinic.org/proxy/mcrfcenters-nfmc-nccrahs-resources-creatingsafeplayareasbooklet.1.pdf.

Farm Safety 4 Just Kids Web site. 2010. Available at: http://www.fs4jk.org. Accessed November 9, 2010.

Farmsafe Australia. 2003. *Safe Play Areas on Farms.* A Resource Package. New South Wales: Farmsafe Australia, Inc.

Forastieri V. 2002. *Children at Work Health and Safety Risks.* 2nd ed. Geneva, Switzerland: International Labour Organization.

Gadomski A, Burdick P, Jenkins P, et al. 2003. Randomized field trial to evaluate the effectiveness of the North American Guidelines for Childhood Agricultural Injury Prevention (NAGCAT). American Public Health Association Abstract No. 64051. Available at: http://apha.confex.com/apha/131am/techprogram/paper_64051.htm. Accessed January 27, 2005.

Gerberich SG, Gibson RW, French LR, et al. 2001. Injuries among children and youth in farm households: regional Rural Injury Study-I. *Inj Prev.* 7:117–122.

Goldcamp M, Hendricks KJ, Myers JR. 2004. Farm fatalities to youth 1995-2000: a comparison by age groups. *J Safety Res.* 35:151–157.

Haddon W. 1972. A logical framework for categorizing highway safety phenomena and activity. *J Trauma.* 12:193–207.

Hard DL, Myers JR. 2006. Fatal work-related injuries in the agriculture production sector among youth in the United States, 1992-2002. *J Agromedicine.* 11:57–65.

Hartling L, Brison RJ, Crumley ET, et al. 2004. A systematic review of interventions to prevent childhood farm injures. *Pediatrics.* 114:483–496.

Heaney CA, Wilkins JR III, Dellinger W, et al. 2006. Protecting young workers in agriculture: participation in tractor certification training. *J Agric Saf Health.* 12:181–190.

Hendricks KJ, Adekoya N. 2001. Non-fatal animal related injuries to youth occurring on farms in the United States. *Inj Prev.* 7:307–311.

Hendricks KJ, Goldcamp M. 2010. Injury surveillance for youth on farms in the U.S., 2006. *J Agric Saf Health.* 16:279–291.

Hendricks KJ, Layne LA, Goldcamp EM, Myers JR. 2004. *Injuries among youth living on farms in the United States, 2001.* (RIP No. 06). Paper presented at the meeting of the National Institute of Farm Safety; June 20–24, 2004; Keystone, CO.

Hillsboro Sentry-Enterprise. 2009. Six-Year-Old Richland County Boy Killed in Farm Accident. (Hillsboro, WI), July 23.

Hutton C. Boy, 12, Dies in Farm Accident. *Wausau Daily Herald* (Wausau, WI), September 6.

Joles A. 2007. Child Killed in Combine Accident. *Tuscola County Advertiser* (Caro, MI), September 25, 2010.

Kidd P, Townley K, Cole H, et al. 1997. The process of chore teaching: implications for farm youth injury. *Fam Community Health.* 19:78–89.

Layne LA, Goldcamp EM, Myers JR, Hendricks KJ. 2009. Youth living on Hispanic-operated farms: injuries and population estimates in the U.S., 2000. *J Agric Saf Health.* 15:377–388.

Lee BC. 2010. Applying agricultural work guidelines from one country in another. In: Fassa AG, Parker DL, Scanlon TJ, editors. *Child Labour: A Public Health Perspective.* NY: Oxford University Press. 229–241.

Lee B, Gallagher S, Marlenga B, Hard D, 2002. *Childhood Agricultural Injury Prevention: Progress Report and Updated National Action Plan from the 2001 Summit.* Marshfield, WI: Marshfield Clinic.

Lee BC, Gunderson PD, 1992. Childhood agricultural injury prevention: issues and interventions from multiple perspectives. Proceedings from the Childhood Agricultural Injury Prevention Symposium. Marshfield, WI: Marshfield Clinic, National Farm Medicine Center.

Lee B, Jenkins L, Westaby J. 1997. Factors influencing exposure of children to major hazards on family farms. *J Rural Health.* 13:206–215.

Lee B, Marlenga B, 1999. *Professional Resource Manual: North American Guidelines for Children's Agricultural Tasks.* Marshfield, WI: Marshfield Clinic.

Lee BC, Westaby JD, Chyou PH, Purschwitz MA. 2007. Agricultural employers' hiring and safety practices for adolescent workers. *J Agric Saf Health.* 13:25–32.

Liller KD, Noland V, Rijal P, et al. 2002. Development and evaluation of the Kids Count Farm Safety Lesson. *J Agric Saf Health.* 8:411–421.

Marlenga B, Brison RJ, Berg RL, et al. 2004. Evaluation of the North American Guidelines for Children's Agricultural Tasks using a case series of injuries. *Inj Prev.* 10:350–357.

Marlenga B, Pickett W, Berg RL. 2002. Evaluation of an enhanced approach to the dissemination of the North American Guidelines for Children's Agricultural Tasks: a randomized controlled trial. *Prev Med.* 35:150–159.

McLaurin J, editor. 2000. *Guidelines For the Care of Migrant Farmworkers' Children.* AAP Committee on Community Health Services and Migrant Clinicians Network. Elm Grove Village: IL: American Academy of Pediatrics.

Merchant JA, Kross B, Donham K, Pratt D, 1989. *A Report to the Nation: Agricultural Occupational and Environmental Health: Policy Strategies for the Future.* Iowa City, IA: The National Coalition for Agricultural Safety and Health.

Miller M, Bush D. 2004. Review of the Federal Child Labor Regulations: updating hazardous and prohibited occupations. *Am J Ind Med.* 45:218–221.

Montgomery County Chronicle. 2009. 2-Year-Old Girl Dies in Gate Mishap. (Caney, KS), October 7.

Murphy DJ. 1992. *Safety and Health for Production Agriculture.* St. Joseph, MI: American Society of Agricultural Engineers.

Murphy DJ. 2003. *Looking Beneath the Surface of Agricultural Safety and Health.* St. Joseph, MI: American Society of Agricultural Engineers.

Myers JR, Hendricks KJ. 2001. *Injuries Among Youth on Farms in the United States 1998.* Publication No. 2001-154. Washington, DC: Department of Health and Human Services/National Institute for Occupational Safety and Health.

National Agricultural Statistics Service. 2008. *2008 Census of Agriculture.* Available at: http://www.naas.usda.gov/compendia/cats/agriculture.html. Accessed October 24, 2010.

National Committee for Childhood Agricultural Injury Prevention. 1996. *Children and Agriculture: Opportunities for Safety and Health.* Marshfield, WI: Marshfield Clinic.

National Institute for Occupational Safety and Health. 2010a. *Injuries to Youth on Farms and Safety Recommendations.* U.S. National Institute for Occupational Safety and Health Publication No. 2009-117. Available at: http://www.cdc.gov/niosh/docs/2009-117. Accessed February 17, 2010.

National Institute for Occupational Safety and Health. 2010b. The NIOSH Childhood Agricultural Injury Surveillance Project. Available at: http://www.cdc.gov/niosh/childag/childagsurvproj.html. Accessed August 10, 2010.

National Institute for Occupational Safety and Health. 2010c. Trends in Childhood Agricultural Nonfatal Injury Rates, 1998 Through 2009. Internal Analysis of the Childhood Agricultural Injury Survey (CAIS) Surveillance System. Morgantown, WV: National Institute for Occupational Safety and Health.

National Safety Council. 2004a. Hazardous Occupations Safety Training in Agriculture (HOSTA) Steering Committee Program Manual. Itasca, IL: National Safety Council.

National Safety Council. 2004b. *Injury Facts, 2004 Edition.* Itasca, IL: National Safety Council.

Neufeld S, Wright SM, Gaut J. 2002. Not raising a "bubble kid": farm parents' attitudes and practices regarding the employment, training and supervision of their children. *J Rural Health.* 18:57–66.

Olson N. Man Shoots, Kills Self in Hospital. *Marshfield News-Herald* (Marshfield, WI), November 5, 2002.

Payne P. Teen Killed in Grain Accident Was Member of Sonoma Farm Family. *The Press Democrat* (Santa Rosa, CA), August 12, 2009.

Petrea RE, editor. 2003. *Using History and Accomplishments to Plan for the Future: A Summary of 15 Years in Agricultural Safety and Health and Action Steps for Future Directions.* Urbana, IL: Agricultural Safety and Health Network.

Pfizer Global Pharmaceuticals, Pfizer Inc. 2004. *Farm Safety Awareness in the Faces of Public Health.* New York, NY:6–11.

Pryor SK, Caruth AK, McCoy CA. 2002. Children's injuries in agriculture related events: the effect of supervision on the injury experience. *Issues Compr Pediatr Nurs.* 25:189–205.

Rasmussen RC, Schermann MA, Shutske JM, Olson DK. 2003. Use of the North American Guidelines for Children's Agricultural Tasks with Hmong Farm Families. *J Agric Saf Health.* 9:265–274.

Reed DB, Claunch DT. 2000. Nonfatal farm injury incidence and disability to children. A systematic review. *Am J Prev Med.* 18:70–79.

Rivara FP. 2002. Prevention of injuries to children and adolescents. *Inj Prev.* 8:iv5–8.

Runyan CW. 1998. Using the Haddon matrix: introducing the third dimension. *Inj Prev.* 4:302–307.

Schuler RT, Skjolaas CA, Purschwitz MA, Wilkinson TL. 1994. Wisconsin youth tractor and machinery certification programs evaluation. ASAE Paper No. 94-5503. St. Joseph, MI: American Society of Agricultural Engineers.

Stallones L, Gunderson P. 1994. Epidemiological perspectives on childhood agricultural injuries within the United States. *J Agromedicine.* 1:3–18.

Stueland DT, Lee BC, Nordstrom DL, et al. 1996. A population based case-control study of agricultural injuries in children. *Inj Prev.* 2:192–196.

Swenson E, 2004. *National Agricultural Tractor and Safety Initiative: A Plan of the NIOSH Agricultural Safety and Health Centers.* Seattle, WA: University of Washington.

U.S. Department of Labor. 1975. *Occupational Safety and Health Standards for Agriculture.* Available at: http://www.osha.gov/pls/oshaweb/owadisp.show_ document?p_table=STANDARDS&p_id=10954. Accessed August 10, 2010.

U.S. Department of Labor. 1991. The Fair Labor Stands Act of 1938, as Amended. WH Publication No. 1318. Washington, DC: U.S. Government Printing Office.

U.S. Department of Labor. 2004a. *Child Labor Requirements in Agricultural Occupations Under the Fair Labor Standards Act.* Child labor bulletin 102. WH Publication No. 1295. Washington, DC: U.S. Government Printing Office.

U.S. Department of Labor. 2004b. Youth Rules. Available at: http://www.youthrules.dol.gov. Accessed February 9, 2005.

U.S. Department of Labor. 2005. Youth in Agriculture. Available at: http://www.osha.gov/SLTC/youth/agriculture/index.html. Accessed February 9, 2005.

U.S. General Accounting Office. 1998. *Child Labor in Agriculture.* General Accounting Office/Health, Education, and Human Services Publication No. 98-193. Washington, DC: U.S. General Accounting Office.

Vela Acosta MS, Lee B, editors. 2001. *Migrant and Seasonal Hired Adolescent Farmworkers: A Plan to Improve Working Conditions.* Marshfield, WI: Marshfield Clinic.

Chapter 9

Sports and Recreational Injuries

Stephen W. Marshall, PhD,[1] *Julie Gilchrist, MD,*[2] *Gitanjali Taneja, PhD,*[3] *and Karen D. Liller, PhD*[4]

Tracy suffered a concussion playing high school basketball in her junior year. Her eyes were focused on reaching for a rebound, and Tracy didn't see the other player before she collided with her and hit her head. "I went to school the next day after the game, but I felt really sick." The feelings of nausea, dizziness, and blurred vision were familiar. As a seventh grader she had a concussion and felt the same way. When a key game came up 2 days later, Tracy felt dizzy and nauseous. "The coach told me to tell the trainer. I didn't want to tell the trainer 'cause he would sit me out of the game. So I kept quiet, but I shouldn't have played." After the game she passed out in the locker room.

"They took me to the hospital and told me I had a concussion, which I knew, but I didn't know that my life was about to change." Tracy continued to feel nauseous, had headaches, balance problems, and difficulty concentrating and reading. "We had to put sheets on the windows to block out the light and I couldn't watch TV because the lights and noise would make me feel sick. My mom also had to help me walk 'cause my vision was blurry and I felt so dizzy all of the time. But the hardest part was not being able to go to school and missing most of my junior and senior years of high school."

Symptoms from the concussion forced Tracy to stay at home. She visits the doctor every month and had to learn how to walk again because of her problems with balance. Several years after the injury, Tracy is beginning to feel better, but she still struggles with symptoms from the concussion, and she will never again participate in any sport that has a risk of head injury. You can watch Tracy and her mom tell their story online (available at http://www.youtube.com/watch?v=yIqZDbk3M40 and http://www.youtube.com/watch?v=uO-ordcPWSU).

Injuries related to sports and recreation seem like a contradiction of sorts. When people think of recreation, they typically associate it with fun and relaxation. However, injuries due to these activities are a substantial public health problem. According to data collected by the National Health Interview Survey, an annual face-to-face survey of over 37,000 households in the United States, nearly seven million Americans each year sought medical care for a sports or recreational injury between 1997 and 1999. This translates to a rate of 26 injury episodes per 1000 persons per year. More than half of these injuries were sustained by youth between the ages of 5 and 24 (Conn, Annest, and Gilchrist 2003). Furthermore, each year an estimated 135,000 5- to 18-year-olds with sports- and recreation-related traumatic brain injuries are treated in U.S. hospital emergency departments (Gilchrist et al. 2007). In boys ages 15–19 years, 52% of all unintentional injury visits to the emergency department are for sports- and recreation-related injuries; for girls in this age group, it is 38% (Gotsch et al. 2002).

[1]Department of Epidemiology, Gillings School of Global Public Health, University of North Carolina, Chapel Hill.
[2]Division of Unintentional Injury Prevention, NCIPC, CDC, Atlanta, Georgia.
[3]National Children's Study, Eunice Kennedy Shriver National Institute of Child, Health and Human Development, NIH, Bethesda, Maryland.
[4]University of South Florida Graduate School and College of Public Health, Tampa, Florida.

Sports injuries are considered by some as "just part of the game." However, these injuries can be disabling and have lasting consequences (e.g., anterior cruciate ligament [ACL], spinal cord, and traumatic brain injuries). Fortunately, similar to other injuries, sports injuries are often preventable. Furthermore, prevention is important because the economic costs associated with sports and recreational injuries are remarkable. The medical costs of sports and recreational injuries to children under age 18 years were over $11 billion in 2003. If you include parents' work losses, pain and suffering, and product liability and legal fees, this societal cost spirals to over $121 billion in 2003 (U.S. Consumer Product Safety Commission 2000a, 2003b). Although much of the morbidity does not ultimately result in hospitalization, children often have to miss school for treatment and/or recovery. According to one study, 20% of injured school children lost one or more days from school due to their injury (Conn, Annest, and Gilchrist 2003). Thus, caregivers have to arrange care for them and they may fall behind in school.

Until recently, sports and recreational injury prevention research has been limited—possibly because many of these injuries tend to be less severe than injuries from other causes. Most people do not die from sports and recreational injuries, and most of these injuries are not catastrophic in nature. There are also many challenges associated with conducting research on these injuries. Because the outcome of most of these injuries is rarely death or even hospitalization, counting these injuries becomes less concrete. In general, there is an absence of data on the functional and emotional outcomes of sports and recreational injuries in children. A great number of sports and recreational injuries are not reported and the injured often do not seek medical care. In cases where victims undergo medical treatment, the manner in which their injuries are classified is limited by which codes are available from the International Classification of Diseases (ICD) manuals. Although these codes have become more refined with each revision, even the most recent version, ICD-10, fails to capture most sports and recreational activities. For example, while bicycling-related deaths are readily identifiable in this coding system, team sports such as basketball and football are not. The lack of codes is a limiting factor in accurately determining the number of sports and recreational injuries associated with specific activities.

Even if it were possible to count all sports and recreational injuries, calculating the risk of injury would still be difficult, as we lack the participation data needed to determine population exposure. For example, the National Center for Catastrophic Sport Injury Research (Mueller and Cantu 2011) collects data on fatal and serious nonfatal injuries among high school and college athletes participating on school-sponsored teams. By determining the number of individuals who participate in team sports, they are able to calculate injury rates for these activities; however, since many injuries occur in less formal, unstructured, and unregulated settings, these rates only provide a partial picture of even the most serious sports injuries. Some researchers have used sporting goods marketing data (American Sports Data's "Superstudy of Sports Participation") as rate denominator (Singh et al. 2008), suggesting that sporting goods industry information, if validated, might be routinely used to track sports participation for the calculation of exposure-based injury rates.

Given the increasing proportion of children and youth who are overweight and obese (U.S. Department of Health and Human Services 2010), the U.S. Surgeon General has recommended that Americans engage in more physical activity and exercise in order to prevent obesity-related disease (U.S. Department of Health and Human Services 1996). According to some estimates, there has been an increase in the number of children participating in organized sports in the last several years (American Academy of Pediatrics Committee on Sports Medicine and Fitness and Committee on School Health 2001); however, decreases in unstructured play and recreation may explain the concomitant increase in obesity (Marshall and Guskiewicz 2003). It may be that the intensity of organized physical activity is increasing for a small proportion of "elite" child athletes at the same time that the overall level of physical activity is declining in the general population of children (Marshall and Guskiewicz 2003; Carlson et al. 2006). Additionally, there are training programs available for preschool-age children and children younger than preschool age (American Academy of Pediatrics Committee on Sports Medicine and Fitness and Committee on School Health 2001; Adirim and Cheng 2003). Increased participation in sports and recreational activities, which results in increased exposure, leads to an increased risk for injury. Thus, it is critical that, as we encourage youth to be more active, we are mindful of the risks associated with these activities, as well as the means by which to reduce them.

Morbidity and Mortality Related to Most Common Injuries

Injuries due to participation in organized sports are in many ways categorically different than recreational injuries. Unstructured play and recreational activities leave the responsibility of safe play up to the individual (or in young children, their caregivers). Organized sports are generally governed by certain rules that are developed to promote fair play and safety. Further, in contrast to play in less structured settings, organized sports have coaches and referees present to enforce rules and encourage players to use the required protective gear.

As can be seen from Figure 9.1, there is a higher rate (per population) of sports and recreational injuries in children and youth than in adults. Of course, this reflects the fact that children and youth have a higher level of participation in sports. According to data from emergency department visits, the eight sports and recreational activities resulting in the highest absolute number of injuries to children ages 5–14 years were as follows: bicycling, all-terrain vehicles (ATVs), playgrounds, football, baseball/softball, basketball, roller sports, and soccer. These activities have high numbers of injuries compared to other activities, but not necessarily high rates of injuries. Large numbers of injuries in one sport over another may simply reflect a

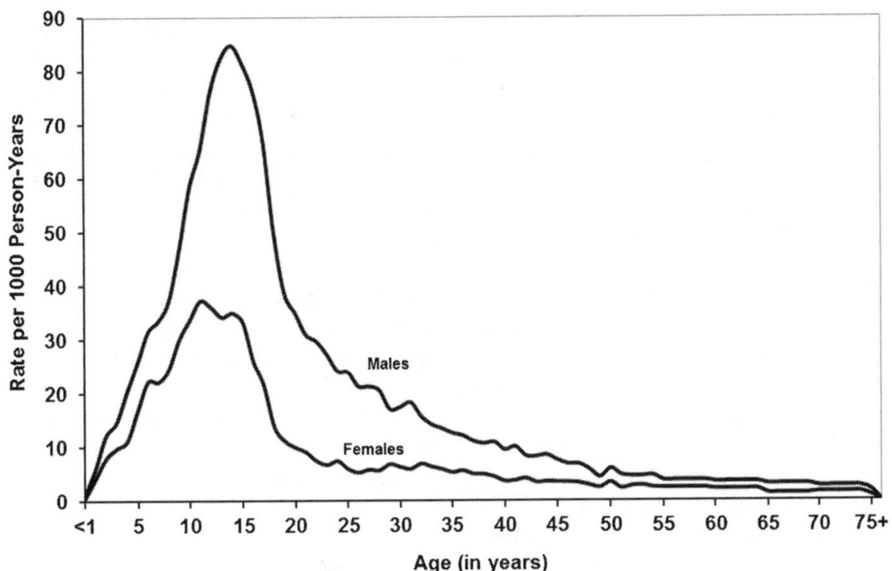

Figure 9.1. Incidence of Emergency Department-Attended Injury From Sports and Recreational Physical Activity, by Age and Sex.

Source: Emergency Department Records (National Electronic Injury Surveillance System All Injury Program), United States, July 2000–June 2001. Reproduced from Gotsch et al. (2002) and Marshall and Golightly (2007).

larger number of participants in that sport. As indicated above, we have limited exposure data for sports and recreational activities. Thus, we are usually unable to calculate rates (or risk) of injury, unless we limit our analysis to injuries as a result of participation in organized sports. Similarly, low numbers of injuries in a sport do not indicate that the sport is safer than other sports. For example, cheerleading and gymnastics have low numbers of injuries overall; however, the rate of catastrophic injury due to these sports is high compared to other sports (Purvis and Burke 2001).

Fatalities

The National Center for Catastrophic Sport Injury Research classifies fatal sports injuries as direct or indirect. Direct injuries refer to those which result directly from participation in the skills of the sport (e.g., direct head trauma or spinal cord injury). Indirect injuries are those that are caused as a result of exertion while participating in a sport, or a secondary complication to a nonfatal injury (e.g., heat-related illness) (Mueller and Cantu 2007). Deaths due to sports and recreation are usually a result of head injuries, heat stroke, or cardiac arrest (Purvis and Burke 2001). In very rare cases, a sudden impact to the chest wall, such as from a baseball or a hockey puck, can trigger cardiac arrest (Link et al. 1998; Maron et al. 1995).

Although fatal events are rare, they have great social significance because they engender enormous grief in the surrounding community. The inherent tragedy of a child who dies playing organized sports makes these injuries highly unacceptable to society. Furthermore, fatal sports injuries sometimes serve as springboards for community-driven prevention activities that may safeguard against similar tragedies and less severe sports injuries in the future.

Nonfatal Injuries

As previously stated, sports injury information is scarce. It is not readily available through current online injury databases of deaths and emergency department visits such as WISQARS (Web-based Injury Statistics Query and Reporting System) because of a lack of available codes for sports and recreational activities and injuries. When data can be gleaned on the burden of sports- and recreation-related injuries, the lack of participation data makes comparisons across years, age groups, gender, or activities difficult. Participation data would allow the calculation of rates of injury and the ability for comparisons. However, there are several resources collecting both injury and participation information from specific groups of athletes to allow valid comparisons to be made.

The state of Florida has funded the Sports Medicine and Athletic Related Trauma (SMART) Institute to improve sports safety (available at http://www.health.usf.edu/nocms/medicine/orthopaedic/smart.htm). Since 2006, SMART-supported certified athletic trainers have collected injury and participation information on more than 5000 high school athletes each year at ten Hillsborough County schools. This type of state-supported initiative is unfortunately rare, but presents a model example for other states wishing to address child and adolescent sports injuries.

At the national level, estimates of injury burden and participation among high school athletes are collected by the Center for Injury Research and Policy at The Research Institute at Nationwide Children's Hospital, Columbus, Ohio, funded in part by the Centers for Disease Control and Prevention (CDC). In 2005, a web-based data system (RIO) (Reporting Injuries Online, or RIO™) was launched to collect injury and participation information from certified athletic trainers caring for high school athletes in nine sports (available at http://www.injuryresearch.net/highschoolrio.aspx) (Comstock et al. 2006). Data have been collected annually on athletes in 100 U.S. high schools nationally representative of geographic location and school size. Schools are randomly selected from among those that agree to participate. In 2009, data collection was expanded to capture injuries and participation in 21 sports. These data have been used by the National Athletic Trainers' Association, the National Federation of State High School Associations, and the National Operating Committee on Standards for Athletic Equipment to drive evidence-based discussions of potential risk management/safety efforts (e.g., rule changes, improved protective equipment, education programs).

The previously described data collection efforts focus on athletes at the high school level. However, the National Collegiate Athletic Association (NCAA) Injury Surveillance System (ISS) has been collecting injury and participation information on collegiate athletes since 1982 (Dick, Agel, and Marshall 2007). Historically, this has been a voluntary reporting system so that captured injuries and calculated rates are representative of only the schools choosing to report. Despite this limitation, the data have supported the efforts of the NCAA Sport Rules Committees and the NCAA Committee on Competitive Safeguards and Medical Aspects of Sports. Data from ISS have been used to support policy and rule changes to enhance player safety. For instance, rules and officiating changes to prevent concussion in men's ice hockey; policy modifications of permissible equipment, contact, or practices in spring and preseason football; and additions of protective eyewear in women's lacrosse were all shaped based on data from ISS (Dick et al. 2007). In 2004, the NCAA ISS developed a web-based reporting system to streamline data collection, and efforts are currently under way to establish a representative sample so that the national burden of sports injuries at the collegiate level can be estimated.

Between these high school and the collegiate systems, we are getting a more detailed picture of the risks of competitive sports and the effectiveness of interventions. However, these data collection efforts do not include the intramural, club, and league play outside of sanctioned school events, or the injuries that occur during recreational activities outside of organized sporting events. Further work is necessary to identify the number and demographics of participants in various activities to allow valid comparisons of risks across genders, age groups, activities, and years. Validation of participation information collected by marketing firms or new data collection of participation through public health surveillance of physical activity might provide the needed information.

Focus on Select Injuries: Concussion, Heat, and Anterior Cruciate Ligament

This section addresses three specific sports and recreational injuries that are of particular concern and are currently the focus of efforts to improve awareness, and to identify, develop, test, and disseminate interventions.

Concussion

Concussions have become a very important topic in youth sports over the past 5 years. Concussions were once considered to be mere "bellringers" or "dings." However, we now know that any concussion—defined as altered neurologic status due to an impact or acceleration/deceleration of the head—is a serious injury and should be managed carefully to prevent a catastrophic outcome or lasting consequences. The American Academy of Pediatrics has recently summarized current knowledge on the diagnosis and management of concussion in children and adolescent athletes (Halstead et al. 2010). In brief, athletes who are symptomatic should be withheld from competition and practice to minimize the risk of another impact to the head. Any youth athlete showing signs of concussion should be removed from the field of play immediately, and should not be allowed to return to the sport until cleared to return by a health professional with experience in diagnosing and managing concussion. Return to play will be determined by the resolution of all symptoms both at rest and when challenged physically and cognitively, which might be a matter of weeks or months after injury (Cantu and Voy 1995). Careful evaluation by a health professional experienced in the diagnosis and management of concussion is required (Halstead et al. 2010). Signs and symptoms of concussion include (but are not limited to) long-term and short-term memory loss, delays in cognitive processing, dizziness and balance problems, nausea and vomiting, visual disturbances, neck pain, and headache. Loss of consciousness, long considered to be the hallmark sign of concussion, is actually rare (Guskiewicz et al. 2003). The cumulative effects of multiple concussions are poorly understood at this time, but there is evidence that youth athletes with a past history of concussion are at increased risk for further concussions (Guskiewicz et al. 2003).

If a second blow to the head occurs while the athlete is still recovering from the first concussion, the consequences can be severe or even fatal (Cantu 1992). Even with appropriate resolution of symptoms and return to play, some youth athletes may sustain multiple concussions close together in time, with each injury exhibiting increasing severity or duration of symptoms. These athletes should potentially be counseled about the dangers of continuing in their sport (Halstead et al. 2010).

Much attention in recent years has focused on the long-term effects of repeated concussion, which has recently been linked to neurodegenerative diseases, depression, and traumatic encephalopathy. The potential for long-term consequences reinforces the importance of concussion prevention, recognition, and response. The brains of children are suspected to be more susceptible to concussion than those of adults. Fortunately, the CDC has done much to increase awareness about the prevention of, recognition of, and response to concussion. Free educational kits targeting athletes, parents, coaches, teachers and school counselors, and physicians are provided online (available at http://www.cdc.gov/concussion). We urge child injury experts and advocates to visit this site and become familiar with these materials, and actively disseminate them through their community networks.

Heat Injury

Among U.S. high school athletes, heat illness is the third leading cause of death during sports participation (Coris, Ramirez, and Van Durme 2004). More than 9000 high school athletes each year are treated for heat-related injury (Gilchrist et al. 2010). These occurred most commonly in football and during the month of August (Gilchrist et al. 2010). Gradual acclimation to hot or humid environments is required in order to minimize the risk of heat injury. Close attention to hydration and appropriate dress is critical. For outdoor sports, consideration of altering or canceling practice or participation in high-risk conditions is important. Organized sporting groups and organizations should develop guidelines for practices and competitions under high-risk conditions. Heat AND humidity should be monitored continuously throughout practice. Copious quantities of ice water should always be on hand as a primary means of rapidly treating any athletes who show signs of heat stress. For large outdoor practices, such as preseason football or long-distance running in hot or humid conditions, trained health care professionals should be present to watch for signs of distress and provide immediate treatment. The National Athletic Trainers' Association has developed guidelines on preventing heat-related illness (Binkley et al. 2002). Additionally, the CDC provides online information regarding the prevention of heat illness (available at http://www.cdc.gov/Features/ExtremeHeat).

Technology can assist in the prevention of heat illness. Recently, small body temperature sensors have become available. These can be swallowed by the athlete prior to practice. These wirelessly transmit core body temperature data from within the digestive tract to data receivers that can be carried or worn on the outside of the body. Fortunately, the damage due to heat injury is almost always reversible if the affected athletes can be rapidly detected and treated.

Anterior Cruciate Ligament Injury

Tears and ruptures of the ACL are devastating injuries. To restore full function after injury often requires surgical reconstruction, followed by 6 to 12 months of rehabilitation. Reconstructions in pediatric populations are now much more common than previously; however, they are a complex and difficult procedure, since the femur and tibia are still growing, making anchoring the graft problematic. Equally concerning is the accelerated progression to osteoarthritis in those with ACL and meniscal tears (Lohmander et al. 2007).

ACL injuries are problematic from a prevention standpoint since they often result from noncontact or indirect contact mechanisms, rather than external contact directly to the knee joint. They typically occur in landing or planting and cutting movements. Athletes frequently comment that they were injured performing an action that they have executed without ill effect thousands of times before. An alteration in the immediate environment—such as an unexpected change in direction by an opposing player—often occurs immediately before the injury.

Curiously, the rate of ACL injury is two to five times higher in female athletes relative to male athletes in comparable sports. Despite more than a decade of intensive research, the reasons for the excess risk in females are still not entirely explained. ACL injuries most likely have multiple interrelated causes, with hormonal levels, anatomy, muscle firing patterns, and neurocognitive factors all playing a role. However, neuromuscular training programs provide the most promising opportunity for prevention, since these programs can be readily incorporated into sports team warm-ups or practices (Griffin 2001; Griffin et al. 2006). An example of a rigorously evaluated intervention program is provided online (available at http://www.aclprevent.com) (Gilchrist et al. 2008). Other plyometric or neuromuscular training programs have also been evaluated (Griffin et al. 2006); however, the benefits of any of these physical training programs are only ensured when athletes use correct biomechanical technique during the training. The required "dose" of neuromuscular training needed to attain an injury prevention effect, and how long the training effects persist, are currently unknown.

Team Sports Injuries

Basketball

Basketball is one of the most common activities among youth in the United States, and perhaps the most popular youth team sport. Although basketball has traditionally been considered a noncontact sport, the sport has evolved such that contact between players has become common (Zvijac and Thompson 1996). Among high school and college basketball players, basketball injuries result in a high number of indirect fatalities compared to other sports (Mueller and Cantu 2007). It is also the team sport associated with the highest absolute number of injuries (Conn, Annest, and Gilchrist 2003; U.S. Consumer Product Safety Commission 2003b). This might be partially explained by the large numbers of people who participate in the sport, rather than an innate danger in the sport itself. Nonetheless, there are ways to make the sport safer, and certain measures have already been shown to effectively decrease the number of injuries.

High school players are more likely to become injured during practice, whereas college athletes are more likely to become injured during competition (Zvijac and Thompson 1996). The most common types of basketball injuries are sprains, fractures, and dislocations (Scanlan et al. 2001). Hands and fingers are commonly injured, as are knees and ankles (Purvis and Burke 2001; Zvijac and Thompson 1996; Scanlan et al. 2001). Eye injuries are common, but most can be prevented with proper eye protection (Zvijac and Thompson 1996). Head and spinal cord injuries are rare.

Randomized controlled trials in college-age military cadets indicate that ankle braces have some effectiveness in preventing ankle injuries in basketball (Sitler et al. 1994). Similarly, mouthguards have been shown to be effective in preventing dental injuries in the college game (Labella, Smith, and Sigurdsson 2002). Whether these interventions have efficacy in younger populations is still unknown. Dentist-fitted mouthguards are recommended; they need to be replaced annually or earlier if damaged or when children outgrow them.

Football

Of the sports that are widely played in the United States, football has the distinction of having the greatest risk of injury. In the early part of the 20th century, when the game was still evolving, the number of deaths and injuries in college football was a matter of national concern. The impetus to reform the sport eventually led to the formation of the National Collegiate Athletic Association (NCAA). The modern game retains the sport's early emphasis on vigorous body contact, body mass, and athletic acceleration, but has invested heavily in protective equipment as a means of controlling injury.

Pioneering research during the 1960s demonstrated that cleat length had an impact on the risk of knee injury, with shorter cleats reducing the risk of injury. Furthermore, maintenance of the playing field was also found to be important to reducing injury risk (Robey, Blyth, and Mueller 1971). As a general recommendation, all protective equipment should be (1) appropriate to the activity or position, (2) in good condition, (3) well fitting, and (4) worn both consistently and correctly. In addition, youth need to be trained to use equipment correctly. This is particularly true of the helmet. When the modern hard-shell helmet was first introduced into the sport in 1970s, it was initially used by some as a battering ram, resulting in an upswing in the incidence of paralysis and other catastrophic injuries. Educational campaigns and rules prohibiting making initial contact with the opponent using the head were introduced to correct this situation (Mueller and Blyth 1987). Concussion in football, as in all sports, poses special risks, since the management of this injury is problematic and requires trained professionals. See the Concussion section under "Particular Injuries of Public Concern."

Baseball/Softball

Baseball enjoys a special place in American culture. The sport has historically claimed to epitomize American values and dominated the sports landscape in the United States during much of the 20th century (Rader 1992). Modern nonprofessional baseball is largely a youth sport. Nearly two thirds of baseball participants are less than 18 years of age; older participants tend to transition into recreational softball leagues (Baseball and Softball Council 1996). Collegiate data indicate that baseball and softball have a similar injury rate, and that their injury rates are lower than in contact/collision sports such as football and soccer. However, the repetitive-motion injuries associated with baseball/softball are of considerable concern.

There has been long-standing interest in reducing the risk of injury to children and adolescents playing these sports (American Academy of Pediatrics Committee on Sports Medicine and Fitness 1994). Breakaway bases have demonstrated effectiveness in youth and recreational adult baseball and softball, and their use should be encouraged throughout baseball and softball at all levels (Janda et al. 1988; Sendre et al. 1994; Janda et al. 1993). Breakaway bases are bases that clip into a support post that is fixed to the ground; the base separates from its post when a sliding athlete hits the base. In addition, studies of protective eyewear indicate that polycarbonate lenses provide excellent protection for batters from the risk of being hit in the eye by a pitched ball (Vinger et al. 1997; American Academy of Pediatrics 1996). Face guards are strongly recommended for batters and reduce the risk of facial injury by 23% to 35% (Danis, Hu, and Bell 2000; Marshall et al. 2003).

Unexpected contact with the ball is the single most frequent proximate cause of injury for youth participants, and thus use of safety balls also has the potential to considerably reduce the overall risk of injury (Kyle 1996; Pasternack, Veenema, and Callahan 1996; Mueller, Marshall, and Kirby 2001). There is a wide range of safety balls used in youth baseball, including tennis balls, rubber balls, cloth balls, and specialized reduced impact balls (also known as RIF balls) and these are effective in preventing injuries from ball contact (Marshall et al. 2003, Pasternack, Veenema, and Callahan 1996).

Pitching a baseball is an ergonomically stressful activity, and youth pitchers that throw a large number of pitches in a short span of time run the risk of incurring repetitive overuse symptoms, particularly in the elbow or shoulder (Andrews and Fleisig 1998; Fleisig et al. 1995). Care should be taken to monitor the number and frequency of pitches thrown by a child or adolescent and restrict the amount of pitching if pain, swelling, or other overuse symptoms appear in the arm, particularly the elbow, or shoulder. USA Baseball recommends that pitchers who are 9 to 10 years old should be limited to no more than 75 pitches per week and no more than 50 pitches in any one game. For 11- to 12-year-old pitchers, the limits are 100 pitches per week and no more than 75 pitches per game, and for 13- to 14-year-old pitchers, it is 125 pitches per week and 75 pitches per game.

Pitchers in fast-pitch softball use an underarm windmill pitch that is also highly stressful to the young arm. However, research on pitching-related arm and shoulder injuries to date has largely focused on baseball. There is a pressing need for basic information about the risks associated with fast-pitch softball (Pollack et al. 2005, Flyger, Button and Rishiraj 2006).

Soccer

Soccer is the most popular sport in the world, for adults and youth. The 2010 FIFA World Cup had a record number of viewers worldwide and was the first soccer World Cup to be held on the African continent. Of the 18 million people who compete in organized soccer in the United States, 75% are under 18 years of age. Participation in soccer for both girls and boys jumped during the 1980s and 1990s (increased 73% overall between 1989 and 1999 at the high school level) (U.S. Consumer Product Safety Commission 1995). The intensity and standard of competition has also risen with increased organization of soccer participation.

The detection of deficits in cognitive processing in professional European soccer stars (Matser et al. 1999) has led to great concern about the potential for heading of the ball to adversely affect academic performance in youth players. In fact, similar deficits do not seem to exist in collegiate players in the United States, and it is highly doubtful that they would exist in youth players (Guskiewicz et al. 2002). Nevertheless, several products—essentially padded headbands—designed to absorb impact forces have been marketed in the United States. The effectiveness of these products has not been examined in epidemiologic studies.

The neurological deficits observed in professional soccer players may not in fact be the result of heading the ball, but rather they may stem from repeated concussions due to impacts with other players or the ground (Kirkendall and Garrett 2001). This suggests that a "fair head rule"—allowing a player who is well positioned to take a header uncontested—would do much to address the safety issues associated with heading.

Knee and ankle injuries are common among soccer players. It has been suggested that training in movement techniques—known as neuromuscular, pylometric, or proprioceptive training—can reduce the risk of ankle and knee injury in soccer and other sports that involve cutting, landing, and jumping (Myklebust et al. 2003; Junge and Dvorak 2004). These training programs typically target prevention of tears and rupture of the ACL, a ligament within the knee that is more prone to rupture in girls than boys. See the ACL section under "Particular Injuries of Public Concern."

From a practical standpoint, all playing fields should be well maintained and in good condition. Goalposts should be padded to limit the risk of injury from goalpost collisions. If movable goals are used, they must be correctly anchored, since death can result if the goals tip over during play (U.S. Consumer Product Safety Commission 1995; DeMarco and Reeves 1994).

Ice Hockey

Ice hockey tends to have a lower number of participants and is more regionally focused than many other sports. However, it has a high rate of injury (Gerberich et al. 1987; Agel et al. 2007; Agel, Dompier, Dick, and Marshall 2007). Approximately one third of collegiate players have previously suffered a dental injury (Sane, Ylipaavalniemi, and Leppanen 1988). This injury is preventable if a face guard that completely covers the lower and upper face is worn. However, the standard helmet face guard has an opening in the lower face that permits the intrusion of the hockey stick. In addition, the face guard is hinged, and players sometimes skate with the face guard in the up position. This alters the impact dynamics of the helmet by repositioning the mass of the helmet on the player's head; thus, it greatly increases the loading on the cervical spine and places the player at risk for spinal cord injury (Reynen and Clancy 1994).

The game is fast-paced, involves body checking, and is played on a slippery surface. As a result, it has a high rate of injury. Among collegiate males, ice hockey game-related injury rates rank fourth behind football, wrestling, and soccer. Among collegiate females, ice hockey game-related injuries rates rank third behind soccer and gymnastics (Hootman, Dick, and Agel 2007). Play should not commence if the ice is not in good condition. Furthermore, parents, administrators, and officials should collaborate to ensure that fighting is strongly discouraged. Players who become overly aggressive should be removed from the game. Helmet telemetry data suggest that youth players who are braced and prepared for an impact do a better job of absorbing the resulting forces than unprepared players (Mihalik et al. 2010). Therefore, a logical focus would be on limiting unanticipated collisions, rather than trying to reduce or eliminate all collisions.

Cheerleading

Over the past two decades, cheerleading has evolved from support-orientated dance routines on the sidelines of the high school football game into a sport in its own right (Hutchinson 1997). Modern cheerleading teams (or, more formally, competitive spirit squads) compete against one another in stand-alone competitions. They perform aerobic routines and gymnastic stunts that sometimes involve high-risk formations such as three-level pyramids. At the high school level, it is the tenth most popular sport for girls nationally, with over 95,000 participants (National Federation of State High School Associations 2010). There is also a burgeoning private gym industry devoted to cheerleading.

As the athletic demands of the sport have increased, so have concerns about safety. The American Association of Cheerleading Coaches and Advisors recommends that teams work slowly toward the more demanding athletic stunts, and that adequate numbers of spotters should be present in both competitions and practices. Aerial tumbling moves and pyramid formations should only be attempted with adequate preparation and under close supervision. Further, high school cheerleading teams are restricted to pyramids no higher than two levels. Floor pads should be used. Poor quality coaching has been identified as a risk factor for cheerleading injury at the high school level (Schulz et al. 2004). Thus, school officials should ensure that coaching staff are experienced and qualified. Cheerleading can present significant risks to the young athlete and ongoing surveillance of this sport should be a high priority.

Individual Sports/Recreational Injuries

Playground Injuries

Injuries related to playground activities account for many of the injuries to youth aged 0–9 years (Gotsch et al. 2002). Although the mortality associated with these activities is not high (four playground deaths in 2001) (Centers for Disease Control and Prevention 2004), morbidity is significant with more than 200,000 children visiting emergency departments for treatment of a playground injury each year (U.S. Consumer Product Safety Commission 2003a). Most injuries on playgrounds are due to falls, and obviously falls from higher elevations generally result in more serious injuries than falls from lower surfaces. Fractures to upper limbs are the most common type of injury (Norton, Nixon, and Sibert 2004). Although less frequent than falls, children can also become injured by colliding with swings or other moving equipment and coming into contact with sharp surfaces or pinch points. From 2001 to 2008, the U.S. Consumer Product Safety Commission (CPSC) investigated reports of 40 deaths involving playground equipment. Over two thirds of all playground equipment-related deaths involved hanging or other asphyxiation, usually on slides or swings (O'Brien 2009). Previous reports suggest that this occurs primarily from ropes, shoestrings, cords, leashes, clothing strings, and other items tied to, or entangled on the equipment (Tinsworth and McDonald 2001). Approximately 75% of playground injuries occur on equipment designed for public use while the rest occur on equipment designed for home use or homemade equipment. In locations where injuries occurred on public equipment, almost 80% had some kind of protective surface under the equipment such as bark mulch or wood chips. In contrast, only about 9% of injuries occurring at home had a protective surfacing, most often sand (Tinsworth and McDonald 2001).

The introduction of softer, impact-absorbing surfaces under playground equipment, combined with ensuring that equipment meets height and maintenance standards (U.S. Consumer Product Safety Commission 2003a), has decreased the number of serious injuries due to falls (Norton, Nixon, and Sibert 2004). The number of head injuries due to falls on playgrounds has also decreased with the implementation of softer surfaces (Norton, Nixon, and Sibert 2004). Children should be limited to playing on playgrounds that follow guidelines set forth by CPSC. This includes ensuring that there are adequate spaces between equipment items so that the flow of children around the equipment does not become congested, creating the potential for collisions, falls, and injuries. Children commonly use equipment in ways that were not initially intended. For example, they will jump off of swings and merry-go-rounds while they are still in motion or slide down slides head first; thus, it is important that there is adequate space and an appropriate surface on which to land safely. Impact-absorbing surfaces reduce the risk of injury on playgrounds, but these surfaces do require maintenance on a regular basis. Wood or bark chips tend to migrate away from high-traffic areas and must be regularly redistributed to ensure a uniform depth across the whole playground. They may also be prone to runoff following a heavy thunderstorm. Synthetic mats can erode over time. Caregivers should walk around the playground, inspect the surfacing, and arrange for repairs if needed. Particular attention is required to high-traffic areas, such as the base of slides.

Other playground injury prevention strategies have been developed. The National Program for Playground Safety, a national clearinghouse of playground information, has developed recommendations based on the "S.A.F.E." model, which includes tips on playground supervision, age-appropriate equipment design, fall-related injury prevention surfacing, and equipment maintenance and repair (National Program for Playground Safety 2005).

Young children grow rapidly and playground equipment varies in size in order to accommodate children of all ages. It is important that caregivers are aware of the physical and developmental capabilities of their children and allow them to only play on equipment that is safe and age/size appropriate. Caregivers should be alert to the potential hazards of playgrounds and should be prepared to intervene when equipment is used inappropriately or children engage in hazardous play.

Bicycle Injuries

Bicycling is one of the most popular recreational activities among children, with an estimated 44.3 million youth under 21 riding bicycles in the United States (Rodgers 2000). In addition to recreation, many youth use bicycles as a means of transportation to school or other activities. Unfortunately, bicycling injuries are one of the most common types of sports and recreational injuries among youth (Gotsch et al. 2002), and the most common for children aged 5–14 years (Conn, Annest, and Gilchrist 2003). In 2001, a total of 185 children aged 0–18 years died from bicycle-related injuries (National Center for Health Statistics 2003). Of these 185 deaths, 122 suffered a head injury, 14 suffered a neck injury, and 10 suffered both a head and neck injury. Further, CPSC estimated 415,000 children experienced a musculoskeletal injury due to cycling in 2000 (Purvis and Burke 2001). Bicycle-related injuries account for more emergency department visits for children and adolescents compared to other sports and recreational injuries, and two thirds of all bicycle-related fatalities are due to traumatic brain injuries (Centers for Disease Control and Prevention 1995).

The most common bicycling injuries result from falls and collisions with immovable objects, but the more serious bicycle crashes typically involve collisions with motor vehicles. One way of preventing bicycles from colliding with motor vehicle traffic is to separate the cyclists from the drivers. Bicycle lanes and paths have become more common, but studies that have been able to measure their effectiveness are scarce. For youth cyclists, the most promising interventions are likely traffic-calming interventions that limit the speed of cars in neighborhoods, such as speed tables and chicanes (Ewing and Brown 2009).

The effectiveness of bicycle helmets has been demonstrated in case-control studies (Thompson, Rivara, and Thompson 1989, 1996). According to the American Academy of Pediatrics Committee on Injury and Poison Prevention, wearing a bicycle helmet is one of the most effective safety measures that a child can take to prevent injury (American Academy of Pediatrics Committee on Injury and Poison Prevention 2001). The percentage of cyclists who wear helmets has steadily increased over the years; however, many children and most adolescents still do not wear helmets regularly or at all (Rivara et al. 1998). Like helmets in football and other sports, it is important that they be (1) appropriate to the activity or position, (2) in good condition, (3) well fitting, and (4) worn both consistently and correctly.

Educational campaigns, helmet subsidies, and local and state legislation have been promoted as means for increasing helmet use and decreasing the number of bicycling injuries (Rivara et al. 1998). Many states have laws in place requiring youth under age 16 to wear helmets. Other states have different age requirements, and several localities require all ages to wear helmets. At this point in time, there are no states that require people of all ages to wear helmets and only about half of America's children under the age of 15 are covered by a helmet law (Bicycle Helmet Safety Institute 2004; Schieber, Gilchrist, and Sleet 2000).

Despite these efforts, use of bicycle helmets by children and adolescents remains at very low levels in many of our states. The fact that a proven intervention exists (the helmet) but it is widely underutilized, is highly concerning. To date, legislation without education and enforcement has apparently been ineffective. Further progress in this area will likely require heightened levels of community awareness and concern regarding head injury from bicycling.

Winter Sports: Skiing and Snowboarding

Skiing and snowboarding are popular winter sports among children and adolescents, with snowboarding gaining in popularity. Fifty-two-thousand children and adolescents are seen in U.S. hospital emergency departments each year for injuries from winter sports (U.S. Consumer Product Safety Commission 2003b). However, these sports have distinct injury patterns with snowboarding responsible for a larger proportion of head injuries, neck and spinal injuries, upper limb fractures, and foot/ankle injuries than skiing. Skiers commonly experience knee, thumb, and shoulder injuries from falling.

Head injuries account for the majority of deaths and serious injuries in both skiing and snowboarding. The rates of head and spinal injuries in these sports have been on the rise with the advent of increased jumping in both sports (Koehle, Lloyd-Smith, and Taunton 2002). The weight of evidence suggests a positive benefit of helmets in skiing and snowboarding (U.S. Consumer Product Safety Commission 1999; Hagel et al. 2005; Mueller et al. 2008; Sulheim et al. 2006), despite earlier suggestions that helmets may increase the rate of neck injuries (Koehle, Lloyd-Smith, and Taunton 2002) or may lead to an increase in risk-taking behavior (Rees-Jones 1999). Evidence-based recommendations are not yet available; however, for those who choose to wear a helmet, it should be one that conforms to a performance standard such as ASTM F2040 or the Snell Foundation's RS98. As with any helmet, fit is critical; one should be prepared to try on multiple helmets when purchasing or renting.

Knee injuries are common among skiers, but less so among snowboarders. With the advent of the bindings that reliably release when properly adjusted for the skier, lower leg and ankle fracture rates have decreased. Leather alpine boots have been replaced by stiff plastic boots that protect the ankle and lower leg. However, this redistributes forces up to the knee with a dramatic increase in ligamentous injuries to the knee (particularly the ACL). Conventional binding systems release in response to twisting or a forward lean. Newer "multi-release" bindings may also release with a lateral twist at the heel or a backward lean; however, no decrease in ACL injuries in association with these newer bindings has yet been demonstrated.

Another key injury prevention tool in winter sports includes the adjustment of bindings to set what force is necessary to release the boot from the ski or snowboard. Standards have been developed and a device to measure release values is available. Unfortunately, these are not routinely used in ski shops. Inappropriately adjusted bindings have been associated with increased rates of injury in children (Finch and Kelsall 1998; Goulet et al. 1999).

In snowboarding, knee injuries are less common, but the rates of wrist, ankle, and spinal injuries are more common than among skiers. There is strong evidence to support the use of wrist guards to prevent wrist injuries in snowboarding (Machold et al. 2002).

Finally, novice skiers and snowboarders tend to have higher rates of injuries than more experienced participants. Two studies of lessons have been unable to demonstrate a decreased risk of injury in those who participated in lessons. However, inexperienced or novice skiers should consider participating in lessons, and should be supervised until they can reliably perform basic skills. All participants should ski within their ability levels, always maintain control, and adhere to the National Ski Patrol's Responsibility Code (Figure 9.2). This code is an example of measures to increase the safety of all participants and is generally the personal responsibility of each individual participant.

Trampolines

Trampolines, though not commonly used, have a high rate of injury. There are an estimated three million backyard trampolines in use today (U.S. Consumer Product Safety Commission 2000b). CPSC estimates that, among children ages 18 years and under, over 209,000 trampoline-related injuries received medical attention in 2003, of which 96% occurred at home. Sprains and strains along with fractures accounted for 60% of the injuries. Injuries to the lower extremities, head and neck, and upper extremities accounted for 36%, 22%, and 30% of the injury estimates, respectively (U.S. Consumer Product Safety Commission 2000b; Schroeder and Ault 2001). The resulting medical costs alone for these injuries was over $260 million (U.S. Consumer Product Safety Commission 2000b). Because of the high rate of serious or fatal head or neck injuries, the American Academy of Pediatrics recommends that trampolines not be used in the home, outdoor playgrounds, or in routine physical education programs (American

- Always stay in control, and be able to stop or avoid other people or objects.
- People ahead of you have the right of way; it is your responsibility to avoid them.
- You must not stop where you obstruct a trail or are not visible from above.
- When starting downhill or merging into a trail, look uphill and yield to others.
- Always use devices to help prevent runaway equipment.
- Observe all posted warning signs; keep off closed trails and out of closed areas.
- Before using any lift, you must have the knowledge and ability to load, ride, and unload safely.
- Source: National Ski Patrol (http://www.nsp.org/slopesafety/respcode.aspx)

Figure 9.2. National Ski Patrol's Responsibility Code.

Academy of Pediatrics Committee on Injury and Poison Prevention and Committee on Sports Medicine and Fitness 1999).

All-Terrain Vehicles

ATVs are three- or four-wheeled vehicles that were initially intended for use in rural environments where off-road travel was necessary for activities such as farming and logging. Since then, their popularity has gained and they are used widely for recreational purposes. CPSC estimates that over 1700 deaths and over 284,000 emergency department treated injuries have occurred related to ATVs from 1999 to 2001. One third (or 94,000) of these injuries occurred among children under the age of 16 (Ingle 2003). The American Academy of Pediatrics has recommended that no one under the age of 16 use an ATV—as either a driver or passenger.

Thirty percent of all hospitalized ATV injury cases involved youth under age 18 (Helmkamp et al. 2008). Youth are often hurt while riding ATVs on their own; however, incidents involving very young children who are riding ATVs as passengers are not unusual (Helmkamp, O'Hara, and David 1999). Legislation requiring helmet use on ATVs is lacking in most places. Enforcement of these laws is another challenge, as ATV use often occurs on private property or in remote areas that are unlikely to be patrolled.

In the late 1980s, ATV manufacturers entered into consent decrees with CPSC. Among other things, the consent decrees stopped the sale by dealers of three-wheel ATVs, placed engine size restrictions on sales intended for children, and implemented driver training programs. The consent decrees expired in 1998; however, features are still in place voluntarily by major manufacturers. The major ATV manufacturers agreed in consent decrees in 1988 and in subsequent voluntary action plans that engine size restrictions would be placed on ATVs sold for use by children less than 16 years of age. Despite the recommended engine size of 90 cubic centimeters or less for children under 16 years of age, 87% of all emergency department treated injuries in 2001 were related to ATVs of a larger engine size for this age group (Levenson 2003).

In recent years, ATV injury estimates have been at or have approached injury levels seen prior to the consent decrees. Nationwide, pediatric hospitalizations for ATV injuries have increased 150% from 1618 in 1997 to 4039 in 2006 (Bowman and Aitken 2010). Across all age groups, hospitalized ATV injury cases increased 90% over the 5-year period from 2000 to 2004 (Helmkamp et al. 2008). Increases in the number of ATV riders, hours of ATV riding, and number of ATVs in use have also increased during this time. However, the increase in exposure to ATVs does not completely account for the rise in injuries (Levenson 2003).

In an attempt to reverse the rising rates of ATV injury, West Virginia enacted legislation in 2004 that regulated ATV use (Haddy et al. 2008). Part of this statute required helmet use and training for ATV riders aged <18 years. However, the ATV-related death rate in the state among children did not decline, and total ATV-related traffic fatalities increased from 0.72 per 100,000 population in 2004, to 1.32 in 2006 (Haddy et al. 2008). It appears that safety recommendations and regulations are widely ignored by ATV users. A survey of 228 children at agricultural fairs revealed that high-risk driving behavior among children operating ATVs is highly prevalent, and safety recommendations were largely ignored (Campbell et al. 2010).

In-Line Skating/Roller Sports

Many children and adolescents participate in roller sports, including skateboarding, riding scooters, roller skating and in-line skating. Much of this activity is recreational in nature, but some is conducted in a team situation, such as in the case of roller hockey. In recent years, in-line skating has gained popularity among people of all ages, as it can be a good form of aerobic exercise as well as a convenient mode of transportation. Skateboarding and riding scooters have recently regained popularity. As with many other sports and recreational activities, the rise in participation has come with a rise in injuries. Scooter and in-line skating injuries tend to occur more often among youth between the ages of 5 and 12 years, whereas skateboarding injuries occur more often among teenage youth (Powell and Tanz 2004).

Some of the injury patterns for roller sports mirror those of bicycling injuries, because both activities involve the possibility of traveling at high speeds. Both activities come with the possibility of falling as well as colliding with other objects, either stationary or moving. Deaths due to in-line skating are rare, and similar to bicycling fatalities, the majority are due to collisions with motor vehicles (American Academy of Pediatrics Committee on Injury and Poison Prevention and Committee on Sports Medicine and Fitness 1998). Separating the skaters from traffic is an obvious step in reducing fatalities and serious injuries. With regard to scooters, a study at a Pittsburgh hospital found that most nonmotorized scooter injuries were due to falls and 26% were due to collisions with motor vehicles (Gaines, Shultz, and Ford 2004). More recently, motorized scooters, which are similar to nonpowered scooters but sport a small gasoline engine or electric motor and a battery, have been gaining in popularity. Although most injury data on scooters focus on nonpowered scooters, CPSC estimates that in 2000, there were over 4000 emergency room visits as a result of motorized scooters. They recommend that children under 12 should not ride motorized scooters (Office of Information and Public Affairs, U.S. Consumer Product Safety Commission 2001).

As with other sports and recreational injuries, the majority of injuries due to roller sports are not fatal. Wrists are most commonly injured, although knees and elbows are common injury sites as well. Wrist guards, knee pads, and elbow pads have proven effective in protecting in-line skaters against injuries (Schieber et al. 1996) and are recommended for all roller activities. The importance of helmets cannot be underestimated.

Equestrian

Equestrian injuries are an important sports- and recreation-related injury among children and young adults. More than 30 million people worldwide ride horses on a regular basis, and 15 million of those individuals are under the age of 13 (Bixby-Hammett 1987). Along with this intense interest in riding horses comes the risk of injury. Many horse owners are under the age of 20. CPSC estimates that there were approximately 78,500 horseback riding injuries seen in hospital emergency departments across the country, of which nearly 40% occurred among individuals between the ages of 0 and 24 years, and 19% occurred among children 0–14 years (U.S. Consumer Product Safety Commission 2009).

Equestrian activities are of particular concern because the horse may weigh up to 500 kg (1100 lbs), move at a speed of 65 km/h (40 mph), kick with a force of nearly 1 ton, and have its rider 3 meters above the ground (Ball et al. 2007). The most serious injuries occur when a rider is thrown from a horse. Riders are also at risk when dismounting. Finally, other activities besides riding, for example, grooming, pose dangers such as being kicked (Ghosh et al. 2000).

The American Academy of Pediatrics has stated that education programs are needed emphasizing risk and preventive methods (such as those offered by the United States Pony Club). Such programs emphasize risks involved in horseback riding and methods to minimize them. Parents need to verify that the horses their children ride are matched with riding capabilities; riding activities should be supervised and commensurate with the skill of the rider.

All riders should wear helmets that meet the 1988 American Society for Testing and Materials (ASTM) standards and are certified by the Safety Equipment Institute (SEI). The helmets should be secured with appropriate chin straps. All organizations and activities (e.g., riding schools, horse shows, rodeos) that promote or sanction horseback riding events should require entrants to use SEI-certified helmets. Riders also should wear properly fitted boots and nonskid gloves, wear tighter clothing, regularly maintain and inspect equipment, replace working parts, and use appropriately sized stirrups (Centers for Disease Control and Prevention 1990). It is also prudent that riders should be trained by experienced instructors who themselves have completed accredited horse safety courses, emphasize safe riding techniques, and wear helmets when around horses.

Risk and Protective Factors

Due to physical, cognitive, and behavioral differences, children are more susceptible to certain kinds of injury than adults. For example, it is widely believed that prior to puberty, children do not adjust to heat as well, putting them at greater risk for heat-related injuries (Adirim and Cheng 2003; Purvis and Burke 2001). Growing cartilage in young children may be more vulnerable to stresses (such as overuse injuries). Children have proportionately bigger heads than adults with a higher center of gravity and possibly immature balance and coordination, which can lead to increased risk of loss of balance and more falls (Adirim and Cheng 2003). Younger children tend to sustain more head injuries and more frequent injuries to upper extremities in general than older children or adults (Purvis and Burke 2001), perhaps due to their higher center of gravity. Given their smaller size/mass, children generate less force than adults in a fall; however, as children grow stronger and heavier, they generate greater acceleration and thus greater forces. This, combined with the increased competitiveness that often comes with higher levels of play, puts older children at greater risk for contact injuries. Appropriate matching of competitors so that children of similar size, strength, and skill are competitors may help reduce injuries in contact sports, but can be challenging to implement, since children do not grow in uniform amounts at predetermined ages and most competition stratification is by age, gender, and skill (Dyment 1991).

Developmental level may play a role in injury risk. In general, children younger than age 10 years have less-developed motor skills than older children (Adirim and Cheng 2003). This, combined with less developed cognitive and perceptive skills, also puts children at greater risk than adults. Children might be less capable than adults of perceiving risks (e.g., less attention to inputs from peripheral vision) and assessing those risks in certain situations (Schieber and Thompson 1996). Young children may not be capable of fully understanding the need for certain rules and skills of a sport, regardless of the fact that they are being taught by a coach (American

Academy of Pediatrics Committee on Sports Medicine and Fitness and Committee on School Health 2001).

Fitness and conditioning also are related to injury risk. Studies in adults demonstrate a relationship between lower levels of physical fitness and injury (Bixler and Jones 1992), although this has not been thoroughly examined in children. Sports or activity-specific skills, regardless of one's level of fitness, may be protective of injury. For instance, appropriate tackling technique is important in preventing injuries in football and soccer. Correct biomechanics also play a role in baseball, softball, and many other activities. However, in several limited studies of bicycle safety education and skiing lessons, there was no demonstrated effect of skills training on injury rates. However, all participants should make use of available resources to learn the necessary skills and to ensure appropriate biomechanics before undertaking activities independently. Furthermore, as skill level rises, so does likely access to higher and more elite levels of competition. These more elite levels generally embody greater intensity of competition, which once again creates the potential for increased injury risk.

Overall, boys have higher rates of injury than girls; however, certain specific injuries (e.g., ACL injuries) have a higher incidence among girls. Children aged 0–4 years have the lowest rate of injuries due to sports and recreation compared to all other age groups (Gotsch et al. 2002). This is likely due to minimal exposure to such activities. Among boys, those aged 15–24 years are at highest risk of sport- and recreation-related injuries, whereas among girls the risk is highest among 5- to 14-year-olds (Gotsch et al. 2002). Overall, unlike other causes of injury, White youth seem to get injured (or seek medical attention) as a result of sports and recreational injuries more often than Black youth (Conn, Annest, and Gilchrist 2003; Ni, Barnes, and Hardy 2002). Additionally, children from nonpoor households have a higher rate of injuries than children from near-poor and poor households (Ni, Barnes, and Hardy 2002).

Finally, intrinsic psychosocial and behavioral characteristics of the individual (risk taking, sensation seeking) may contribute to injury risk. Those prone to engaging in risky behaviors, such as extreme sports, might be more likely to place themselves in situations that expose them to higher risks. Sports and recreational activities certainly allow participants to push their physical limits; the amount that each participant is willing to push forward contributes to injury risk.

Interventions to Reduce Injuries, Including Research Endeavors

Most injury prevention interventions have focused on behavioral, environmental, or policy change. Behavioral interventions are those that involve a participant making a change to decrease risk of injury, such as improving conditioning, wearing protective gear appropriately and consistently, or choosing activities or locations to minimize risk of injury (e.g., riding on a bicycle path rather than in the road with traffic). Environmental interventions are those that alter the environment in which athletes participate. Examples include building bicycle paths, improving field conditions and padding, or removing obstacles near the area of play. Finally, policy changes can have broad effects in encouraging changes to reduce injury risks. Policy changes may be limited to a particular team or group (e.g., all bicycle club members must wear helmets on club rides), or may include legislation that includes all members of the population (e.g., state or local bicycle helmet laws). A refinement of a previously developed Haddon Matrix (a useful conceptual tool for organizing intervention activities) for youth sports injury is shown in Table 9.1.

In organized sports, coaching quality and behavioral characteristics are widely assumed to be important. Coaches at the youth level should emphasize building the skills of the sport and enjoyment of participation over winning. Most organized sports have training and certification programs for coaches.

Table 9.1. Haddon Matrix for Youth Recreational and Sports Injury

	Host (Athlete)	Agent/Vehicle (Energy)	Physical Environment (Playing Field)	Social Environment (Team/Coach/School/Parents)
Pre-event (before the injury)	Appropriateness of the activity to the skills of the child Recognition of injury risk factors	Visibility of child (reflective materials)	Condition, design, maintenance, and lighting of playing surfaces	Support for defined play areas (skateboard parks, playgrounds) Attitudes toward competition Restriction of dangerous play Neuromuscular training programs
Event (during the injury event)	Physical characteristics (joint laxity, physique) Response time during the event	Energy-absorbing equipment and surfaces Protective equipment appropriate to the activity	Surfacing (artificial or natural) Padding (e.g., on goalposts)	Monitoring of children by parents and others Financial support for certified athletic trainers at all sporting events
Post-event (after the injury)	Conditioning Adherence to rehabilitation Parental management of rehabilitation compliance	Reporting and replacing faulty equipment	Ensure emergency medical personnel have access to environment	Quick and appropriate response Access to appropriate clinicians trained in sports and recreational injuries (team physician, certified athletic trainer) Careful management of concussions Information to make return-to-play decisions and parental support

Source: Adapted from Weaver, Marshall, Miller (2002).

Behavioral Interventions

Behavioral interventions often occur at the level of the individual. These are interventions that each participant can choose whether or not to adopt. Appropriate decisionmaking can be influenced by parents, coaches, social norms, educational campaigns, policies, and legislation. For instance, research in football and soccer shows that strengthening, conditioning, and balance training can reduce injuries (MacKay et al. 2004; Gilchrist et al. 2008). However, it is not clear how to effectively promote the use of these interventions and encourage their adoption by coaches and other adults. Behavioral research is needed in this area.

Additionally, research in military basic trainees demonstrates that those with higher levels of aerobic physical fitness are less likely to be injured compared to those who are less fit (Bixler and Jones 1992; National Research Council 2006, pp. 80–85). Again, behavioral research on how to promote physical fitness and conditioning as a safety intervention in physically active children is needed.

Other effective behavioral interventions include the use of certain protective equipment. This is particularly relevant in recreational activities or unorganized sporting activities where policies and regulations may not be present to require the appropriate use of gear. For instance, bicycle helmets are extremely effective in preventing head and brain injuries (Rivara et al. 1998). This evidence has led to state laws covering many or most of the children in 21 states and the District of Columbia, and many other cities and counties, as of November 2010 (available at http://www.bhsi.org/mandator.htm). However, enforcement of these laws has been historically weak or nonexistent. Thus, youth riders still essentially choose whether or not to wear a helmet each time they ride, even in the regions where it is mandated.

Other equipment such as elbow pads and wrist guards are recommended for those participating in small-wheeled sports such as roller skating, in-line skating, and skateboarding (Schieber et al. 1996; Schieber, Branche-Dorsey, and Ryan 1994). Most sports with an organized component have recommended or required protective equipment which participants, even in unorganized settings, should be encouraged to wear. Social support and social norms play an important role in motivating and reinforcing safety behaviors (Weaver, Marshall, and Miller 2002). For example, youth are influenced by seeing their parents or peers using protective gear, such as bicycle helmets. Further, they are more likely to engage in behaviors that they perceive as socially desirable (Thompson, Sleet, and Sacks 2002). Thus, parents should communicate positive messages about safety and role model safe behavior. Rewarding children for good behavior can be effective as well.

All protective equipment should be appropriate to the sport and player, be maintained in good condition, fit the player correctly, and be used consistently. In organized sports, use of protective equipment needs to be regulated if it is to be universally implemented. Simply making the equipment available typically does not work, since social pressure inhibits the voluntary usage of protective equipment in sports and recreation. It is very important that children should be properly fitted for protective equipment. Some children may be too small for certain equipment. If the gear does not fit properly or is uncomfortable, children will be less likely to wear it consistently. Additionally, poor-fitting equipment might not offer the proper protection (Adirim and Cheng 2003) and might even endanger the child. Parents and coaches can reduce injury risks for children and youth by ensuring that protective equipment is available, in good condition, fits well, and is used consistently and correctly.

Promotion of skills acquisition can be important in the prevention of injuries. However, studies to assess the injury prevention effects of taking lessons to improve skills have had mixed results. Ski lessons and bicycle skills education have not been associated with a decrease in injury risk in research studies (MacKay et al. 2004). However, football coaches who instruct in proper technique, are older, have advanced degrees, have collegiate playing experience, and utilize assistant coaches have teams with lower injury rates (MacKay et al. 2004; Blyth and Mueller 1974).

Advocating for the principles of sportsmanship and fair play, when combined with good refereeing to ensure compliance with safety rules, can decrease injuries. Studies in football demonstrate the benefit of rules preventing spearing, face tackling, and butt blocking (Mueller and Blyth 1987; Torg et al. 1979; Torg, Vegso, and Sennett 1987), and in hockey, prevention of checking from behind (Watson, Singer, and Sproule 1996).

Finally, participants should take personal responsibility to learn the appropriate skills necessary to participate safely in their chosen activities. For instance, as shown earlier, the National Ski Patrol has a Responsibility Code which is posted on most ski and snowboarding slopes (Figure 9.2). This delineates the tenets that participants must abide by to decrease injury risk for all participants.

Environmental Interventions

Environmental interventions decrease injuries by altering how a participant encounters their surroundings. For instance, many of the serious and fatal injuries suffered by recreational cyclists and pedestrians (such as walkers, joggers, and participants in small-wheeled sports) occur when they encounter motor vehicle traffic. Separation of these participants from the traffic through the use of bike lanes, sidewalks, and walking trails is effective in decreasing injury rates (Retting, Ferguson, and McCartt 2003).

In organized sports, environmental interventions can also reduce injuries. Ensuring that safe and well-maintained sports facilities are available is a fundamental environmental intervention. This includes providing dedicated park areas for children to ride bicycles and skateboards, providing good facilities with adequate lighting for evening and night events (such as evening baseball games), and installing and maintaining quality surfaces for playgrounds and playing fields. Breakaway bases are effective in reducing sliding injuries in male and female athletes at the recreational, collegiate, and professional levels (Janda et al. 1990; Sendre et al. 1994). Other simple interventions include ensuring that the playing fields and courts are free from holes, obstacles, or other tripping hazards; ensuring that goalposts are padded and secured; and providing a space between the legal field of play and seats, bleachers, fences, walls, and other obstacles.

Playing surface is an aspect of the environment that has seen technological progress in recent years. Ground hardness has been identified as a risk factor for lower extremity injuries (Nigg and Segesser 1988; Orchard 2002; Orchard and Powell 2003; Takemura et al. 2007). It appears that the most recent type of artificial surfaces may offer some injury prevention advantage, since they are more yielding than natural grass surfaces, especially in hot, dry conditions (Meyers 2010; Meyers and Barnhill 2004).

Advocating for Policy/Legislation Interventions

Policies and legislation can help ensure that covered groups conform to injury prevention recommendations. These can occur at a variety of levels from rules and policies required to participate with recreational teams and activities to comprehensive legislation mandating certain behaviors under penalty of law. Injury prevention policies and legislation are powerful tools to change the social norm regarding injury prevention behaviors.

The most commonly studied injury prevention policy in sports and recreation is bicycle helmet legislation. Following studies demonstrating the benefit of helmet use, local and state officials began mandating helmet use in some groups through legislative action. The first mandatory helmet use law was passed in 1990 in Victoria, Australia. During the previous decade, safety advocates had conducted multifaceted school and community-based education programs to encourage helmet use, resulting in observed helmet use of 31%. One year after enacting the legislation, observed helmet use increased to 75%; however, bicycle use in children and teens decreased (Centers for Disease Control and Prevention 1993). This experience, and others to follow, suggested several tenets of successful injury prevention programs. Policy and legislative actions should be accompanied by education and enforcement. If these are overlooked, understanding of the necessity of the policy/rule/legislation and the consequences of inaction will be lacking and may result in less than optimal compliance.

In addition to state and local legislative mandates, school and community policies are also important (Barrios et al. 2001). Currently, 97% of middle schools and 99% of high schools have policies in place regarding the appropriate use of gear in interscholastic sports and activities; however, only 79% of middle schools and 86% of high schools have similar policies covering these same sports when played in a physical education class (Kolbe, Kann, and Brener 2001). Increasingly, children are participating in sports and recreational activities outside of the school setting and appropriate policies are necessary to protect the participants.

Recently some states have enacted laws requiring that athletes be removed from participation in sports if they are suspected of having a concussion. Washington was the first state to pass one of these laws, following a tragic event in which a boy named Zackery Lystedt suffered a catastrophic head injury during a middle school football game. Between July 2009 and September 2010, a total of nine states had enacted such laws (Sportsconcussions.org 2011). Although the net effect of such laws is likely to be positive, concern has been expressed that these laws might have the negative effect of discouraging reporting of concussion symptoms by youth athletes. Despite this concern, the trend toward such legislation appears to be accelerating. At the time of writing, federal legislation requiring that schools provide education and training on concussions, and support for recovery of concussed athletes, was under consideration in the U.S. House of Representatives' Committee on Education and Labor.

Strategies for Advocating for Safer Sports and Recreational Activities

Establishing healthy, regular physical activity and exercise at an early age is important in order to prevent obesity-related diseases and other negative health effects in later life (U.S. Department of Health and Human Services 1996g). Increasing the physical fitness and level of physical activity in the population is an important health goal (Office of Disease Prevention and Health Promotion, U.S. Department of Health and Human Services 2009). In general, the risk of physical activity through sports and recreation is greatly outweighed by the benefits. However, as Americans attempt to become more active, they should become more cognizant of the risks associated with the activities in which they choose to engage. They should also be given guidance as to what activities would benefit them the most while minimizing the risk for injury. Injury is a major barrier to the maintenance of physical activity, so it makes sense not just to promote physical activity, but to promote safe physical activity. The public health message should be to exercise safely, not just to exercise. One objective of the federal government's Healthy People 2020 plan is to reduce medically attended sports and recreational injuries by 10% (Office of Disease Prevention and Health Promotion, U.S. Department of Health and Human Services 2009). This is true among young children as well. A serious childhood injury can later impact overall health and fitness through adulthood, both through discouraging maintenance of regular physical activity, and through long-term sequelae of injury such as osteoarthritis.

As we have noted throughout the chapter, many interventions geared at sports and recreational safety have been successfully implemented, which has resulted in safer play for youth and countless saved lives. Football athletes have been outfitted from head to toe, with helmets on their heads and shorter cleats on their shoes. Many public playgrounds all over the country now have softer surfaces

Table 9.2. Resources on Youth Sports Safety

Organization	Web Site	What's There?
CDC	http://www.cdc.gov/concussion	Information toolkits on concussion for athletes, coaches, parents, and teachers
STOP	http://www.stopsportsinjuries.org	Prevention resources for youth sports injury for athletes, parents, and coaches
RIO	http://injuryresearch.net/rio.aspx	Data on high school sports injury
Datalys Center	http://www.datalyscenter.org	Data on collegiate sports injury
SMART	http://www.health.usf.edu/nocms/ medicine/orthopaedic/smart.htm	Youth sports safety in Florida
National Athletic Trainers' Association	http://www.nata.org/health-issues	Information on concussion, heat illness, ACL injury, and back pain
National Center for Catastrophic Sports Injury Research	http://www.unc.edu/depts/nccsi	Data on sports injuries resulting in death and permanent disability
American Academy of Pediatrics	http://www.aappolicy.aappublications.org	Recommendations on the following: Injuries in youth soccer Heat stress Trampolines Youth ice hockey In-line skating injuries Baseball and softball Protective eyewear
National Youth Sports Safety Foundation	http://www.nyssf.org	Newsletter and fact sheets
American Orthopaedic Society for Sports Medicine	http://www.sportsmed.org Under "AOSSM library"	Sports medicine updates: a free downloadable bimonthly newsletter featuring articles on sports medicine
CPSC	http://www.cpsc.gov Under "CPSC Publications"	Reports on the following: ATVs, playgrounds, bicycles, and recreational and sports injuries
National Safe Kids Campaign	http://www.safekids.org	Information on sports, playground, and bicycle injuries

(*continued on next page*)

Table 9.2. *(continued)*

Organization	Web Site	What's There?
National Federation of State High School Associations	http://www.nfhs.org	Data on the numbers of participants in high school sports, by sport and state
National Program for Playground Safety	http://www.uni.edu/playground	Information on safety tips, educational materials, equipment distributors and standards

underneath equipment. All of these interventions began with efforts by individuals who advocated for safety.

For example, in 1990, Howard County, Maryland, became the first jurisdiction in the United States to mandate the use of bicycle helmets for bicyclists younger than 16 years old. This was prompted by the death of two individuals who were students at the same school and were killed as a result of bicycle crashes in two separate incidents. Neither of the victims was wearing a helmet (Scheidt, Wilson, and Stern 1992). After the deaths of their students and classmates, students and teachers at the school became committed to improving bicycle safety in Howard County. They met with lawmakers in their community who worked to draft a bill that required all youth under 16 to wear an approved bicycle helmet while riding in that county. Those who failed to follow the law would be fined. With great support of the community, the bill was passed (Scheidt, Wilson, and Stern 1992). Prior to the law being passed, law enforcement officers worked to educate youth about safety and the importance of helmet use (Cote et al. 1992). Together, the community worked to enact legislation that has led to Howard County having the highest rate of bicycle helmet use in the United States (Cote et al. 1992).

Parents of children are often very concerned about the risk of sports and recreational activities. Currently, no uniform agency exists for distributing risk information on sports and recreational activities to parents. Information comes piecemeal from a variety of agencies and organizations. Parents of injured children have generally been neither vocal nor organized in advocating for increased resources for prevention of sports and recreational injury. Thus, there is a need for professionals in the community to connect the many disparate threads in this area. Schools are a good place to teach and advocate safe behavior. A CDC-sponsored School Health Task Force has made several recommendations on what schools can do to develop, teach, implement, and enforce safety rules (Barrios et al. 2001). Advocacy groups such as the Consumer Federation of America are currently lobbying for a ban on youth ATV use and stricter safety standards at playgrounds. Change often begins with grassroots efforts and a few committed citizens.

There is an urgent need to build the advocate base for youth sports and recreational injury. Parents should be cognizant of their children's activities and seek out information from reputable sources to help their children participate safely. In addition, parents, injury prevention professionals, and other interested parties can work at the local level to encourage local schools, parks, clubs leagues, and other groups to provide the safest possible environment for all participants. Finally, these parties can encourage agencies and organizations at the local, state, and national level to support further prevention research and dissemination efforts.

Building a climate of safety around youth sports and recreation is a delicate balancing act. On the one hand, we want to encourage and promote physical activity in youth. On the other hand, it must be recognized that there are inherent risks in all physical activity, but that these can be minimized through the use of injury control strategies. There are a large number of organizations that actively work to promote safety in youth sports and recreational activities (Table 9.2). These organizations often do not have input from injury prevention professionals and would welcome involvement from this community. Injury prevention professionals can assist these organizations in locating and using data to support the need for change and to evaluate the effects of changes. Additionally, injury prevention professionals should provide guidance to ensure that promoted efforts are scientifically supported.

Conclusion

In the 21st century, it is more important than ever to promote sports and recreational activities for youth and children. Areas of current action include (but are not limited to) education about concussion identification and management, rule changes to protect child and youth athletes, advocacy for bicycle helmets, better regulation of ATV hazards, and improvements in playground design. Through the incorporation of safety messages and injury control measures into these activities, much can be done to ensure that children truly enjoy sports and recreational pastimes and continue to participate in physically active recreational pursuits as they mature into adults.

Acknowledgment

Thanks to Karen Roos, MSPT, ATC, for her assistance in preparing this chapter.

References

Adirim TA, Cheng TL. 2003. Overview of injuries in the young athlete. *Sports Med.* 33:75–81.

Agel J, Dick R, Nelson B, et al. 2007. Descriptive epidemiology of collegiate women's ice hockey injuries: National Collegiate Athletic Association Injury Surveillance System, 2000–2001 through 2003–2004. *J Athl Train.* 42:255–260.

Agel J, Dompier TP, Dick R, Marshall SW. 2007. Descriptive epidemiology of collegiate men's ice hockey injuries: National Collegiate Athletic Association Injury Surveillance System, 1988–1989 through 2003–2004. *J Athl Train.* 42:247–254.

American Academy of Pediatrics. 1996. Protective eyewear for young athletes. *Pediatrics.* 98:311–313.

American Academy of Pediatrics Committee on Injury and Poison Prevention. 2001. Bicycle helmets. *Pediatrics.* 108:1030–1032.

American Academy of Pediatrics Committee on Injury and Poison Prevention and Committee on Sports Medicine and Fitness. 1998. In-line skating injuries in children and adolescents. *Pediatrics.* 101:720–722.

American Academy of Pediatrics Committee on Injury and Poison Prevention and Committee on Sports Medicine and Fitness. 1999. Trampolines at home, school, and recreational centers. *Pediatrics.* 103:1053–1056.

American Academy of Pediatrics Committee on Sports Medicine and Fitness. 1994. Risk of injury from baseball and softball in children 5 to 14 years of age. *Pediatrics.* 93:690–692.

American Academy of Pediatrics Committee on Sports Medicine and Fitness and Committee on School Health. 2001. Organized sports for children and preadolescents. *Pediatrics.* 107:1459–1462.

Andrews J, Fleisig GS. 1998. Preventing throwing injuries. *J Orthop Sports Phys Ther.* 27:187–188.

Ball CG, Ball JE, Kirkpatrick AW, et al. 2007. Equestrian injuries: incidence, injury patterns, and risk factors for 10 years of major traumatic injuries. *Am J Surg.* 193:636–640.

Barrios LC, Desai S, Sleet DA, Sosin DM. 2001. School health guidelines to prevent unintentional injuries and violence. *MMWR Morb Mortal Wkly Rep.* 50:1–46.

Baseball and Softball Council. 1996. *Baseball: A Report on Participation in America's National Pastime.* North Palm Beach, FL: Sporting Goods Manufacturers Association.

Bicycle Helmet Safety Institute. 2004 [rev. September 10, 2011]. *Helmet Laws for Bicycle Riders.* Available at: http://www.helmets.org/mandator.htm. Accessed September 19, 2011.

Binkley HM, Beckett J, Casa DJ, et al. 2002. National Athletic Trainers' Association position statement: exertional heat illnesses. *J Athl Train.* 37:329–343. Available at: http://www.nata.org/NR070810. Accessed September 19, 2011.

Bixby-Hammett DM. 1987. Accidents in equestrian sports. *Am Fam Physician.* 36:209–214.

Bixler B, Jones RL. 1992. High school football injuries: effects of a post-halftime warm-up and stretching routine. *Fam Pract Res J.* 12:131–139.

Blyth CS, Mueller FO. 1974. Football injury survey 3. injury rates vary with coaching. *Phys Sportsmed.* 2:45–50.

Bowman SM, Aitken ME. 2010. Still unsafe, still in use: ongoing epidemic of all-terrain vehicle injury hospitalizations among children. *J Trauma.* [Epub ahead of print].

Campbell BT, Kelliher KM, Borrup K, et al. 2010. All-terrain vehicle riding among youth: how do they fair? *J Pediatr Surg.* 45: 925–929.

Cantu RC. 1992. Cerebral concussion in sport, management and prevention. *Sports Med.* 14:64–74.

Cantu RC, Voy R. 1995. Second impact syndrome: a risk in any contact sport. *Phys Sportsmed.* 23:27–34.

Carlson SA, Hootman JM, Powell KE, et al. 2006. Self-reported injury and physical activity levels: United States 2000 to 2002. *Ann Epidemiol.* 16:712–719.

Centers for Disease Control and Prevention. 1990. Current trends injuries associated with horseback riding—United States, 1987 and 1998. *MMWR Morb Mortal Wkly Rep.* 39:329–332.

Centers for Disease Control and Prevention. 1993. Mandatory bicycle helmet use—Victoria, Australia. *MMWR Morb Mortal Wkly Rep.* 42 (18):359–363.

Centers for Disease Control and Prevention. 1995. Injury-control recommendations: bicycle helmets. *MMWR Morb Mortal Wkly Rep.* 44:1–17.

Centers for Disease Control and Prevention (CDC), Division of Public Health Surveillance and Informatics, Epidemiology Program Office. 2004. CDC Wonder Database. Atlanta, GA: CDC. Available at: http://wonder.cdc.gov. Accessed September 19, 2011.

Comstock RD, Knox C, Yard E, Gilchrist J. 2006. Sports-related injuries among high school athletes—United States, 2005–06 school year. *MMWR Morb Mortal Wkly Rep.* 55:1037–1040.

Conn J, Annest JL, Gilchrist J. 2003. Sports and recreation related injury episodes in the US population, 1997–99. *Inj Prev.* 9:117–123.

Coris E, Ramirez AM, Van Durme DJ. 2004. Heat illness in athletes: the dangerous combination of heat, humidity and exercise. *Sports Med.* 34:9–16.

Cote TR, Sacks JJ, Lambert-Huber DA, et al. 1992. Bicycle helmet use among Maryland children: effect of legislation and education. *Pediatrics.* 89:1216–1220.

Danis RP, Hu K, Bell M, 2000. Acceptability of baseball faceguards and reduction of oculofacial injury in receptive youth league players. *Inj Prev.* 6:232–234.

DeMarco J, Reeves C. 1994. Epidemiologic notes and reports injuries associated with soccer goalposts—United States, 1979–1993. *MMWR Morb Mortal Wkly Rep.* 43:153–155.

Dick R, Agel J, Marshall SW. 2007. National Collegiate Athletic Association Injury Surveillance System commentaries: introduction and methods. *J Athl Train.* 42:173–179.

Dyment PG, editor. 1991. *Sports Medicine: Health Care for Young Athletes.* 2nd ed. Elk Grove Village, IL: American Academy of Pediatrics.

Ewing R, Brown S. 2009. *U.S. Traffic Calming Manual.* Washington, DC: APA Planners Press and American Society of Civil Engineers.

Finch CF, Kelsall HL. 1998. The effectiveness of ski bindings and their professional adjustment for preventing alpine skiing injuries. *Sports Med.* 25:407–416.

Fleisig GS, Andrews JR, Dillman CJ, Escamilla RF. 1995. Kinetics of baseball pitching with implications about injury mechanisms. *Am J Sports Med.* 23:233–239.

Flyger N, Button C, Rishiraj N. 2006. The science of softball: implications for performance and injury prevention. *Sports Med.* 36:797–816.

Gaines BA, Shultz BL, Ford HR. 2004. Nonmotorized scooters: a source of significant morbidity in children. *J Trauma.* 57: 111–113.

Gerberich SG, Finke R, Madden M, et al. 1987. An epidemiological study of high school ice hockey injuries. *Childs Nerv Syst.* 3:59–64.

Ghosh A, Di Scala C, Drew C, et al. 2000. Horse-related injuries in pediatric patients. *J Pediatr Surg.* 35:1766–1770.

Gilchrist J, Haileyesus T, Murphy M, et al. 2010. Heat illness among high school athletes—United States, 2005–2009. *MMWR Morb Mortal Wkly Rep.* 59:1009–1013.

Gilchrist J, Mandelbaum BR, Melancon H, et al. 2008. A randomized controlled trial to prevent noncontact anterior cruciate ligament injury in female collegiate soccer players. *Am J Sports Med.* 36.8:1476–1483.

Gilchrist J, Thomas KE, Wald M, Langlois J. 2007. Nonfatal traumatic brain injuries from sports and recreation activities—United States, 2001–2005. *MMWR Morb Mortal Wkly Rep.* 56:733–737.

Gotsch K, Annest JL, Holmgreen P, Gilchrist J. 2002. Nonfatal sports- and recreation-related injuries treated in emergency departments, United States, July 2000–June 2001. *MMWR Morb Mortal Wkly Rep.* 51:736–740.

Goulet C, Régnier G, Grimard G, et al. 1999. Risk Factors associated with alpine skiing injuries in children: a case-control study. *Am J Sports Med.* 27:644–650.

Griffin L, editor. 2001. *Prevention of Noncontact ACL Injuries.* Rosemont, IL: American Academy of Orthopaedic Surgeons.

Griffin LY, Albohm MJ, Arendt EA, et al. 2006. Understanding and preventing non-contact ACL injuries: a review of the Hunt Valley II Meeting, January 2005. *Am J Sports Med.* 34:1512–1532.

Guskiewicz KM, Marshall SW, Broglio SP, et al. 2002. No evidence of impaired neurocognitive performance in collegiate soccer players. *Am J Sports Med.* 30:157–162.

Guskiewicz KM, McCrea M, Marshall SW, et al. 2003. Cumulative effects associated with recurrent concussion in collegiate football players: the NCAA Concussion Study. *JAMA.* 290:2549–2555.

Haddy L, Light T, Thayer C, et al. 2008. All-terrain vehicle fatalities—West Virginia, 1999–2006. *MMWR Morb Mortal Wkly Rep.* 57:312–315.

Hagel BE, Pless IB, Goulet C, et al. 2005. Effectiveness of helmets in skiers and snowboarders: case-control and case crossover study. *BMJ.* 330:281 [errata 345].

Halstead ME, Walter KD, and The Council on Sports Medicine and Fitness Sport-Related Concussion in Children and Adolescents. 2010. Sport-related concussion in children and adolescents. *Pediatrics.* 126:597–615.

Helmkamp JC, Furbee PM, Coben JH, Tadros A. 2008. All-terrain vehicle-related hospitalizations in the United States, 2000–2004. *Am J Prev Med.* 34:39–45.

Helmkamp JC, O'Hara FJ, David J. 1999. All-terrain vehicle-related deaths—West Virginia, 1985–1997. *MMWR Morb Mortal Wkly Rep.* 48:1–4.

Hootman JM, Dick R, Agel J. 2007. Epidemiology of collegiate injuries for 15 sports: summary and recommendations for injury prevention initiatives. *J Athl Train.* 42:311–319.

Hutchinson M.R. 1997. Cheerleading injuries: patterns, prevention, case reports. *Phys Sportsmed.* 25:83–90.

Ingle R. 2003. *2002 Annual Report of ATV Deaths and Injuries.* Washington, DC: U.S. Consumer Product Safety Commission.

Janda DH, Mackesy D, Maguire R, et al. 1993. Sliding-associated injuries in college and professional baseball—1990–1991. *MMWR Morb Mortal Wkly Rep.* 42:229–230.

Janda DH, Wojtys EM, Hankin FM, Benedict ME. 1988. Softball sliding injuries. a prospective study comparing standard and modified bases. *JAMA.* 259:1848–1850.

Janda DH, Wojtys EM, Hankin FM, et al. 1990. A three-phase analysis of the prevention of recreational softball injuries. *Am J Sports Med.* 18:632–635.

Junge A, Dvorak J. 2004. Soccer injuries: a review on incidence and prevention. *Sports Med.* 34:929–938.

Kirkendall DT, Garrett WE Jr. 2001. Heading in soccer: integral skill or grounds for cognitive dysfunction. *J Athl Train.* 36:328–333.

Koehle MS., Lloyd-Smith R, Taunton JE. 2002. Alpine ski injuries and their prevention. *Sports Med.* 32:785–793.

Kolbe LJ, Kann L, Brener ND. 2001. Overview and summary of findings: School Health Policies and Programs Study 2000. *J Sch Health.* 71:253–259.

Kyle S.B. 1996.*Consumer Product Safety Commission Youth Baseball Protective Equipment Project Final Report.* Washington, DC: U.S. Consumer Product Safety Commission, Office of Information and Public Affairs.

Labella CR, Smith BW, Sigurdsson A. 2002. Effect of mouthguards on dental injuries and concussions in college basketball. *Med Sci Sports Exerc.* 34:41–44.

Levenson, M. 2003. *All-Terrain Vehicle 2001 Injury and Exposure Studies.* Washington, DC: U.S. Consumer Product Safety Commission.

Link MS, Wang PJ, Pandian NG, et al. 1998. An experimental model of sudden death due to low-energy chest-wall impact (comotio cordis). *New Engl J Med.* 339:1805–1811.

Lohmander LS, Englund PM, Dahl LL, Roos EM. 2007. The long-term consequence of anterior cruciate ligament and meniscus injuries: osteoarthritis. *Am J Sports Med.* 35:1756–1769.

Machold W, Kwasny O, Eisenhardt P, et al. 2002. Reduction of severe wrist injuries in snowboarding by an optimized wrist protection device: a prospective randomized trial. *J Trauma.* 52:517–520.

MacKay M, Scanlan A, Olsen L, et al. 2004. Looking for the evidence: a systematic review of prevention strategies addressing sport and recreational injury among children and youth. *J Sci Med Sport.* 7:58–73.

Maron BJ, Poliac LC, Kaplan JA, Mueller FO. 1995. Blunt impact to the chest leading to sudden death from cardiac arrest during sports activities. *New Engl J Med.* 333:337–342.

Marshall SW, Golightly YM. 2007. Sports injury and arthritis. *N C Med J.* 68:430–433.

Marshall SW, Guskiewicz KM. 2003. Sports and recreational injury: the hidden cost of a healthy lifestyle. *Inj Prev.* 9:100–102.

Marshall SW, Mueller FO, Kirby DT, Yang J. 2003. Evaluation of safety balls and face guards to prevent injury in youth baseball. *JAMA.* 289:568–574.

Matser EJ, Kessels AG, Lezak MD, et al. 1999. Neuropsychological impairment in amateur soccer players. *JAMA.* 282:971–973.

Meyers MC. 2010. Incidence, mechanisms, and severity of game-related college football injuries on FieldTurf versus natural grass: a 3-year prospective study. *Am J Sports Med.* 38:687–697.

Meyers M, Barnhill BS. 2004. Incidence, causes, and severity of high school football injuries on FieldTurf versus natural grass: a 5-year prospective study. *Am J Sports Med.* 32:1626–1638.

Mihalik JP, Blackburn JT, Greenwald RM, et al. 2010. Collision type and player anticipation affect head impact severity among youth ice hockey players. *Pediatrics.* 125:e1394–e1401.

Mueller BA, Cummings P, Rivara FP, et al. 2008. Injuries of the head, face, and neck in relation to ski helmet use. *Epidemiology.* 9:270–276.

Mueller FO, Blyth CS. 1987. Fatalities from head and cervical spine injuries occurring in tackle football: 40 years' experience. *Clin Sports Med.* 6:185–196.

Mueller FO, Cantu RC. 2007. National Center for Catastrophic Sport Injury Research. *National Center for Catastrophic Sport Injury Research 21st Annual Report. January 5*. Chapel Hill: University of North Carolina.

Mueller FO, Cantu RC. 2011. National Center for Catastrophic Sport Injury Research. Available at: http://www.unc.edu/depts/nccsi. Accessed March 1, 2011.

Mueller FO, Marshall SW, Kirby D. 2001. Injuries in Little League Baseball 1987–1996. *Phys Sportsmed.* 29:41–48.

Myklebust G, Engebretsen L, Braekken IH, et al. 2003. Prevention of anterior cruciate ligament injuries in female team handball players: a prospective intervention study over three seasons. *Clin J Sport Med.* 1:71–78.

National Center for Health Statistics. 2003. *2001 Multiple Cause-of-Death File.* Hyattsville, MD: U.S. Department of Health and Human Services, Centers for Disease Control and Prevention, National Center for Health Statistics.

National Federation of State High School Associations. 2010. High school participation data. Available at: http://www.nfhs.org/content.aspx?id=3282&linkidentifier=id&itemid=3282. Accessed December 1, 2010.

National Program for Playground Safety. 2005. *Keep Your Children Safe: A Checklist for Parents.* Available at: http://www.uni.edu/playground. Accessed September 19, 2011.

National Research Council, Committee on Youth Population and Military Recruitment. 2006. *Assessing Fitness for Military Enlistment: Physical, Medical, and Mental Health Standards.* Sackett PR, Mavor AS, editors. Board on Behavioral, Cognitive, and Sensory Sciences, Division of Behavioral and Social Sciences and Education. Washington, DC: National Academies Press.

Ni H, Barnes P, Hardy AM. 2002. Recreational injury and its relation to socioeconomic status among school aged children in the US. *Inj Prev.* 8:60–65.

Nigg BM, Segesser B. 1988. The influence of playing surfaces on the load on the locomotor system and on football and tennis injuries. *Sports Med.* 5:375–385.

Norton C, Nixon J, Sibert JR. 2004. Playground injuries to children. *Arch Dis Child.* 89:103–108.

O'Brien CW. 2009. *Injuries and Investigated Deaths Associated With Playground Equipment, 2001–2008.* Washington, DC: U.S. Consumer Product Safety Commission. Available at: http://www.cpsc.gov/LIBRARY/FOIA/FOIA10/os/playground.pdf. Accessed September 19, 2011.

Office of Disease Prevention and Health Promotion, U.S. Department of Health and Human Services-Healthy People 2020, November 3, 2009. Healthy People 2020 Objective Topic Areas. http://healthypeople.gov/2020/topicsobjectives2020/pdfs/HP2020objectives.pdf, Accessed March 1, 2011.

Office of Information and Public Affairs, U.S. Consumer Product Safety Commission. Motorized scooter use increases and injuries climb [released August 22, 2001]. Washington, DC: News from CPSC, U.S. Consumer Product Safety Commission.

Orchard J. 2002. Is there a relationship between ground and climatic conditions and injuries in football? *Sports Med.* 32:419–532.

Orchard JW, Powell JW. 2003. Risk of knee and ankle sprains under various weather conditions in American football. *Med Sci Sports Exerc.* 35:1118–1123.

Pasternack JS, Veenema KR, Callahan CM. 1996. Baseball injuries: a Little League survey. *Pediatrics.* 98:445–448.

Pollack KM, Canham-Chervak M, Gazal-Carvalho C, et al. 2005. Interventions to prevent softball related injuries: a review of the literature. *Inj Prev.* 11:277–281.

Powell EC, Tanz RR. 2004. Incidence and description of scooter-related injuries among children. *Ambul Pediatr.* 4:495–499.

Purvis JM, Burke RG. 2001. Recreational injuries in children: incidence and prevention. *J Am Acad Orthop Surg.* 9:365–374.

Rader BG. 1992. *Baseball: A History of America's Game.* Urbana, IL: University of Illinois Press.

Rees-Jones A. 1999. Skiing helmets. 1999. *Br J Sports Med.* 33:3.

Retting RA, Ferguson SA, McCartt AT. 2003. A review of evidence-based traffic engineering measures designed to reduce pedestrian–motor vehicle crashes. *Am J_Public Health.* 93:1456–1463.

Reynen PD, Clancy JG. 1994. Cervical spine injury, hockey helmets, and face masks. *Am J Sports Med.* 22:167–170.

Rivara FP, Thompson DC, Patterson MQ, Thompson RS. 1998. Prevention of bicycle related injuries: helmets, legislation, and education. *Annu Rev Public Health.* 19:293–318.

Robey JM, Blyth CS, Mueller FO. 1971. Athletic injuries: application of epidemiologic methods. *JAMA.* 217:184–189.

Rodgers GB. 2000. Bicycle and bicycle helmet use patterns in the United States in 1998. *J Safety Res.* 31:149–158.

Sane J, Ylipaavalniemi P, Leppanen H. 1988. Maxillofacial and dental ice hockey injuries. *Med Sci Sports Exerc.* 20:202–207.

Scanlan A, MacKay A, Reid D, et al. 2001. *Sports and Recreation Injury Prevention Strategies: Systematic Review and Best Practices.* Ottawa, Ontario: Children's Hospital of Eastern Ontario Research Institute. Available at: http://www.injuryresearch.bc.ca/Publications/Reports/SportSystematicReport.pdf. Accessed September 19, 2011.

Scheidt P, Wilson MH, Stern MS. 1992. Bicycle helmet law for children: a case study of activism in injury control. *Pediatrics.* 89:1248–1250.

Schieber RA, Branche-Dorsey CM, Ryan GW. 1994. Comparison of in-line skating injuries with roller-skating and skateboarding injuries. *JAMA.* 271:1856–1858.

Schieber RA, Branche-Dorsey CM, Ryan GW, et al. 1996. Risk factors for injuries from in-line skating and the effectiveness of safety gear. *New Engl J. Med.* 335:1630–1635.

Schieber RA, Gilchrist J, Sleet DA. 2000. Legislative and Regulatory Strategies to Reduce Childhood Unintentional Injuries. *Future Child.* 10:111–136.

Schieber RA, Thompson NJ. 1996. Developmental risk factors for childhood pedestrian injuries. *Inj Prev.* 2:228–236.

Schroeder T, Ault K. 2001. *The NEISS Sample (Design and Implementation) From 1997 to the Present.* Washington, DC: U.S. Consumer Product Safety Commission.

Schulz MR, Marshall SW, Yang J, et al. 2004. A prospective cohort study of injury incidence and risk factors in North Carolina high school competitive cheerleaders. *Am J Sports Med.* 32:396–405.

Sendre RA, Keating TM, Hornak JE, Newitt PA. 1994. Use of the Hollywood impact base and standard stationary base to reduce sliding and base-running injuries in baseball and softball. *Am J Sports Med.* 22:450–453.

Singh S, Smith GA, Fields SK, McKenzie LB. 2008. Gymnastics-related injuries to children treated in emergency departments in the United States 1990–2005. *Pediatrics.* 121:e954–e960.

Sitler M, Ryan J, Wheeler B, et al. 1994. The efficacy of a semirigid ankle stabilizer to reduce acute ankle injuries in basketball. A randomized clinical study at West Point. *Am J Sports Med.* 22:454–461.

Sportsconcussions.org. Available at: http://www.sportsconcussions.org. Accessed March 1, 2011.

Sulheim S, Holme I, Ekeland A, Bahr R. 2006. Helmet use and risk of head injuries in alpine skiers and snowboarders. *JAMA.* 295:919–924.

Takemura M, Schneiders AG, Bell ML, et al. 2007. Association of ground hardness with injuries in rugby union. *BR J Sports Med.* 41:582–587.

Thompson DC, Rivara FP, Thompson RS. 1996. Effectiveness of bicycle safety helmets in preventing head injuries. A case-control study. *JAMA.* 276:1968–1973.

Thompson NJ, Sleet D, Sacks JJ. 2002. Increasing the use of bicycle helmets: lessons from behavioral science. *Patient Educ Couns.* 46:191–197.

Thompson RS, Rivara FP, Thompson DC. 1989. A case-control study of the effectiveness of bicycle safety helmets. *New Engl J Med.* 320:1361–1367.

Tinsworth DK, McDonald JE. 2001. *Special Study: Injuries and Deaths Associated With Children's Playground Equipment.* Washington, DC: U.S. Consumer Product Safety Commission.

Torg JS, Truex R Jr, Quedenfeld TC, et al. 1979. The National Football Head and Neck Injury Registry: report and conclusions 1978. *JAMA.* 241:1477–1479.

Torg JS, Vegso JJ, Sennett B. 1987. The National Football Head and Neck Injury Registry: 14-year report on cervical quadriplegia (1971–1984). *Clin Sports Med.* 6:61–72.

U.S. Consumer Product Safety Commission. 1995. *Guidelines for Movable Soccer Goal Safety.* Washington, DC: U.S. Consumer Product Safety Commission.

U.S. Consumer Product Safety Commission. 1999. *Skiing Helmets: An Evaluation of the Potential to Reduce Head Injury.* Washington, DC: U.S. Consumer Product Safety Commission.

U.S. Consumer Product Safety Commission, Directorate for Economic Analysis. 2000a. *The Consumer Product Safety Commission's Revised Injury Cost Model.* Washington, DC: U.S. Consumer Product Safety Commission.

U.S. Consumer Product Safety Commission. 2000b. *Trampolines.* Washington, DC: U.S. Consumer Product Safety Commission.

U.S. Consumer Product Safety Commission. 2003a. *Handbook for Public Playground Safety.* Washington, DC: U.S. Consumer Product Safety Commission.

U.S. Consumer Product Safety Commission. 2003b. *NEISS Coding Manual, 2003: National Electronic Injury Surveillance System.* Washington, DC: U.S. Consumer Product Safety Commission.

U.S. Consumer Product Safety Commission. 2010. *NEISS Data Highlights—2009.* Washington, DC: U.S. Consumer Product Safety Commission. Available at: http://www.cpsc.gov/neiss/2009highlights.pdf. Accessed December 1, 2010.

U.S. Department of Health and Human Services. 1996. *Physical Activity and Health. A Report of the Surgeon General.* Atlanta, GA: Centers for Disease Control and Prevention, National Center for Chronic Disease Prevention and Health Promotion. Available at: http://www.cdc.gov/nccdphp/sgr/sgr.htm. Accessed September 19, 2011.

U.S. Department of Health and Human Services. 2010. *Trends in the Prevalence of Obesity, Dietary Behaviors, and Weight Control Practices. National YRBS: 1991–2009.* Atlanta, GA: Centers for Disease Control and Prevention, National Center for Chronic Disease Prevention and Health Promotion, Division of Adolescent and School Health. Available at: http://www.cdc.gov/healthyYouth/yrbs/pdf/us_physical_trend_yrbs.pdf. Accessed September 19, 2011.

Vinger PF, Leonard P, Alfaro DV, et al. 1997. Shatter resistance of spectacle lenses. *JAMA.* 277:142–144.

Watson RC, Singer CD, Sproule JR. 1996. Checking from behind in ice hockey: a study of injury and penalty data in the Ontario University Athletic Association Hockey League. *Clin J Sport Med.* 6:108–111.

Weaver NL, Marshall SW, Miller MD. 2002. Preventing sports injuries: opportunities for intervention in youth athletics. *Patient Educ Couns.* 46:199–204.

Zvijac J, Thompson W. Basketball. 1996. In:Caine DJ, Caine CG, Lindner KJ, editors. *Epidemiology of Sports Injuries.* Champaign, IL: Human Kinetics. 86–97.

Chapter 10

Water-Related Injuries of Children and Adolescents

Linda Quan, MD,[1] Karen D. Liller, PhD,[2] and Elizabeth Bennett, MPH, MCHES[3]

The Tragedy That Befell Preston Thomas de Ibern[4]

Of all the unexpected twists and turns that life presents, none could have been more amazing, more thrilling, or more unexpected than finding out I was pregnant for the first time (after 18 years of marriage)! We named our precious son Preston Thomas de Ibern.

Returning to work and a new career as Preston was soon to start kindergarten, I was invited to a co-worker's barbeque party on the July 4th weekend of 1995. What could be better than a dip in the pool, a fresh-grilled burger, and making new friends on a sultry Florida day like this? Who would have thought that everything in our lives was about to change?

Soon everyone was leaving. The lady of the house invited me for a tour of their new home before we left. I told my boys to go change their clothes so off they went, along with the owner's children.

Everyone had come inside; no one was outside by the pool. The lady of the house showed me the bedroom furniture and their new roman tub, then we walked across the house, past the husbands chatting in the dining room, and over to the kids room. My older son Josh and the owner's little boy were getting ready to play a Nintendo game. I didn't see Preston with the boys. Immediately, I called, "where is Preston?" Suddenly, I felt panicky and started to scan the surroundings, calling frantically. In horror and total dismay, my eyes fell upon what appeared to be something floating out in the pool. I screamed and Preston's dad leaped from the chair, lunged into the pool and handed up our son. His eyes and lips were blue and his little body was limp and lifeless. The neighbors all heard my screams and someone called 911. Preston's father and a nurse who lived nearby performed CPR, to no avail. The paramedics were there within minutes. Everyone peered at the paramedics as they worked feverishly. Frozen in place, I watched the oxygen mask go on, needles injected into his arms and legs and finally he was shocked with paddles several times. Minutes became an eternity until . . . finally . . . they had a breath!

By now there were people everywhere as the stretcher was rushed to the waiting helicopter. Stunned, I stood glaring as the helicopter lifted off. The world seemed to move in slow motion as we made the long trek to the children's hospital. Like robots in motion, our bodies moved but no words were spoken. Suddenly, everything that was important in life no longer mattered. I felt as if I were in a long, dark, empty tunnel with a million of my own thoughts rushing through my mind. How did this happen? Why did this happen? Would Preston survive . . . would he be normal?

[1]University of Washington School of Medicine, Seattle, Washington.

[2]University of South Florida Graduate School and College of Public Health, Tampa, Florida.

[3]Seattle Children's Hospital, Seattle, Washington.

[4]As told by his mother, Carole Y. de Ibern.

We arrived at the hospital to find Preston in a room with machines beeping, attached by wires to his body. He lay there motionless, eyes closed. I had to remind myself to breathe. We were informed that he was in a coma and was not expected to live more than 72 hours. The doctors tried their best to encourage us to shut off the machines but I could not. I promised God that if He allowed Preston to live, I would do everything possible to help him have the best life he could have. I would love him unconditionally and I would find a way to give his life purpose and meaning.

At the age of 5, Preston had a whole world of opportunities ahead of him. All of that changed in the 3 to 5 minutes that doctors estimate he was under water. There was a swollen, bruised area above his left eyebrow. It appears that he ran out to put a toy in the toy box, where he slipped and fell, bumped his head and rolled into the water, unconscious. Preston survived but his brain was devastated. He would never walk again nor would he utter a single word for the rest of his life. He would never again eat by mouth. It took nearly 6 months of therapy for vision to return though he eventually could see well enough to enjoy watching movies on TV. His body was racked with posturing, seizures, severe respiratory problems, and a multitude of other complex problems. He required total care around the clock. I quit my job to stay at his side and care for him.

Having endured seven and a half years of numerous hospitalizations, as many as 21 medications daily, constant therapies, and 15 pneumonias, his tired weak body could no longer fight. On December 2, 2000, the angels carried Preston to Heaven. He was 12 years old.

I never forgot the promise I made to God that day. It wasn't long after Preston's accident that I started finding out that there were many other near-drowning victims, all of them profoundly handicapped. I discovered that an average of 75 perfectly healthy, normal children, under the age of 5, were drowning and nearly four times that many were near-drowning victims every year. I realized that there was no turning back or changing what happened. All I could do was to try to stop it from happening to other children and spare their families the suffering and grief that my family knew so intimately. I could not believe that Florida could have well over a million backyard pools and no statewide legislation to protect our children. In 1996, with Preston by my side, I started to research and pursue legislation. I had never been involved in politics and had no clue that there could possibly be such adversity in trying to save the lives of little children. Appalled at the apathy I had encountered, I became driven. In 1997, I was introduced to Representative Debbie Wasserman Schultz, a Florida congresswoman who was working on pool safety legislation. Together, we began lobbying the legislature to adopt a bill that would address pool safety. The controversial bill met with a great deal of adversity and was almost immediately diluted. With perseverance and determination, Representative Wasserman Schultz, Preston and I, Kathy Ward (whose only grandchild, MacKenzie Merriam, drowned at age 1), and others worked diligently to finally get the bill passed on May 5, 2000. Each time that I testified before the House and/or Senate, Preston was by my side. The bill was given the name "Preston de Ibern/MacKenzie Merriam Residential Pool Safety Act."

Now that you have had a glimpse into the personal life of Preston and his family, my hope is that you will walk away and never forget his story. I want you to realize that this can happen to anyone wherever there are unprotected swimming pools. The fact is that until and unless we have constant and continuing awareness programs, more stringent legislation which addresses all pools and spas (including those built before October 2000), and until we change the attitudes of consumers, we will continue to lose our most precious resources . . . our children. Please do all that you can to keep our children safe![5]

[5]*Editor's Note:* We decided to once again publish the above injury scenario in this second edition, because of its poignant and moving depiction of the tragedy of child drowning and of how resulting advocacy can lead to successful and uplifting outcomes.

Overview of Mortality and Morbidity

Worldwide, drowning is the major cause of injury death to children (Peden and McGee 2003). Drowning is defined as the process of experiencing respiratory impairment from submersion/immersion in liquid (Idris et al. 2003). In the United States, it is the second major cause of unintentional death in children younger than 15 years, third in unintentional deaths among those aged 15 to 34 years, and remains in the top ten causes of unintentional deaths of those over 35 years (Centers for Disease Control and Prevention 2010b).

The most common "vehicle" involved in drowning is water. In a review of 496 unintentional childhood drowning deaths submitted to the National SAFE KIDS Campaign, 39% occurred in pools, 37% occurred in open bodies of water (such as lakes, rivers, and ponds), and 18% occurred in and around the home, in places such as bathtubs, buckets, and spas (Cody et al. 2004). In one review, 32% of drownings among those younger than 18 years occurred while playing near the water and 19% involved boats, rafts, or inner tubes (Washington State Department of Health 2004). Twenty-eight percent were swimming right before they drowned and 19% were playing in the water (Smith et al. 2001).

Drowning rates vary in different bodies of water. This variance may be attributable to the age, gender, predrowning activity, and supervision of the victim in that setting. Bathtub drowning death rates are highest in those younger than 1 year of age. Drowning death rates are highest in swimming pools in those younger than 5 years of age and highest in rivers, lakes, and salt water for those aged 5 through 65 years (Quan and Cummings 2003; Brenner et al. 2001). However, confounders such as water clarity, current, and temperature of different bodies of water may also affect rescue and thus outcome.

Death rates from drowning remain highest in those 1 to 4 years of age in all countries except Africa. Drowning death rates are second highest in those aged 15 to 24 years (Bierens, Knape, and Gelissen 2002). In the United States, 1124 persons younger than 19 years drowned in 2007, with the highest drowning rate (2.6) among children younger than 5 years of age and the second highest rate (1.6) among those aged 15 to 19 years (Centers for Disease Control and Prevention 2010b). The lowest drowning rates occur in school-aged children.

Drowning as a method of suicide or homicide is also a cause of intentional deaths. It is difficult to determine whether drownings are intentional and some drownings are classified as "undetermined." In addition, in small communities, coroners are often unwilling to label such deaths because of the stigma of intentional death. Thus, intentional drowning deaths are probably underestimated (Smith and Howland 1999).

Most children who survive a drowning event that involved medical care survive intact. Pearn initially noted young pediatric survivors had an average IQ of 114 and no other abnormalities (Pearn 1977). While the premorbid condition of his patient population was skewed, consisting of children with home swimming pools, their post-drowning function was good.

Approximately 7 to 13% of drowning victims (Bierens, Knape, and Gelissen 2002; Quan et al. 1989) and most of those who survive a cardiac arrest following a drowning are devastated neurologically by the hypoxia incurred during the drowning and subsequent cardiac arrest (American Academy of Pediatrics Committee on Injury, Violence, and Poison Prevention 2003). Unable to ambulate and respond in a purposeful manner, or in a persistent vegetative state, the economic and emotional toll they represent are enormous. In fact, analyses for some communities have shown positive benefit in terms of cost ratios for prevention programs by reducing medical and public program expenses, lost productivity, and quality adjusted life years saved (Zaloshnja et al. 2003).

The ratios of children surviving hospitalization to those dying vary by state. They vary consistently by age group, with high survival-to-death ratios in children younger than 5 years and inversely low ratios in adolescents and adults (Centers for Disease Control and Prevention 2004; Quan and Cummings 2003). Among injuries, drowning has the highest fatality ratios reported.

Risk Factors and Disparities

Risk factors that have been clearly shown to increase risk for drowning are those that impair the victim's abilities, a history of seizure disorder, and alcohol use. Host, or victim, related risk factors include age, gender, use of alcohol, ethnicity, and seizure history. As with most other injuries, males drown more commonly than females. Once admitted to a hospital following a drowning, males were more likely to die (Graf et al. 1995).

The remarkable preponderance of males older than 1 year involved in drowning incidents, especially among those older than 15 to 24 years, may in part be explained by behaviors. Males report engaging in more water activities than females and are more likely than females to consume alcohol when doing so (Howland et al. 1990, 1993). Howland and colleagues attributed the higher alcohol use by males as a major contributor to their increased drowning risk (Howland et al. 1993).

Alcohol increases the risk for drowning death. Unfortunately, alcohol use is very prevalent in water activities (Howland et al. 1993). Blood alcohol levels are positive among 20 to 30% of adolescent drowning deaths (Howland and Hingson 1988). A case-controlled study of alcohol-related drowning showed that a positive blood alcohol level increased the risk of boater drowning death, and as blood alcohol levels increased the risk of drowning death increased (Smith et al. 2001). In one region, decreasing fatal drowning rates were associated with decreasing rates of positive blood alcohol levels among drowning victims (Cummings and Quan 1999).

In addition, when surveyed, men reported less use of injury prevention practices than women (Saluja et al. 2004). In Canada and the United States, females were more likely than men to use life jackets in boats and powered watercrafts (Quan et al. 1998; Browne, Lewis-Michl, and Stark 2003; Nguyen et al. 2002; Mangione et al. 2010).

Adolescent males compared to females in New Zealand reported lower levels of risk appreciation, increased risk taking, decreased use of safe practices around water activities, and greater belief in their abilities (McCool et al. 2009). These behaviors with increased exposure may explain their greater risk for fatal drowning (Howland et al. 1996).

In the United States, non-Whites have higher fatal drowning rates than Whites. African American children have the highest rates (Centers for Disease Control and Prevention 2010b; Quan and Cummings 2003; Brenner et al. 2001). In Washington State, Asian/Pacific Islanders had the highest drowning death rates, accounting for 18% of drowning deaths although they represented only 7% of the state's population (Washington State Department of Health 2004). Similar disproportionate drowning risk in minority groups in other countries suggest that culture-based knowledge, awareness, experience, or lack thereof with water activities may contribute to drowning risks (Garssen, Hoogenboezem, and Bierens 2008). African Americans reported less swimming ability than Whites and Vietnamese American families reported low awareness and use of safe water practices (Siano et al. 2010; Quan et al. 2006).

Seizures are the most common cause of injury death among epileptics (Mayes 2009). Epilepsy-related drownings accounted for 5 to 7% of drowning deaths in Canada and western Washington (Quan and Cummings 2003). Children and adolescents with epilepsy and no other disability have greatly increased relative risks for both drowning injury (9.9%) and death from drowning (10.4%) compared to those without epilepsy (Diekema, Quan, and Holt 1993; Barooni, Thambirajah Balachandra, and Lee 2007). Among children with epilepsy, risks for drowning and fatal drowning were highest in 5- to 19-year-olds and those in bathtubs.

Environmental and Behavioral Aspects of Risk

Bathtubs

Bathtub drownings involve three different groups of victims: the inadequately supervised infant or toddler, the child or adolescent with a seizure disorder, and the victim of homicide. Neglect or child abuse should always be considered in bathtub drowning (Lavelle et al. 1995). The great majority of children who drowned in bathtubs were placed therein by a caregiver, and more than half of these children were left in the bath with another child (Sweet 2002). Bathtub rings and seats have been associated with drownings of infants younger than 1 year who have been left unattended in the bathtub. Their use may increase the likelihood that the parent will leave the infant unsupervised (Rauchschwalbe, Brenner, and Smith 1997). What is clear is that they should not be used as a substitute for "arm's reach" supervision.

Swimming Pools

Although drowning ranks second or third behind motor vehicles and fires as a leading cause of unintentional injury death to children younger than 15 years, drowning in residential pools is the leading cause of death for children between the ages of 1 and 4 years in most states and resulted in 4200 emergency department visits annually between 2005 and 2007 (U.S. Consumer Product Safety Commission 2010b). In Florida, children between the ages of 1 and 4 have an unintentional drowning rate in residential pools of 4.6/100,000. In a review of child deaths nationally, 39% occurred in pools (14% residential, 7% community, and 18% of unknown type). Swimming pools were the site for 44% of the drownings among 1- to 4-year-olds. Lapses in supervision and breaching pool barriers allow these injuries. In reviewed deaths where barriers were breached, 63% of victims entered through an open or unlocked gate. Of victims whose supervision was known, 39% were alone (Cody et al. 2004).

Open Bodies of Water

As of 2002, ICD-10 codes allow better identification of the dominating role of open water in drownings. Open water is the most likely drowning site for those older than age 4 years in most countries (Bierens, Knape, and Gelissen 2002; Brenner et al. 2001). Geography and accessibility of water determine the type of water involved; in Washington State child death reviews showed that 36% of drownings occurred in a lake or pond, 28% in rivers, and only 4% in the ocean or sound (Washington State Department of Health 2004). In contrast, most drownings involving children over 11 years of age in a coastal community in Florida occurred in natural bodies of salt water (Nichter and Everett 1989). However, almost all involve males who were swimming or boating recreationally. Weather and water conditions may contribute to the risk.

Current Research Findings and Prevention Efforts

Recommendations for the prevention of child and adolescent drownings have been developed by the American Academy of Pediatrics, Safe Kids USA, U.S. Consumer Product Safety Commission, Centers for Disease Control and Prevention, and the World Congress on Drowning (Centers for Disease Control and Prevention 2010b; Cody et al. 2004; Sweet 2002; American Academy of Pediatrics 2010a, 2010b, 2010c; U.S. Consumer Product Safety Commission 2010a; American Academy of Pediatrics Committee on Injury, Violence, and Poison Prevention 2010).

Prevention has focused on multiple aspects of the Haddon matrix, including giving the child the skill of knowing how to swim; decreasing risk by avoiding alcohol use; improving supervision by recreating under lifeguard supervision; and placing four-sided fencing, pool alarms, and covers to remove the environmental hazard from the child's purview.

Prevention of drowning requires a comprehensive approach, not only in terms of what kind of prevention, such as supervision or swimming, but also in the strategies that are used. The Spectrum of Prevention outlines multiple levels of intervention that need to be considered (Figure 10.1). It serves as a template in developing effective programs and helps practitioners to identify gaps in approaching the prevention of drowning. The six levels of the Spectrum are influencing policy and legislation, changing organizational practices, fostering coalitions and networks, educating providers, promoting community education, and strengthening individual knowledge and skills.

Pool Barriers

The injury prevention tactic to prevent swimming pool drownings has been to preclude young children's unsupervised access to water by modifying the environment with barriers. To be effective, pool fences need to be at least 4 feet high, unclimbable, with spacing no more than 4 inches, so small children cannot squeeze through. Gates need to be self-closing and self-latching. Thus, pool fencing is a passive-environmental intervention in that the fence and gate must be appropriately used and maintained. Most fencing laws require public and semipublic pools such as motels and swim clubs to have four-sided, isolation fencing. However, until recently legislation for residential pools has only required three-sided fencing, allowing the house to be the fourth side of the fence, protecting neighborhood children, but not those residing in the house from pool access.

LEVEL OF SPECTRUM	DEFINITION OF LEVEL
6. Influencing Policy and Legislation	Developing strategies to changes laws and policies to influence outcomes
5. Changing Organizational Practices	Adopting regulations and shaping norms to improve health and safety
4. Fostering Coalitions and Networks	Convening groups and individuals for broader goals and greater impact
3. Educating Providers	Informing providers who will transmit skills and knowledge to others
2. Promoting Community Education	Reaching groups of people with information and resources to promote health and safety
1. Strengthening Individual Knowledge and Skills	Enhancing an individual's capability of preventing injury or illness and promoting safety

Figure 10.1. The Spectrum of Prevention.
Source: Cohen and Swift (1999).

The Cochrane Collaboration identified studies that evaluated pool fencing in a defined population and objectively measured the risk of drowning or provided rates of these outcomes in fenced and unfenced pools (Thompson and Rivara 2000). Their review of three case-controlled studies showed that pool fencing significantly reduced the risk of drowning. The odds ratio for fatal and nonfatal drowning risk in a fenced pool compared to an unfenced pool was 0.27 (95% confidence interval [CI]: 0.16–0.47). Isolation fencing (four-sided) was superior to perimeter fencing because perimeter or property fencing allowed access to the pool from the house. The odds ratio for pools with isolation fencing in comparison to three-sided fencing was 0.17 (95% CI: 0.07–0.44). Based on these findings, the report concluded the following: (1) pool fences should have a dynamic and secure gate and isolate (four-sided fencing) the pool from the house (2) legislation should require isolation fencing with secure, self-latching gates for all pools—public, semipublic, and private.

Pool Fencing Laws

Australia and New Zealand have pioneered drowning prevention to address their high toddler pool drowning rates. Their data, legislative approach, and efforts to maintain their laws to address obstacles and evaluate the effect over 20 years provide many useful lessons about legislation in injury prevention.

Unfortunately, residential pool fencing laws have not eliminated toddler pool drownings. Early reports of a 50% decrease in numbers of pool drownings following pool fencing laws in Arizona were encouraging; however, pool drowning rates have only decreased 30% since 1976, and toddler drowning death rates have not changed in New Zealand, Australia, and the United States (Logan et al. 1998; Pearn et al. 2008). Some of the lack of change in rates may be explained by increased exposure as the number of pools has increased (Pearn et al. 2008; Mitchell, Williamson, and Olivier 2010). Exposure data are needed to better evaluate the effects of the laws.

The content of the laws has been part of the problem. Most legislation applies only to newly constructed pools since there are usually building code ordinances that involve permits enforced by building code inspectors at the time of construction. Rarely does legislation apply to existing residential pools. For example, in 2000, Florida amended its originally proposed pool barrier legislation that required a child-resistant fence 5 feet high surrounding residential swimming pools on any new residential swimming pool built after October 1, 1998, and on any private swimming pool before the act when the dwelling was sold, leased, or rented after October 1, 1998 (Chapter 515, F.S., November 25, 1997). The bill was changed in 2000 to apply to only new residential pools, spas, and hot tubs and requires pool owners to have one of four safety features to supplement and complement the requirement for constant adult supervision of young children and medically frail elderly persons around such aquatic environments. These safety features include a pool barrier (4 feet high) that isolates the pool from the home, the use of an approved safety pool cover, all doors and windows providing direct access from the home to the pool must be equipped with an exit alarm that has a minimum sound pressure rating of 85 dBA at 10 feet, or all doors providing direct access from the home to the pool must be equipped with a self-closing, self-latching device with a release mechanism placed no lower than 54 inches above the floor. Although four-sided fencing is the only barrier method that has been studied and has been shown to work, various states and the U.S. Consumer Product Safety Commission have adopted legislation to include other barrier adjuncts, such as pool covers and alarms (U.S. Consumer Product Safety Commission 2010a). Standardized wording and requirements across regions would improve application and enforcement of these laws.

Inevitably, the incomplete success of pool fencing laws lies with pool owners. Unfortunately, although pool fencing is primarily a passive intervention, pool owners must maintain the fence and gate and ensure the gate functions properly. In-depth reviews of residential pool drownings show parental failure to do so (Franklin, Scarr, and Pearn 2010; Quan et al. 2011). This is not surprising, for when surveyed, Australian pool owners did not perceive that the pool was a hazard and that a childproof fence was important, regardless of whether or not they had children (Fisher and Balanda 1997). In California, a state with high toddler drowning rates, only 35% of those who endorsed four-sided fencing around pools actually had a fence surrounding their own pool (Wintemute and Wright 1991). This phenomenon, called the *knowledge-user gap*, is a well-described hurdle in changing human behaviors.

The failure of pool fencing laws to greatly reduce toddler deaths primarily lies in failure to implement or enforce the laws. Despite long-standing national pool fencing laws, only 44% of New Zealand authorities reported complying with the law (Morrison et al. 1999). In the United States, most fencing laws are county-based ordinances for new pool construction; few statewide laws exist. Fewer apply to existing pools. A national law is needed coupled with a commitment to enforcement. Many opportunities exist to enforce the laws, such as requiring home pool inspections whenever the house is rented, sold, or repaired. Furthermore, efforts should focus on increasing compliance.

To prevent toddler drownings, the disturbing complacencies among pool owners must be overcome. Clearly, universal pool fencing laws and their enforcement are needed. Care provider disbelief and the failure of pool fencing to protect children also highlight the need for new behavioral approaches to preventing pool drownings.

Life Jackets

Life jackets (also known as personal flotation devices [PFDs] or life vests) have been made of various materials and used for centuries to enhance flotation. The U.S. Coast Guard developed standards for varying types of use. Only life jackets designated "U.S. Coast Guard approved" should be considered effective. The U.S. Coast Guard, boating organizations, and the American Academy of Pediatrics recommend wearing life jackets when on a boat (American Academy of Pediatrics Committee on Injury, Violence, and Poison Prevention 2003).

Though life jacket use is high among young children, it remains low among teen and adult boaters. Observation studies show continued low usage of life jackets among U.S. boaters (Mangione et al. 2010). The average life jacket wear rate for 2009 on all boats (including personal watercraft [PWC]) was only 22.3%, down from the 2008 wear rate of 23.4%. For adults (≥18 years) and youth combined on boats (0–17 years of age), not including PWCs, the wear rate was only 17.4%, down slightly from the wear rate of 17.9% in 2008. This continues a downward national trend. Males, persons more than 14 years of age, and motor boaters were the highest nonusers of life jackets. Another study showed that children younger than 15 years were more likely to wear a life jacket if an adult in the boat was wearing one (Quan et al. 1998). Following statewide efforts to increase life jacket use, wear rates increased 21% among Washington State children (Treser, Trusty, and Yang 1997). The media promotes these unsafe behaviors. In a study of G-rated and PG-rated movies, only 17% of boaters wore life jackets (Pelletier et al. 2000).

In Canada and the United States, 85% or more of persons who died while boating were not wearing life jackets (U.S. Department of Transportation 2010; Groff and Ghadiali 2003). One study of PWC crashes surmised that life jackets saved the lives of persons who were ejected from the PWC (Jones 1999). Recently, a matched control study showed that boaters wearing life jacket had half the drowning rate of those who did not (relative risk: 0.51; 95% CI: 0.35–0.74). Use of life jackets by children when playing in or near the water has increased survival rates in Chinese youth and saves have been reported at life jacket loaner sites (Yang et al. 2007; Delaney 2002; Bennett and Bernthal 2001).

Many communities have implemented life jacket loan programs to make life jackets available to boaters, swimmers, and for other types of water recreation. Loaner programs may increase use. In Alaska, 75% of children under 18 used life jackets at loaner sites compared to 50% at nonloaner sites (Delaney 2002). Loaner programs in Washington State and by the BoatU.S. Foundation loan anywhere from a few dozen to over 500 jackets and have documented saves from drowning (BoatU.S. Foundation 2010).

Although long associated with boating safety, life jackets have failed to become the boating world's seat belt equivalent. Expanding their use to those playing by and in the water is a concept new to users, manufacturers, and advertisers. Ignorance remains an important barrier to their use for swimming. Parents mistake the effectiveness of swimming aids; 19% believed that water wings protect children (Cody et al. 2004). Clear, consistent, and expanded messaging for life jacket use while in and next to the water is needed for parents, teenagers, and boaters.

Barriers to wearing life jackets on boats fall into five broad categories based on boater perception that there is a low risk of drowning; wearing a life jacket restricts movement and interferes with performance of activities; wearing a life jacket is uncomfortable; life jackets are unattractive or unfashionable; and wearing a life jacket is a sign of fear (Bennett et al. 1999).

Parents of children who did not always wear life jackets on boats cited reasons for nonuse including how close they are to the child, having a life jacket available nearby if needed, and the child's swimming ability. Children 8 to 12 years old reported they did not wear life jackets because they could swim, they could grab the life jacket easily if needed, or life jackets were unavailable. In addition, 23% of parents reported that they themselves don't wear life jackets on a boat. Parents' confidence in their ability to choose and fit a life jacket, life jacket ownership, and the perception that children could swim well were also factors that influenced reported life jacket use (Bennett et al. 1999, 109–113). In other research, teen males were particularly concerned that a life jacket might negatively affect their desire to present an image of fearlessness and believed that life jackets are a sign of being afraid (Groff and Ghadiali 2003, 1–287). In fact, the swimming community has given mixed messages about life jacket use. Many swim sites prohibit their use stating that life jacket use prevents acquisition of swimming skills. However, as of 2009, American Red Cross swim programs include water safety (including the importance of life jackets) teaching in all levels of swim lessons for swim participants and promote parent education in water safety (American Red Cross 2009).

In recent years, more colorful, lightweight, and less bulky life jackets have been developed to address the issue of bulk and discomfort and the perceived "ugly" factor. Present U.S. Coast Guard approved life jackets include inflatable life jackets for ages 16 and older, including a suspender style. Unfortunately, these newer styles have not increased life jacket use.

Campaigns to increase life jacket use have increased ownership rates and use by boaters (Treser, Trusty, and Yang 1997). Any promotion of life jacket use should address parent's efficacy by including information on how to fit a life jacket (Bennett and Bernthal 2001). In addition, promotions should focus on adult life jacket use in addition to use by children since adult role modeling affects use (Quan et al. 1998; Bennett et al. 1999).

Life jacket use is mandated for children on boats in the United States. State laws vary by age of child, boat length, and boating activities such as being underway or not. A federal rule requires any child under 13 to wear a life jacket when on any type and size of recreational boating vessel. However, it does not replace state legislation. Another federal rule requires appropriately sized life jackets be available, not worn, for anyone in a boat (U.S. Coast Guard 2002). There has not been a clear mandate for life jacket use among adolescents and adults, the victims of most boating-related drownings. National observational data show that life jacket use decreases with age, from 94% in those younger than 5 years to 38.9% in 13- to 17-year-olds and 8% in those older than 17 years (Mangione et al. 2010).

Not surprisingly, it is difficult to demonstrate an association between life jacket laws and significant decreases in drowning deaths. In Washington state, prior to a state law requiring children younger than 13 years to wear life jackets, 63% of those younger than 15 years were already wearing life jackets in small boats. After the law, 77% were wearing them (Christoffel 2000). Although the 22% increase was encouraging, it was not statistically significant.

Supervision

Inadequate supervision is cited as a primary contributing factor in most drowning studies (Landen, Bauer, and Kohn 2003; Rimsza et al. 2002; Brenner 2003). In a national child death review, 88% of drownings occurred while the child was being supervised (Cody et al. 2004). However, misperceptions about supervision abound. Drownings can occur when a child is left under the supervision of an "older" sibling, usually younger than 4 years of age (Byard et al. 2001). Many parents believe a drowning is a noisy event, allow themselves to be distracted or out of sight of the child for extended periods of time, expecting to be warned of sounds of distress (Byard et al. 2001; Simon, Tamura, and Colton 2003). Parents may be more likely to allow their child to swim without supervision if the child is perceived to be an excellent swimmer, if the child swims with a buddy, or if the child has had several years of swimming lessons. Parents become overconfident about their children's safety and abilities around water. In one study, 55% of parents said that they do not worry much or at all about their child drowning (Cody et al. 2004).

What constitutes adequate supervision has not been well defined. Saluja defined three domains—proximity, continuity, and attention—for drowning situations (Saluja et al. 2004). Adult supervision, being at hand, and being continuously present are needed for children bathing and in open water. Adults should be within an arm's length, providing "touch supervision" for young children and poor swimmers. They should focus all attention on the child and should not be engaged in other distracting activities including using alcohol or drugs (American Academy of Pediatrics Committee on Injury, Violence, and Poison Prevention 2010). However, supervision requires additional, unique skills not required for prevention of other injuries. These include being able to recognize a drowning in progress, know how to respond safely and provide safe rescue without putting one's self in danger, and how to provide cardiopulmonary resuscitation (CPR). All these require education and practice.

Nowhere has the role of supervision been more contentious than in swimming pools. The fact that 80% of toddler swimming pool drownings occur in residential homes, usually their own, and under parental supervision has been interpreted differently. Some deduce that parental supervision should be improved. However, most injury prevention specialists say the data illustrate the predictable failure of relying on supervision, an active intervention, since no one could be more invested in their child's safety than a parent. Second, it shows the need for a more passive and proven intervention (isolation fencing).

Recently an international task force developed guidelines for parents, families, and individuals recreating around open water. These guidelines begin to further define appropriate supervision by identifying knowledge, skills, and the planning needed before going to recreate and when at the water site. These guidelines also address a critical aspect of supervision unique to drowning injury, that of responsivity or the skills needed when a drowning is in progress to prevent progression to death (Quan, Moran, and Bennett 2010).

Supervision is an even more challenging prevention tactic among adolescents. The majority of adolescent drownings occur while swimming, playing, or boating with peers in open water such as lakes and rivers. Using a conceptual framework for adolescent risk behavior, adolescent drowning prevention must consider both risks and protective factors that take into account a combination of biology/genetics, social environment, perceived environment, personality, and behavior (National Center for Injury Prevention and Control 2006). For example, social risk factors might include lack of adult supervision or a party with alcohol that precedes water activity. Protective factors might include adult role models for life jacket use and family life with clear rules and consequences. Making good decisions about where and when to swim are important factors (Quan, Moran, and Bennett 2010; National Center for Injury Prevention and Control 2006).

The Developmental Asset framework, developed by the Search Institute, should be considered in designing adolescent drowning prevention interventions (Benson et al. 1999). The framework acknowledges the research-based associations of 40 qualities, attitudes, and behaviors—called "developmental assets"—with success and safety among young people. The assets are categorized into two groups. External assets identify important roles that families and communities play in promoting healthy development. Internal assets identify those characteristics and behaviors that reflect positive internal growth and development of young people. The internal assets help young people make thoughtful and positive choices and, in turn, be better prepared for challenging situations. Several assets are directly applicable to drowning risk and prevention:

- Adult role models who demonstrate positive responsible behavior
- Positive peer influence
- Responsibility for choices
- Planning and decisionmaking
- Resistance skills
- Youth programs such as teen swimming lessons

Development of these assets may help protect adolescents from drowning and also establish a foundation for other kinds of success (Seattle Children's Hospital 2010). However, since adolescent risk taking and perceptions of risk involving drowning vary so clearly based on gender, ethnicity, and educational levels, these approaches need to address and target specific groups (McCool et al. 2009, 360–366; Moran 2008, 68–71).

Swimming Lessons

Recent data show that swimming lessons given to children <5 years of age may lower their drowning risk. Although most children are not developmentally ready for formal swimming lessons until their fourth birthday, swimming lessons improved their swimming abilities and decreased risk behaviors around pools (Asher et al. 1995, 228–233; Parker and Blanksby 1997, 83–87). However, swimming lessons without adequate parental education can induce a false sense of security leading parents to supervise their children less around water or allow children to take more risks around water (Moran and Stanley 2006a, 139–143). Fortunately, water safety education can successfully instill appropriate attitudes to parents of toddlers in swim programs (Moran and Stanley 2006b, 254–256). Most drowning studies report that 20 to 50% of fatalities were known swimmers. Thus, the swimmer's perceived ability may not match the water conditions. Knowing how to swim is helpful but not the only answer to preventing drowning.

Recognizing the limitations of swimming lessons, the American Academy of Pediatrics and American Red Cross recommended in 2010 that aquatic programs should not be promoted as a means to prevent drownings, and that parents must continually supervise children around water regardless of past or present swimming instruction (American Academy of Pediatrics Committee on Injury, Violence, and Poison Prevention 2010, 178–185). All aquatic programs should teach parents "touch" supervision for the nonswimmer, the cognitive and motor limitations of infants, children, and teenagers, the inherent risks of water, the layers of protection needed for drowning prevention, and the key role of adults in supervision and monitoring of the safety of children in and around water. Furthermore, lessons should focus on water safety and teach specific water survival skills such as floating (American Red Cross 2009).

Lifeguarding

Lifeguards provide classic prevention in that they can prevent drownings from occurring and provide rescue and resuscitation (Branche and Stewart, 2001). Lifeguard presence has been shown to decrease activities and behaviors among pool users that would probably increase the risk of drowning (Harrell 2001, 327–330). While no study has conclusively proven that lifeguard presence decreases drowning, drownings at public and semipublic pools decreased dramatically when lifeguard supervision was improved (Quan and Gomez 1990, 344–346). Drowning risk is estimated to be one in eight million visits at lifeguarded sites (U.S. Lifesaving Association 2010).

Reduction of Alcohol Use

All 50 U.S. states have boating under the influence (BUI) legislation. The content of the laws varies as does the type of penalty. In 13 states the BUI legislation also applies to motor vehicle licenses. A 1990 study conducted by the National Association of State Boating Law Administrators found a greater percent decline in boating fatalities in states with more stringent BUI laws (National Transportation Safety Board 1993). However, because the logistics of commandeering the boat of a drunken operator are difficult and time-consuming, enforcement remains the major barrier to efficacy of these laws. This may help explain why increasing the drinking age did not affect the drowning rate of teenagers (Howland et al. 1998, 288–291). However, several states have decreased the acceptable alcohol level and increased enforcement by linking BUI incidents with drivers' licenses, increasing fines, and removing boater registration cards.

Messaging to improve the quality of supervision occasionally advises parents not to consume alcohol while supervising children in the water.

Recommendations for Research, Practice, Advocacy

Research needs abound in the epidemiology, behavioral aspects, and intervention of drowning. Denominator data are needed for exposure to water activities, swimming ability, and supervision. Research needs to address various ethnic groups to explain their increased risk and how to address them. The attitudes and barriers to safe practice around water activities need to be explored in adolescent males, motor boaters, and diverse communities. Ways to improve supervision, safe bathing, and swimming practices among these groups and those with epilepsy need exploration. A water safety awareness/risk perception schema needs to be developed to identify and prioritize those at risk and the effects of interventions to increase awareness. Among the intervention studies needed, the efficacy of life jackets, swimming lessons and survival swimming, lifeguard presence, and boating safety education should be prioritized (Quan, Moran, and Bennett 2010).

While drowning prevention must be perceived by the individual, advocacy for drowning prevention requires multiple levels and types of involvement. Christoffel has provided a conceptual framework for understanding the advocacy process that includes stages of gathering information, developing strategies, and taking action (Christoffel 2000, 722–726). Although the stages are sequential, they may also occur simultaneously so that adjustments based on findings from each stage are continually made. Successful advocacy efforts require involvement of many participants, including drowning prevention and Safe Kids coalitions, community and boating safety groups, health service providers, health provider organizations, journal editors, legal experts, legislators, the private sector, researchers and academicians, research funding agencies, and victims' families (Christoffel 2000, 722–726). The leaders of the advocacy effort need to identify participating individuals whose skills will differ and develop complementary, interacting, and distinct roles for each of them.

Existing laws need to be reviewed for content and enforcement. Pool fencing laws need to apply to all pools, public and private, established and new, and be enforced. Ways to enforce existing legislation need reevaluation. Some will be opportunistic; others require concerted policy change to the culture of water-related recreation. Alcohol use is an example of the latter. Promotion of a cultural change around alcohol and water use might achieve successful changes in alcohol and driving norms and result in decreased drowning fatalities. Restricting or prohibiting alcohol consumption in specific aquatic environments warrants consideration (Diplock and Jamrozik 2006, 314–317). Efforts to decrease boat-related drownings center around increasing life jacket use and safe boating practices. Mandatory life jacket use must be considered for all age groups. Over half the states have in place laws requiring boating safety courses for boaters. The effectiveness of these courses needs better evaluation.

Given that the majority of adolescents and adults drown in open water, prevention of open water drownings needs emphasis. Efforts should address the underestimation of the risk of water, of combining alcohol with water, the need for lifeguards, and the use of life jackets. Efforts to increase use should target parents as adult life jacket use increases the likelihood of child use (Quan et al. 1998, 203–205).

Open-water drowning will increase as these sites are increasingly used by lower socioeconomic and diverse populations who are unfamiliar with open water. Furthermore, global warming will increase waterside recreational water use. However, in many states, state budget cuts ended lifeguarding in state parks. The concerning numbers of drowning deaths in these unsupervised swim areas warrant evaluation and close surveillance (Loss Prevention Review Team 2005). Decreasing safe swim opportunities could increase drowning as populations either fail to acquire familiarity with water activities and safe practices and/or swim in unsupervised or poorly maintained swim sites.

Efforts are needed to make open-water swim sites safer (Franklin, Scarr, and Pearn 2010, 123–126). The concept of "safe open-water sites" should be developed using approaches used to make swimming pools safer. Prevention of swimming pool-related drowning evolved through development of standards for design and construction, improved supervision, and availability of safety and rescue equipment at pools. Specifically, this would include physical modification of sites to minimize hazards and open-water training standards for lifeguards.

Drowning prevention is very much predicated on involving communities to address local risks, populations, resources, and solutions. Advocacy efforts will be required to keep, promote, and even require swimming lessons for children in risky communities. Unfortunately, recent budget cuts have led to the closing and selling of public, community pools, thereby decreasing opportunities for development of water safe behaviors and skills.

How can we apply all of this information to practice? Awareness of risks and prevention strategies as well as supervisory and rescue skills for drowning prevention are needed. When the number of hours of exposure (to water activities) have been estimated in Australia, the risk of drowning is strikingly higher than previously thought (Mitchell, Williamson, and Olivier 2010, 261–266). Risk perception plays a major role in drowning prevention. The public underestimates the risk and overestimates treatment outcomes (Michalsen 2003, 201–204). Protective hypothermia, the dive reflex, and resuscitation are concepts that are perceived as leading to good outcomes; however, success with these is not supported by fact. Practitioners and educators need to better inform the public of the risks and prevention opportunities. Drowning prevention history shows clearly that success cannot be achieved without individual compliance. Important messages to impart include the following:

- Improve and increase supervision around water using lifeguards and parents who constantly watch their children and are prepared for an emergency.
- Change the culture of life jacket use to be associated with water rather than just boats. Life jackets should be introduced where and when children learn to swim. Local pools need to welcome life jacket use as do lifeguarded beach areas.
- Include water survival, such as floating, as part of swim lesson instruction. Swimming lessons should address use of life jackets, the differences between pool and open-water swimming including identifying some of the dangers of open water, and safe swimming practices.
- Educate families who have children with seizures about ongoing risks. Children and adolescents with seizure disorders need to recognize the lifetime risk of drowning, especially in a bathtub. Changing to a lifestyle of showering, not bathing should be encouraged by health care practitioners.
- Provide adolescents with safe swimming environments and skills to make appropriate decisions around the water. Being able to identify water risks, stand up to peer pressure, plan ahead for going out on the water, take personal responsibility, and be able to apply resistance skills may be useful strategies to prevent adolescent drowning (Search Institute 2006). Changing current norms around adult life jacket use and alcohol will impact adolescent behavior.
- Target messages to adolescents and young adults, fishermen, and motor boaters to influence their risk perception and behaviors around use of prevention technology such as life jackets and alcohol avoidance.
- Develop culturally tailored messaging and programs to address the attitudes, beliefs, and skills of different racial and ethnic groups.
- Increase the number of pool owners trained in CPR and water rescue as bystander CPR increases the likelihood of survival following a drowning event (Kyriacou et al. 1994, 137–142).
- Develop comprehensive community efforts to increase life jacket use employing behavioral theories and adapt campaigns that have increased the use of booster seats and bicycle helmets (Yang et al. 2007, 178–182; Bennett et al. 1999, 109–113). Social marketing campaigns may be very useful to explore.

In addition to drowning, other water injuries can be very serious. Unfortunately, a recent review study of nonsubmersion injuries in aquatic sporting and recreational activities showed a lack of adequate descriptive studies for swimming, diving, boating, surf sports, fishing, water polo, and water sliding (Chalmers and Morrison 2003, 745–770). Well-designed studies are needed that accurately describe the injuries, their incidence, and risk factors. There is much inconsistency in inclusion criteria and reporting of incidence rates. Although the incidence rates for these injuries overall were low (i.e., fractures, wounds, and dislocations), catastrophic disabling injuries occurred with diving (spinal cord injuries) and amputation from boat propeller strikes. Several large retrospective studies showed that traumatic injuries were rare in children and adolescents who drowned; cervical spine injury was the most prominent of these injuries, related to a history of diving- or motor vehicle-related drowning, and occurred mostly in adolescent males (Hwang et al. 2003, 50–53; Watson et al. 2001, 658–662).

For children and adolescents, serious diving injuries occur when striking one's head on the bottom of the pool or other body of water following miscalculation of water depth. Recreational diving spinal cord injuries occur more frequently in males younger than 25 years of age with the highest incidence in males between the ages of 11 and 15 years. Most of these injuries occur in private residential pools (Blanksby et al. 1997, 228–246). Diving injuries are likely to be underestimated due to the victim's drowning and the report of death being drowning only (Kluger et al. 1994, 349–351).

To prevent diving-related spinal cord injuries, water depth, the angle of the dive entry, and the diver's velocity are very important (Blanksby et al. 1997, 228–246). Recommendations include water depths for recreational diving are not less than 1.52 m; pools that are deep at one end and quickly and suddenly decline in depth in the shallow end should be avoided. Reports suggest that the best time to teach safe diving is when one is learning how to swim. This instruction should include not only the dangers of diving in shallow water, but also how to position the arms and head before entering the water, steering up to the water surface after the dive, and jumping in feet first instead of diving or sliding into the water (Watson et al. 2001, 658–662).

Recently, the National Electronic Injury Surveillance system was used to perform a retrospective analysis of diving-related injuries from 1990 through 2006 to children <20 years of age. The results showed that 111, 341 children were treated for diving-related injuries in emergency departments during the 17 years of the study. Those mostly affected were between the ages of 10 and 14 (36%). Injuries mostly occurred to the head and/or neck and face. The leading cause of injuries was collision with a diving board and/or platform. Children experienced greater injuries as they performed a flip and/or handstand or a backward dive (Day et al. 2008, e388–e394).

Another concern is pool and spa entrapment injuries. These injuries occur when part of the child's body becomes attached to a drain as the result of the powerful suction of the water circulation system, or a leg or arm is inserted into the drain that has a missing or broken cover (Quraishi et al. 2006). This calls for the need for supervision, barriers, and tying up children's long hair and removing items that may be trapped when swimming. The Graham-Baker Act requires installing anti-entrapment drain covers and safety vacuum release systems, or even more than one drain. All drain covers must be maintained (U.S. Consumer Product Safety Commission 2010b).

The Role of Physician Advocacy

Health care providers are in a powerful role for advising parents. However, a 1996 national survey of 560 pediatricians showed that very few (4.1%) were involved in community and/or legislative efforts to prevent childhood drowning, and less than half provided written materials about drowning prevention to their patients (40%). Even more disturbing was that only 18% of pediatricians received formal education on drowning prevention during their pediatric residency training (O'Flaherty and Pirie 1996, 169–174). Surprisingly, Los Angeles County pediatricians, family physicians, and pediatric nurse practitioners showed that about two thirds of the sample did not know that drowning deaths were more common than deaths due to toxic ingestions or firearm injuries for young children (Barkin and Gelberg 1999, 1217–1219). The American Academy of Pediatrics does not mention swimming pool hazards or recommend swimming lessons in their guide to age-related injury prevention counseling for 2- to 4-year-olds, or life jackets or swim lessons for 8 year olds (American Academy of Pediatrics 2010b, 2010c). Emergency departments provide an opportunity to reach large numbers of patients and families. Surprisingly, parents of children visiting a pediatric emergency department valued drowning prevention messages included in their written discharge instructions. In fact, 35% said they would consider buying a life jacket because of the messages (Quan et al. 2001, 382–385). Distribution of water safety equipment might be successful in the emergency department setting too.

Physician counseling should address identification of risks, such as exposure to pools, open water, and boating, prevention modalities including use of life jackets for water-related activities including playing near water, swimming/water safety lessons, and quality of supervision.

Seizure patients need specific counseling. The Epilepsy Foundation recommends not swimming when anticonvulsant medications have not been taken, wearing a life jacket, informing lifeguards and teachers of the seizure risk, swimming with someone who could provide rescue, and never leaving a child unattended (Epilepsy Foundation 2010). Moreover, patients of all ages with seizure disorders should be encouraged to shower and not bathe, since their drowning risk continues through adulthood (Quan and Cummings 2003, 163–168).

A Final Note: Personal Watercraft Injuries

PWC injuries, though generally not causing drowning, represent a unique set of water-related injuries. PWCs are designed to be operated by a person or persons sitting, standing, or kneeling on the craft, rather than within the confines of the hull. It is also designed to carry between one and three persons. In 2008, Americans owned one million PWCs (Research and Innovative Technology Administration, Bureau of Transportation Statistics 2009). In 2009, PWCs ranked second in terms of number of total injuries and deaths (N = 920), behind open motorboats (N = 2173) (U.S. Department of Transportation 2010). Age of PWC operators was a major risk factor with approximately 34% (296/878) of PWC-related injuries involving youth under 20 years of age.

PWCs are the ONLY type of recreational watercraft where the leading cause of death is not drowning but blunt trauma. The most common injury mechanism is collision with another PWC, boat, or fixed object. Injuries of children in Florida admitted to a local trauma center for jet ski injuries were more serious than those that occur in small boats (Beierle et al. 2002, 535–538; discussion 538). Most injury diagnoses involve the head, face, and/or neck (55%) and included lacerations, contusions, fractures, maxillofacial, arterial, and brain injuries (Branche, Conn, and Annest 1997, 663–665; Shatz et al. 1998, 198–201). In a 10-year retrospective review of 66 children between the ages of 5 and 19 hospitalized for PWC injuries, 4 died and 28 incurred disabilities (Rubin et al. 2003, 1525–1529).

Improved technology represents a major injury prevention opportunity as jet skis are maneuverable only when the throttle is open (American Academy of Pediatrics Committee on Injury and Poison Prevention 2000, 452–453). They can avoid an obstacle, not by slowing and changing direction as other vehicles do, but by increasing speed and turning direction. Also, stopping is only achieved by cutting the throttle—this leads to coasting and loss of steering ability. While newer models now incorporate off-throttle steering capacity, many older models will continue to be used for years.

Legislation has been passed to mitigate some of the risk factors. To operate PWC in Florida, one must be >14 years of age; to rent PWC, one must be 18 years of age. Some states, including Florida, require every PWC operator to take an educational course. However, efficacy of these courses has not been evaluated.

Areas for safety promotion include having safety equipment, educational training requirements, a citizen complaint provision, and at least a minimum of prohibited operations. To improve safety for children, the American Academy of Pediatrics continues to recommend the following: (1) no one younger than 16 should operate PWC; (2) the operator and passengers should wear U.S. Coast Guard approved PFDs; (3) alcohol and other drug use should be avoided before and while operating PWCs; (4) operators should participate in a safe boating course; (5) safe operating practices should always be followed; (6) PWCs should not be operated when swimmers are in the water;(7) if PWC is used to tow another person on skis, knee boards, tubes, or other devices, a second person must face the rear to monitor the person being towed; (8) all persons who rent PWCs should comply with all recommendations; and (9) protective equipment such as wet suits, gloves, boots, eyewear, and helmets may be important to wear (American Academy of Pediatrics Committee on Injury and Poison Prevention 2000, 452–453).

Personal watercraft injuries treated in U.S. emergency departments have increased fourfold (Branche, Conn, and Annest 1997, 663–665). It is likely that without the support of better regulations and related legislation PWC injuries will increase. The speeds of these crafts continue to increase as does their overall use. The American Academy of Pediatrics recommended additional PWC safety research, work within communities to pass legislation that support the recommendations, and funding to support enforcement of all regulations (American Academy of Pediatrics Committee on Injury and Poison Prevention 2000, 452–453).

In conclusion, a resonating theme throughout this chapter has been not only the importance of water-related injuries, but the opportunities and need for better research, practice, and advocacy, involving active and passive measures. Research, practice, and advocacy must work in concert to prevent needless water-related injuries and deaths among children and adolescents. Preston's story certainly illustrates that no more time can be wasted in pursuing the answers.

References

American Academy of Pediatrics (AAP). 2010a. *The Injury Prevention Program.* Elk Grove Village, IL: AAP. Available at: http://www.aap.org/family/tippmain.htm. Accessed November 18, 2010.

American Academy of Pediatrics (AAP). 2010b. *Safety for Your Child: 2 to 4 Years.* Elk Grove Village, IL: AAP. Available at: http://www.healthychildren.org/English/tips-tools/Pages/Safety-for-Your-Child-2-to-4-Years.aspx. Accessed November 18, 2010.

American Academy of Pediatrics (AAP). 2010c. *Safety for Your Child: 8 Years.* Elk Grove Village, IL: AAP. Available at: http://www.healthychildren.org/English/tips-tools/Pages/Safety-for-Your-Child-8-Years.aspx. Accessed November 18, 2010.

American Academy of Pediatrics Committee on Injury and Poison Prevention. 2000. Personal watercraft use by children and adolescents. *Pediatrics.* 105:452–453.

American Academy of Pediatrics Committee on Injury, Violence, and Poison Prevention. 2003. Prevention of drowning in infants, children, and adolescents. *Pediatrics.* 112:437–439.

American Academy of Pediatrics Committee on Injury, Violence, and Poison Prevention. 2010. Prevention of drowning. *Pediatrics.* 126:178–185.

American Red Cross. 2009. *Water Safety Instructor's Manual.* Yardley, PA: Staywell.

Asher KN, Rivara FP, Felix D, et al. 1995. Water safety training as a potential means of reducing risk of young children's drowning. *Inj Prev.* 1:228–233.

Barkin S, Gelberg L. 1999. Sink or swim—clinicians don't often counsel on drowning prevention. *Pediatrics.* 104:1217–1219.

Barooni S, Thambirajah Balachandra A, Lee L. 2007. Death in epileptic people: a review of Manitoba's medical examiner's cases. *J Forensic Leg Med.* 14:275–278.

Beierle EA, Chen MK, Langham MR Jr, et al. 2002. Small watercraft injuries in children. *Am Surg.* 68:535–538; discussion 538.

Bennett E, Bernthal T. 2001. *Life Vest Loan Program Guide.* Seattle, WA: Children's Hospital and Regional Medical Center.

Bennett E, Cummings P, Quan L, Lewis FM. 1999. Evaluation of a drowning prevention campaign in King County, Washington. *Inj Prev.* 5:109–113.

Benson PL, Scales PC, Leffert N, Roehlkepartain EC. 1999. *A Fragile Foundation: The State of Developmental Assets Among American Youth.* Minneapolis, MN: Search Institute.

Bierens JJ, Knape JT, Gelissen HP. 2002. Drowning. *Curr Opin Crit Care* 8:578–586.

Blanksby BA, Wearne FK, Elliott BC, Blitvich JD. 1997. Aetiology and occurrence of diving injuries: a review of diving safety. *Sports Med.* 23:228–246.

BoatU.S. Foundation. *Life Jacket Loaner Program.* 2010. Alexandria, VA: BoatU.S. Foundation. Available at: http://www.boatus.com/foundation/ljlp. Accessed November 15, 2010.

Branche C, Stewart S, editors. 2001. *Lifeguard Effectiveness: A Report of the Working Group.* Atlanta, GA: Centers for Disease Control and Prevention, National Center for Injury Prevention and Control.

Branche CM, Conn JM, Annest JL. 1997. Personal watercraft-related injuries. a growing public health concern. *JAMA.* 278:663–665.

Brenner RA. 2003. Prevention of drowning in infants, children, and adolescents. *Pediatrics.* 112:440–445.

Brenner RA, Trumble AC, Smith GS, et al. 2001. Where children drown, United States, 1995. *Pediatrics.* 108:85–89.

Browne ML, Lewis-Michl EL, Stark AD. 2003. Watercraft-related drownings among New York State residents, 1988–1994. *Public Health Rep.* 118:459–463.

Byard R, de Koning C, Blackbourne B, et al. 2001. Shared bathing and drowning in infants and young children. *J Paediatr Child Health.* 37:542–544.

Centers for Disease Control and Prevention. 2004. Nonfatal and fatal drownings in recreational water settings—United States, 2001–2002. *MMWR Morb Mortal Wkly Rep.* 53:447–452.

Centers for Disease Control and Prevention (CDC). 2010a. *Injury Prevention and Control: Data and Statistics.* Atlanta, GA: CDC. Available at: http://www.cdc.gov/injury/wisqars/index.html. Accessed November 18, 2010.

Centers for Disease Control and Prevention (CDC). 2010b. *Unintentional Drowning: Fact Sheet.* Atlanta, GA: CDC. Available at: http://www.cdc.gov/HomeandRecreationalSafety/Water-Safety/waterinjuries-factsheet.html. Accessed November 15, 2010.

Chalmers D, Morrison L. 2003. Epidemiology of non-submersion injuries in aquatic sporting and recreational activities. *Sports Med.* 33:745–770.

Christoffel KK. 2000. Public health advocacy: process and product. *Am J Public Health.* 90:722–726.

Cody B, Quraishi A, Dastur M, Mickalide A. 2004. *Clear Danger: A National Study of Childhood Drowning and Related Attitudes and Behaviors.* Washington, DC: National SAFE KIDS Campaign.

Cohen L, Swift S. 1999. The spectrum of prevention: developing a comprehensive approach to injury prevention. *Inj Prev.* 5:203–207.

Cummings P, Quan L. 1999. Trends in unintentional drowning: the role of alcohol and medical care. *JAMA.* 281:2198–2202.

Day C, Stolz U, Mehan TJ, et al. 2008. Diving-related injuries in children <20 years old treated in emergency departments in the United States: 1990–2006. *Pediatrics.* 122:e388–e394.

Delaney, M. 2002. *Loaner Life Jackets Saving Alaskan children's Lives.* Kodiak, AK: U.S. Coast Guard 17th District.

Diekema DS, Quan L, Holt VL. 1993. Epilepsy as a risk factor for submersion injury in children. *Pediatrics.* 91:612–616.

Diplock S, Jamrozik K. 2006. Legislative and regulatory measures for preventing alcohol-related drownings and near-drownings. *Aust N Z J Public Health.* 30:314–317.

Epilepsy Foundation. 2010. *Fact sheet on seizure-related causes of death and preventative measures.* Landover, MD: Epilepsy Foundation. Available at: http://www.epilepsyfoundation.org. Accessed November 18, 2010.

Fisher KJ, Balanda KP. 1997. Caregiver factors and pool fencing: an exploratory analysis. *Inj Prev.* 3:257–261.

Franklin RC, Scarr JP, Pearn JH. 2010. Reducing drowning deaths: the continued challenge of immersion fatalities in Australia. *Med J Aust.* 192:123–126.

Garssen MJ, Hoogenboezem J, Bierens JJ. 2008. Reduction of the drowning risk for young children, but increased risk for children of recently immigrated non-westerners. *Ned Tijdschr Geneeskd.* 152:1216–1220.

Graf WD, Cummings P, Quan L, Brutocao D. 1995. Predicting outcome in pediatric submersion victims. *Ann Emerg Med.* 26:312–319.

Groff P, Ghadiali J. 2003. Will it Float? Mandatory PFD Legislation: *A Background Research Paper.* Toronto, ON: SMARTRISK.

Harrell WA. 2001. Does supervision by a lifeguard make a difference in rule violations? Effects of lifeguards' scanning. *Psychol Rep.* 89:327–330.

Howland, J, Birckmayer J, Hemenway D, Cote J. 1998. Did changes in minimum age drinking laws affect adolescent drowning (1970–90)? *Inj Prev.* 4:288–291.

Howland J, Hingson R. 1988. Alcohol as a risk factor for drownings: a review of the literature (1950–1985). *Accid Anal Prev.* 20:19–25.

Howland J, Hingson R, Heeren T, Mangione T. 1993. Alcohol use and aquatic activities—United States, 1991. *MMWR Morb Mortal Wkly Rep.* 42:675–682.

Howland J, Hingson R, Mangione TW, et al. 1996. Why are most drowning victims men? Sex differences in aquatic skills and behaviors. *Am J Public Health.* 86:93–96.

Howland J, Mangione T, Hingson R, et al. 1990. A pilot survey of aquatic activities and related consumption of alcohol, with implications for drowning. *Public Health Rep.* 105: 415–419.

Hwang V, Shofer FS, Durbin DR, Baren JM. 2003. Prevalence of traumatic injuries in drowning and near drowning in children and adolescents. *Arch Pediatr Adolesc Med.* 157:50–53.

Idris AH., Berg RA, Bierens J, et al. 2003. Recommended guidelines for uniform reporting of data from drowning: the "Utstein style." *Circulation.* 108:2565–2574.

Jones CS. 1999. Drowning among personal watercraft passengers: the ability of personal flotation devices to preserve life on arkansas waterways, 1994–1997. *J Ark Med Soc.* 96:97–98.

Kluger Y, Jarosz D, Paul DB, et al. 1994. Diving injuries: a preventable catastrophe. *J Trauma.* 36:349–351.

Kyriacou DN, Arcinue EL, Peek C, Kraus JF. 1994. Effect of immediate resuscitation on children with submersion injury. *Pediatrics.* 94:137–142.

Landen MG, Bauer U, Kohn M. 2003. Inadequate supervision as a cause of injury deaths among young children in Alaska and Louisiana. *Pediatrics.* 111:328–331.

Lavelle JM., Shaw KN, Seidl T, Ludwig S. 1995. Ten-year review of pediatric bathtub near-drownings: evaluation for child abuse and neglect. *Ann Emerg Med.* 25:344–348.

Logan P, Branche CM, Sacks JJ, et al. 1998. Childhood drownings and fencing of outdoor pools in the United States, 1994. *Pediatrics.* 101:E3.

Loss Prevention Review Team. 2005. *Drowning Prevention.* Report to the Director of the Office of Financial Management. Olympia, WA: Washington State Parks and Recreation Commission. Available at: http://www.ofm.wa.gov/rmd/lprt/reports/parksfinalrpt.pdf. Accessed November 12, 2010.

Mangione TW, Lisinski, HE, Higgins-Biddle M, et al. 2009 *Life Jacket Wear Rate Observation Study.* Boston, MA: JSI Research and Training Institute. Available at: http://www.uscgboating.org/assets/1/workflow_staging/publications/380.pdf. Accessed November 15, 2010.

Mayes BN. 2009. Review: People with epilepsy have higher risk of death by drowning than the general population. *Evid Based Med.* 14:21.

McCool, J, Ameratunga S, Moran K, Robinson E. 2009. Taking a risk perception approach to improving beach swimming safety. *Int J Behav Med.* 16:360–366.

Michalsen A. 2003. Risk assessment and perception. *Inj Control Saf Promot.* 10:201–204.

Mitchell R J, Williamson AM, Olivier J. 2010. Estimates of drowning morbidity and mortality adjusted for exposure to risk. *Inj Prev.* 16:261–266.

Moran K. 2008. Taking the plunge: diving risk practices and perceptions of New Zealand youth. *Health Promot J Austr.* 19:68–71.

Moran K, Stanley T. 2006a. Parental perceptions of toddler water safety, swimming ability and swimming lessons. *Int J Contr Saf Promot.* 13:139–143.

Moran K, Stanley T. 2006b. Toddler drowning prevention: teaching parents about water safety in conjunction with their child's in-water lessons. *Int J Contr Saf Promot.* 13:254–256.

Morrison L, Chalmers DJ, Langley JD, et al. 1999. Achieving compliance with pool fencing legislation in New Zealand: a survey of regulatory authorities. *Inj Prev.* 5:114–118.

National Center for Injury Prevention and Control. 2006. *CDC Injury Fact Book.* Atlanta GA: Centers for Disease Control and Prevention.

National Transportation Safety Board. 1993. *Recreational Boating Safety.* Washington, DC: National Transportation Safety Board.

Nguyen MN, Poupart G, Normandeau J, et al. 2002. Comportements et croyances des amateurs d'activites nautiques et de plein air: Etude sur les comportements et les perceptions des risques a la santé. *Revue Canadienne De Santé Publique [Can J Public Health]* 93:208–212.

Nichter MA, Everett PB. 1989. Profile of drowning victims in a coastal community. *J Fla Med Assoc.* 76:253–256.

O'Flaherty J, Pirie P. 1996. Prevention of Pediatric drowning and near-drowning: a survey of members of the American Academy of Pediatrics. *Pediatrics.* 99:169–174.

Parker HE, Blanksby BA. 1997. Starting age and aquatic skill learning in young children: mastery of prerequisite water confidence and basic aquatic locomotion skills. *Aust J Sci Med Sport.* 29:83–87.

Pearn J. 1977. Neurological and psychometric studies in children surviving freshwater immersion accidents. *Lancet.* 1:7–9.

Pearn JH, Nixon JW, Franklin RC, Wallis B. 2008. Safety legislation, public health policy and drowning prevention. *Int J Contr Saf Promot.* 15:122–123.

Peden MM, McGee K. 2003. The epidemiology of drowning worldwide. *Inj Control Saf Promot.* 10:195–199.

Pelletier AR, Quinlan KP, Sacks JJ, et al. 2000. Injury prevention practices as depicted in G-rated and PG-rated movies. *Arch Pediatr Adol Med.* 154:283–286.

Quan L, Bennett E, Cummings P, et al. 1998. Are life vests worn? A multiregional observational study of personal flotation device use in small boats. *Inj Prev.* 4:203–205.

Quan L, Bennett E, Cummings P, Henderson P, Del Beccaro MA. 2001. Do parents value drowning prevention information at discharge from the emergency department? *Ann Emerg Med.* 37:382–385.

Quan L, Crispin B, Bennett E, Gomez A. 2006. Beliefs and practices to prevent drowning among Vietnamese-American adolescents and parents. *Inj Prev.* 12:427–429.

Quan L, Cummings P. 2003. Characteristics of drowning by different age groups. *Inj Prev.* 9:163–168.

Quan L, Gomez A. 1990. Swimming pool safety—an effective submersion prevention program. *J Environ Health.* 52:344–346.

Quan L, Gore EJ, Wentz K, et al. 1989. Ten-year study of pediatric drownings and near-drownings in King County, Washington: lessons in injury prevention. *Pediatrics.* 83:1035–1040.

Quan L, Bennett E, Moran K, Bierens J. Use of a consensus-based process to develop international guidelines to decrease recreational open water drowning deaths. *Int Health Promot Educ* (in press).

Quan L, Pilkey D, Gomez A, Bennett E. 2011. Analysis of paediatric drowning deaths in Washington State using the Child Death Review (CDR) for surveillance: what CDR does and does not tell us about lethal drowning injury. *Inj Prev.* 17(Suppl 1):i28–i33.

Quraishi AY, Morton S, Cody B, Wilcox R. 2006. Pool and Spa Drowning: A National Study of Drain Entrapment and Pool Safety Measures.Washington, DC: Safe Kids Worldwide.

Rauchschwalbe R, Brenner RA, Smith GS. 1997. The role of bathtub seats and rings in infant drowning deaths. *Pediatrics.* 100:E1.

Research and Innovative Technology Administration, Bureau of Transportation Statistics. 2009. *Personal Watercraft Safety Data.* Washington, DC: U.S. Department of Transportation. Available at: http://www.bts.gov/publications/national_transportation_statistics/html/table_02_44.html. Accessed November 15, 2010.

Rimsza ME, Schackner RA, Bowen KA, Marshall W. 2002. Can child deaths be prevented? The Arizona child fatality review program experience. *Pediatrics.* 110:e11.

Rubin LE, Stein PB, DiScala C, Grottkau BE. 2003. Pediatric trauma caused by personal watercraft: a ten-year retrospective. *J Pediatr Surg.* 38:1525–1529.

Saluja G, Brenner R, Morrongiello BA, et al. 2004. The role of supervision in child injury risk: definition, conceptual and measurement issues. *Inj Control Saf Promot.* 11:17–22.

Search Institute. 2006. The Asset Approach: 40 Elements of Healthy Development. Search Institute, Minneapolis, MN. http://www.search-institute.org/content/asset-approach. Accessed November 17, 2011.

Seattle Children's Hospital. Water Safety Tips for Families. 2010. Available at: http://www.seattlechildrens.org/pdf/CE423.pdf. Accessed November 17, 2011.

Shatz DV, Kirton OC, McKenney MG, et al. 1998. Personal watercraft crash injuries: an emerging problem. *J Trauma.* 44:198–201.

Siano CJ, Messiah SE, Banan L, et al. 2010. Swimming proficiency in a multiethnic sample in a high-risk area for drowning. *Arch Pediatr AdolescMed.* 164:299–300.

Simon HK, Tamura T, Colton K. 2003. Reported level of supervision of young children while in the bathtub. *Ambul Pediatr.* 3:106–108.

Smith GS, Howland J. 1999. Declines in drowning: exploring the epidemiology of favorable trends [Comment]. *JAMA.* 281:2245–2247.

Smith GS, Keyl PM, Hadley JA, et al. 2001. Drinking and recreational boating fatalities: a population-based case-control study. *JAMA.* 286:2974–2980.

Sweet D. 2002. Memorandum: Fatality Information for the "In-Home Drowning Prevention Campaign. Washington DC: U.S. Consumer Product Safety Commission.

Thompson DC, Rivara FP. 2000. Pool fencing for preventing drowning in children. *Cochrane Database Syst Rev.* no. 2:CD001047.

Treser CD, Trusty MN, Yang PP. 1997. Personal flotation device usage: do educational efforts have an impact? *J Public Health Policy.* 18:346–356.

U.S. Coast Guard (USCG), U.S. Department of Transportation (DOT). 2002. *Wearing of Personal Flotation Devices (PFD) by Certain Children Aboard Recreational Vessels*. Washington, DC: USCG, DOT.

U.S. Consumer Product Safety Commission. 2010a. *Pool and Spa Safety.* Bethesda, MD: U.S. Consumer Product Safety Commission. Available at: http://www.poolsafely.gov/pool-spa-safety. Accessed November 15, 2010.

U.S. Consumer Product Safety Commission. 2010b. *Pool or Spa Submersion: Estimated Injuries and Reported Fatalities, 2010 Report.* Bethesda, MD: U.S. Consumer Product Safety Commission. Available at: http://www.cpsc.gov/library/foia/foia10/os/poolsub2010.pdf. Accessed November 15, 2010.

U.S. Department of Transportation (DOT). 2010. *Recreational Boating Statistics 2009.* Washington, DC: DOT. Available at: http://www.uscgboating.org/assets/1/workflow_staging/Publications/394.PDF. Accessed November 12, 2010.

U.S. Lifesaving Association. 2010. *United States Lifesaving Association Data.* Available at: http://www.usla.org/statistics/public.asp. Accessed March 1, 2010.

Washington State Department of Health. 2004. *Child Death Review State Committee Recommendations on Child Drowning Prevention.* Olympia, WA: Washington State Department of Health.

Watson RS, Cummings P, Quan L, et al. 2001. Cervical spine injuries among submersion victims. *J Trauma.* 51:658–662.

Wintemute GJ, Wright MA. 1991. The attitude-practice gap revisited: risk reduction beliefs and behaviors among owners of residential swimming pools. *Pediatrics.* 88:1168–1171.

Yang L, Nong QQ, Li CL, et al. 2007. Risk factors for childhood drowning in rural regions of a developing country: a case-control study. *Inj Prev.* 13:178–182.

Zaloshnja E, Miller TR, Galbraith MS, et al. 2003. Reducing injuries among Native Americans: five cost-outcome analyses. *Accid Anal Prev.* 35:631–639.

Chapter 11

Child Physical Abuse and Neglect

David DiLillo, PhD,[1] Rosalita C. Maldonado, MA,[1] and Laura E. Watkins, MA[1]

Putting a Face on Injury: The True Case of Little Sebastian Duffek[2]

In the early morning after Christmas of 2008, Josie Trine asked her husband, Christopher Duffek, aged 22 years, to watch over their 5-week-old infant son, Sebastian (henceforth referred to as "Little Sebastian"), when he awoke that morning. She then went back to sleep. Approximately 1.5 hours later, Josie was awakened to Christopher telling her he had choked their baby. Josie immediately called 911 to report that her son was having difficulty breathing, but when authorities arrived they found the baby lifeless with bruises on his neck and shoulders. Christopher was overheard saying that he had murdered something or someone. Efforts to resuscitate Little Sebastian were unsuccessful, and he was pronounced dead at the hospital.

According to records, when police arrived, Christopher described how he had severely shaken and choked his 5-week-old infant son after becoming frustrated when he would not stop crying. He reported that he shook his son by the neck and hit his baby's chest once with his fist. Christopher also stated that Little Sebastian's head may have hit his knee. Police believe that Christopher shook his baby by the neck for as long as half an hour until Little Sebastian stopped breathing, and then waited approximately an hour before waking his wife, Josie. An autopsy revealed that Little Sebastian had suffered a skull fracture, bleeding in his brain, and blunt force trauma.

Upon arrest for child abuse, Christopher's competency came into question, because he had been recently released from psychiatric treatment for a mental illness. Records and reports from family members indicated that Christopher had a long history of struggling with mental health issues, including bipolar disorder, schizophrenia, depression, and Asperger's syndrome. Court records revealed that before 2007, Christopher was under guardianship as an adult because he was incapable of taking care of himself, and that he had spent several stays at local psychiatric facilities. Christopher eventually made enough progress to move into an independent supervised apartment for people living with a mental illness, which is where he met his wife. Records show Christopher had a history of responding aggressively; he once punched his wife in the face after she expressed wanting to end their relationship.

After Christopher was arrested, he received treatment at the state psychiatric hospital and ultimately was found competent to stand trial. Christopher pled no contest to a reduced charge of attempted second-degree murder. Although the judge recognized that Christopher suffered from serious mental health issues, he did not believe it justified the brutality endured by Little Sebastian, and sentenced Christopher to 25 to 40 years in prison for murdering his infant son.

[1]Department of Psychology, University of Nebraska–Lincoln, Nebraska.

[2]The case presented is an actual occurrence of severe child abuse. The facts described are drawn from various local, regional, and national media accounts of this case appearing between December 2008 and May 2010.

Putting It Into Context: Advocacy

Although all child abuse is disturbing, the story of Little Sebastian represents a particularly horrific example—one involving extreme brutality that resulted in the death of a young infant. Although death is not the most common consequence of abuse, it is the most tragic and unacceptable outcome. What can be gleaned from this case that might prove useful in preventing similar incidents of abuse in the future? In considering this question, three factors emerge that may shed light on important directions for child abuse advocacy. These factors include the unique challenges faced by parents living with a mental illness, the need for increased awareness concerning unintentional childhood injuries, and the need for increased intervention efforts for families with a history of violence within the home.

Living with a mental illness can be quite demanding for a parent, contributing to increased stress that may adversely affect family functioning. Although mental illness does not usually lead parents to abuse their children, increased severity of mental illness and lack of another competent caregiver in the home are associated with loss of custody of a child (Sands 1995). In the present case, it is reasonable to wonder whether Christopher was experiencing severe symptoms at the time of the incident, given that he received psychiatric care shortly before Little Sebastian's death. Unfortunately, it does not appear that Christopher or his wife were receiving specialized services for parents with mental illness at the time of the incident. How can professionals work together to provide services to parents struggling with a mental illness that may place them at greater risk for child maltreatment? Can mental health community agencies or psychiatric care facilities provide support for these families? It seems vital that child abuse advocates increase efforts to provide at-risk families with easy access to social services.

A second area in which increased awareness is needed concerns unintentional childhood injuries. Before Little Sebastian was shaken to death, his father described how he became frustrated that Little Sebastian would not stop crying. When parents attempt to physically control their children without harmful intent, children may unintentionally suffer minor to severe injuries or even death. In attempting to quiet a crying baby, parents sometimes resort to shaking without intending to harm the child. However, this behavior can quickly escalate into a violently abusive act, known as "shaken baby syndrome," a well-known risk for severe injuries, including permanent disabilities and death. It is important to increase awareness of how physical actions intended to control a child, such as shaking a baby, can quickly escalate to abuse and have lasting detrimental effects.

Finally, there is a need to increase intervention efforts for families with a history of assaultive behavior in the home. Christopher had previously shown aggressive behavior toward his wife, by punching her in the face during an argument. Although partner abuse is not always predictive of child abuse, there is a significant relationship between these two types of family violence (Kelleher et al. 2006). Given this co-occurrence, partner abuse should be seen as a possible marker of other forms of violence in the home—including child physical abuse—signaling the need for outside intervention.

Conceptual Issues

Child maltreatment is a term that encompasses many forms of caregiver mistreatment of children, including physical abuse, sexual abuse, neglect, and emotional abuse. Although not a new phenomenon, the maltreatment of children has not always been recognized as a social problem. In fact, research, practice, and advocacy efforts in this field were slow to develop until the early 1960s, when Henry Kempe and colleagues (1962) coined the term "battered child syndrome" to describe traumatic injury inflicted on children by parents. Kempe and colleagues directed much of their efforts at describing the syndrome of child abuse in terms of the injury and physical impairments caused to children, and focused on parental factors (e.g., psychopathology) as contributing factors. Although the efforts of Kempe and colleagues sparked an interest in the study of child maltreatment that continues today, professionals still struggle with how to define the phenomena. In fact, as noted by the National Research Council (1993), little progress has been made in generating a clear and consistent definition of child abuse and neglect in the past several decades. Furthermore, professionals may shape their definitions to fit their agenda (Miller-Perrin and Perrin 2007). For example, the definition a researcher uses may be influenced by his or her theoretical orientation, whereas legal professionals may focus on documentation of abusive acts (Miller-Perrin and Perrin 2007). Regardless of one's definitional goal, researchers acknowledge that child physical abuse and neglect are complex and heterogeneous problems (Cicchetti 1988; Wolfe and McGee 1991; Zuravin 1991) that are difficult to define (Wolfe 1999).

Determining whether an act is abusive involves consideration of a variety of factors surrounding the behavior. In regard to physical abuse, for example, Zuravin (1991) acknowledged the importance of taking into account the potential for severe consequences of an act (e.g., slapping vs. scalding). Other important factors deserving consideration include the prevalence, severity, chronicity, duration, and age of onset of abuse (Hecht and Hansen 2001; Widom 2000; Wolfe 1999; Zuravin 1991), as well as the impact of cultural and community values on parents' socialization practices (Wolfe 1999). Moreover, although data suggest that 75% to 90% of children in the United States have experienced corporal punishment (e.g., spanking, slapping) at some point (Graziano and Namaste 1990; Straus et al. 1998; Straus 2001), there is lack of consensus regarding whether this form of discipline should be considered abusive. Views among even prominent child abuse experts vary on this issue. Some propose that corporal punishment has harmful effects for children (e.g., antisocial behavior), is no more effective than other forms of discipline, and should never be used (Straus 2005), whereas others question the link between spanking and detrimental effects, suggesting that corporal punishment may be as effective as other means of discipline (Larzelere 2000). Thus, distinguishing between acts that constitute an extreme form of physical discipline and those that qualify as abuse is problematic and quite controversial (Hansen, Sedlar, and Warner-Rogers 1999; Kolko 2002).

Not only is it difficult to establish a consistent operational definition of child physical abuse, some researchers propose that the current conceptual divide between unintentional child injury and intentional child injury is a false dichotomy (Liller 2001; Peterson and Brown 1994). More specifically, these researchers argue that the two areas of research are likely part of a larger, multifaceted phenomenon, noting that both fields have much in common (Peterson and Brown 1994). For example, Peterson and Brown (1994) note that virtually all serious injuries to children could be prevented. Thus, the label of neglect becomes meaningless (Peterson and Brown 1994). Moreover, although some make the distinction that unintentional injuries are accidental and that intentional injuries involve intent to harm, investigators have reported that the risk factors for both categories of injury are similar, regardless of intent (Liller 2001). Consequently, as noted by Liller (2001), the continued distinction between these types of injury to children may preclude collaborative prevention and intervention efforts that could apply to the broader field of violence to children. Thus, it has been argued that, rather than classifying abuse as unintentional or nonaccidental, both child physical abuse and neglect are better conceptualized as a violation of standards of care for children (Garbarino, Guttmann, and Seeley 1986).

Although neglect is the most frequently reported form of child maltreatment (U.S. Department of Health and Human Services 2006) and some consider it to be the central feature of all maltreatment (Erickson and Egeland 2002), neglect has been the focus of far fewer investigative efforts than has physical or sexual abuse. The difficulties of operationalizing neglect may be one reason it has received less attention. First, and possibly most problematic, is the complexity of determining the range and specificity of children's needs and which parental behaviors constitute minimum standards of care. This task is challenging because it involves making a subjective judgment of what adequate parenting/caregiver behavior involves (National Clearinghouse on Child Abuse and Neglect [NCCAN] 2001). Further, harm due to neglect is seldom externally observable, particularly in the short-term (Miller-Perrin and Perrin 2007). Thus, many professionals have suggested that definitions of neglect should not be contingent on the presence of short-term sequelae because in many cases, the effects of neglect do not emerge until later in life (Erickson and Egeland 2002).

Definitions of Child Physical Abuse and Neglect

Despite difficulties in formulating cohesive definitions of child physical abuse and neglect, several concepts have converged to provide some consistency. The Child Abuse Prevention and Treatment Act mandates states to incorporate the following into determinations of child maltreatment: (1) any recent act or failure to act on the part of a parent or caretaker that results in death, serious physical or emotional harm, sexual abuse or exploitation; or (2) an act or failure to act that presents an imminent risk of serious harm (NCCAN 2003a, 2004).

The Centers for Disease Control and Prevention recently put forth a set of definition recommendations for child maltreatment, which was defined as any act or series of acts of commission or omission by a parent or other caregiver that results in harm, potential for harm, or threat of harm to a child (Leeb et al. 2008). Acts of commission include words or overt actions, such as physical abuse, sexual abuse, or psychological abuse (Leeb et al. 2008; Warner-Rogers, Hansen, and Hecht 1999). Conversely, acts of omission (child neglect) are failures to provide for a child's basic needs (Leeb et al. 2008) or failures to provide for a child in a manner that promotes healthy growth and development (NCCAN 2001; Warner-Rogers, Hansen, and Hecht 1999; Zuravin 1991).

Consistent with this perspective, in 2004 the National Clearinghouse on Child Abuse and Neglect (NCCAN) defined child physical abuse as physical injury (ranging from minor bruises to severe fractures or death) as a result of punching, beating, kicking, biting, shaking, throwing, stabbing, choking, hitting (with a hand, stick, strap, or other object), burning, or otherwise harming a child (NCCAN 2004). Moreover, any behavior that results in injury to a child qualifies as abuse, regardless of the caregiver's intent. In addition, the NCCAN defines neglect as a failure to provide for a child's basic needs in one or more of the following areas: physical, medical, educational, and emotional (NCCAN 2004). Supplementary categories of neglect have been identified, such as medical, emotional, and educational neglect, as well as inadequate supervision. Thus, in determining neglectful behaviors, one must consider providing proper nutrition and shelter; protection from harm; appropriate medical, mental health, and educational services for children; and attention to a child's physical, psychological, and emotional needs (DePanfilis 2006; Erickson and Egeland 2002).

Physical Injury and Death

Data from the Fourth National Incidence Study of Child Abuse and Neglect suggest that between 2005 and 2006, approximately 1,256,600 children experienced maltreatment, which is 1 child of every 58 in the United States (Sedlak et al. 2010). An estimated 553,300 children experienced abuse, including physical (323,000), sexual (135,300), and emotional (148,500) abuse, and an estimated 772,700 children were neglected (Sedlak et al. 2010). In addition, the annual report of the National Child Abuse and Neglect Data System reported that during 2008, approximately 772,000 children were determined to be victims of abuse or neglect by Child Protective Services (U.S. Department of Health and Human Services 2010). However, databases that include only reported incidents of abuse underestimate the actual prevalence of child maltreatment. Surveys including nonreported abuse incidents suggest considerably higher rates of child maltreatment (Straus et al. 1998).

Injuries sustained from acts of physical abuse range from minor physical injuries (e.g., bruises) to serious disfigurement and disability. Common injuries sustained by abused children are burns, chest and abdominal injuries, and fractures (Myers 1992). In addition, neglect may result in growth and developmental delays, lead or other poisoning, and failure to thrive (Ricci 2000). Obviously, the most severe consequence of child abuse is death. According to Daro (1988), deaths related to child abuse are a leading cause of both infant and child mortality. In 2008, an estimated 1740 children died of some form of child abuse or neglect (U.S. Department of Health and Human Services 2010). Approximately 30% of these deaths were related to child neglect, and 40% were caused by multiple maltreatment types (U.S. Department of Health and Human Services 2010). However, many injuries classified as unintentional may be due to physical abuse or neglect. As many as 50% to 60% of deaths that are a result of abuse or neglect are not recorded as such (Crume et al. 2002). Thus, it is likely that mortality rates are higher than estimated (Wiese and Daro 1995). Children who sustain physical force or violent shaking often suffer head injury, which is one of the most life-threatening injuries related to maltreatment (Committee on Child Abuse and Neglect 2001). In fact, head injuries are the most common cause of death in maltreated children (Dias et al. 2005), and it has been estimated that approximately 20% to 25% of infants who suffer from shaken baby syndrome die as a result of their injuries (U.S. Advisory Board on Child Abuse and Neglect 1995).

Short- and Long-Term Psychological Consequences

In general, maltreated children may experience a variety of detrimental abuse-related outcomes, including intellectual difficulties and impaired physical, social, and psychological development. In particular, child physical abuse has been linked to a variety of difficulties, such as depression, anxiety, and suicide attempts (Johnson et al. 2002; Silverman, Reinherz, Giaconia 1996), impaired language and cognitive development, poor academic achievement (NCCAN 2004), and externalizing behaviors (e.g., heightened oppositionality and aggression) (Trickett and Kuczynski 1986). Research specifically examining neglect has suggested that neglected children experience disruptions in attachment and various psychological factors, such as low self-esteem (Egeland 1991; Kaufman and Cicchetti 1989) and cognitive deficits (Mackner, Starr, and Black 1997). Neglected children also exhibit impaired social interactions and are seen as dependent and distractible in classroom settings (NCCAN 2003b).

Physically abused and neglected children experience not only short-term cognitive, emotional, and behavioral difficulties but also detrimental effects that extend beyond childhood. For example, research has demonstrated that physical abuse is associated with multiple internalizing and externalizing mental health diagnoses in both children and adolescents (Flisher et al. 1997). In fact, adolescence may be a particularly troublesome time for physically abused and neglected children, because maltreatment is associated with higher rates of delinquency among this age group (Kelley, Thornberry, and Smith 1997; Widom 1989a). Even beyond adolescence, the effects of physical abuse have been found to extend into adulthood. For example, prior abuse is associated with an increased likelihood of violence in subsequent dating relationships (Wolfe et al. 2001) and greater rates of perpetrating abuse against one's children (Ertem, Leventhal, and Dobbs 2000). Widom (1989b) also documented longitudinal associations between child physical abuse and adult violence, which she terms a "cycle of violence." Furthermore, adults who were abused as children display greater rates of substance abuse (Malinosky-Rummell and Hansen 1993) and are four times more likely to experience personality disorders during early adulthood (Johnson et al. 1999).

Costs

Although children bear the overwhelming personal costs of physical abuse and neglect, the financial toll of these acts extends far beyond the boundaries of the child and family. For example, child physical abuse exacts an indirect toll on society through its relationship to special education, juvenile delinquency, mental health and health care, violent crime, and job productivity loss (Wang and Holton 2007). The total costs of child abuse and neglect in the United States alone have been estimated conservatively at $103.8 billion per year (Wang and Holton 2007). Direct costs to society include those incurred through the child welfare system, which investigates potential incidents of abuse and neglect, as well as costs to mental and medical healthcare, legal, and judicial systems (NCCAN 2004; Wang and Holton 2007). The cost of providing services to maltreated families has been estimated to be more than $33 billion per year (Wang and Holton 2007).

Risk Factors

Physical abuse and neglect cut across all racial/ethnic groups and socioeconomic strata. Nevertheless, certain factors are associated with a higher risk of maltreatment. The presence of one or two factors does not inevitably signal the presence of abuse or neglect. However, as risk factors accumulate and interact with each other, the likelihood of abuse or neglect occurring greatly increases. Outlined below are some of the major child, parent, and family risk factors associated with physical abuse and neglect.

Child Factors

Investigations to determine individual child risk factors for abuse and neglect often produce inconsistent or contradictory results (National Research Council 1993). Difficulties in such research include disentangling those factors that contribute to risk of abuse from those that are consequences of abuse. Despite such differences, these research efforts provide insight into potential child-related factors that may place children at increased risk for physical abuse and neglect. For example, data suggest that child fatalities are more common among young children, particularly those aged less than 3 years (U.S. Department of Health and Human Services 2006). Further, health status (e.g., physical and emotional disabilities) and difficult temperament/behavior (e.g., increased oppositionality) have also been linked to an increased risk for maltreatment (Kolko 2002). For example, children with physical or developmental challenges experience greater rates of reported abuse and neglect (Crosse, Kaye, and Ratnofsky 1992). The NCCAN (2003b) suggests that childhood trauma, birth-related difficulties (e.g., premature birth, exposure to toxins), and involvement with antisocial peer groups are all risk factors for child abuse and neglect. However, it is also important to note that investigators have suggested that child risk factors may play a greater role in the maintenance of abusive and neglectful behaviors than in the onset of such behaviors (Ammerman 1991; Wolfe 1985).

Parent Factors

A number of factors related to caregivers also place children at an increased risk for physical abuse and neglect. With regard to fatalities, those resulting from child physical abuse are more often caused by male caregivers (including fathers), whereas those associated with neglect are more often caused by mothers (U.S. Advisory Board on Child Abuse and Neglect 1995). Furthermore, data suggest that younger parents are more likely than older parents to physically abuse their children (Brown et al. 1998), and that abusive mothers often report decreased social support networks (Bishop and Leadbeater 1999). Kolko (2002) summarizes a number of parental factors associated with child maltreatment, including a history of abuse, increased stress, maladaptive coping strategies (e.g., anger management difficulties, emotion-focused coping), and psychological factors (e.g., depression). In addition, parental substance abuse and parenting styles that are inconsistent, overly controlling, or critical have been linked to physical abuse and neglect (Kolko 2002). Caregivers who have inappropriate developmental expectations of their children and those who make negative attributions about their children's behaviors are also at an increased risk for child maltreatment.

Family Factors

Certain family characteristics, such as single parenthood, the presence of domestic violence in the home, and family stressors (e.g., financial), are associated with increased rates of abuse and neglect (Connell-Carrick 2003; Shepard and Raschick 1999). However, ecologically based models of child maltreatment suggest that abuse is a product not only of the immediate family context but also of the family's relationship with surrounding environmental influences (Belsky 1993). Indeed, although maltreatment occurs within the context of the parent–child relationship, it is a complex phenomenon that arises from an interaction of child, parent, and larger societal factors (Belsky 1993). Thus, a number of family variables, including family interactions within broader community and societal contexts, may place a child at increased risk of abuse or neglect. More specifically, coercive parent–child interactions and poor family relationships (e.g., limited cohesion and satisfaction), unemployment, poverty, marital discord, exposure to domestic violence, and lack of social support have all been implicated as risk factors for maltreatment (Kolko 2002). Furthermore, the NCCAN (2003b) reported that low socioeconomic status, homelessness, community violence, poor schools, life stressors, divorce, and domestic violence are all family variables that increase the probability that maltreatment will occur. Poverty, substance abuse, maternal depression, social isolation, and living in a dangerous neighborhood have all been identified as risk factors for neglect specifically (Ernst, Meyer, and DePanfilis 2004).

Up-To-Date Research Findings and Recommendations for Practice

Prevention of Abuse

Because of the potential risk factors associated with physical abuse and neglect, as well as the deleterious sequelae of maltreatment, efforts at preventing child maltreatment are of enormous importance. Prevention efforts can be classified as primary, secondary, and tertiary (Commission on Chronic Illness 1957) or similarly as universal, selected, and indicated (Guterman 2004; Mirazek and Haggerty 1994). Because tertiary or indicated prevention efforts include interventions after abuse has occurred (e.g. the majority of treatment approaches), this section will focus on primary and secondary or universal and selected preventions (e.g. efforts aimed to prevent abuse before it occurs).

Prevention efforts have shifted away from the pathologic view of abusive and neglectful families toward efforts targeting parenting skills and education, as well as reducing parenting related stress (Wekerle and Wolfe 1998). Consequently, similar to many treatment approaches, specific prevention efforts are aimed at assisting, supporting, and educating parents. Home visitation programs are one such approach and often involve targeting new parents or at-risk families to provide education and shape parent–child interactions (Daro and Donnelly 2002; Miller-Perrin and Perrin 2007). Many in-home approaches involve nurse visitation programs, which have demonstrated efficacy in improving caregiving behaviors (i.e., reduced rates of maltreatment, as well as medical encounters related to injury), and maternal health care (Eckenrode et al. 2001; Korfmacher, Kitzman, and Olds 1998; Olds et al. 1998). In addition, these programs provide both support and education for parents (Roberts et al. 1991) and are recommended in the prevention of child physical abuse and neglect (Krug et al. 2002).

Related interventions, such as Project SafeCare (Gershater-Molko, Lutzker, and Wesch 2003), target families at risk for abuse or neglect and may be classified as a secondary/selected effort. This in-home approach has been shown to improve child health care and home safety, and to strengthen the parent–child relationship (Edwards and Lutzker 2008; Gershater-Molko, Lutzker, and Wesch 2003). Alternative universal prevention approaches are parent education programs and parent support groups, which both provide parents with the opportunity to gain support and knowledge from one another, and are often successful in providing motivation to commit to services because of the support network inherent in the group (Daro and Donnelly 2002). Such interventions are provided outside of the home, commonly through local schools or community-based programs (e.g., Head Start). These groups have been linked to positive outcomes, such as increased parental functioning, positive parent–child interactions, and a strengthened social support network (Daro and Donnelly 2002).

Rather than target parents specifically, some prevention efforts adopt a broader focus by targeting society in an attempt to prevent child maltreatment. These approaches aim to educate the public, often using the media to publicize child abuse awareness campaigns. The argument behind this approach is that increasing knowledge about child maltreatment will help reduce the amounts of child abuse in society (Miller-Perrin and Perrin 2007). Several organizations, both nationwide and at state and local levels, have attempted to increase public awareness regarding the problem of child abuse for several decades. For example, Prevent Child Abuse America promoted public service announcements depicting the horrors of abuse beginning in the 1970s (Daro and Donnelly 2002). Such campaigns have been associated with increased public awareness, as well as an increase in reports of child abuse (McCurdy and Daro 1994). Statewide approaches to alert society to the tragedy of child abuse include such efforts as the Blue Ribbon Campaign to Prevent Child Abuse in Virginia and the Nebraska Health and Human Services public awareness campaign entitled, "You Have the Power to Protect a Child." The former campaign includes television and radio spots highlighting child maltreatment, as well as newspaper advertisements.

Treatment Approaches

Interventions after the occurrence of physical abuse include those that target the individual child and those that focus on the parent, family treatment, and multisystemic approaches. For neglectful families, interventions primarily focus on caregivers' parenting behaviors. Such interventions are typically time intensive and involve multiple providers. What follows is a brief overview of some of the main treatment approaches for child physical abuse and neglect.

Child-Focused Interventions

The treatment of abused and neglected children can be challenging because there is no consistent clinical picture of an abused child. Thus, as noted by Wurtele (1998), there are several potential domains of intervention (e.g., physical, cognitive, behavioral, socioemotional); effective treatment must involve comprehensive assessment across these domains to determine the necessary targets for intervention. Comprehensive interventions also must take into account the broader systemic context of maltreatment, including issues of family preservation/reunification and foster care placement. In the case of physical abuse, initial intervention may involve medical practitioners to treat physical injury and to set the foundation for later psychological, psychosocial, and legal intervention (Ricci 2000). For neglected children, initial intervention will likely also involve efforts to establish a stable environment and determine the developmental, educational, and medical and emotional health status of the child (Ricci 2000). Psychological interventions for maltreated children are designed to assist them in managing the emotional and behavioral sequelae of physical abuse and neglect. Such interventions include day treatment programs, individual therapy, and play therapy sessions. Although studies have demonstrated the effectiveness of child-focused interventions (Oates and Bross 1995; Wolfe and Wekerle 1993), continued research in this area is necessary, because most of these investigations have involved young children and have not differentiated between types of abuse.

One of the more recent projects to evaluate the evidence for interventions for maltreated children and their families comes from a report by the National Crime Victims Research and Treatment Center, which summarized treatment approaches with empirical support of both efficacy and effectiveness (Saunders, Berliner, and Hanson 2004). Although some treatments in the report received the highest rating, indicating an empirically supported, efficacious treatment, the majority of the treatments were classified only as supported and acceptable (see Chambless and Ollendick 2000 for details of effective and efficacious classification criteria). The majority of interventions for abused and neglected children are tertiary approaches.

One approach noted in the National Crime Victims Research and Treatment Center report (Saunders, Berliner, and Hanson 2004) is cognitive behavioral therapy (CBT), which involves helping children identify and alter abuse-related cognitions, teaching new coping skills to manage the emotional and behavioral symptoms related to abuse, and increasing social competence (Bonner 2004) in an effort to decrease the interpersonal outcomes related to maltreatment. Several CBT approaches have demonstrated empirical support and are considered acceptable treatments for maltreated children, including an individual child physical abuse-focused CBT protocol by Kolko and Swenson (2002) that consists of child components that involve addressing views of family violence, coping strategies, interpersonal skills, and the use of role-play, feedback, and homework exercises. CBT approaches for children may also target trauma-related symptoms (Cohen and Mannarino 1993; Deblinger and Heflin 1996). Such interventions are designed to reduce the emotional outcomes related to abuse, as well as address cognitive distortions and negative, abuse-related schemas. Neglected children may evidence a variety of developmental delays; thus, intervention efforts may include therapeutic school settings that focus on addressing cognitive, motor, and social delays, or in the case of severe neglect, hospitalization and medical management (DePanfilis 2006). Although there is evidence that interventions are effective for some of these domains (Fantuzzo et al. 1996), well-designed studies of interventions for neglected children are limited and difficult to conduct (Allin, Wathen, and MacMillan 2005).

Parent-Focused Interventions

As noted, child physical abuse may stem, in part, from increasingly coercive parent–child interactions (Wolfe and Wekerle 1993). More specifically, abusive parents often maintain negative attributions about their children's actions (e.g., seeing innocuous behaviors as defiant) and perceive that the only effective discipline techniques are those involving physical punishment (Chaffin et al. 2004). Interventions have been used to help maltreating caregivers alter these perceptions and interrupt the coercive patterns that develop with their children. In general, these interventions target children who display behavioral problems and involve teaching parents skills to increase child compliance, decrease disruptive behaviors, and increase positive parent–child interactions (Brestan and Payne 2004).

One model that is widely used with physically abusive parents is Parent–Child Interaction Therapy (PCIT; Herschell and McNeil 2005), which has received support as an acceptable treatment. When applied to physical abuse, PCIT targets child behavior and emotional problems associated with physical abuse, as well as deficits in the parent–child relationship that can lead to violence (Urquiza 2004). PCIT has been shown to reduce child behavior problems and increase positive parent–child interactions (Kolko and Swenson 2002). It has also been shown to reduce the incidence of future child abuse reports (Chaffin et al. 2004). Furthermore, PCIT has demonstrated effectiveness across a variety of ethnic minority populations (Butler and Eyberg 2006), with treatment gains having been shown to generalize across time (Eyberg et al. 2001), settings (McNeil et al. 1991) and even to untreated siblings (Brestan et al. 1997). Several other parent training interventions used with maltreating families include *Living With Children: New Methods for Parents and Teachers* (Patterson and Gullion 1968), *Helping the Noncompliant Child: A Clinician's Guide to Parent Training* (Forehand and McMahon 1981), and *Defiant Children: A Clinician's Manual for Assessment and Parent Training* (Barkley 1997).

Family-Focused and Multisystemic Interventions

Although the line between parent and family-focused interventions can be fuzzy, family-focused interventions tend to target parent–child relationships and various family issues (e.g., boundaries; Ralston and Sosnowski 2004). For example, intensive family preservation programs provide interventions that are tailored to a family's needs and may involve crisis intervention and behavior modification to address a variety of family risk factors (Haapala and Kinney 1988). These interventions are designed to prevent the out-of-home placement of abused and neglected children. Although initial studies suggested these programs reduce out-of-home placements (Bath and Haapala 1993) and improve family functioning (e.g., communication, behavior problems) (Blythe, Jiordano, and Kelly 1991), some have raised serious questions about these findings on the basis of methodological limitations of studies evaluating such programs (Lindsey, Martin, and Doh 2002). An additional family treatment program is the Parent–Child Education Program (Wolfe 1991), which targets the use of power in discipline and aims to establish positive parent–child interactions. This program involves the use of effective parenting strategies, increasing compliance, strengthening the parent–child relationship, and learning new coping strategies to deal with parenting stress (Wolfe 2004). Another family-focused intervention is physical abuse-informed family therapy (Kolko 1996), in which family members participate in parallel CBT to address understanding of coercive behavior, problem-solving, and communication skills. This treatment has been shown to improve parental distress, abuse risk, and family cohesion and conflict when compared with traditional community services (Kolko 1996).

According to the multisystemic perspective approaches, abusive behaviors are maintained through interactions among a variety of factors within the broader social–ecological framework surrounding the behavior (e.g., family, school, peer, society) (Brunk, Henggeler, and Whelan 1987). Therefore, these treatment approaches are aimed at a number of factors, including systemic problems, which may aid families in maintaining motivation to change (Ayoub, Willett, and Robinson 1992), as well as reducing the stress level of abusive parents so that therapeutic concerns can be addressed. Abusive families may display a wide variety of dysfunction that requires the provision of multiple services, and multisystemic and societal approaches emphasize this need. A well-known approach for abusive and neglectful families is multisystemic therapy (Henggeler et al. 1998). Although created to target antisocial behavior in youth, multisystemic therapy has been adapted for use with maltreating and neglectful families. This intervention has been shown to improve parent–child interactions when compared with parent training approaches (Brunk, Henggeler, and Whelan 1987). It is also one of the few approaches to demonstrate effectiveness in addressing a variety of youth and parent-related risk factors for abused and neglected adolescents (Swenson et al. 2010).

Role and Importance of Advocacy

Advocacy has been defined as the pursuit of influencing outcomes—including public policy and resource allocation decisions within political, economic, and social systems and institutions—that directly affect people's lives (Advocacy Institute n.d.). Children, as a constituency, are lacking in the ability to advocate for themselves, as are those with severe mental illnesses. They must instead depend on others to work on their behalf toward the prevention of abuse and neglect and to serve as a voice for their interests when maltreatment does occur. As noted previously, child abuse advocacy might be said to have started with Kempe and colleagues' (1962) exposure of the battered child syndrome more than 40 years ago. It was this exposure that brought attention to what had previously been considered private family matters and precipitated scientific and public interest in the physical abuse of children. Today, child abuse advocacy is not a highly organized or integrated movement. Rather, it is a conglomeration of various entities, including specialized organizations, professional associations, and legal and policy groups that work in various ways to reduce the prevalence and impact of child abuse and neglect. Discussed next will be some of the most visible entities representing these groups. To aid readers in learning about child abuse advocacy, Web addresses for relevant organizations are provided.

Specialized Organizations

A fundamental belief of many advocacy groups is that increased societal awareness of abuse can help reduce its prevalence. With this goal in mind, there are several national organizations that focus on public education campaigns about specific abuse issues. The National Center on Shaken Baby Syndrome (at http://www.dontshake.com), for example, has a mission of educating parents and childcare providers about the dangers of shaking babies and promoting research on the prevention of shaken baby syndrome. The center also works to train professionals to prevent and identify cases of shaken baby syndrome. Likewise, the National Organization on Fetal Alcohol Syndrome (at http://www.nofas.org) works through communities to help local advocates evaluate and address the prevalence of fetal alcohol syndrome.

There are also organizations with broader objectives that subsume issues related to abuse and neglect. The Child Welfare League of America (at http://www.cwla.org), for example, is a membership organization dedicated to the overall well-being of children. This organization's advocacy agenda is broad, dealing with a host of interrelated issues, ranging from childcare, to teen pregnancy, to youth substance abuse issues. Child abuse and neglect are also included in this agenda. Within this realm, the league supports community-based approaches to preventing abuse and neglect by strengthening families, as well as improving child protective service's ability to address maltreatment. The league also draws attention to specific abuse-related issues, such as baby abandonment.

As does the Child Welfare League, the Children's Defense Fund (at http://www.childrensdefense.org) pursues a broad child-oriented agenda that includes the problems of undereducation, poverty, and illness. One of their policy priorities is to protect every child from abuse and neglect. Their efforts in doing so are based on the belief that partnerships among public child protection agencies, other agencies and organizations serving children, and families themselves can be most effective in combating abuse. An example of such partnerships is the Early Childhood Home Visitation Program, which provides support and education to families of young children to foster development, increase academic preparedness, and reduce child abuse and neglect. The Children's Defense Fund works at national, state, and local levels.

A third organization, Prevent Child Abuse America (at http://www.preventchildabuse.org), also works to advocate for children by influencing policies, increasing education and awareness, and promoting programs to address child abuse and neglect. This national organization also seeks funding for ongoing research geared toward preventing child abuse and neglect.

Professional Membership Associations

Membership associations are multidisciplinary groups consisting of professionals who have a vested interest in reducing the incidence and effects of child abuse and neglect. These nonprofit groups contain members of various fields that span the areas of research, service provision, and policy related to child maltreatment. The American Professional Society on the Abuse of Children (at http://

www.apsac.org) is one such group, dedicated to identifying, treating, and preventing child abuse. The group also seeks to educate the public and impact policy on multiple levels. The American Professional Society on the Abuse of Children pursues this agenda in part through local chapters in several states. The International Society for the Prevention of Child Abuse and Neglect (at http://www.ispcan.org) is another prominent organization of mixed disciplines that promotes training, provides resources, and facilitates the exchange of information related to child maltreatment, with an explicitly global focus. Both of these professional organizations foster communication through the publication of newsletters, official society journals that provide outlets for empirical research, and regular conferences to facilitate exchange of information and ideas relevant to maltreatment.

Legal and Policy Groups

The Court Appointed Special Advocate (CASA; at http://www.nationalcasa.org) program represents a significant and growing source of advocacy for abused children within the legal system. Although CASA operates with several different models, the essence of the program consists of volunteers serving as advocates for child abuse and neglect victims who are involved in judicial proceedings. These volunteers (70,000 nationally) are appointed by the court to familiarize themselves with the facts of a case (through interviews with the child, parents, and involved professionals), to develop a relationship with the child victim, and to advocate for that child during legal proceedings. CASA is able to make official reports to the court regarding recommendations for placing children in permanent, safe living situations. One strength of the CASA program is that data supporting its effectiveness are starting to emerge. For example, there is evidence that CASA is at least as affective as attorney guardian ad litems in achieving several goals, including being more likely to make face-to-face contact with children and to file written briefs with the court, and, most important, having more cases that result in adoption and fewer that involve repeated stints in foster care (Youngclarke, Ramos, and Granger-Merkle 2004).

Other law and policy-related groups are also involved in child abuse advocacy on both the national and local levels. The American Bar Association Center for Children and the Law (at http://www.abanet.org/child/home.html) was formed in the late 1970s exclusively to focus on issues of child abuse and neglect. Although its purview has expanded, the center remains involved in abuse and neglect issues, ranging from improving the judicial processes related to abuse and neglect, to developing alternative techniques for the forensic interviewing of child victims, and to influencing public policy that affects the well-being of children.

On more of a state than national level are law and policy centers that seek to monitor legal and policy matters related to abuse and neglect, and to empirically evaluate their implementation and effectiveness. Staffed primarily by attorneys and behavioral and social scientists, these centers attempt to link research to the legislative and policy issues that affect families, such as poverty, domestic violence, unwanted pregnancy, and matters related to abuse and neglect, including child welfare reform, the foster care system, and juvenile justice. One such center is the Center for Children, Families, and the Law at the University of Nebraska-Lincoln (http://ccfl.unl.edu). Established in 1987, the center fulfills it mission through a combination of research, outreach, and training activities, which include competency-based case management training for child protection and safety workers in the state of Nebraska.

Future Research, Practice, and Advocacy Directions

Research

Researchers have typically divided child maltreatment into different subtypes, including child physical abuse, sexual abuse, neglect, psychological abuse, and exposure to domestic violence.

Traditionally, research has been conducted independently in each of these realms. This work has been tremendously helpful in understanding individual forms of abuse. At the same time, traditional divisions between abuse types—and those who research them—may sometimes limit progress in understanding abuse and neglect. Households in which one type of abuse occurs are often fraught with other forms as well (Clemmons et al. 2003). Consider, for example, the inextricable associations between the physical abuse and the emotional abuse that so often accompanies it (Claussen and Crittenden 1991). Understanding the co-occurrence of abuse types can help, for example, with the development of more efficient interventions that address a few key risk factors associated with multiple forms of abuse.

A related issue is the need to develop more comprehensive etiologic models of child abuse and neglect. Most studies to date have investigated single factor theories of the causes and effects of abuse. Although the study of individual contributors is worthwhile, the complex nature of maltreatment calls for models that take into account multiple contributing factors. Conceptual models that consider transactions among various levels of risk factors have been proposed (Cicchetti and Lynch 1993). However, from both a methodological and resource standpoint, it is difficult to account for the many factors—societal, cultural, family, individual—that play a role in the development of abuse. Longitudinal studies, which follow abused and matched nonabused controls prospectively to evaluate adjustment across time, hold promise for illuminating the complex nature of abuse and neglect. Although a few such studies exist, greater use of longitudinal approaches would shed light on important questions about the cause, consequences, and mechanisms of abuse.

Finally, definitional inconsistencies have long plagued this area of research, limiting generalization of findings and making comparisons across studies difficult. Neglect, in particular, has been difficult to define, probably because of the inherent challenges in measuring the absence of parental behaviors, rather than the more salient acts of commission that constitute physical abuse. The field would benefit from greater consensus regarding what constitutes various abuse types.

Practice

There are several directions in which the prevention and treatment of abuse issues could go in the future. Most important, perhaps, is the need for interventionists to use current scientific knowledge in the course of practice with maltreated children. As noted previously, prevention and treatment approaches for physically abused and neglected youth are still in the relatively early stages of development. Development of these programs is challenging, however, because of the vast array of potential causes and consequences of abuse and neglect. Nevertheless, in recent years there has been an increase in randomized controlled trials to evaluate interventions. As these findings are realized, it will be incumbent on practitioner and state and local agencies to stay abreast of them to use the most empirically supported approaches. Although initiatives to disseminate evidence-based interventions are under way (Cohen and Mannarino 2008), too often there has been a disconnect between those producing the empirical research on abuse and neglect and the practitioners for whom those findings are most relevant. It will be important for both researchers and practitioners to reach across this divide to offer more coordinated services to those in need.

To date, most empirically supported interventions are aimed at younger children, often preschool age. There is need, however, to extend treatment gains made with younger populations to older victims because many victims are in late childhood or early adolescence when abuse occurs, or there is a delay in the emergence of symptoms.

Advocacy

Advocates have long led the way in increasing awareness about cutting-edge issues related to abuse and neglect. From this standpoint, the advocacy movement is in an excellent position to keep child maltreatment in the public consciousness. Topics such as shaken baby syndrome have come to the attention of medical professionals and the public largely through advocacy efforts. Nevertheless, advocacy organizations must continually strive to keep issues of abuse and neglect at the top of policymakers' agendas, so that their cause is not adversely affected by the usual dips in political attention that affect so many social issues. In contrast with other, well-funded interests, child advocates must rely on the gravity of the issues more than financial support of politicians when advancing policy initiatives. Therefore, the movement must continually draw attention to the problem of abuse and neglect on behalf of children who do not have an independent voice.

References

Advocacy Institute (n.d.). Available at: http://www.advocacyinstitute.org. Accessed October 7, 2011.

Allin HC, Wathen N, MacMillan H. 2005. Treatment of child neglect: a systematic review. *Can Child Adolesc Psychiatr Rev.* 50:497–504.

Ammerman RT. 1991. The role of the child in physical abuse: a reappraisal. *Violence Vict.* 6:87–101.

Ayoub C, Willett JB, Robinson DS. 1992. Families at risk of child maltreatment: entry-level characteristics and growth in family functioning during treatment. *Child Abuse Negl.* 16:495–511.

Barkley RA. 1997. *Defiant Children: A Clinician's Manual for Assessment and Parent Training.* New York: Guilford.

Bath H, Haapala DA. 1993. Intensive family preservation services with abused and neglected children: an examination of group differences. *Child Abuse Negl.* 17:213–225.

Belsky J. 1993. Etiology of child maltreatment: a developmental-ecological analysis. *Psychol Bull.* 114:413–434.

Bishop SJ, Leadbeater BJ. 1999. Maternal social support patterns and child maltreatment: comparison of maltreating and nonmaltreating mothers. *Am J Orthopsychiatry.* 69:172–181.

Blythe BJ, Jiordano MJ, Kelly SA. 1991. Family preservation with substance abusing families: help that works. *Child, Youth, and Family Services Quarterly.* 14:12–13.

Bonner B. 2004. Cognitive-behavioral and dynamic play therapy for children with sexual behavior problems and their caregivers. In: Saunders BE, Berliner L, Hanson RF, editors. *Child Physical and Sexual Abuse: Guidelines for Treatment (Revised Report: April 26, 2004).* Charleston, SC: National Crime Victims Research and Treatment Center. 34–36.

Brestan EV, Eyberg SM, Boggs SR, Algina J. 1997. Parent-child interaction therapy: parents' perceptions of untreated siblings. *Child Fam Behav Ther.* 19:13–28.

Brestan E, Payne H. 2004. Behavioral parent training interventions for conduct-disordered children. In: Saunders BE, Berliner L, Hanson RF, editors. *Child Physical and Sexual Abuse: Guidelines for Treatment (Revised Report: April 26, 2004),* Charleston, SC: National Crime Victims Research and Treatment Center. 61–65.

Brown J, Cohen P, Johnson J, Salzinger S. 1998. A longitudinal analysis of risk factors for child maltreatment: findings of a prospective study of officially recorded and self-reported child abuse and neglect. *Child Abuse Negl.* 22:1065–1079.

Brunk M, Henggeler SW, Whelan JP. 1987. Comparison of multisystemic therapy and parent training in the brief treatment of child abuse and neglect. *J Consult Clin Psychol.* 55:171–178.

Butler AM, Eyberg SM. 2006. Parent-child interaction therapy and ethnic minority children. *Vulnerable Children Youth Stud.* 1:246–255.

Chaffin M, Silovsky JF, Funderburk B, et al. 2004. Parent-child interaction therapy with physically abusive parents: efficacy for reducing future abuse reports. *J Consult Clin Psychol.* 72:500–510.

Chambless DL, Ollendick TH. 2000. Empirically supported psychological interventions: controversies and evidence. *Ann Rev Psychol.* 52:685–716.

Cicchetti D. 1988. The organization and coherence of socioemotional, cognitive, and representational development: illustrations through a developmental psychopathology perspective on Down syndrome and child maltreatment. In: Thompson RA, editor. *36th Annual Nebraska Symposium on Motivation: Socioemotional Development.* Lincoln, NE: University of Nebraska Press. 259–366.

Cicchetti D, Lynch M. 1993. Toward an ecological/transactional model of community violence and child maltreatment: consequences for children's development. *Psychiatry.* 56:96–118.

Claussen AH, Crittenden PM. 1991. Physical and psychological maltreatment: relations among types of maltreatment. *Child Abuse Negl.* 15:5–18.

Clemmons JC, DiLillo D, Martinez IG, et al. 2003. Co-occurring forms of child maltreatment and adult adjustment reported by Latina college students. *Child Abuse Negl.* 27:751–767.

Cohen JA, Mannarino AP. 1993. A treatment model of sexually abused preschoolers. *J Interpers Violence.* 8:115–131.

Cohen J, Mannarino AP. 2008. Disseminating and implementing trauma-focused CBT in community settings. *Trauma Violence Abuse.* 9:214–226.

Commission on Chronic Illness. 1957. *Chronic Illness in the United States, Vol. 1.* Cambridge, MA: Harvard University Press.

Committee on Child Abuse and Neglect. 2001. Shaken-baby syndrome: rotational cranial injuries technical report. *Pediatrics.* 108:206–210.

Connell-Carrick K. 2003. A critical review of the empirical literature: identifying correlates of child neglect. *Child Adolesc Social Work J.* 20:389–342.

Crosse SB, Elyse Kaye E, Ratnofsky A. 1992. *A Report on the Maltreatment of Children with Disabilities.* Washington, DC: U.S. Department of Health and Human Services, National Clearinghouse on Child Abuse and Neglect Information.

Crume TL, DiGuiseppi C, Byers T, et al. 2002. Underascertainment of child maltreatment fatalities by death certificates, 1990-1998. *Pediatrics.* 110:1–6.

Daro D. 1988. Confronting Child Abuse Research for Effective Program Design. New York: Free Press.

Daro D, Donnelly AC. 2002. Child abuse prevention: accomplishments and challenges. In: Myers JEB, Berliner LA, Briere J, et al., editors. *The APSAC Handbook on Child Maltreatment.* 2nd ed. Thousand Oaks, CA: Sage Publications. 431–488.

Deblinger E, Heflin AH. 1996. *Treatment for Sexually Abused Children and Their Non-Offending Parents: A Cognitive-Behavioral Approach.* Thousand Oaks, CA: Sage Publications.

DePanfilis D. 2006. *Child Neglect: A Guide for Prevention, Assessment, and Intervention.* Washington, DC: U.S. Department of Health and Human Services, Administration on Children and Families, Administration for Children, Youth, and Families, Children's Bureau, Office on Child Abuse and Neglect.

Dias MS, Smith K, deGuehery K, et al. 2005. Preventing abusive head trauma among infants and young children: a hospital-based, parent education program. *Pediatrics.* 115:470–477.

Eckenrode J, Zielinski D, Smith E, et al. 2001. Child maltreatment and the early onset of problem behaviors: can a program of nurse home visitation break the link? *Dev Psychopathol.* 13:873–890.

Edwards A, Lutzker JR. 2008. Iterations of the SafeCare Model: an evidence-based child maltreatment prevention program. *Behav Modif.* 32:736–756.

Egeland B. 1991. A longitudinal study of high-risk families: issues and findings. In: Starr RH Jr, Wolfe DA, editors. *The Effects of Child Abuse and Neglect: Issues and Research.* New York: Guilford. 33–56.

Erickson MF, Egeland B. 2002. Child neglect. In: Myers JEB, Berliner LA, Briere J, editors. *The APSAC Handbook on Child Maltreatment.* 2nd ed. Thousand Oaks, CA: Sage Publications. 21–54.

Ernst JS, Meyer M, DePanfilis D. 2004. Housing characteristics and adequacy of the physical care of children: an exploratory analysis. *Child Welfare.* 83:437–452.

Ertem IO, Leventhal JM, Dobbs S. 2000. Intergenerational continuity of child physical abuse: how good is the evidence? *Lancet.* 356:814–819.

Eyberg SM, Funderburk BW, Hembree-Kigin TL, et al. 2001. Parent-child interaction therapy with behavior problem children: one and two year maintenance of treatment effects in the family. *Child Fam Behav Ther.* 23:1–20.

Fantuzzo J, Sutton-Smith B, Atkins M, et al. 1996. Community-based resilient peer treatment of withdrawn maltreated preschool children. *J Consult Clin Psychol.* 64:1377–1386.

Flisher AJ, Kramer RA, Hoven CW, et al. 1997. Psychosocial characteristics of physically abused children and adolescents. *J Am Acad Child Adolesc Psychiatry.* 36:123–131.

Forehand RL, McMahon RJ. 1981. *Helping the Noncompliant Child: A Clinician's Guide to Parent Training.* New York: Guilford.

Garbarino J, Guttmann E, Seeley JW. 1986. *The Psychologically Battered Child: Strategies for Identification, Assessment, and Intervention.* San Francisco: Jossey-Bass.

Gershater-Molko RM, Lutzker JR, Wesch D. 2003. Project SafeCare: improving health, safety, and parenting skills in families reported for, and at-risk for child maltreatment. *J Fam Violence.* 18:377–389.

Graziano AM, Namaste KA. 1990. Parental use of physical force in child discipline: a survey of 679 college students. *J Interpers Violence.* 5:449–463.

Guterman NB. 2004. Advancing prevention research on child abuse, youth violence, and domestic violence: emerging strategies and issues. *J Interpers Violence.* 19:299–321.

Haapala DA, Kinney JM. 1988. Avoiding out-of-home placement of high-risk status offenders through the use of intensive family preservation services. *Crim Justice Behav.* 15:334–348.

Hansen DJ, Sedlar G, Warner-Rogers JE. 1999. Child physical abuse. In: Ammerman RT, Hersen M, editors. *Assessment of Family Violence: A Clinical and Legal Sourcebook.* New York: Wiley. 127–156.

Hecht DB, Hansen DJ. 2001. The environment of child maltreatment: contextual factors and the development of psychopathology. *Aggress Violent Behav.* 6:433–457.

Henggeler SW, Schoenwald SK, Borduin CM, et al. 1998. *Multisystemic Treatment of Antisocial Behavior in Children and Adolescents.* New York: Guilford.

Herschell AD, McNeil CB. 2005. Theoretical and empirical underpinnings of parent-child interaction therapy with child physical abuse populations. *Educ Treat Children.* 28:142–162.

Johnson JG, Cohen P, Brown J, et al. 1999. Childhood maltreatment increases risk for personality disorders during early adulthood. *Arch Gen Psychiatry.* 56:600–606.

Johnson RM, Kotch JB, Catellier DJ, et al. 2002. Adverse behavioral and emotional outcomes from child abuse and witnessed violence. *Child Maltreat.* 7:179–186.

Kaufman J, Cicchetti D. 1989. Effects of maltreatment on school-age children's socioemotional development: assessments in a day-camp setting. *Dev Psychol.* 25:516–524.

Kelleher K, Gardner W, Coben J, et al. 2006. Co-occurring intimate partner violence and child maltreatment: local policies/practices and relationships to child placement, family services and residence. Washington, DC: National Institute of Justice. Doc. 213503.

Kelley BT, Thornberry TP, Smith CA. 1997. *In the Wake of Childhood Maltreatment.* Washington, DC: National Institute of Justice.

Kempe CH, Silverman FN, Steele BF, et al. 1962. The battered child syndrome. *JAMA.* 181:17–24.

Kolko DJ. 1996. Individual cognitive behavioral therapy and family therapy for physically abused children and their offending parents: a comparison of clinical outcomes. *Child Maltreat.* 1:322–342.

Kolko DJ. 2002. Child physical abuse. In: Myers JEB, Berliner LA, Briere J, et al. editors. *The APSAC Handbook on Child Maltreatment.* 2nd ed. Thousand Oaks, CA: Sage Publications. 21–54.

Kolko DJ, Swenson CC. 2002. *Assessing and Treating Physically Abused Children and Their Families: A Cognitive-Behavioral Approach.* Thousand Oaks, CA: Sage Publications.

Korfmacher J, Kitzman H, Olds D. 1998. Intervention processes as predictors of outcomes in a preventive home-visitation program. *J Commun Psychol. Special Issue: Home Visitation II.* 26:49–64.

Krug EG, Mercy JA, Dahlberg LL, Zwi AB. 2002. *World Report on Violence and Health.* Geneva (Switzerland): World Health Organization.

Larzelere RE. 2000. Child outcomes of nonabusive and customary physical punishment by parents: an updated literature review. *Clin Psychol Rev.* 3:199–221.

Leeb RT, Paulozzi LJ, Melanson C, et al. 2008. *Child Maltreatment Surveillance: Uniform Definitions for Public Health and Recommended Data Elements, Version 1.0.* Atlanta, GA: Centers for Disease Control and Prevention, National Center for Injury Prevention and Control.

Liller KD. 2001. The importance of integrating approaches in child abuse/neglect and unintentional injury prevention efforts: implications for health educators. *Int J Health Educ.* 4:283–289.

Lindsey D, Martin S, Doh J. 2002. The failure of intensive casework services to reduce foster care placements: an examination of family preservation studies. *Children Youth Serv Rev.* 24:743–775.

Mackner LM, Starr RH Jr, Black MM. 1997. The cumulative effect of neglect and failure to thrive on cognitive functioning. *Child Abuse Negl.* 21:691–700.

Malinosky-Rummell R, Hansen DJ. 1993. Long-term consequences of childhood physical abuse. *Psychol Bull.* 114:68–79.

McCurdy K, Daro D. 1994. Current trends in child abuse reporting and fatalities. *J Interpers Violence.* 9:75–94.

McNeil CB, Eyberg S, Eisenstadt TH, et al. 1991. Parent-child interaction therapy with behavior problem children: generalization of treatment effects to the school setting. *J Child Clin Psychol.* 20:140–151.

Miller-Perrin CL, Perrin RD. 2007. *Child Maltreatment: An Introduction.* 2nd ed. Thousand Oaks: Sage Publications.

Mirazek PB, Haggerty RJ. 1994. *Reducing Risks for Mental Disorders.* Washington, DC: National Academy Press.

Myers JEB. 1992. *Legal Issues in Child Abuse and Neglect.* Thousand Oaks, CA: Sage Publications.

National Clearinghouse on Child Abuse and Neglect. 2001. *Acts of Omission: An Overview of Child Neglect.* Washington, DC: US Department of Health and Human Services.

National Clearinghouse on Child Abuse and Neglect. 2003a. *Child Abuse and Neglect State Statute Series Statutes-at-a-Glance: Definitions of Child Abuse and Neglect.* Washington, DC: US Department of Health and Human Services.

National Clearinghouse on Child Abuse and Neglect. 2003b. *Recognizing Child Abuse and Neglect: Signs and Symptoms.* Washington, DC: US Department of Health and Human Services.

National Clearinghouse on Child Abuse and Neglect. 2004. *What Is Child Abuse and Neglect?* Washington, DC: US Department of Health and Human Services.

National Research Council. 1993. *Understanding Child Abuse and Neglect.* Washington, DC: National Academy Press.

Oates RK, Bross DC. 1995. What have we learned about treating child physical abuse? A literature review of the last decade. *Child Abuse Negl.* 19:463–473.

Olds D, Henderson C Jr, Kitzman H, et al. 1998. The promise of home visitation: results of two randomized trials. *J Community Psychol.* 26:5–21.

Patterson GR, Gullion ME. 1968. *Living With Children: New Methods for Parents and Teachers.* Champaign, IL: Research Press.

Peterson L, Brown D. 1994. Integrating child injury and abuse-neglect research: common histories, etiologies, and solutions. *Psychol Bull.* 116:293–315.

Ralston ME, Sosnowski PB. 2004. Family focused, child centered treatment interventions in child maltreatment. In: Saunders BE, Berliner L, Hanson R, editors. *Child Physical and Sexual Abuse: Guidelines for Treatment (Revised Report: April 26, 2004).* Charleston, SC: National Crime Victims Research and Treatment Center. 66–68.

Ricci LR. 2000. Initial medical treatment of the physically abused child. In: Reece RM, editor. *Treatment of Child Abuse: Common Ground for Mental Health, Medical, and Legal Practitioners.* Baltimore: The Johns Hopkins University Press. 81–94.

Roberts RN, Wasik BH, Casto G, Ramey CT. 1991. Family support in the home: programs, policy, and social change. *Am Psychol.* 46:131–137.

Sands, Roberta G. 1995. The parenting experience of low-income single women with serious mental disorders. *Families in Society: The Journal of Contemporary Human Services* 76:86–89.

Saunders BE, Berliner L, Hanson RF. 2004. *Child Physical and Sexual Abuse: Guidelines for Treatment (Revised Report: April 26, 2004).* Charleston, SC: National Crime Victims Research and Treatment Center.

Sedlak AJ, Mettenburg J, Basena M, et al. 2010. *Fourth National Incidence Study of Child Abuse and Neglect (NIS-4): Report to Congress.* Washington, DC: U.S. Department of Health and Human Services, Administration for Children and Families.

Shepard M, Raschick M. 1999. How child welfare workers assess and intervene around issues of domestic violence. *Child Maltreat.* 4:148–156.

Silverman AB, Reinherz HZ, Giaconia RM. 1996. The long-term sequelae of child and adolescent abuse: a longitudinal community study. *Child Abuse Negl.* 20:709–723.

Straus MA. 2001. *Beating the Devil Out of Them: Corporal Punishment in American Families and Its Effects on Children.* New Brunswick, NJ: Transaction Publishers.

Straus MA. 2005. Children should never, ever, be spanked no matter what the circumstances. In: Loseke DR, Gelles RJ, Cavanaugh MM, editors. *Current Controversies on Family Violence.* 2nd ed. Thousand Oaks, CA: Sage Publications. 137–157.

Straus MA, Hamby SL, Finkelhor D, et al. 1998. Identification of child maltreatment with the parent-child conflict tactics scales: development and psychometric data for a national sample of American parents. *Child Abuse Negl.* 22:249–270.

Swenson CC, Schaeffer CM, Henggeler SW, et al. 2010. Multisystemic therapy for child abuse and neglect: a randomized effectiveness trial. *J Fam Psychol.* 24:497–507.

Trickett PK, Kuczynski L. 1986. Children's misbehaviors and parental discipline strategies in abusive and nonabusive families. *Dev Psychol* 22:115–123.

U.S. Advisory Board on Child Abuse and Neglect. 1995. *A Nation's Shame: Fatal Child Abuse and Neglect in the United States.* Washington, DC: US Department of Health and Human Services.

U.S. Department of Health and Human Services, Administration on Children Youth and Families. 2006. *Child Maltreatment 2004.* Washington, DC: US Government Printing Office.

U.S. Department of Health and Human Services, Administration for Children and Families, Administration on Children, Youth and Families, Children's Bureau. 2010. *Child Maltreatment 2008.* Washington, DC: US Government Printing Office.

Urquiza AJ. 2004. Parent–child interaction therapy (PCIT). In: Saunders BE, Berliner L, Hanson R, editors. *Child Physical and Sexual Abuse: Guidelines for Treatment (Revised Report: April 26, 2004).* Charleston, SC: National Crime Victims Research and Treatment Center. 81–83.

Wang C-T, Holton J. 2007. *Total Estimated Cost of Child Abuse and Neglect in the United States.* Chicago, IL: Prevent Child Abuse. Available at: America.http://www.preventchildabuse.org/about_us/media_releases/pcaa_pew_economic_impact_study_final.pdf. Accessed July 15, 2010.

Warner-Rogers JE, Hansen DJ, Hecht DB. 1999. Child physical abuse and neglect. In: Van Hasselt V, Hersen M, editors. *Handbook of Psychological Approaches with Violent Offenders: Contemporary Strategies and Issues.* New York: Kluwer Academic/Plenum Publishers. 329–356.

Wekerle C, Wolfe DA. 1998. The role of child maltreatment and attachment style in adolescent relationship violence. *Dev Psychopathol.* 10:571–586.

Widom CS. 1989a. Does violence beget violence? A critical examination of the literature. *Psychol Bull.* 106:3–28.

Widom CS. 1989b. Child abuse, neglect and adult behavior: research design and findings on criminality, violence, and child abuse. *Am J Orthopsychiatry.* 58:260–270.

Widom CS. 2000. Motivation and mechanisms in the cycle of violence. In: Hansen DJ, editor. *Motivation and Child Maltreatment Vol 46.* Lincoln, NE: University of Nebraska Press. 1–37.

Wiese D, Daro D. 1995. *Current Trends in Child Abuse Reporting and Fatalities: The Results of the 1994 Annual Fifty State Survey.* Chicago, IL: National Committee to Prevent Child Abuse.

Wolfe DA. 1985. Child-abusive parents: an empirical review and analysis. *Psychol Bull.* 97:462–482.

Wolfe DA. 1991. *Preventing Physical and Emotional Abuse of Children.* New York: Guilford.

Wolfe DA. 1999. *Child Abuse: Implications for Child Development and Psychopathology.* 2nd ed. Thousand Oaks, CA: Sage Publications.

Wolfe DA. 2004. Parent-child education program for physically abusive parents. In: Saunders BE, Berliner L, Hanson R, editors. *Child Physical and Sexual Abuse: Guidelines for Treatment (Revised Report: April 26, 2004).* Charleston, SC: National Crime Victims Research and Treatment Center. 78–80.

Wolfe DA, McGee R. 1991. Assessment of emotional status among maltreated children. In: Starr RH Jr, Wolfe DA, editors. *The Effects of Child Abuse and Neglect: Issues and Research.* New York: Guilford. 257–277.

Wolfe DA, Scott K, Wekerle C, Pittman A-L. 2001. Child maltreatment: risk of adjustment problems and dating violence in adolescence. *J Am Acad Child Adolesc Psychiatry.* 40:282–289.

Wolfe DA, Wekerle C. 1993. Treatment strategies for child physical abuse and neglect: a critical progress report. *Clin Psychol Rev.* 13:473–500.

Wurtele S. 1998. Victims of child maltreatment. In: Singh N, editor. *Applications in Diverse Populations.* New York: Elsevier. 341–358.

Youngclarke D, Ramos KD, Granger-Merkle L. 2004. Trends & developments in the juvenile court: a systematic review of the impact of court appointed special advocates. *J Cent Famil Child Court.* 5:109–126.

Zuravin SJ. 1991. Research definitions of child physical abuse and neglect: current problems. In: Starr RH Jr, Wolfe DA, editors. *The Effects of Child Abuse and Neglect: Issues and Research.* New York: Guilford. 100–128.

Chapter 12

Firearm Injuries

Shannon Frattaroli, PhD, MPH,[1] Katherine A. Vittes, PhD, MPH,[2] Sara B. Johnson, PhD, MPH,[3] and Stephen P. Teret, JD, MPH[4]

Anthony, at age 13 years, had little reason to believe that his father's semiautomatic pistol was loaded when he pointed it at his best friend, Eric, age 14 years, and pulled the trigger.

Earlier that afternoon, when the two boys left school, they went to Anthony's house for a snack and to play. Anthony's mother had an appointment that took her away from home, so the boys fended for themselves. After eating, Anthony said to Eric "Come with me. I want to show you something." They went upstairs to Anthony's parent's bedroom, where Anthony opened the door to his father's closet, reached up to the shelf, and pulled down the loaded pistol that his father kept there for protection. Anthony removed from the pistol the magazine or clip that held the ammunition, and thinking that the gun was then unloaded, took it downstairs and outside the home where he and Eric could play with it. In the yard, Anthony pointed the gun at Eric's head, saying "BAM!" as he pulled the trigger. The pistol discharged the round that had remained in the chamber, and the bullet entered Eric's face to the left of his nose. Eric fell to the ground, unconscious; Anthony ran back into the house, replaced the gun in his father's closet, and called 911. By the time the first responders got to Anthony's home, Eric had died.[5]

The story of Anthony and Eric represents a common tragedy that underscores the need to apply effective injury prevention strategies to the firearm injury problem. Over the past few decades, researchers, advocates, and practitioners have advanced the science and practice of injury prevention principles to address the needs of gun violence prevention. In this chapter, we summarize the lessons learned from this work and suggest directions for advancing the accomplishments to date. Although the complex nature of firearm injury presents a formidable challenge for the injury prevention field, it is a challenge that we are well equipped to face.

The Nature of Firearm Injury in the United States

Mortality

In 2007, 3067 youth 19 years of age and younger died of firearm injuries. Of these deaths, 71% were homicides, 22% were suicides, 4% were unintentionally inflicted, and 2% were of

[1]Johns Hopkins Bloomberg School of Public Health, Center for Injury Research and Policy, Center for Gun Policy and Research, Baltimore, MD.
[2]Johns Hopkins Bloomberg School of Public Health, Center for Gun Policy and Research, Baltimore, MD.
[3]Johns Hopkins School of Medicine, Department of Pediatrics; Johns Hopkins Bloomberg School of Public Health, Department of Population, Family & Reproductive Health, Baltimore, MD.
[4]Johns Hopkins Bloomberg School of Public Health, Center for Law and the Public's Health, Baltimore, MD.
[5]The names used in this story are fictional, and the facts are an amalgam taken from actual, similar incidents. Some readers may notice that this story also began this chapter in the first edition of this book. Although time may have passed, this experience continues to be a relevant and powerful example of the need for injury prevention professionals to continue to engage in research, practice, and advocacy to prevent firearm injuries.

undetermined intent. Eighty-eight percent of young people who were killed by gunfire were male. The disproportionate burden of gun death falls on adolescents between the ages of 15 and 19 years, who accounted for 87% of people aged less than 20 years who died in 2007 as a result of firearm injuries.

Although 48% of those who died were White, Black youth were disproportionately affected. For mortality per 100,000 population, Black youth were 4.9 times more likely than White youth to die by gunfire. The racial differences in gun homicides, specifically, are even more alarming: Black youth are 8.1 times more likely than White youth to die from gun homicide (National Center for Injury Prevention and Control 2010a).

Youth gun violence began to increase rapidly in the mid-1980s and reached a peak in the early 1990s. In 1993, young people were killed by guns at a rate of 8 per 100,000, more than twice the 2007 rate (3.7/100,000). In recent years, the number and rate of gun deaths among youth have declined, but remain high, especially for teenage youth of color (Fingerhut and Christoffel 2002; National Center for Injury Prevention and Control 2010a).

Morbidity

Firearm injuries are among the most lethal types of injury, so the ratio of fatal to nonfatal injuries is small in comparison with many other mechanisms of childhood injury. Nonetheless, for every youth killed by gunfire, more than five others are injured. In total, 17,566 children and adolescents aged less than 20 years survived gunshot injuries in 2007 at a rate of 21 per 100,000. Seventy-three percent of these nonfatal injuries resulted from assault, 24% resulted from unintended gunfire, and 3% resulted from suicide attempts. The small proportion of nonfatal firearm suicide attempts reflects the lethality of the method. As with fatal gun injuries, the majority of victims of nonfatal injuries are male (91%) and aged 15 to 19 years (89%) (National Center for Injury Prevention and Control 2010b).

Costs of Gun Violence

Using 1994 data, Cook et al. (1999) estimated the lifetime medical cost of gunshot injuries at $2.3 billion annually, approximately half of which is paid for by the public with tax dollars. Approximately three quarters of the gun-related hospitalizations examined were due to assaults. However, the direct medical costs of gun violence are only a fraction of their total cost to society. Other costs include lost productivity, reduced quality of life, and other intangible costs. With a "willingness to pay" analysis (i.e., the amount people are willing to pay or sacrifice to get something they want), Cook and Ludwig (2000, 2002) estimated that gun violence costs society approximately $100 billion per year. They attribute $15 billion of these costs to youth gun violence. The authors also found that gun violence reduces the quality of life for all children in the United States by influencing housing choices and mobility, instilling fear, and restricting freedom of movement (Cook and Ludwig 2002).

Risk Factors

The risk factors associated with firearm injuries reveal important differences between guns and other agents of injury. Unlike other consumer products for which injury is an unintended consequence, firearms are designed to inflict harm. The ease with which a shooter can discharge a force that is destructive to humans is one important reason that firearms are the most lethal method of suicide and homicide. Despite their danger, the Consumer Product Safety Commission (CPSC) has no jurisdiction over firearms because of a decision by Congress in which the CPSC was explicitly forbidden from regulating guns (15 U.S.C. Sec. 2052(a)(1)(E)

1982). As a result, unlike every other consumer product that is legally sold in the United States, the design of guns is not regulated by the federal government to protect the public's health and safety.

Firearms are dangerous products to have in the home. Researchers have documented associations between rates of household firearm ownership and firearm homicide, suicide, and unintentional firearm deaths (Miller et al. 2001, 2002a, 2002b) and established that the presence of a gun in the home increases the risk of injury to household residents (Kellermann et al. 1992, 1993; Wiebe 2003a, 2003b). One study described the burden of living in a gun-owning home by tracing the source of guns used in unintentional or self-inflicted injuries to children and youth. Fifty-seven percent of the self-inflicted gun injuries and 19% of the unintentional gun injuries examined were caused by guns from the victims' parents' homes. Those numbers increased to 90% and 72%, respectively, when the researchers expanded the gun sources to include the homes of relatives and friends, in addition to parents (Grossman, Reay, and Baker 1999).

The risk to children associated with guns in the home is modified by many factors, including gun storage. Approximately one third of homes with children in the United States have a gun (Schuster et al. 2000; Smith 2001). In 43% of these homes, parents store their guns unlocked; in 9%, parents store their guns unlocked and loaded (Schuster et al. 2000). Anecdotal evidence and experimental research findings offer vivid evidence of children's curiosity with regard to guns. Researchers who observed young boys playing in a room with a planted, hidden gun documented that when the boys found the gun, 76% of the time they handled it, and in almost half of those instances, they pulled the trigger (Jackman et al. 2001). The American Academy of Pediatrics (AAP) recommends that parents keep homes with children gun-free. However, for parents who choose to bring a gun into the home, the AAP advises parents to lock the gun unloaded and store ammunition separately (Committee on Injury and Poison Prevention 2000).

The home is a place where too many children and youth can access guns, but the presence of a gun in the home is a risk that parents can eliminate or control. Parents' decisions to keep their homes gun-free do not affect the risks to their children associated with guns accessible outside the home. Indeed, older children and adolescents find their access to guns relatively unfettered should they seek out guns for protection or perpetration. In the United States, guns are plentiful and subject to minimal regulation. Cook and Ludwig (1996) estimate that the United States is home to at least 200 million privately owned firearms. Youth report obtaining firearms through corrupt licensed dealers, straw purchasers, unlicensed street dealers, friends, family, acquaintances, and theft (Ash et al. 1996; Braga and Kennedy 2001; Cook, Molliconi, and Cole 1995; Webster et al. 2002). How best to address these risks in light of available research is the focus of much of the remainder of this chapter.

The New Policy Environment for Gun Violence Prevention in the United States

In 2008 and 2010, the Supreme Court issued two opinions that reverse more than 125 years of case law on the meaning and reach of the Second Amendment to the U.S. Constitution. In 2008 the Supreme Court ruled that the District of Columbia's long-standing handgun ban was unconstitutional and established for the first time that the Second Amendment confers an individual right to own a handgun (District of Columbia v. Heller 2008). The *District of Columbia v. Heller* opinion did recognize this right as subject to reasonable limitations. In the 2010 *McDonald v. Chicago* decision, the Court extended the right established in Heller to affect laws enacted by states and localities, and reiterated the limitations on its new interpretation of the Amendment (McDonald v. Chicago 2010). Although the precise impact of these court decisions on gun violence prevention policies in a post-McDonald era is unknown, there is little doubt that the Court's rulings in *Heller* and *McDonald* will be a factor in state and local gun policy considerations for many years to come.

Application of Research to Practice and Advocacy

Strategies for Changing Individual Behavior: Education

Given the dangerous nature of firearms, their prevalence in society, and the many opportunities for children and youth to access guns, strategies that aim to change individuals' behavior to minimize or eliminate the risks previously described offer a seemingly logical approach to preventing gun injuries among youth. Several programs exist that are designed to teach children to avoid guns they may encounter during play, and their sponsoring organizations promote these curricula as effective. An evaluation measuring the impact of firearm safety education programs on children's knowledge gain showed promising results (Liller et al. 2003). However, most evaluations that assess whether such programs confer the skills children need to avoid injury demonstrate that such behavior change is not achieved by completing the programs (Hardy et al. 1996; Hardy 2002a; Himle et al. 2004). These findings may not represent the potential of all firearm safety education programs for all children. One evaluation assessed the efficacy of a behavioral skills training program and found that the 6- and 7-year-old participants were able to demonstrate the gun avoidance behaviors they were taught when tested in a simulated real-world setting. The study's authors note that Himle et al. (2004) did not find the same intervention to be effective with a sample of younger children and that their own efficacy test was limited both by a lack of long-term follow-up and by the challenges associated with simulating a real-world environment (Gatheridge et al. 2004). Two more recent studies evaluated the efficacy of behavioral skills training of children by peers (i.e., 6- and 7-year-olds training 4- and 5-year-olds) and parents (Gross et al. 2007; Jostad et al. 2008). Although the results of both evaluations were somewhat promising, the small sample sizes (only six peer–peer pairs and four parent–child pairs) limit their utility. These findings should be interpreted with caution. Given the allure of guns to naturally curious children, the cognitive limitations that characterize childhood, and the established challenges associated with teaching gun safety to children, there are good reasons to pursue alternative strategies to those that seek to gun-proof children (Hardy 2002b, 2003).

Parent-oriented educational interventions provide an appealing alternative to those aimed at children. However, evaluations of clinic-based educational programs fail to show an adequately positive impact on gun storage practices among patients of a primary care pediatrics practice (Grossman et al. 2000; Oatis et al. 1999) or on parents' decisions to remove firearms from the homes of suicidal adolescents (Brent et al. 2000). The disappointing results of parent-focused educational programs are not surprising in light of the evidence that parents tend to overestimate their children's ability to act safely in the presence of guns (Baxley and Miller 2006; Connor and Wesolowski 2003; Farah, Simon, and Kellermann 1999; Webster et al. 1992a). In addition, the viability of pediatrician firearm counseling models is questionable. Although pediatricians and pediatric residents express high levels of support for counseling parents about the risk of firearms in the home, a majority failed to report providing such counseling (Solomon et al. 2002; Webster et al. 1992b).

Clinic-based educational interventions aimed at parents have not translated into the safe gun storage behaviors intended by the interventions' developers. Findings from North Carolina suggest that a safe storage message *alone* is insufficient to prompt the desired behavior change; interventions must also provide direct access to the safety equipment they counsel families to use. After a community intervention that included firearm safety counseling and free gun locks, researchers reported increases in self-reported safe firearm storage practices among a cohort of participating gun owners (Coyne-Beasley, Schoenbach, and Johnson 2001). An Alaskan program that provided gun safes and trigger locks to gun-owning families demonstrated an increase in the use of safes on follow-up (Horn et al. 2003). More recently, an evaluation of a pediatric clinic-based firearm safety counseling program that provided firearm cable locks also revealed a significant improvement in participants' safe storage of firearms at the 6-month follow-up (Barkin et al. 2008). Research findings from gun safety interventions parallel findings from other areas of injury prevention that have documented improved effectiveness from combining low- or no-cost safety products with injury prevention messages in clinical settings (Gielen et al. 2002). Although evaluations of these message/product distribution interventions are promising, the long-term effect on behavior change remains untested. Furthermore, whether these interventions result in the repeated safe behaviors (e.g., replacing a trigger lock after every gun use) needed for safe storage practices to affect firearm injury rates is also unanswered.

Educational strategies aimed at communities as a whole are an alternative to clinic-based interventions that target individuals and families. An evaluation of a media campaign to encourage the use of gun lock boxes and trigger locks in King County, Washington, demonstrated no difference between the intervention and control counties in safe gun storage (Sidman et al. 2005). Although other media campaigns promoting safe gun storage exist, few have been rigorously evaluated. Thus, whether these campaigns are effective remains to be seen.

Educational strategies for preventing firearm injuries are plentiful. As is the case for other areas of injury prevention, the logic and seeming simplicity of strategies that aim to teach people to act safely are a powerful lure. However, evaluations of several educational interventions reveal that attempts to teach children gun avoidance skills may only be effective among certain ages of children and may require more skill-focused training than exists with the most commonly used programs. Furthermore, the tendency of parents to underestimate the risks to their children associated with guns in the home also calls into question the value of parental education and counseling to reduce firearm injury among children. Programs that provide access to the safety products referenced in educational messages do show promise, and any future parent-focused educational efforts should invest the resources needed to provide parents with the information and means to reduce the risks posed to their children by keeping guns in the home. The disappointing impact of interventions designed to gun-proof children suggests that real progress on this issue will only result when interventions cease relying on children to keep themselves safe from weapons intended for use by adults.

Strategies for Changing Individual Behavior: Reducing Demand

For adolescents, strategies that aim to reduce the demand for guns offer an alternative behavior change strategy that does not rely on the safe behavior messages previously described. Demand strategies are important to consider for adolescents because the pattern of gun injury includes more intentional gun use (self-protection, assault, suicide) during the adolescent years relative to young children. Youth report that fear of arrest and incarceration influences their decision-making about whether to acquire and carry guns (Freed et al. 2001). How and the extent to which such fears affect youth gun behaviors are not known. The literature concerning adult fear of incarceration and guns suggests harsh sentencing policies do not deter criminal gun activity. An evaluation of the effect of enhanced penalties for felons charged with illegal gun possession concluded that one program, Project Exile, failed to reduce gun homicide (Raphael and Ludwig 2003). Interventions that seek to capitalize on adolescent fear of incarceration, such as the Scared Straight program, have also failed to demonstrate a positive impact on youth criminal behavior (Finckenauer and Gavin 1999).

Although programs that rely solely on punishment and incarceration as a strategy for deterring youth gun involvement are ineffective, interventions that threaten punishment in the context of more comprehensive, community-based campaigns are encouraging. In Boston, a community gun violence prevention initiative that included participation from law enforcement (police, prosecutors, parole and probation, and the Bureau of Alcohol, Tobacco, Firearms and Explosives), the faith community, and gang outreach through street workers resulted in dramatic declines in youth gun homicides (Kennedy, Piehl, and Braga 1996). The intervention included strategies to reduce the supply of guns to Boston youth in targeted neighborhoods and Boston youth's demand for guns. Several other communities have experimented with variations on the law enforcement–community partnership approach to identify, deter, and punish those involved with youth gun violence (Fagan 2002).

Another notable youth gun violence prevention initiative is CeaseFire Chicago. Although CeaseFire differs from the Boston campaign in that it places greater emphasis on prevention than deterrence, like the Boston campaign, CeaseFire relies on the faith community and outreach workers to mentor high-risk youth and connect them with community resources. CeaseFire also uses highly trained "violence interrupters," many of whom are themselves former gang members and convicts, to provide would-be shooters and victims with real-time behavioral alternatives to the use of violence in conflicts. A recent evaluation of the program demonstrated a 16% to 34% reduction in shootings directly attributable to the CeaseFire intervention in five of the seven neighborhoods studied (Skogan et al. 2008). In addition, four program areas experienced a decrease in retaliatory homicides after the implementation of CeaseFire, a particularly noteworthy finding given that 40% of the conflicts mediated by violence interrupters involved threats of retribution for prior shootings.

Given CeaseFire's success, several other communities have implemented programs using the same or a similar model. Findings from an evaluation of Baltimore's program, called "Safe Streets," show mixed results (Webster, Mendel, and Vernick 2009). Fatal shootings decreased in two of the four Baltimore neighborhoods but increased in the other two neighborhoods. Notably, the successful neighborhoods had three times as many conflict mediations as the unsuccessful neighborhoods. A recent evaluation of Pittsburgh's version of CeaseFire showed an increase in gun assaults in all three of the intervention neighborhoods and an increase in the number of homicides in one of the three locations (Wilson, Chermak, and McGarrell 2010). The evaluation's authors cite difficulty in selecting adequate comparison communities, problems with program implementation, and the program's failure to focus on gang violence as possible explanations for these findings.

The success of community-based youth gun violence prevention programs like those in Boston and Chicago depends largely on sufficient, long-term funding. Inadequate funding, which is partly to blame for high turnover among outreach workers and violence interrupters in Chicago, has resulted in clients left without outreach workers, sites being understaffed, and the program losing credibility in the community (Skogan et al. 2008). In the worst cases, funding cuts can result in program closure. A temporary funding crisis in 2007 that forced most CeaseFire Chicago locations to close their doors was accompanied by a sharp increase in shootings in these districts. In contrast, shootings continued to decline in the two districts in which CeaseFire remained in operation (CeaseFire 2010). Thus, it seems that once the interventions end, the associated decreases in youth gun violence revert to preprogram levels.

The Role of Advocacy and Practice

Evaluations of individual behavior change interventions are instructive with regard to how best to use prevention resources. Interventions that rely solely on educational messages to teach children safe gun behavior or fear tactics to discourage juvenile delinquency have not been demonstrated effective. There is a need for advocates and practitioners to discourage efforts that rely solely on children's ability to make safe decisions about guns to reduce firearm violence. This is a heavy burden that children are ill equipped to bear.

The individual education model is similarly disappointing when applied to parents. However, more comprehensive approaches that deliver individual behavior change messages in combination with safe storage products have led to changes in gun storage practices. Although fear-based admonitions aimed at dissuading children from engaging in criminal gun behaviors alone are unlikely to affect their decisionmaking, penalties for gun involvement that are certain and swift, and supported by a community-based infrastructure have yielded impressive results. The challenge for advocates and practitioners, therefore, is to resist the surface appeal associated with individual behavior change strategies in favor of more comprehensive models that target both individual behavior and the settings in which children make decisions about guns (Johnson and Jones 2011).

Strategies for Designing Safer Guns

Guns are designed to inflict serious or fatal injury. Perhaps it is this fact that has delayed progress on safer gun designs. In 2007, 138 gun deaths and 4165 gun injuries involving children and youth resulted from unintentionally fired guns. These injuries, often referred to by the media as "accidents," are in fact events that occur regularly, with a strikingly similar fact pattern: A child finds an unlocked gun, and in the course of play, the gun discharges, injuring (often fatally) a sibling or playmate (Ismach et al. 2003; Wintemute et al. 1987). The injury profile that began this chapter is a more detailed example of such incidents.

Why guns are operable by children is a question without a reasonable answer. Beginning in the late 1970s, injury prevention researchers began advocating for changes in the design of guns that would render them inoperable in a child's hand (Baker, Teret, and Dietz 1980). "Childproof" gun designs actually date back to the late 1800s, when, in response to a child's injury as a result of unintentional gun fire, legend has it that D.B. Wesson of Smith & Wesson fame charged one of his designers to develop a gun that could not be fired by a child (Jinks 1977). Early designs relied on mechanical impediments to prevent unintended gunfire. As this design strategy evolved, the preference for personalized guns, or guns that could only be fired by an authorized user, took hold. High-technology radio frequency transponders, fingerprint recognition systems, and computer chips became the technologies of choice for the modern personalized gun. The realization that technology could offer the public a gun that is both inoperable by children and operable only by authorized users expanded the potential impact of personalized guns. The availability of such a gun has implications for adolescent suicide prevention, as well as the prevention of assaults and homicides committed with stolen guns (Freed, Vernick, and Hargarten 1998; Teret and Wintemute 1993; Teret et al. 1998).

As of this writing, personalized gun technology is not generally available to consumers. Two less sophisticated safety devices, the magazine safety and the loaded chamber indicator, have long been available on select gun models. (A magazine safety is a built-in feature on some pistols that prevents the gun from firing once the magazine is removed. This feature is important because people often incorrectly believe that a gun has no ammunition when the magazine has been removed. A loaded chamber indicator is a device designed to indicate whether the gun is loaded and ready to fire.) Although the preventive potential of these devices is more modest than personalized gun technology, their lifesaving potential is well documented (General Accounting Office 1991; Vernick et al. 2003). Had the gun that fired the fatal bullet to Eric's head included either a magazine safety or a loaded chamber indicator, the play of Anthony and Eric described at the start of this chapter would have been a reckless footnote to an otherwise typical day in the lives of two adolescent boys.

The Role of Advocacy and Practice

To date, progress toward increasing the availability of safer guns has been realized through advocacy and practice efforts. In California, advocates organized in support of State Senator Jack

Scott's bill, which became law in 2007, requiring that new semiautomatic handguns sold in the state be equipped with a magazine safety and a loaded chamber indicator (Cal. Penal Code 2003). The Massachusetts legislature enacted into law a bill that requires all handguns sold in the state to meet certain childproofing standards (Massachusetts Gen. Laws 2000). Under Maryland's Responsible Gun Safety Act of 2000, only handguns with an approved integrated locking mechanism can be sold new in the state. The law also mandates that the state's Handgun Roster Board produce an annual report on the status of personalized gun technology (Md. Public Safety Code 2000). In 2002, New Jersey passed a law that will permit only personalized guns to be sold in the state once their Attorney General deems the technology ready for public use (New Jersey Rev. Stat. 2002). Several other state and local governments, as well as the U.S. Congress, have considered variations of these safer gun design bills. Continued advances on designing safer guns and assuring their availability to consumers will likely occur only with support and action from advocates and practitioners. A model personalized gun bill, developed by the Johns Hopkins Center for Gun Policy and Research, is available for advocates' and legislators' use (DeFrancesco et al. 2000).

Regulatory strategies to encourage safer gun design offer an alternative to the legislative approaches previously described. In 1997, Massachusetts Attorney General Scott Harshbarger promulgated the nation's first consumer protection regulations for handguns. This application of executive power established a precedent for translating the consumer safety responsibility of Attorneys General into design safety standards for firearms. Although the reach of consumer protection authority by Attorneys General varies among the states, a report issued by a national gun violence prevention organization identifies 20 states with the apparent legal authority needed to regulate gun design using consumer protection powers (Center to Prevent Handgun Violence 2001). This strategy is an important, yet underused approach to influencing the safety design features available to gun purchasers.

Efforts to bring safer gun designs to consumers include the use of litigation (Association of Trial Lawyers and the Johns Hopkins Center for Gun Policy and Research 1995; Mair, Teret, and Frattaroli 2005; Teret and Wintemute 1983; Vernick and Teret 1999). Whereas legislators may be more susceptible to the influence of the powerful lobbies that oppose calls to mandate safer gun designs, the courts are generally viewed as more independent. Before October 2005, lawsuits initiated by victims of tragedies similar to Anthony and Eric's story could seek monetary damages from gun manufacturers to raise the cost of ignoring safety technology and encourage the investment needed to bring safer gun designs to the market. However, the decision by Congress and the President in 2005 to grant the firearm industry broad immunity from such lawsuits through the Protection of Lawful Commerce in Arms Act effectively closed the courthouse doors to most victims whose injuries could have been prevented if the guns that caused their injuries were safer by design (Vernick, Rutkow, and Salmon 2007).

Strategies for Changing the Environment

Firearm injuries to children and youth are a by-product of individuals and guns mixing in a particular setting. Interventions aimed at reducing these injuries by adjusting individuals' behaviors and those that focus on gun design grapple with the human and product factors. Interventions aimed at changing the environment in which firearm injury occurs offer another approach. With an estimated 200 million privately owned guns (Cook and Ludwig 1996) and a timid regulatory system for minimizing the foreseeable harms that are likely to result from this massive civilian arms stockpile, the United States provides an environment where young people and guns too often collide.

Federal oversight of the gun industry and gun sales is perpetually underfunded, undervalued, and under threat of elimination (Vizzard 1997). The weak system of federal oversight contributes to the availability and accessibility of guns to youth (Cook, Molliconi, and Cole 1995; Wintemute 2002). In response to the shortcomings at the federal level, some states have enacted laws to control gun commerce within their borders (Vernick and Hepburn 2003). Evaluations of state policies that require licensing of gun owners and registration of guns, place limits on the number of guns that can be purchased by an individual, and ban the sale of Saturday night special guns all demonstrate positive impacts on measures of illegal gun trafficking and easy accessibility (Webster and Starnes 2000; Webster, Vernick, and Hepburn 2001; Weil and Knox 1996).

Other strategies seeking to change the environment in which firearm injuries occur focus directly on gun possession. In response to citizen reports or law enforcement intelligence, St. Louis police officers visited the homes of youth allegedly in possession of firearms. Police asked parents for permission to search for and remove firearms believed to be in their child's possession. To encourage participation, police removed firearms from the home without pressing charges. The program resulted in police seizing more than 1300 guns in 3 years (Office of Juvenile Justice and Delinquency Prevention 1999). In Kansas City, police identified areas where concentrated, high rates of violent crime were occurring, and targeted people in these "hot spots" for aggressive weapons searches. The effect of working with the community to develop this intervention that targeted law enforcement resources on a violent part of the city was to gain the support of the community and reduce gun crime and homicide during the intervention period (Sherman, Shaw, and Rogan 1995).

Microstamping is a relatively recent technology that equips firearms with the ability to imprint multiple, unique, microscopic codes on the cartridge casings that are expelled when a gun is fired. Unlike guns, expended cartridge casings often are left behind at crime scenes and can be recovered by law enforcement. Microstamping technology allows forensic experts to obtain information from the recovered cartridge casings (e.g., the manufacturer, model, and serial number of the gun) and use this information to trace the gun to its original retail purchaser (Ohar and Lizotte 2009). Even when the original purchaser is not the shooter, his or her identity can be a valuable clue to solving a case. Law enforcement officers often rely on crime gun tracing to help them identify firearm traffickers who supply firearms to adolescents and others who are prohibited from having them (Veen et al. 1997). Laws mandating that all new semiautomatic pistols have microstamping capability have been passed in California and the District of Columbia (Cal. Penal Code 2007; DC Code 2009). Several other states are working on passing similar laws. The California law was scheduled to go into effect in January of 2010, but has yet to be implemented because of patent restrictions imposed by the inventors of the microstamping technology (Vernick, Webster, and Vittes 2010).

In an attempt to encourage safer gun storage, 18 states have enacted child access prevention laws that specify criminal penalties for adults whose guns are accessible to youth. Such laws are enforceable only after an incident resulting from a child's access to firearms occurs. This postincident threat of criminal prosecution is based on the notion that such penalties will raise the stakes associated with keeping an unlocked gun accessible to children, increase the proportion of gun owners who safely store their guns, and reduce youth access to guns. Evaluations of such laws have yielded a modest positive effect on suicide (Webster et al. 2004) and mixed results with regard to the impact on unintentional firearm deaths (Cummings et al. 1997; Webster and Starnes 2000).

The Role of Advocacy and Practice

Legislative initiatives to control the illicit market that supplies guns to youth is a focus of several gun violence prevention advocacy organizations. Licensing and registration, and one gun a month laws are two examples of such policies (DeMarco and Schneider 2000). Gun shows are another focus of advocacy efforts to control the illicit gun market. Gun shows are a source of guns for prohibited purchasers, including youth (Wintemute 2007), and as such are a logical target for interventions aimed at changing the environment in which youth are able to access firearms.

Policy strategies to affect the environment in which youth acquire firearms are not limited to legislative bodies. Creative use of executive authority by one local health commissioner led to the temporary closure of a hardware store known to sell ammunition to youth illegally, suggesting that in some jurisdictions, executive authority to address the environmental conditions that support and profit from youth gun violence can be addressed through public health agencies (Lewin et al. 2005).

The Asking Saves Kids (ASK) Campaign of the PAX organization is based on the idea that changes in social norms regarding guns are needed to achieve reductions in youth gun violence prevention. The ASK Campaign encourages parents to "ASK" other parents if a gun is present in their home before sending their children to play. By establishing the ASK norm, PAX intends to increase awareness and action concerning the dangers associated with keeping guns in homes where children play. Perhaps such a discussion would have motivated Anthony's parents to lock away the pistol that fired the fatal shot to Eric's head in the injury profile that began this chapter.

SPEAK UP, another campaign of the PAX organization, also aims to change social norms around young people and guns. SPEAK UP encourages youth to report threats of gun violence in their schools and communities. The campaign is composed of lesson plans, educational wallet cards and posters, and a national public awareness campaign about the importance of reporting weapon-related threats. SPEAK UP also staffs a 24-hour national hotline for students to anonymously report threats by calling or sending a text message.

Despite the recent Supreme Court rulings establishing a limited individual right to gun ownership, and poor and underfunded federal oversight of gun laws, more than 500 mayors from cities and towns across the United States have joined Mayors Against Illegal Guns (MAIG). New York Mayor Michael Bloomberg and Boston Mayor Thomas Menino founded MAIG in 2006 to support legislative initiatives intended to curtail illegal gun acquisition and use while defending the ownership rights of law-abiding citizens (Mayors Against Illegal Guns, Coalition History 2010). MAIG supports a variety of federal, state, and local initiatives, including gun dealer employee background checks, microstamping, and mandated reporting of lost and stolen firearms. The coalition has also partnered with Walmart, the nation's largest firearm retailer, to institute a set of responsible sales policies. MAIG has an active Web site, has produced several policy reports, and has convened several national conferences and summits.

Future Research, Advocacy, and Practice

Research

Social Norms

Several public health campaigns have sought to change individual behavior by changing collective attitudes and the social acceptability of health risk behaviors. "Social norms" campaigns have been applied, with varying degrees of success, to such injury risk factors as seat belt use and binge drinking (Cohn et al. 2002; Glider et al. 2001; Haines and Spear 1996; Wechsler et al. 2003, 2004). The ASK Campaign is one example of a social norms approach to gun violence prevention. By enlisting parents to inquire about guns and gun storage in the homes where their children play, the ASK Campaign may influence gun storage norms. Research is needed to establish how social norms approaches can best be applied to youth gun violence prevention efforts and to evaluate the impact of such interventions.

Whereas some programs target broader social norms, there is evidence of the need for more focused social norms change in communities where youth gun violence is pervasive. For example,

Rich and Stone (1996) identified a widespread sentiment among young men in urban Boston. Specifically, these men felt pressure to engage in retaliatory violence in response to their own victimization to avoid being labeled "suckers." This norm fueled cycles of shootings and stabbings (Rich and Stone 1996). Prevention programs can be used to their best advantage by acknowledging and addressing social norms supportive of gun violence in various communities.

Community-based youth gun violence preventions, such as CeaseFire Chicago, emphasize the importance of social norm changes in the long-term, while addressing shorter-term behavioral solutions to gun violence. Unfortunately, CeaseFire and campaigns like it are often undermined by limited funding and high rates of staff turnover. A violence prevention program in Lowell, Massachusetts, might provide instruction on ways to reduce the loss of valued outreach workers (Frattaroli et al. 2010). Lowell outreach workers are involved in the hiring of other outreach workers, are provided with ongoing structured training, attend weekly meetings that offer a safe place to discuss challenges, have biannual retreats, and are given the opportunity to advance within the program (e.g., managers are former outreach workers).

Organizing and Advocating for Gun Violence Prevention

Gun violence prevention efforts are heavily dependent on advocates to help mobilize the grass roots, encourage research funding, and focus the political debate about firearms. The field would benefit from more systematic study of how to effectively organize and advocate for gun violence prevention. During the 1990s, the number of gun violence prevention advocacy groups increased and the issue gained visibility. There are many lessons to be learned from the experiences of advocacy organizations in the gun violence prevention community and in other issue areas that face similar challenges. As we look forward, opportunities for advocates to respond to the recent court decisions that restrict the scope of state and local gun violence prevention laws will be important. Research that documents and explains the changes that occur in response to the *Heller* and *McDonald* decisions will also be important. Evaluations that monitor the impacts of these changes on gun-related morbidity and mortality will provide valuable contributions to the growing literature about the relationship among guns, policy, and the public's health.

Adolescent Development Research

Understanding youth development, and the particular developmental vulnerabilities to injury that exist throughout childhood and adolescence, is critical to crafting effective youth gun violence prevention strategies. Knowledge of early childhood development has been used to promote age-appropriate interventions designed to prevent unintentional injuries in young children. For example, childproof caps for medicines are now recognized as an effective strategy for preventing curious youngsters from poisoning (Christoffel and Gallagher 1999). This kind of developmental approach to prevention should be extended into adolescence (Johnson and Jones 2011).

Adolescents' access to firearms in their homes and communities, and through their peer networks, comes at a time when they are particularly developmentally vulnerable to injury. In the last several years, the process of brain development has received increased attention in the research literature. Adolescence is a time when the brain undergoes a wave of major development and remodeling. "Executive functions" of the brain that govern impulse control, planning, foresight, understanding of cause and effect relationships, and emotional regulation are still developing until approximately 25 years of age (Giedd et al. 1999; Sowell et al. 1999a, 1999b, 2001). Thus, adolescents' brains may not yet be capable of fully processing and evaluating the consequences of their decisions. This has implications for education and policy strategies related to youth gun violence prevention, because adolescents' ability to resist firearms and other potentially seductive items is questionable.

Because adolescents may not be able to act unfailingly in accordance with health education messages, environmental modification may provide a "safety net" for adolescents who make poor decisions (Johnson and Jones 2011). Because adolescence is a time of increasing autonomy (and decreasing supervision), the high prevalence of guns in the United States means that youth are gaining their independence in an environment where guns are accessible to them and when they are developmentally ill equipped to consider the consequences of misusing a gun. This research is in its infancy, but should be further explored in the context of youth violence prevention.

Policy Implementation

Policies that prevent access to firearms, alter the way they are sold or marketed, or mandate safer designs are among the most potentially effective tools for preventing youth violence (Wintemute 2002). However, research demonstrates that gun violence prevention policies are not always implemented, or implemented in a way that fails to achieve the greatest public health gain (Frattaroli 1999). Additional attention to the implementation phase of the policy process is needed, particularly in the area of gun violence prevention, in which policies are subject to passionate social and political debate. By understanding how best to translate written policies into effective preventive actions, gun violence prevention researchers can provide advocates and practitioners with the tools needed to ensure the lifesaving impact policymakers intend.

Surveillance

The need for systematic collection of firearm injury data has long been advocated to better understand the nature of the problem and to craft appropriate prevention strategies (Mercy, Ikeda, and Powell 1998; Rosenberg and Hammond 1995; Teret, Wintemute, and Beilenson 1992). Unlike motor vehicle crashes and other unintentional injury issues, until recently there have been few detailed data on firearm deaths. In response to this need, an increasing number of state and local violent injury reporting systems are being developed (Barber et al. 2000). The National Violent Death Reporting System (NVDRS) links data on homicides and suicides from law enforcement, coroners, vital statistics, and crime laboratories. The NVDRS is modeled in part on the National Highway Traffic Safety Administration's Fatality Analysis Reporting System and is designed to inform violence prevention research and policy. Seventeen states currently provide data to the NVDRS (Hemenway et al. 2009), but the Centers for Disease Control and Prevention expect to include all 50 states and the District of Columbia in the future (Karch, Dahlberg, and Patel 2010).

Advocacy and Practice

Several high-profile school shootings in the late 1990s have brought gun violence "closer to home" for many Americans. This, coupled with the broader public concern that gun violence has disproportionately affected the nation's youth, has contributed to a proliferation of gun violence prevention and advocacy organizations in the last decade (Frattaroli 2003). In 2000, several hundred thousand people gathered in Washington, D.C., to take part in the "Million Mom March," arguably the nation's most successful public gun violence prevention event (Wallack, Winett, and Nettekoven 2003). The March aimed to promote "sensible gun laws," demonstrate the political counterpoint to gun-rights organizations, and hold Congress accountable for gun violence prevention legislation (Wallack, Winett, and Nettekoven 2003).

Despite the success of the Million Mom March, advocacy groups have struggled to harness the power of their grassroots supporters in a sustained way (Frattaroli 2003; Wallack, Winett, and Nettekoven 2003). There are several strategies that could help advocates maximize the impact of their resources. Gun violence prevention advocates tend to focus their policy efforts on enacting legislation. However, greater attention also should be paid to how the policies they support are implemented. Policies with poor (or no) implementation threaten to squander both the hard-won gains of the movement and the political will necessary to achieve them.

Gun violence prevention advocates would benefit from expanding to include groups of people who have traditionally not been active on the issue but may be disproportionately affected by guns, such as people of color and youth. By expanding the field and focusing on diversity, advocacy organizations can build broader appeal. In addition, the effectiveness of gun violence prevention advocates is somewhat hindered by a lack of cooperation within the field, because differing perspectives on strategies and goals have at times been barriers to a more unified movement (Frattaroli 2003). Strategies to increase cooperation would likely prove beneficial. Finally, partnerships with officials in health departments and law enforcement would likely strengthen existing advocacy efforts and provide valuable insight into the government systems responsible for preventing, treating, and controlling youth gun violence (Frattaroli 2003). To best advocate for prevention, the gun violence prevention movement needs to keep the "grass roots" involved and energized, promote unity within the movement, foster diversity, and identify political opportunities to effect change and promote careful policy implementation.

New opportunities for advocacy could also serve to recharge gun violence prevention advocacy efforts. New information about gun shows and the ease with which prohibited purchasers can access guns (Wintemute 2009) may move advocates and elected officials to address the gun show loophole that continues to provide ready access to guns for youth. The Supreme Court's recent decisions on the Second Amendment will likely lead to reanalyses of existing state and local laws and new case law on the topic. How courts respond to the new cases that arise will have implications for future approaches to advancing gun violence prevention policies.

Conclusions

The combined efforts of researchers, practitioners, and advocates working in the field of injury prevention hold great promise for reducing the toll of unnecessary deaths from trauma. Hundreds of thousands of lives have already been saved by modifying products such as automobiles. The greatest savings of lives lost by gunfire remain in our future. Although changes in violent or careless behaviors need to occur, and methods for achieving those behavioral changes should be perfected, we can also save lives in the immediate future by modifying the design and availability of guns. These injury prevention strategies are within our technologic grasp; however, the critical question is whether they are within our political grasp. It is for this reason that injury prevention researchers, practitioners, and advocates need to work collaboratively at the federal, state, and local levels to translate promising ideas into lifesaving reality.

References

Ash P, Kellermann AL, Fuqua-Whitley D, Johnson A. 1996. Gun acquisition and use by juvenile offenders. *JAMA.* 275:1754–1758.

Association of Trial Lawyers of America and the Johns Hopkins Center for Gun Policy and Research. 1995. *Conference Report: Guns, A Public Health Approach.* Baltimore: The Association of Trial Lawyers of America and the Johns Hopkins Center for Gun Policy and Research.

Baker SP, Teret SP, Dietz PE. 1980. Firearms and the public health. *J Public Health Policy.* 1:224–229.

Barber C, Hemenway D, Hargarten S, et al. 2000. A "call to arms" for a national reporting system on firearm injuries. *Am J Public Health.* 90:1191–1193.

Barkin SL, Finch SA, Ip EH, et al. 2008. Is office-based counseling about media use, timeouts, and firearm storage effective? Results from a cluster-randomized controlled trial. *Pediatrics.* 122:e15–25.

Baxley F, Miller M. 2006. Parental misperceptions about children and firearms. *Arch Pediatr Adolesc Med.* 160:542–547.

Braga A, Kennedy D. 2001. The illicit acquisition of firearms by youth and juveniles. *J Crim Justice.* 29:379–388.

Brent DA, Baugher M, Birmaher B, et al. 2000. Compliance with recommendations to remove firearms in families participating in a clinical trial for adolescent depression. *J Am Acad Child Adolesc Psychiatry.* 39:1220–1226.

Cal. Penal Code. 12130. 2003.

Cal. Penal Code. 12126. 2007.

CeaseFire. 2010. *Increase in Shootings after CeaseFire Funding Is Interrupted.* Available at: http://www.ceasefirechicago.com/budget_07.shtml. Accessed May 27, 2010.

Center to Prevent Handgun Violence. 2001. *Targeting Safety: How State Attorneys General Can Act Now to Save Lives.* Washington, DC: Center to Prevent Handgun Violence.

Christoffel T, Gallagher SS. 1999. *Injury Prevention and Public Health: Practical Knowledge, Skills, and Strategies.* Sudbury: Jones and Bartlett Publishers.

Cohn LD, Hernandez D, Byrd T, Cortes M. 2002. A program to increase seat belt use along the Texas-Mexico border. *Am J Public Health.* 92:1918–1920.

Committee on Injury and Poison Prevention. 2000. Firearm-related injuries affecting the pediatric population. *Pediatrics.* 105:888–895.

Connor SM, Wesolowski KL. 2003. "They're too smart for that": predicting what children would do in the presence of guns. *Pediatrics.* 111:E109–E114.

Cook PJ, Lawrence BA, Ludwig J, Miller TR. 1999. The medical costs of gunshot injuries in the United States. *JAMA.* 282:447–454.

Cook PJ, Ludwig J. 1996. *Guns in America: Results of a Comprehensive Survey of Gun Ownership and Use.* Washington, DC: Police Foundation.

Cook PJ, Ludwig J. 2000. *Gun Violence: The Real Costs.* New York: Oxford University Press.

Cook PJ, Ludwig J. 2002. The costs of gun violence against children. *Future Child.* 12:86–99.

Cook PJ, Molliconi S, Cole T. 1995. Regulating gun markets. *J Crim Law Criminol.* 86:59–92.

Coyne-Beasley T, Schoenbach VJ, Johnson RM. 2001. "Love our kids, lock your guns": a community-based firearm safety counseling and gun lock distribution program. *Arch Pediatr Adolesc Med.* 155:659–664.

Cummings P, Grossman DC, Rivara FP, Koepsell TD. 1997. State gun safe storage laws and child mortality due to firearms. *JAMA.* 278:1084–1086.

DeFrancesco S, Lester KJ, Teret SP, Vernick JS. 2000. *A Model Handgun Safety Standard Act.* Baltimore: The Johns Hopkins Center for Gun Policy and Research.

DeMarco V, Schneider GE. 2000. Elections and public health. *Am J Public Health.* 90:1513–1514.

DC code §7-2505.03. 2009.

District of Columbia v. Heller, 554 U.S. 2008.

Fagan J. 2002. Policing guns and gun violence. *Future Child.* 12:133–151.

Farah MM, Simon HK, Kellermann AL. 1999. Firearms in the home: parental perceptions. *Pediatrics.* 104:1059.

Finckenauer JO, Gavin PW. 1999. *Scared Straight: The Panacea Phenomenon Revisited.* Prospect Heights: Waveland Press.

Fingerhut LA, Christoffel KK. 2002. Firearm-related death and injury among children and adolescents. *Future Child.* 2002;12:24–37.

Frattaroli S. 1999. *The Implementation of the 1996 Maryland Gun Violence Act: A Case Study.* Baltimore: The Johns Hopkins School of Hygiene and Public Health.

Frattaroli S. 2003. Grassroots advocacy for gun violence prevention: a status report on mobilizing a movement. *J Public Health Policy.* 24:332–354.

Frattaroli S, Pollack KM, Jonsberg K, et al. 2010. Streetworkers, youth violence prevention, and peacemaking in Lowell Massachusetts: lessons and voices from the community. *Prog Community Health Partnersh.* 4:171–179.

Freed LH, Vernick JS, Hargarten SW. 1998. Prevention of firearm-related injuries and deaths among youth. A product-oriented approach. *Pediatr Clin North Am.* 45:427–438.

Freed LH, Webster DW, Longwell JJ, et al. 2001. Factors preventing gun acquisition and carrying among incarcerated adolescent males. *Arch Pediatr Adolesc Med.* 155:335–341.

Gatheridge BJ, Miltenberger RG, Huneke DF, et al. 2004. Comparison of two programs to teach firearm injury prevention skills to 6- and 7-year-old children. *Pediatrics.* 114:e294–e299.

General Accounting Office. 1991. *Accidental Shooting: Many Deaths and Injuries Caused by Firearms could be Prevented.* Washington, DC: U.S. General Accounting Office.

Giedd J, Blumenthal J, Jeffries NO, et al. 1999. Brain development during childhood and adolescence: a longitudinal MRI study. *Nat Neurosci.* 2:861–863.

Gielen AC, McDonald EM, Wilson MEH, et al. 2002. Effects of improved access to safety counseling, products, and home visits on parents' safety practices: results of a randomized trial. *Arch Pediatr Adolesc Med.* 156:33–40.

Glider P, Midyett SJ, Mills-Novoa B, et al. 2001. Challenging the collegiate rite of passage: a campus-wide social marketing media campaign to reduce binge drinking. *J Drug Educ.* 31:207–220.

Gross A, Miltenberger RG, Knudson P, et al. 2007. Preliminary evaluation of a parent training program to prevent gun play. *J Appl Behav Anal.* 40:691–695.

Grossman DC, Cummings P, Koepsell TD, et al. 2000. Firearm safety counseling in primary care pediatrics: a randomized, controlled trial. *Pediatrics.* 106:22–26.

Grossman DC, Reay DT, Baker SA. 1999. Self-inflicted and unintentional firearm injuries among children and adolescents: the source of the firearm. *Arch Pediatr Adolesc Med.* 153:875–878.

Haines M, Spear SF. 1996. Changing the perception of the norm: a strategy to decrease binge drinking among college students. *J Am Coll Health.* 45:134–140.

Hardy MS. 2002a. Teaching firearm safety to children: failure of a program. *J Dev Behav Pediatr.* 23:71–76.

Hardy MS. 2002b. Behavior-oriented approaches to reducing youth gun violence. *Future Child.* 12:100–117.

Hardy MS. 2003. Effects of gun admonitions on the behaviors and attitudes of school-aged boys. *J Dev Behav Pediatr.* 24:352–358.

Hardy MS, Armstrong FD, Martin BL, Strawn KN. 1996. A firearm safety program for children: they just can't say no. *J Dev Behav Pediatr.* 17:216–221.

Hemenway D, Barber CW Gallagher SS, Azrael DR. 2009. Creating a national violent death reporting system: a successful beginning. *Am J Prev Med.* 37:68–71.

Himle MB, Miltenberger RG, Gatheridge BJ, Flessner CA. 2004. An evaluation of two procedures for training skills to prevent gun play in children. *Pediatrics.* 113:70–77.

Horn A, Grossman DC, Jones W, Berger LR. 2003. Community based program to improve firearm storage practices in rural Alaska. *Inj Prev.* 9:231–234.

Ismach RB, Reza A, Ary R, et al. 2003. Unintended shootings in a large metropolitan area: an incident-based analysis. *Ann Emerg Med.* 41:10–17.

Jackman GA, Farah MM, Kellermann AL, Simon HK. 2001. Seeing is believing: what do boys do when they find a real gun? *Pediatrics.* 107:1247.

Jinks RG. 1977. *History of Smith & Wesson: Nothing of Importance Will Come Without Effort.* North Hollywood: Beinfeld Publishing Company.

Johnson SB, Frattaroli S. 2003. The adolescent brain as a work in progress: a new way of thinking about kids and guns. Poster presented at the 9th Annual Citizens' Conference to Stop Gun Violence; February 21, 2003; Arlington, VA.

Johnson SB, Jones V. 2011. Adolescent development and risk of injury: using developmental science to improve interventions. *Inj Prev.* 17:50–54.

Jostad CM, Miltenberger RG, Kelso P, Knudson P. 2008. Peer tutoring to prevent firearm play. *J Appl Behav Anal.* 41:117–123.

Karch DL, Dahlberg LL, Patel N. 2010. Surveillance for violent deaths—national violent death reporting system, 16 States, 2007. *MMWR Surveill Summ.* 59(SS04)1–50.

Kellermann AL, Rivara FP, Rushforth NB, et al. 1993. Gun ownership as a risk factor for homicide in the home. *N Engl J Med.* 329:1084–1091.

Kellermann AL, Rivara FP, Somes G, et al. 1992. Suicide in the home in relation to gun ownership. *N Engl J Med.* 327:467–472.

Kennedy D, Piehl A, Braga A. 1996. Youth violence in Boston: gun markets, serious youth offenders, and a use reduction strategy. *Law Contemp Probl.* 59:147–198.

Lewin NL, Vernick JS, Beilenson PL, et al. 2005. The Baltimore Youth Ammunition Initiative: a model application of local public health authority in preventing gun violence. *Am J Public Health.* 95:762–765.

Liller KD, Perrin K, Nearns J, et al. 2003. Evaluation of the "Respect Not Risk" firearm safety lesson for 3rd-graders. *J Sch Nurs.* 19:338–343.

Mair JS, Teret SP, Frattaroli S. 2005. A public health perspective on gun violence prevention. In: Lytton TD, editor. *Suing the Gun Industry: A Battle at the Crossroads of Gun Control and Mass Torts.* Ann Arbor: University of Michigan Press. 39–61.

Massachusetts Gen. Laws. ch. 140 sec. 12130. 2000.

Mayors Against Illegal Guns, Coalition History. 2010. Available at: http://www.mayorsagainstillegalguns.org/html/home/home.shtml. Accessed June 28, 2010.

McDonald v. Chicago, 561 U.S. 2010.

Md. Public Safety Code. sec. 5-132(d)(1). 2000.

Mercy JA, Ikeda R, Powell KE. 1998. Firearm-related injury surveillance. An overview of progress and the challenges ahead. *Am J Prev Med.* 15:6–16.

Miller M, Azrael D, Hemenway D. 2001. Firearm availability and unintentional firearm deaths. *Accid Anal Prev.* 33:477–484.

Miller M, Azrael D, Hemenway D. 2002a. Rates of household firearm ownership and homicide across US regions and states, 1988-1997. *Am J Public Health.* 92:1988–1993.

Miller M, Azrael D, Hemenway D. 2002b. Household firearm ownership and suicide rates in the United States. *Epidemiology.* 13:517–524.

National Center for Injury Prevention and Control. 2010a. *WISQARS Fatal Injury Reports 2007.* WISQARS. http://webappa.cdc.gov/sasweb/ncipc/mortrate10_us.html. Accessed May 27, 2010.

National Center for Injury Prevention and Control. 2010b. *WISQARS Nonfatal Injury Reports 2007.* WISQARS. http://webappa.cdc.gov/sasweb/ncipc/nfirates2001.html. Accessed May 27, 2010.

New Jersey Rev. Stat. 2C:39-1dd. 2002.

Oatis PJ, Fenn Burderer NM, Cummings P, Fleitz R. 1999. Pediatric practice based evaluation of the Steps to Prevent Firearm Injury program. *Inj Prev.* 5:48–52.

Office of Juvenile Justice and Delinquency Prevention. 1999. *Promising Strategies to Reduce Gun Violence.* Washington, DC: National Institute of Justice.

Ohar OP, Lizotte TE. 2009. Extracting ballistic forensic intelligence: microstamped firearms deliver data for illegal firearm traffic mapping: technology, implementation, and applications. *Proceedings of SPIE.* 7434:74340G.

Raphael S, Ludwig J. 2003. Prison sentence enhancements: the case of Project Exile. In: Ludwig J, Cook PJ, editors. *Evaluating Gun Policy: Effects on Crime and Violence.* Washington, DC: The Brookings Institution Press. 251–277.

Rich JA, Stone DA. 1996. The experience of violent injury for young African-American men: the meaning of being a "Sucker." *J Gen Intern Med.* 11:77–82.

Rosenberg M, Hammond WR. 1995. Surveillance: the key to firearm injury prevention. *Am J Prev Med.* 15:1.

Schuster MA, Franke TM, Bastian AM, et al. 2000. Firearm storage patterns in US homes with children. *Am J Public Health.* 90:588–594.

Sherman L, Shaw JW, Rogan DP. 1995. *The Kansas City Gun Experiment.* Research in Brief. Washington, DC: National Institute of Justice.

Sidman EA, Grossman DC, Koepsell TD, et al. 2005. Evaluation of a community-based handgun safe-storage campaign. *Pediatrics.* 115:E654–E661.

Skogan WG, Harnett SM, Bump N, Dubois J. 2008. *Evaluation of CeaseFire Chicago.* Chicago: Institute for Policy Research, Northwestern University.

Smith TW. 2001. *2001 National Gun Policy Survey of the National Opinion Research Center: Research Findings.* Chicago: National Opinion Research Center.

Solomon BS, Duggan AK, Webster DW, Serwint JR. 2002. Pediatric residents' attitudes and behaviors related to counseling adolescents and their parents about firearm safety. *Arch Pediatr Adolesc Med.* 156:769–775.

Sowell ER, Thompson PM, Holmes CJ, et al. 1999a. In vivo evidence for post-adolescent brain maturation in frontal and striatal regions. *Nat Neurosci.* 2:859–861.

Sowell ER, Thompson PM, Holmes CJ, et al. 1999b. Localizing age-related changes in brain structure between childhood and adolescence using statistical parametric mapping. *NeuroImage.* 9:587–597.

Sowell ER, Thompson PM, Tessner KD, Toga AW. 2001. Mapping continued brain growth and gray matter density reduction in dorsal frontal cortex: inverse relationships during post-adolescent brain maturation. *J Neurosci.* 21:8819–8829.

Teret SP, DeFrancesco S, Hargarten SW, Robinson K. 1998. Making guns safer. *Issues Sci Technol.* Summer:37–40.

Teret SP, Wintemute GJ. 1983. Handgun injuries: the epidemiologic evidence for assessing legal responsibility. *Hamline Law Review.* 6:341–350.

Teret SP, Wintemute GJ. 1993. Policies to prevent firearm injuries. *Health Aff.* 12:96–108.

Teret SP, Wintemute GJ, Beilenson PL. 1992. The Firearm Fatality Reporting System. A proposal. *JAMA.* 267:3073–3074.

U.S.C. Sec.2052(a)(1)(E). 1982.

Veen J, Dunbar S, Reuland M, Stedman J. 1997. The BJA firearms trafficking program: demonstrating effective strategies to control violent crime. Police Executive Research Forum. Series: BJA Bulletin. Washington, DC: Bureau of Justice Assistance.

Vernick JS, Teret SP. 1999. New courtroom strategies regarding firearms: tort litigation against firearm manufacturers and constitutional challenges to gun laws. *Houston Law Review.* 36:1713–1753.

Vernick JS, Hepburn LM. 2003. State and federal gun laws: trends for 1970–1999. In: Ludwig J, Cook PJ, editors. *Evaluating Gun Policy.* Washington, DC: Brookings Institution Press. 345–402.

Vernick JS, O'Brien M, Hepburn LM, et al. 2003. Unintentional and undetermined firearm related deaths: a preventable death analysis for three safety devices. *Inj Prev.* 9:307–311.

Vernick JS, Rutkow L, Salmon DA. 2007. Availability of litigation as a public health tool for firearm injury prevention: comparison of guns, vaccines, and motor vehicles. *Am J Public Health.* 97:1991–1997.

Vernick JS, Webster DW, Vittes KA. 2010. Law and policy approaches to keeping guns from high risk people. In: Culhane JG, editor. *Reconsidering Law and Policy Debates: A Public Health Perspective.* Cambridge, UK: Cambridge University Press. 153–184.

Vizzard WJ. 1997. In the Cross Fire: A Political History of the Bureau of Alcohol, Tobacco and Firearms. Boulder: Lynne Rienner Publishers.

Wallack L, Winett L, Nettekoven L. 2003. The Million Mom March: engaging the public on gun policy. *J Public Health Policy.* 24:355.

Webster DW, Freed LH, Frattaroli S, Wilson MH. 2002. How delinquent youths acquire guns: initial versus most recent gun acquisitions. *J Urban Health.* 79:60–69.

Webster DW, Mendel JS, Vernick JS. 2009. Interim Evaluation of Baltimore's Safe Streets Initative: Effects on Violence. Presented at the American Public Health Association annual meeting; November 9; Philadelphia, PA.

Webster DW, Starnes M. 2000. Reexamining the association between child access prevention gun laws and unintentional shooting deaths of children. *Pediatrics.* 106:1466–1469.

Webster DW, Vernick JS, Hepburn LM. 2001. Relationship between licensing, registration, and other gun sales laws and the source state of crime guns. *Inj Prev.* 7:184–189.

Webster DW, Vernick JS, Zeioli AM, Manganello JA. 2004. Association between youth focused firearm laws and youth suicide. *JAMA.* 292:594–601.

Webster DW, Wilson ME, Duggan AK, Pakula LC. 1992a. Parents' beliefs about preventing gun injuries to children. *Pediatrics.* 89:908–914.

Webster DW, Wilson ME, Duggan AK, Pakula LC. 1992b. Firearm injury prevention counseling: a study of pediatricians' beliefs and practices. *Pediatrics.* 89:902–907.

Wechsler H, Nelson TE, Lee JE, et al. 2003. Perception and reality: a national evaluation of social norms marketing interventions to reduce college students' heavy alcohol use. *J Stud Alcohol.* 64:484–494.

Wechsler H, Seibring M, Liu IC, Ahl M. 2004. Colleges respond to student binge drinking: reducing student demand or limiting access. *J Am Coll Health.* 52:159–168.

Weil DS, Knox RC. 1996. Effects of limiting handgun purchases on interstate transfer of firearms. *JAMA.* 275:1759–1761.

Wiebe DJ. 2003a. Firearms in U.S. homes as a risk factor for unintentional gunshot fatality. *Accid Anal Prev.* 35:711–716.

Wiebe DJ. 2003b. Homicide and suicide risks associated with firearms in the home: a national case control study. *Ann Emerg Med.* 4:771–782.

Wilson JM, Chermak S, McGarrell EF. 2010. *Community-Based Violence Prevention: An Assessment of Pittsburgh's One Vision One Life Program.* Santa Monica: The RAND Corporation.

Wintemute GJ. 2002. Where the guns come from: the gun industry and gun commerce. *Future Child.* 12:54–71.

Wintemute GJ. 2007. Gun shows across a multistate American gun market: observational evidence of the effects of regulatory policies. *Inj Prev.* 13:150–155.

Wintemute GJ. 2009. *Inside Gun Shows: What Goes On When Everybody Thinks Nobody's Watching.* Davis, CA: Violence Prevention Research Program.

Wintemute GJ, Teret SP, Kraus JF, et al. 1987. When children shoot children: 88 unintended deaths in California. *JAMA.* 257:3107–3109.

Chapter 13

Youth Suicide

Lloyd Potter, PhD, MPH[1]

On Tuesday, a 15-year-old boy killed himself. He was a friend of a 14-year-old girl whose body was found 2 weeks ago. According to the medical examiner's office, both teens died of asphyxia. Both youth belonged to the same social group. School administrators identified approximately ten students belonging to the social group, and counselors have been contacting these students and their parents to offer services. Services were also offered to all high school students. The 15-year-old had been expelled from high school and was attending a juvenile justice program.

The story above, begs a simplistic explanation for the boy's suicide. His friend had died by suicide two weeks before, and he was in trouble with the law and had been expelled from school. However, the boy had had a difficult emotional life and had suffered from depression since he was young. It becomes less clear that these two events alone are what led to his suicide compared with the influence of a number of other more long-term issues. The boy's birth parents had an acrimonious divorce when he was 9 years old, which evolved from a history of intense conflict, occasionally erupting into physical violence. After a difficult custody battle, he and his younger brother lived with his mother. His mother's boyfriend moved in with them when he was 11 years old, and he rarely saw his birth father. The boy never felt attachment to his mother's boyfriend, and they moved to another city because her boyfriend's job was transferred. At 13 years of age, the boy became noticeably withdrawn and depressed. His school referred him to psychotherapy, but after a few visits he never went back. His new friends used alcohol and occasionally used marijuana, and soon he did also. At 14 years of age, he was arrested for shoplifting beer and was put on juvenile probation. He was frequently truant from school and barely passing his courses. At 15 years of age, he was arrested for vandalism and possession of marijuana a few days after his friend died by suicide.

Introduction

Youth suicide is a significant but preventable public health problem facing every community in the nation today. The consequences associated with suicidal behavior and suicide are serious to individuals, families, and society. Suicide imposes a substantial burden on communities, health care, and other service systems. Suicidal behavior takes many forms. Those covered in this chapter are forms of self-directed violence that includes suicidal thoughts, attempted suicides, and completed suicides. Suicidal behavior is defined as the intentional use of physical force, threatened or actual, against oneself that either results in or has a high likelihood of resulting in injury, death, psychologic harm, maldevelopment, or deprivation (Krug et al. 2002).

Before the application of a public health approach to the prevention of suicide, the approach to addressing suicide was reactive. This involved giving attention and resources to the psychiatric treatment of suicidal individuals and, all too often, medical treatment of injured victims. During

[1]Department of Demography and Institute for Demographic and Socioeconomic Research, University of Texas at San Antonio.

the past four decades, a public health approach has increasingly been applied, bringing an emphasis and commitment to identifying policies and programs to prevent youth suicide. The public health approach derives from a tradition of collaboration among a broad spectrum of scientific disciplines, organizations, and communities to solve the problem. In particular, the health sector, including emergency departments and community health agencies, plays a prominent role as a source of information about the problem and provides potential sites for interventions to prevent the occurrence of suicidal behavior. The public health approach emphasizes the utility of applying a variety of scientific tools (e.g., epidemiology, behavioral and social sciences, and engineering) toward understanding the causes of the issue and identifying effective prevention strategies. The perspective and methods of public health work to understand and prevent injury and death from suicidal behavior.

Significant advances have been made in understanding suicide as a public health issue. In 1996, the World Health Organization (WHO) issued the "Prevention of Suicide: Guidelines for the Formulation and Implementation of National Strategies" (United Nations/World Health Organization 1996). In recognition of the growing problem of suicide worldwide, the WHO urged member nations to address this issue. In the United States, an innovative public/private partnership to seek a national strategy for the United States was established, including agencies in the U.S. Department of Health and Human Services, encompassing the Centers for Disease Control and Prevention (CDC), the Health Resources and Services Administration, the Indian Health Service, the National Institute of Mental Health, the Office of the Surgeon General, the Substance Abuse and Mental Health Services Administration, and the Suicide Prevention Advocacy Network, a public grassroots advocacy organization composed of suicide survivors (persons close to someone who completed suicide), attempters of suicide, community activists, and health and mental health clinicians. In 1999, the U.S. Surgeon General's office issued a brief report, *The Surgeon General's Call to Action to Prevent Suicide* (U.S. Public Health Service 1999), and in 2002, the Institute of Medicine published a report on the causes of suicide, recommending prevention strategies (Goldsmith et al. 2002). The 2001 release of the *National Strategy for Suicide Prevention,* developed with public and private sector partners with leadership and support from the Surgeon General, created a framework with specific goals and objectives that have guided the development of many state plans' strategy (U.S. Public Health Service 2001).

Mortality and Morbidity Information

Despite the declining rates in recent years, suicide continues to be one of the leading causes of death among youth aged 15 to 24 years. Suicide was the third leading cause of death among youth aged 10 to 24 years in 2007. The 4320 suicides in 2007 accounted for more than 11.5% of all deaths in this age group (Centers for Disease Control and Prevention [CDC] 2010a). Overall, the deaths from suicide in 2007 resulted in more than 1.3 million years of potential young life lost from the future of the United States.

Youth suicide rates have also declined slightly in recent years. Since 2000, the suicide rate among those aged 10 to 24 years declined 1.4%, from 7.0 to 6.9 per 100,000 in 2007. During this period, rates of suicide using firearms and poisoning declined slightly, and suicides by suffocation increased.

Suicide rates vary substantially by sex and across racial/ethnic groups. Suicide is substantially more likely for males. The suicide rate in 2007 for young (10–24 years) males in 2007 (11.2 per 100,000) was 4.8 times higher than the rate for females (2.3 per 100,000). Suicide rates are highest among American Indian/Alaskan Native youth (19.0 per 100,000) and non-Hispanic White youth (7.9 per 100,000) and lower among non-Hispanic Asian and Pacific Island youth (6.3 per 100,000), Hispanic youth (4.8 per 100,000), and Non-Hispanic Black youth (4.6 per 100,000).

Data from a nationally representative sample of U.S. emergency departments collected by the National Electronic Injury Surveillance System–All Injury Program (CDC 2010b) provide an estimate of the number of nonfatal injuries due to self-directed violence that are treated in U.S. emergency departments. An estimated 134,866 injuries among youth aged 10 to 24 years were attributed to self-directed violence in 2008. Females (88,252) were almost twice as likely as males (46,615) to be treated for injuries because of self-directed violence. Given that males are far more likely to die by suicide than females, the ratio of nonfatal injuries to suicides among youth (10–24 years) is far lower in males (13 to 1) than in females (124 to 1).

To fully understand the prevalence of youth suicide, it is necessary to look beyond incidents that are brought to the attention of a coroner or physician. Self-report data allow us to estimate the proportion of youth who engage in a variety of behaviors that put them or others at risk for suicidal behavior. For example, data from CDC's Youth Risk Behavior Survey are collected every other year from a large nationally representative sample of high school students. These data indicate that suicidal behavior among high school students has been declining slightly over the past 8 to 9 years. The percent of students who reported a suicide attempt in the past 12 months declined from 8.8% in 2008 to 6.3% in 2009 (CDC 2010c).

In 2009, approximately 1 in 13 female high school students (8.1%) reported attempting suicide at least once in the past 12 months. Compared with females, slightly more than half as many males (4.6%) reported attempting suicide. Suicidal ideation was more common, with 17.4% of females and 10.5% of males reporting having seriously considered suicide in the past 12 months (Eaton et al. 2010).

Risk and Protective Factors

No single factor or combination of factors can contribute or protect a young individual from suicidal behavior. Rather, multiple factors combine to contribute to and shape behavior over the course of adolescent development. Risk and protective factors exist in every area of life—individual, relationship (family, peer group), community, and societal/environmental. Individual characteristics interact in complex ways with people and conditions in the environment to produce (and protect from) violent behavior. Risk factors do not operate in isolation—the more risk factors a child or young person is exposed to, the greater the likelihood that he or she will become suicidal. Longitudinal research has demonstrated how risk and protective factor influences will differ depending on when they occur in the course of a young person's development, with the influence of some factors increasing or decreasing as a child moves from infancy to early adulthood.

An ecologic framework is useful for public health efforts to prevent youth violence and attain a deeper understanding of how the varied environments that children and youth inhabit affect their development. First introduced in the late 1970s, this ecologic model was initially applied to child abuse and subsequently to youth violence (Bronfenbrenner 1979). The model explores the relationship between individual and contextual factors and considers suicidal behavior as the product of multiple levels of influence on behavior. It recognizes that each person functions within a complex network of individual, family, peer, and community contexts that affect his or her capacity to avoid risk. Health and injury practitioners who understand the interplay of these varied influences on youth are more likely to be able to identify those who are vulnerable and will have an increased chance of successfully intervening to reduce and prevent suicidal behavior.

An ecologic systems model of human development provides a useful framework for understanding the risk and protective factors for suicidal behavior and potentially identifying opportunities for intervention. A simplified version of this model has the individual existing and developing within the context of close interpersonal relationships (family and peers). Individuals, family, and peers exist and develop in the context of their community, and all of these exist within a broader social, cultural, economic macrosystem. Each level influences and is influenced by other levels. There are several implications of this ecologic model for understanding suicidal behavior. First, it allows for the direct influence of environmental factors (familial, societal, and physical) on behavior. The model also explicitly acknowledges the multilevel determinants of behavior. By fitting the model to suicidal behavior, it is not just family or community or societal factors but all of these that contribute to the development of suicidal behavior. Moreover, these factors interact with one another to influence whether or not individuals engage in suicidal behavior.

Most etiologic research into suicidal behavior occurs at one level of analysis. Studies that are limited to one level of analysis are easier to conduct, although, at higher levels of aggregation, they suffer from potential problems when attempting across-level interpretation (Glick and Roberts 1984; Iversen 1991; Richards, Gottfredson, and Gottfredson 1990). A classic example of an ecologic analysis is that of Emile Durkheim's (1951) study of suicide. He explored ecologic associations between suicide rates and population characteristics (e.g., religion and marital status). Although Durkheim was able to say there was an association between suicide rates of a population and population characteristics, he was not able to make statements of causation at the individual level of analysis. The discussion that follows uses the basic framework of the ecologic model (individual, family and peers, community, macrosystem) as the basis for discussing research at each level.

Individual

At the individual level, there are biological and behavioral characteristics that have been associated with suicide. A number of studies have implicated hereditary factors and biological factors influencing the propensity for suicidal behavior (Mann 1987; Rainer 1984; Roy 1993). Substantial evidence has suggested that deficiencies in the serotonergic system are associated with suicidal behavior (Lowther et al. 1997; Mann, Arango, and Underwood 1990; Ohmori, Arora, and Meltzer 1992). A feeling of hopelessness is one characteristic that has been generally associated with this behavior (Beck, Brown, and Steer 1997; Shaffer et al. 1996; Weishaar and Beck 1992). A number of psychiatric disorders have been associated with suicidal behavior, such as depression (Beck et al. 1985; Brent and Perper 1995; Wolk and Weissman 1996), bipolar affective disorder (Ahrens et al. 1995; Tondo, Jamison, and Baldessarini 1997; Tondo et al. 1998), conduct disorder (Brent et al. 1995; Shaffer et al. 1996; Shafii et al. 1988), and alcoholism and substance abuse (Bryant et al. 1995; Porsteinsson et al. 1997; Windle and Windle 1997).

Sexual orientation has emerged as a significant issue in relation to risk for suicide. Numerous news stories have noted cases of suicide among persons who identified as being lesbian, gay, bisexual, or transgender (LBGT), especially in the context of them experiencing bullying behavior from peers. Some evidence indicates that LBGT youth experience greater emotional distress as a function of perceived discrimination (Almeida et al. 2009). Assessing whether or not there is elevated risk among LGBT youth for suicide is difficult because postmortem assessment of sexual orientation is difficult. However, evidence that there is elevated risk of suicidal ideation and behavior among LGBT youth is becoming well established, and the need to incorporate prevention efforts sensitive to the needs of LGBT youth is clear (Suicide Prevention Resource Center 2008).

Family and Close Relationships

Characteristics of, and behavior within, the family environment have significant influence on the development of individuals. A number of family environment characteristics have been associated with suicide and suicidal behavior, including family conflict or discord (Bertera 2007; Brent 1995; Campbell et al. 1993), parental attachment (DeJong, Virkkunen, and Linnoila 1992;

Herba et al. 2008), poor family functioning (Adams, Overholser, and Lehnert 1994), childhood separation from parents (Bagley and Ramsay 1985), child abuse and neglect (Bryant and Range 1995; Molnar et al. 1998), intimate partner abuse/conflict (Deykin, Alpert, and McNamara 1985), and loss of a peer (Brent et al. 1992, 1996). Larger family size has also been associated with lower rates of suicide (Denney et al. 2009).

Among persons in the teen years, peers have significant influence on behavior. Bullying behavior has been linked to suicidal behavior in the media and by a number a studies. Some research indicates that the potential influence of bullying on the development of suicidal behavior may be mediated by characteristics of the victim in relationship to characteristics of their parents (Herba et al. 2008). For example, victims of bullying would be more likely to experience suicidal ideation if they also experienced rejection at home that resulted from victim characteristics and negative parental reactions to those characteristics.

Another factor that may operate at the level of family and peers, although it is clearly linked to community characteristics, is access to means. A number of studies have indicated with varying degrees of rigor that access to firearms increases risk of completed suicide (Beautrais, Joyce, and Mulder 1996; Cummings et al. 1997).

Bertera (2007) found that negative exchanges with family were associated with increased suicide ideation scores in younger (15–17 years) but not older (18–19 years) adolescents. It was also found that positive support provided a buffering effect that was age-specific and independent of gender, income, or mood disorders.

Community and Societal

Suicide rates vary substantially internationally (Krug, Dahlberg, and Powell 1996), suggesting cultural differences in suicidal behavior. These cultural differences seem to result in variation of method selected (Burvill 1995; Canetto and Lester 1998; Ko and Kua 1995). Various indicators of economic factors have been explored in relation to suicide rates (Burvill 1995; Ko and Kua 1995; Reinfurt, Stewart, and Weaver 1991; Yang and Clum 1995; Yang and Lester 1995). Studies generally support an association between economic factors and suicide, although several have not found an association.

There are a number of key concepts at several levels of aggregation (individual, family/peer, community, and macrosystem) that seem to be central for understanding the causes of suicide. Unfortunately, there are no research findings that have been able to simultaneously link all these levels together to provide an understanding of the causes of suicide that would allow us to develop and implement highly effective multisystemic interventions for the prevention of suicidal behavior. This highlights the issue of taxonomy. In reviewing the literature on suicide, few studies use the same definitions. Variables and constructs that we use as predictors occupy a vast range, as do variables and constructs that actually measure some form of suicidal behavior. Thus, although there have been limited efforts to articulate taxonomy of suicide (O'Carroll et al. 1996), we are left with a rapidly developing field of research that is struggling for both a more refined taxonomy and a more developed framework for understanding the causes.

Current Research, Prevention, and Intervention Strategies

The CDC has reviewed and summarized a range of strategies intended to prevent suicidal behavior (O'Carroll, Potter, and Mercy 1994). A review of suicide prevention efforts listed in the guide suggests that most suicide prevention programs embrace the high-risk model of prevention where the goal is case finding and referral (Rose 2001). Screening and referral, crisis centers, and community organization are common examples of this high-risk approach. Suicide awareness or education activities, media guidelines, and means restriction are examples of population-based interventions. Currently, neither the high-risk nor the population prevention approach can be said to be more effective than the other. However, it is reasonable to expect that a combination of these approaches would be a more effective way to affect suicide rates and suicide-related morbidity than only one approach. Implementation of efforts to reduce suicide risk with a focus on a population or a population segment combined with more intensive efforts to identify and provide services for those at greatest risk should lead to more positive outcomes.

There are a number of programmatic strategies for suicide prevention that schools and communities might consider implementing. Regardless of the strategies a school may use, it is important that it develops a comprehensive plan for preventing suicide, safely managing a student who may be suicidal, and responding appropriately and effectively after a suicide occurs. Other strategies include providing gatekeeper training, prevention education, screening, peer support programs, and crisis intervention; restricting access to means; providing aftercare to those who experience significant loss; and educating families.

Gatekeeper Training

Gatekeeper training in schools is a type of program designed to help school staff (e.g., teachers, counselors, and coaches) identify and refer students at risk for suicide. These programs teach staff how to respond to suicide or other crises in the school. This is a commonly implemented strategy, and it makes sense to ensure that key school staff members know how to respond to someone in crisis or someone who is thinking about suicide. There are a number of different programs available, and some communities have developed their own programs. Most gatekeeper models tend to include training individuals to ask if a person has concerns about or is thinking about suicide. They also tend to emphasize listening, being supportive, and transferring care of persons who are considering suicide to an appropriate professional. The logic of the gatekeeper model is that adults who come in contact with youth should know clearly what they should do if they encounter a youth who they think might be suicidal. There are several assumptions inherent in the model that should be considered. It assumes that appropriate services are available and that a system is in place to enable the gatekeeper to make an appropriate referral and transfer care. The gatekeeper model assumes that youth who are at risk for suicide will be more likely to be identified and more likely to receive effective care if a person trained as a gatekeeper has contact with them.

Results from evaluations of gatekeeper training programs suggest that persons trained are more likely to believe they would act to prevent youth suicide, demonstrate greater confidence in suicide assessment and intervention knowledge, and have higher levels of comfort, competence, and confidence in helping at-risk youth (Isaac et al. 2009; Matthieu et al. 2008; Reis and Cornell 2008; Wyman et al. 2008). One effort to evaluate application of gatekeeper training in schools conducted a group-based randomized trial and found that suicide identification behaviors increased most for staff already communicating with students about suicide and distress and that increased knowledge and appraisals were not sufficient to increase suicide identification behaviors (Wyman et al. 2008). The authors suggest that skill training for staff already serving as "natural gatekeepers" and efforts to modify students' help-seeking behaviors are likely to have the greatest impact.

The concept behind suicide prevention education is that students learn about suicide and its warning signs, and how to seek help for themselves or others. These programs often incorporate a variety of activities that develop self-esteem and social competency. An educational approach is relatively popular. Substantial numbers of people can be reached, and the programs are usually delivered with limited duration and exposure. Studies indicate that an educational approach can increase knowledge of warning signs and sources of help and referral. There is little evidence to suggest that an educational strategy will result in changing attitudes toward suicide or willingness to seek help. There is evidence from one study that youth who had attempted suicide in the past had negative reactions to an education program (Shaffer et al. 1991). Thus, caution should be taken in implementing this strategy, and resources should be in place to recognize persons who may be at risk and to provide appropriate care and referrals. As with any curricula being considered, suicide prevention education programs should be evaluated in terms of the practicality of the content and duration for achieving intended outcomes. If the content and duration are limited, achieving desired outcomes may be limited as well.

Screening Programs

Screening programs usually involve administering a questionnaire or other screening instrument to identify high-risk adolescents and young adults and provide further assessment and treatment. Repeated assessment can be used to measure changes in attitudes or behaviors over time, to test the effectiveness of a prevention strategy, and to detect potential suicidal behavior.

Screening strategies are focused on identifying underlying characteristics associated with suicidal behavior. Behaviors and symptoms associated with major depression are usually the factors that are focused on. Not all persons who attempt or complete suicide exhibit behaviors or symptoms consistent with a diagnosis of major depression. Although there is a fair amount of evidence that many, if not most, persons exhibiting suicidal behavior have some form of diagnosable mood disorder. Screening only for indicators of mood disorder will miss some percentage of persons who will go on to attempt or complete suicide. This may be a small number.

In one study, the Diagnostic Interview Schedule for Children had a high rate of sensitivity (identified all cases) for major depression and a specificity of less than 1 (0.88, which is, by most standards, good) (Lucas et al. 2001). The result of lack of specificity in a screening program is that more youth with low risk would need to be seen by a clinician. This increases the cost of screening.

Another issue in screening is that not all persons who are depressed or have a psychiatric disorder will attempt or complete suicide. In many ways, a strategy of screening for psychiatric disorders and case management through treatment is expected to result in reducing suicide rates. The logic is sound, but there does not appear to be experimental or quasi-experimental evaluations conducted to conclude that this strategy will reduce suicidal behavior.

The American Academy of Pediatrics (AAP) recommends screening for suicide risk (Gould et al. 2009) and asking all adolescents about suicidal thoughts when taking a routine medical history. The *AMA Guidelines for Adolescent Preventive Services (GAPS): Recommendations and Rationale* (Elster and Kuznets 1994) and *Bright Futures: Guidelines for Health Supervision of Infants, Children, and Adolescents* (Green and Palfrey 2002) recommend that providers screen adolescents annually to identify those at risk for suicide. However, *Screening for Suicide Risk* (U.S. Preventive Services Task Force 2004) does not recommend screening for suicide because there were no valid or reliable instruments for suicide risk at the time the guide was written.

Mental health screening should probably be part of any school health program. This may be a resource-intensive endeavor, however, because it requires that the system is prepared to provide and manage services for those identified. In any effort to provide services across agencies and organizations, coordination is essential. Coordination must occur among the youth, school, referral agency, and home. Many youth who have been identified as being at risk for suicide using screening tools do not seek or receive mental health treatment (Gould et al. 2009). It is also essential that all youth know to whom they can go if they or a friend needs help. Having a designated coordinator for youth mental health services would facilitate coordination of services and follow up with at-risk youth. A coordinator could also provide leadership in the event of a suicide within the school's population.

Identifying and treating depression have long been at the foundation of efforts to prevent suicide. Millions of Americans have relied on selective serotonin reuptake inhibitors (SSRIs) to treat depression or anxiety. For most adults, SSRIs effectively treat these symptoms, although the Food and Drug Administration (FDA) has released an advisory regarding the risk of suicide in adults taking SSRIs. There is also some debate about research suggesting that in some patients, and youth in particular, SSRIs are associated with increases in suicidal ideation and behavior. This debate has culminated in the review of evidence on this topic by the FDA. The FDA reviewed clinical trials of SSRIs and found that no completed suicides occurred among approximately 2200 children treated with SSRI medications. However, the rate of suicidal thinking or behavior, including actual suicidal attempts, was 4% for those taking SSRI medications, twice the rate of those taking inert placebo pills. This led the FDA to adopt a "black-box" label warning that antidepressants were found to increase the risk of suicidal thinking and behavior in children and adolescents with major depressive disorder. A black-box warning is the most serious type of warning in prescription drug labeling. A more recent review of observational studies had findings consistent with that of the FDA, in that among adolescents, use of SSRIs may increase suicidality (Barbui, Esposito, and Cipriani 2009). Yet another assessment of research found that several large nonindustry studies indicated rates of suicide and suicidal behavior were lower in children who used antidepressants (Bostwick 2006).

The black-box warning states that children and adolescents who start to take SSRI medications should be closely monitored for any worsening in depression, emergence of suicidal thinking or behavior, and in general for any unusual changes in behavior, such as sleeplessness, agitation, or withdrawal from normal social situations. Monitoring for these behaviors and symptoms is especially important during the first 4 weeks of treatment. The publicity associated with the FDA review and action has resulted in concern by some that persons diagnosed with depression will be less likely to treat their symptoms with SSRI medications, which conceivably may lead to overall increases in suicidal ideation and behavior.

Peer Support Programs

Peer support programs can be conducted in or outside of school and are designed to foster peer relationships and competency in social skills among high-risk adolescents and young adults. Peer support programs attempt to provide a setting where young people who may be at risk for suicide can receive support from their peers and develop positive interpersonal relationships. One of the most extensively evaluated peer-support programs is Reconnecting Youth (Eggert et al. 1994, 1995, 2001). The program incorporates social support and life skills training with the following components: a semester-long, daily class designed to enhance self-esteem, decision-making, personal control, interpersonal communication, social activities and school bonding, drug-free social activities and friendships, and a teenager's relationship to school, as well as a school system crisis response plan to address suicide prevention approaches. Another program that uses a peer support model is called "Natural Helpers." This program was implemented in a Native American community and was associated with a decline in suicide rates (CDC 1998). Other more recent research has also found that a peer support approach has significant potential for suicide prevention (Walker et al. 2009). The peer support model is one to consider for primary prevention of suicide and, if implemented well, may actually result in positive outcomes for a number of health issues affecting youth.

Crisis Intervention

In crisis centers and on hotlines, trained volunteers and paid staff provide telephone counseling and other services for suicidal persons. Such programs also may offer a "drop-in" crisis center and referral to mental health services. The function of these services relies on the presumption that suicide attempts are often impulsive and contemplated with ambivalence. Hotlines are designed to deter the caller from self-destructive behaviors until the immediate crisis has passed. The anonymity afforded by hotline calls allows the caller to feel secure and in control. Many hotlines are linked to schools and mental health services.

Research on crisis centers and hotlines indicates they may be beneficial toward reducing suicidality of most suicidal callers (Kalafat et al. 2007). Although variability in training and consistency of persons answering calls may impinge on the overall effectiveness of this strategy (Mishara et al. 2007). The effectiveness of hotlines and crisis centers might be improved by increasing outreach to at-risk groups, requiring consistent training of volunteer staff and taking steps to improve follow-up with those who call (Draper 2007; Joiner et al. 2007).

Restriction of Access to Lethal Means

Activities are designed to restrict access to handguns, drugs, and other common means of suicide. Impulsiveness and ambivalence are important factors in suicidal behaviors among young people (Simon et al. 2001). Therefore, means restriction has the potential for preventing suicides. At least some portion of impulsive decisions to attempt suicide might never be acted on if substantial efforts were needed to arrange for a method of suicide. Means restriction has proven to be a controversial approach to prevention. This is mostly true for firearms, but efforts to promote constructing barriers on bridges, to modify the design of automobiles, and to impose restrictions on dispensing of medication have also resulted in controversy. Efforts to educate parents of youth about risks associated with access to firearms and lethal doses of drugs may be one way that schools can use this strategy for prevention. Also, when a youth is considered to be at risk for suicide, some assessment of their access to means may be called for and some effort to restrict access to means should be implemented.

Intervention After a Suicide

There is evidence that youth who have experienced the loss of a peer to suicide are more likely to consider suicide compared with youth who have not experienced such a loss (Feigelman and Gorman 2008). One strategy for preventing suicide has been to focus on friends and relatives of persons who have died by suicide. The strategy is partially designed to help prevent or contain suicide clusters and to help adolescents and young adults cope effectively with the feelings of loss that follow the sudden death or suicide of a peer. As part of their crisis response plan, schools should have a concerted effort to identify persons who witness a traumatic event or who experienced significant loss as a result of the event. This plan should include provision of appropriate counseling and means to refer and follow up with those affected.

Family Education and Involvement

Parents and caregivers of youth are important to consider when developing and implementing a suicide prevention effort. Family members are often most aware of the mood states and issues troubling children. However, all too frequently, family members are not aware of signs and symptoms of mood disorders or suicide until the situation of a child has evolved into a crisis. Educating parents and caregivers about how to recognize possible symptoms and what to do when they are concerned may be an effective strategy to prevent suicide.

Future Research, Practice, and Advocacy

Identifying and implementing effective interventions with the goal of reducing the incidence of suicidal behavior is an important and resource-intensive step in addressing youth suicide. The research on risk and protective factors suggests that one promising prevention strategy is to promote overall mental health among school-aged children by reducing early risk factors for depression, substance abuse, and aggressive behaviors and building resiliency. In addition to the potential for saving lives, youth benefit from an overall enhancement of academic performance and a reduction in peer and family conflict. A second positive approach is to detect youth most likely to be suicidal by confidentially screening for depression, substance abuse, and suicidal ideation. If a youth reports any of these, further evaluation of the youth can take place by professionals, followed by referral for treatment as needed. Efforts should be made to develop and implement strategies to reduce the stigma associated with accessing mental health, substance abuse, and suicide prevention treatments. Adequate treatment of mental disorders among youth, whether they are suicidal or not, has important academic, peer, and family relationship benefits.

In addition, efforts to limit young people's access to lethal agents, including firearms and medications, may hold great suicide prevention value. Media education is also important, because the risk for suicide contagion as a result of media reporting can be minimized by limited, factual, and concise media reports of suicide. Finally, after exposure to suicide or suicidal behaviors within one's family or peer group, suicide risk can be minimized by having family members, friends, peers, and colleagues of the victim evaluated by a mental health professional. Persons deemed at risk for suicide should then be referred for additional mental health services.

Caution should be used in the development of suicide prevention programs for youth, because researchers have found that some types of suicide prevention efforts may be counterproductive. For example, some school-based youth suicide awareness and prevention programs have had unintended negative effects. Because of the tremendous effort and cost involved in starting and maintaining programs, we should be certain that they are safe and effective before they are further used or promoted.

Although progress is being made toward developing a knowledge base from which we can make programmatic decisions, the need for outcome evaluation of interventions is imperative. There is simply insufficient quality, scientifically based information that we can use to make decisions about where to spend precious intervention resources. The balance between service delivery and research involves difficult choices, but it is important to note that effective service delivery often lies on a foundation of well-planned and executed interventions that have been carefully evaluated.

Advocacy on the part of survivors (those who have lost loved ones to suicide) has been an essential element to moving the field of suicide prevention ahead. *The Surgeon General's Call to Action to Prevent Suicide* (U.S. Public Health Service 1999) came about, in part, in response to the work of survivors advocating for public health to take on and address suicide as a public health issue. This led to development of the *National Strategy for Suicide Prevention: Goals and Objectives for Action* (U.S. Public Health Service 2001), which had been one of the major intermediary outcomes for which advocates had pressed. Clinicians, researchers, persons who care for persons with mental illness, and persons who attempted suicide, among others, have also made significant advocacy efforts. Over the past 10 years, national, state, and local advocacy efforts have grown and influenced the resolve of public officials to begin or expand efforts to address suicide prevention. The U.S. Congress recently passed and funded the Garrett Lee Smith Memorial Act, which provides support to states, colleges, and universities to develop and deliver suicide prevention program efforts. The Garret Lee Smith Memorial Act Grantees have been engaged in significant suicide prevention efforts that have strong evaluation components (Goldston et al. 2010). Advocacy efforts most certainly supported advancing this legislation and are pressing efforts toward additional suicide prevention legislation. The future of suicide prevention in the United States is largely dependent on the ability and resolve of advocates to continue and expand efforts to convince public officials that suicide is a true public health priority.

Developing an Integrated Research, Practice, and Advocacy Agenda

Research has begun to describe youth involvement in multiple forms of violent behavior, documenting the involvement in varied forms of peer violence and suicidal behaviors. One of the few studies that have specifically examined the overlap between physical peer violence and suicidal behaviors was based on the 1997 New York State Youth Risk Behavior Survey. This study found that 11% of high school students reported both suicidal and violent behavior in the past year (Cleary 2000). Research based on the 2001 National Youth Risk Behavior Survey found that adolescents who report suicidal behavior are more likely to report involvement in physical fighting (Swahn, Lubell, and Simon 2004). More specifically, high school students who reported attempting suicide were more likely to have been in a physical fight than students who reported not attempting suicide (61.5% vs. 30.3%) (Swahn, Lubell, and Simon 2004). Higher proportions of both boys and girls who had attempted suicide (77.8% and 54.0%, respectively) reported fighting than those boys and girls who had not attempted suicide (41.2% and 19.8%, respectively). Moreover, among those students who reported attempting suicide, the proportion that reported fighting was highest among ninth graders (64.5%) and decreased with each subsequent grade.

Research has also found that youth who have attacked others with a weapon (Evans et al. 2001; Flannery, Singer, and Wester 2001); engaged in dating violence, particularly for males (Coker et al. 2000); or perpetrated sexual violence (Borowsky, Hogan, and Ireland 1997) have been shown to be at higher risk for suicidal behavior. Research with adults suggests that peer violence and suicide are strongly linked; however, the strength of this association among adolescents and the degree to which it changes by age remain unclear. Also, the extent to which risk for participation in single versus multiple types of violence varies for adolescent boys and girls is generally not well understood. In particular, we have a limited understanding of the role that gender, age, or developmental stage or race and ethnicity may have on the associations of different violent behaviors. Additional information on the linkages among forms of youth violence and how these linkages differ by gender and age is needed to guide the selection, timing, and focus of prevention strategies.

Advancing a complementary ecologic model to think more clearly about how to create communities with a rich network of nurturing supportive relationships has been advocated by some neuroscientists, research scholars, pediatricians, and youth service professionals (Eccles and Gootman 2002). Reviews of new research on the brain, human behavior, and social trends report that networks of enduring, nurturing relationships have shown that positive experiences and exposure to these components significantly strengthen brain development and diminish the likelihood of aggression, depression, and substance abuse. The work of providing this nurture is done largely by families, neighborhoods, community groups, and religious organizations—what the Commission on Children at Risk calls "authoritative communities" (Commission on Children at Risk 2008). The characteristics of social groups, whether of families or other social groups, that will produce good outcomes for children have begun to be identified and can be incorporated into community programs (Eccles and Gootman 2002). This approach does not replace the focus on preventing problems, but provides a broader view of helping youth and undergirds a wide array of activities, such as community service, school to work transition programs, parenting, mentoring, and arts and recreation activities. More collaborative comprehensive and longitudinal research is needed to evaluate which features of community programs influence development, which processes within each activity are related to these outcomes, and which combination of features are best for particular outcomes to supplement family-based, school-setting prevention efforts.

Starting early and advocating for a comprehensive approach will likely yield a large prevention dividend. These efforts should begin during infancy and continue through adolescence. Our best science and practice tell us that we need to begin during infancy with home visitation and parenting programs that promote healthy development. During the childhood years, investments should be made to teach problem-solving skills in schools and other settings, such as in churches. Parenting programs should be continued through childhood and adolescence. As children move into adolescence, mentoring programs and intensive efforts to keep adolescents in school and on track with their education should be emphasized. These programs need to be supported by healthy environments; therefore, community-level efforts are needed to strengthen and empower communities, build trust in and connectedness of youth to their communities, and change norms that do not support development and expression of suicidal behavior.

The greater public health injury community can play an important role in helping to advance a broad suicide prevention policy. At a national level, suicide prevention and mental health promotion associations can promote collective, educational, scholarly, and dissemination activities among their members and allied groups. This can be done through a broad range of research, program and policy development, teaching, and other activities that synthesize expertise from multiple disciplines, settings, and perspectives. Efforts to build bridges between the injury and mental health communities and those sectors that work directly with children and youth (including educational and youth development institutions, criminal justice and social services networks, youth advocates, organizations and researchers, youth leaders, victims, survivors groups, and other interested persons) can further the coordination of findings, address specific youth suicide prevention issues, and develop a more inclusive suicide prevention agenda.

The Substance Abuse and Mental Health Services Administration has recently announced efforts to form the National Action Alliance for Suicide Prevention. The Action Alliance was a key recommendation of the *National Strategy for Suicide Prevention: Goals and Objectives for Action* (U.S. Public Health Service 2001) and will build on noteworthy achievements reached thus far in national suicide prevention. These achievements include federal and state legislation that has advanced suicide prevention planning and programming; programs to improve detection of suicide risk and access to care; the establishment of the national Suicide Prevention Resource Center, a national Best Practices Registry for Suicide Prevention, the Suicide Prevention Lifeline (1-800-273-TALK); and development of the National Violent Death Reporting System. The Action Alliance will focus on updating and advancing the *National Strategy for Suicide Prevention: Goals and Objectives for Action.* It will also work to develop effective public awareness and social marketing campaigns, including targeted messages for specific segments of the population that can change attitudes and norms and reduce suicidal behaviors.

Public health and injury professionals can strengthen ongoing efforts to reduce suicide and suicidal behaviors by fostering community-level change through working with local and national youth development organizations to address the contributing factors of availability of alcohol and other drugs, access to means, insufficient access to health and mental health care, and social isolation faced by many of today's youth.

Resources

American Association of Suicidology: http://www.suicidology.org
American Foundation for Suicide Prevention: http://www.afsp.org
Centers for Disease Control and Prevention: http://www.cdc.gov/injury
Children's Safety Network: http://www.ChildrensSafetyNetwork.org
National Registry of Effective Programs and Practices: http://www.nrepp.samhsa.gov
National Suicide Prevention Lifeline: http://www.suicidepreventionlifeline.org
National Suicide Prevention Resource Center: http://www.sprc.org
The Guide to Community Preventive Services: Systematic Reviews and Evidence Based Recommendations: http://www.thecommunityguide.org

References

Adams DM, Overholser JC, Lehnert KL. 1994. Perceived family functioning and adolescent suicidal behavior. *J Am Acad Child Adolesc Psychiatry.* 33:498–507.

Ahrens B, Grof P, Moller HJ, et al. 1995. Extended survival of patients on long-term lithium treatment. *Can J Psychiatry.* 40:241–246.

Almeida J, Johnson RM, Corliss HL, et al. 2009. Emotional distress among LGBT youth: the influence of perceived discrimination based on sexual orientation. *J Youth Adolesc.* 38:1001–1014.

Bagley C, Ramsay R. 1985. Problems and priorities in research on suicidal behaviours: an overview with Canadian implications. *Can J Commun Ment Health.* 4:15–49.

Barbui C, Esposito E, Cipriani A. 2009. Selective serotonin reuptake inhibitors and risk of suicide: a systematic review of observational studies. *CMAJ.* 180:291–297.

Beautrais AL, Joyce PR, Mulder RT. 1996. Access to firearms and the risk of suicide: a case control study [see comments]. *Aust N Z J Psychiatry.* 30:741–748.

Beck AT, Brown GK, Steer RA. 1997. Psychometric characteristics of the Scale for Suicide Ideation with psychiatric outpatients. *Behav Res Ther.* 35:1039–1046.

Beck AT, Steer RA, Kovacs M, Garrison B. 1985. Hopelessness and eventual suicide: a 10-year prospective study of patients hospitalized with suicidal ideation. *Am J Psychiatry.* 142:559–563.

Bertera E. 2007. The role of positive and negative social exchanges between adolescents, their peers and family as predictors of suicide ideation. *Child Adolesc Social Work J.* 24:523–538.

Borowsky IW, Hogan M, Ireland M. 1997. Adolescent sexual aggression: risk and protective factors. *Pediatrics.* 100:E7.

Bostwick JM. 2006. Do SSRIs cause suicide in children? The evidence is underwhelming. *J Clin Psychol.* 62:235–241.

Brent DA. 1995. Risk factors for adolescent suicide and suicidal behavior: mental and substance abuse disorders, family environmental factors, and life stress. *Suicide Life Threat Behav.* 25(Suppl):52–63.

Brent DA, Moritz G, Bridge J, et al. 1996. Long-term impact of exposure to suicide: a three-year controlled follow-up. *J Am Acad Child Adolesc Psychiatry.* 35:646–653.

Brent DA, Perper JA. 1995. Research in adolescent suicide: implications for training, service delivery, and public policy. [Review]. *Suicide Life Threat Behav.* 25:222–230.

Brent DA, Perper J, Moritz G, et al. 1992. Psychiatric effects of exposure to suicide among the friends and acquaintances of adolescent suicide victims. *J Am Acad Child Adolesc Psychiatry.* 31:629–639.

Brent DA, Perper JA, Moritz G, Baugher M. 1995. Stressful life events, psychopathology, and adolescent suicide: a case control study. *Suicide Life Threat Behav.* 23:179–187.

Bronfenbrenner U. 1979. *The Ecology of Human Development: Experiments by Nature and Design.* Cambridge, MA: Harvard University.

Bryant ES, Garrison CZ, Valois RF, Rivard JC. 1995. Suicidal behavior among youth with severe emotional disturbance. *J Child Fam Stud.* 4:429–443.

Bryant SL, Range LM. 1995. Suicidality in college women who were sexually and physically abused and physically punished by parents. *Violence Vict.* 10:195–201.

Burvill PW. 1995. Suicide in the multiethnic elderly population of Australia, 1979-1990. Special Issue: suicide and aging: international perspectives. *Int Psychogeriatr.* 7:319–333.

Campbell NB, Milling L, Laughlin A, Bush E. 1993. The psychosocial climate of families with suicidal pre-adolescent children. *Am J Orthopsychiatry.* 63:142–145.

Canetto SS, Lester D. 1998. Gender, culture, and suicidal behavior. *Transcult Psychiatry.* 35:163–190.

Centers for Disease Control and Prevention. 1998. Suicide prevention evaluation in a Western Athabaskan American Indian Tribe—New Mexico, 1988-1997. *MMWR Morb Mortal Wkly Rep.* 47:257–261.

Centers for Disease Control and Prevention. 2010a. *Web-based Injury Statistics Query and Reporting System (WISQARS) Fatal Injury Data* [online] [cited September 14, 2010]. Available at: http://www.cdc.gov/injury/wisqars/fatal.html

Centers for Disease Control and Prevention. 2010b. *Web-based Injury Statistics Query and Reporting System (WISQARS) - National Electronic Injury Surveillance System - All Injury Program (NEISS-AIP)* [cited September 14, 2010]. Available at: http://www.cdc.gov/injury/wisqars/nonfatal.html. Accessed July 11, 2011.

Centers for Disease Control and Prevention. 2010c. *Trends in the Prevalence of Suicide-Related Behaviors: National YRBS: 1991–2009* [cited August 27, 2010]. Available at: http://www.cdc.gov/HealthyYouth/yrbs/pdf/us_suicide_trend_yrbs.pdf. Accessed July 11, 2011.

Cleary SD. 2000. Adolescent victimization and associated suicidal and violent behaviors. *Adolescence.* 35:671.

Coker AL, McKeown RE, Sanderson M, et al. 2000. Severe dating violence and quality of life among South Carolina High School students. *Am J Prev Med.* 19:220–227.

Commission on Children at Risk. 2008. Hardwired to connect: the new scientific case for authoritative community. In: Kline KK, editor. *Hardwired to connect: the new scientific case for authoritative community.* New York: Springer. 3–68.

Cummings P, Koepsell TD, Grossman DC, et al. 1997. The association between the purchase of a handgun and homicide or suicide. *Am J Public Health.* 87:974–978.

DeJong J, Virkkunen M, Linnoila M. 1992. Nervous and mental disease: factors associated with recidivism in a criminal population. *J Nerv Ment Dis.* 180:543–550.

Denney JT, Rogers RG, Krueger PM, Wadsworth T. 2009. Adult suicide mortality in the United States: marital status, family size, socioeconomic status, differences by sex. *Soc Sci Q.* 90:1167–1185.

Deykin EY, Alpert JJ, McNamara JJ. 1985. A pilot study of the effect of exposure to child abuse or neglect on adolescent suicidal behavior. *Am J Psychiatry.* 142:1299–1303.

Draper J. 2007. Preventing suicide minute by minute. *Behav Healthc.* 27:29–31.

Durkheim E. 1951. *Suicide: A Study in Sociology.* New York, NY: The Free Press.

Eaton DK, Kann L, Kinchen S, et al. 2010. Youth risk behavior surveillance—United States, 2009. *MMWR.* 59(SS-5):1–142.

Eccles J, Gootman JA, editors. 2002. *Community Programs to Promote Youth Development.* Washington, DC: National Academies Press.

Eggert LL, Thompson EA, Herting JR, Nicholas LJ. 1994. Prevention research program: reconnecting at-risk youth. Special Issue: mental health nursing 2000: issues and challenges. *Issues Ment Health Nurs.*15:107–135.

Eggert LL, Thompson EA, Herting JR, Nicholas LJ. 1995. Reducing suicide potential among high-risk youth: tests of a school-based prevention program. *Suicide Life Threat Behav.* 25:276–96.

Eggert LL, Thompson EA, Herting JR, Randell BP. 2001. Reconnecting youth to prevent drug abuse, school dropout and suicidal behaviors among high-risk youth. In: Wagner EF, Waldron HB, editors. *Innovations in Adolescent Substance Abuse Interventions.* Amsterdam, Netherlands: Pergamon/Elsevier. 51–84.

Elster AB, Kuznets NJ. 1994. *AMA Guidelines for Adolescent Preventive Services (GAPS): Recommendations and Rationale.* Baltimore, MD: Williams & Wilkins.

Evans WP, Marte RM, Betts S, Silliman B. 2001. Adolescent suicide risk and peer-related violent behaviors and victimization. *J Interpers Violence.* 16:1330.

Feigelman W, Gorman BS. 2008. Assessing the effects of peer suicide on youth suicide. *Suicide Life Threat Behav.* 38:181–194.

Flannery DJ, Singer MI, Wester K. 2001. Violence exposure, psychological trauma, and suicide risk in a community sample of dangerously violent adolescents. *J Am Acad Child Adolesc Psychiatry.* 40:435.

Glick WH, Roberts KH. 1984. Hypothesized interdependence, assumed independence. *Acad Manage Rev.* 9:722–735.

Goldsmith SK, Pellmar TC, Kleinman AM, Bunney WE, Committee on Pathophysiology and Prevention of Adolescent and Adult Suicide, and Board of Neuroscience and Behavioral Health, editors. 2002. *Reducing Suicide: A National Imperative.* Washington, DC: National Academies Press.

Goldston DB, Walrath CM, McKeon R, et al. 2010. The Garrett Lee Smith Memorial Suicide Prevention Program. *Suicide Life Threat Behav.* 40:245–256.

Gould MS, Marrocco FA, Hoagwood K, et al. 2009. Service use by at-risk youths after school-based suicide screening. *J Am Acad Child Adolesc Psychiatry.* 48:1193–1207.

Green M, Palfrey JS, editors. 2002. *Bright Futures: Guidelines for Health Supervision of Infants, Children, and Adolescents.* 2nd ed. Arlington, VA: National Center for Education in Maternal and Child Health.

Herba CM, Ferdinand RF, Stijnen T, et al. 2008. Victimisation and suicide ideation in the TRAILS study: specific vulnerabilities of victims. *J Child Psychol Psychiatry.* 49:867–876.

Isaac M, Elias B, Katz LY, et al. 2009. Gatekeeper training as a preventative intervention for suicide: a systematic review. *Can J Psychiatry.* 54:260–268.

Iversen GR. 1991. *Contextual Analysis. Quantitative Applications in the Social Sciences, No. 81.* Newbury Park, CA: Sage Publications, Inc.

Joiner T, Kalafat J, Draper J, et al. 2007. Establishing standards for the assessment of suicide risk among callers to the national suicide prevention lifeline. *Suicide Life Threat Behav.* 37:353–365.

Kalafat J, Gould MS, Munfakh JL, Kleinman M. 2007. An evaluation of crisis hotline outcomes part 1: nonsuicidal crisis callers. *Suicide Life Threat Behav.* 37:322–337.

Ko SM, Kua EH. 1995. Ethnicity and elderly suicide in Singapore. Special Issue: suicide and aging: international perspectives. *Int Psychogeriatr* 7:309–317.

Krug EG, Dahlberg LL, Mercy JA, et al, editors. 2002. *World Report on Violence and Health.* Geneva: World Health Organization.

Krug EG, Dahlberg LL, Powell KE. 1996. Childhood homicide, suicide, and firearm deaths: an international comparison. *World Health Stat Q.* 49:230–235.

Lowther S, De Paermentier F, Cheetham SC, et al. 1997. 5-HT1A receptor binding sites in post-mortem brain samples from depressed suicides and controls. *J Affect Dis.* 42:199–207.

Lucas CP, Zhang Haiying Z, Fisher PW, et al. 2001. The DISC Predictive Scales (DPS): efficiently screening for diagnoses. *J Am Acad Child Adolesc Psychiatry.* 40:443.

Mann JJ. 1987. Psychobiologic predictors of suicide. *J Clin Psychiatry.* 48(Suppl):39–43.

Mann JJ, Arango V, Underwood MD. 1990. Serotonin and suicidal behavior. *Ann N Y Acad Sci.* 600:476–485.

Matthieu MM, Cross W, Batres AR, et al. 2008. Evaluation of gatekeeper training for suicide prevention in veterans. *Arch Suicide Res.* 12:148–154.

Mishara BL, Chagnon F, Daigle M, et al. 2007. Comparing models of helper behavior to actual practice in telephone crisis intervention: a silent monitoring study of calls to the U.S. 1-800-SUICIDE Network. *Suicide Life Threat Behav.* 37:291–307.

Molnar BE, Shade SB, Kral AH, et al. 1998. Suicidal behavior and sexual/physical abuse among street youth. *Child Abuse Negl.* 22:213–222.

O'Carroll PW, Berman AL, Maris RW, et al. 1996. Beyond the Tower of Babel: a nomenclature for suicidology. *Suicide Life Threat Behav.* 26:237–252.

O'Carroll PW, Potter LB, Mercy JA. 1994. Programs for the prevention of suicide among adolescents and young adults. *MMWR Morbid Mortal Wkly Rep.* 43(RR-6):1–7.

Ohmori T, Arora RC, Meltzer HY. 1992. Serotonergic measures in suicide brain: the concentration of 5-HIAA, HVA, and tryptophan in frontal cortex of suicide victims. *Biol Psychiatry.* 32:57–71.

Porsteinsson A, Duberstein PR, Conwell Y, et al. 1997. Suicide and alcoholism. Distinguishing alcoholic patients with and without comorbid drug abuse. *Am J Addict.* 6:304–310.

Rainer JD. 1984. Genetic factors in depression and suicide. *Am J Psychother.* 38:329–340.

Reinfurt DW, Stewart JR, Weaver NL. 1991. The economy as a factor in motor vehicle fatalities, suicides, and homicides. Special Issue: theoretical models for traffic safety. *Accid Anal Prev.* 23:453–462.

Reis C, Cornell D. 2008. An evaluation of suicide gatekeeper training for school counselors and teachers. *Sch Couns.* 11:386–394.

Richards JM, Gottfredson DC, Gottfredson GD. 1990. Units of analysis and item statistics for environmental assessment scales. *Curr Psychol.* 9:407–413.

Rose G. 2001. Sick individuals and sick populations. *Bull World Health Org.* 79:990.

Roy A. 1993. Genetic and biologic risk factors for suicide in depressive disorders. Special Issue: Fifth Annual New York State Office of Mental Health Research Conference. *Psychiatric Q.* 64:345–358.

Shaffer D, Garland A, Vieland V, et al. 1991. The impact of curriculum-based suicide prevention programs for teenagers. *J Am Acad Child Adolesc Psychiatry.* 30:588–596.

Shaffer D, Gould MS, Fisher P, et al. 1996. Psychiatric diagnosis in child and adolescent suicide. *Arch Gen Psychiatry.* 53:339–348.

Shafii M, Steltz-Lenarsky J, Derrick AM, et al. 1988. Comorbidity of mental disorders in the post-mortem diagnosis of completed suicide in children and adolescents. Special Issue: childhood affective disorders. *J Affect Disord.* 15:227–233.

Simon TR, Swann AC, Powell KE, et al. 2001. Characteristics of impulsive suicide attempts and attempters. *Suicide Life Threat Behav.* 39(Suppl):49–59.

Suicide Prevention Resource Center. 2008. *Suicide Risk and Prevention for Lesbian, Gay, Bisexual, and Transgender Youth.* Newton, MA: Education Development Center, Inc. Available at: http://www.sprc.org/library/SPRC_LGBT_Youth.pdf. Accessed July 7, 2011.

Swahn MH, Lubell KM, Simon TR. 2004. Suicide attempts and physical fighting among high school students—United States, 2001. *JAMA.* 292:428–430.

Tondo L, Baldessarini RJ, Hennen J, et al. 1998. Lithium treatment and risk of suicidal behavior in bipolar disorder patients. *J Clin Psychiatry.*59:405–414.

Tondo L, Jamison KR, Baldessarini RJ. 1997. Effect of lithium maintenance on suicidal behavior in major mood disorders. In: Stoff DM, Mann JJ, editors. *The Neurobiology of Suicide: From the Bench to the Clinic (Annals of the New York Academy of Sciences).* New York: New York Academy of Sciences. 339–351.

United Nations/World Health Organization. 1996. *Prevention of Suicide: Guidelines for the Formulation and Implementation of National Strategies (ST/ESA/245).* Geneva: World Health Organization.

U.S. Preventive Services Task Force. 2004. *Screening for Suicide Risk.* Rockville, MD: USPSTF Program Office. Available at: http://www.uspreventiveservicestaskforce.org/uspstf/uspssuic.htm. Accessed July 7, 2011.

U.S. Public Health Service. 1999. *The Surgeon General's Call to Action to Prevent Suicide.* Washington, DC: Office of the Surgeon General, Department of Health and Human Services.

U.S. Public Health Service. 2001. *National Strategy for Suicide Prevention: Goals and Objectives for Action.* Rockville, MD: U.S. Department of Health and Human Services.

Walker RL, Ashby J, Hoskins OD, Greene FN. 2009. Peer-support suicide prevention in a non-metropolitan U.S. community. *Adolescence.* 44:335–346.

Weishaar ME, Beck AT. 1992. Hopelessness and suicide. *Int Rev Psychiatry.* 4:177–184.

Windle RC, Windle M. 1997. An investigation of adolescents' substance use behaviors, depressed affect, and suicidal behaviors. *J Child Psychol Psychiatry.* 38:921–929.

Wolk SI, Weissman MM. 1996. Suicidal behavior in depressed children grown up: preliminary results of a longitudinal study. *Psychiatr Ann.* 26:331–335.

Wyman PA, Brown CH, Inman J, et al. 2008. Randomized trial of a gatekeeper program for suicide prevention: 1-year impact on secondary school staff. *J Consult Clin Psychol.* 76:104–115.

Yang B, Clum GA. 1995. Measures of life stress and social support specific to an Asian student population. *J Psychopathol Behav Assess.* 17:51–67.

Yang B, Lester D, editors. 1995. Suicidal behavior and employment. In: Canetto SS, Lester D, editors. *Women and Suicidal Behavior. Focus on Women.* New York, NY: Springer Publishing Co, Inc. 97–108.

Chapter 14

A Global Perspective on Injuries Among Children and Adolescents

Andrés Villaveces, MD, PhD, MPH[1] and Catherine Vladutiu, MPH[2]

Two Stories

The 13 Surgeries of Anand

On November 14, 2009, at 8:30 A.M., Anand, a child only five-years-old, was standing by the gasoline stove of his house. A neighbor friend of his mother was taking care of him because she was buying food. Suddenly, in a few seconds, the stove exploded and the flames caught Anand's clothing. Her mother's friend tried to take the clothes off as they were burning, but the flames were too strong and burnt Anand's entire body. When his mother arrived, she found Anand, who has a mild cognitive impairment, in very bad condition.

Anand was taken to the hospital in Mumbai, where he received medical care, but his injuries were so severe that currently he cannot turn his head without having to turn his entire body. He cannot speak because his mouth was severely burned, as were his legs and chest. His family sought help from a person they know in the local police force. He helped them contact specialists who will be able to perform corrective plastic surgeries. On evaluation, the specialists have offered to conduct five surgeries for free. But after that, the remaining eight surgeries needed will have to be paid by the family. They are a poor family, and the father is the sole breadwinner. The family is desperately seeking help from the community.

Marcela and Leila: An Example of Child Labor in Bogotá

Internal displacement and lack of education are the main causes of exploitation of children for work. It is 6:45 P.M., and while the majority of people who work in the neighborhood are returning to their homes, 16-year-old Marcela's workday is only beginning. Marcela, who is a single mother, 5 feet 8 inches tall, with black hair and a svelte body, is one of many young adolescents who work from Monday to Sunday in one of the many illegal bars of the barrio Teusaquillo in this city, providing sexual services. She has an average of three clients per day and charges between $20 and $50, depending on the requested service. There are approximately 14 more young women who work with her, but she is the youngest. She says she started when she was 14 years old. She works 6 days per week because she needs to bring food for her young girl, aged 2 years. She states that her work is sometimes dangerous because men can become violent, especially when drinking alcohol. A few blocks from her, toward the north, Leila, aged 16 years, sells garbage bags in the street. She comes from the southwest of the country, where she had to escape because of violence. She works in the street with her two children

[1]Department of Epidemiology, Gillings School of Global Public Health, and UNC Injury Prevention Research Center, University of North Carolina at Chapel Hill.
[2]Department of Epidemiology, Gillings School of Global Public Health, University of North Carolina at Chapel Hill.

(1-year-old twins). She cannot leave them home alone because it is too dangerous. She works every day from 8:00 A.M. to 4:00 P.M. Bogotá receives approximately 40 to 50 internally displaced families every week, many of whom have to work in the streets. Local authorities have linked this type of child labor with lower education levels and are trying to address the problem. Approximately 32% of the 7 million inhabitants of the city are children and adolescents. Many are poor, and most of their problems are related to unintended pregnancies, malnourishment, injuries, and street labor. The city government wants to eliminate child labor exploitation practices by 2012.

Global Contexts of Childhood Injury

In virtually every country, injuries primarily affect the younger populations. Children and adolescents are a special group. The risks of injury increase as children become adolescents and then young adults. Interventions aimed at preventing injuries in adults do not necessarily work among children for a variety of reasons, including differences in child development that affect cognitive and emotional capacity, differences in biological maturity, and differences in activities and overall interests.

Morbidity and Mortality

Unintentional injuries and violence account for approximately 950,000 fatalities among children and adolescents worldwide, and approximately 88% of injury fatalities among children are unintentional. The most common unintentional fatal injuries among children in order of magnitude are road traffic injuries (22.3%), drowning (16.8%), fire-related injuries (9.1%), falls (4.2%), and poisoning (3.9%). Approximately one third of unintentional injuries are categorized as other, including animal bites, natural disasters, and several mechanisms that impair breathing (i.e., asphyxiation). In regard to intentional injuries, most deaths are due to homicide (5.8%), self-inflicted injuries (4.4%), and war (2.3%) (Peden et al. 2008). However, there is wide geographic variability, and in some regions certain mechanisms of injury predominate over others. Approximately 95% of all fatal injuries occur in low- or middle-income countries. In high-income countries, injuries, although lower in magnitude, still account for 40% of all child fatalities (Peden et al. 2008).

Once children reach five years of age and until they become young adults, they will likely experience injuries and violence as their main cause of morbidity and mortality. Overall, the rate of injuries among children is 3.4 times higher in low- and middle-income countries compared with high-income countries. The magnitude of injuries is similar for children of both sexes until the age of five years. From there onward, injuries are consistently higher among males relative to females. In the case of adolescents, injuries have a similar sex distribution as that of young adults; male fatalities account for approximately 86% of all injury fatalities (Peden et al. 2008).

The available global information provides a general view of the trends and risk groups most affected by injuries. Most of the available information globally refers to mortality; however, there are many gaps in information in several countries. The quality of the data collected varies greatly between nations and sometimes within countries; thus, the current global picture of injuries we have is incomplete and likely underestimates the actual magnitude of the problem.

Global Challenges

The most basic source of information about mortality comes from vital statistics reports. According to the World Health Organization (WHO) of the 193 Member Countries, only 109 provide usable vital registration data that follow the *International Classification of Diseases and Injuries* (Peden et al. 2008). The larger the injury problem, the weaker the data information infrastructures tend to be. The scarce information available is usually about mortality. The data quality of nonfatal events is even worse. This makes it more challenging to identify priorities and evaluate interventions and policies aimed at preventing or controlling injuries. Poor infrastructure for data collection is further hampered by the lack of adequate policies aimed at preventing injuries, scarce overall funding, and limited human capacity to promote preventative measures, control injuries, or evaluate interventions.

Institutional isolation and lack of collaboration within societies prevent governments and communities from more efficiently responding to these public health challenges. No matter what income level a country has, there can be considerable differences between and within nations, in terms of the implementation of policies and practices aimed at preventing injuries among children. Philippakis and colleagues (2004) presented estimates that indicate that if the entire United States implemented the same policies adopted in the northeast of that country, approximately one third more of child injury deaths could be prevented as a whole.

There are multiple factors that modulate the occurrence of injuries globally, such as economic globalization processes, rapid urbanization and motorization, and social, political, and environmental instability. The interactions between these factors affect children and adolescents in different ways. These different contexts also provide new elements for research and the implementation of novel practices. The following sections address, topic by topic, the nature of the problem and some of the known solutions from the perspective of research, policy, and advocacy.

Violence-Related Injuries

Child Maltreatment

Risk and Protective Factors

Child maltreatment is a serious public health issue that affects the lives of thousands of children and youth worldwide. In 2002, approximately 31,000 children and youth aged 14 years or less died as the result of homicide; the majority of these deaths occurred among infants and children aged 0 to 4 years (World Health Organization [WHO] and International Society for Prevention of Child Abuse and Neglect 2006). In addition to deaths, child maltreatment has a considerable impact on childhood morbidity. Although estimates of child maltreatment are likely underreported, it is estimated that millions of children worldwide experience some form of nonfatal child abuse and neglect each year (WHO and International Society for Prevention of Child Abuse and Neglect 2006). Several countries have conducted studies to assess the prevalence of child maltreatment. For example, in 2005, the overall prevalence of child maltreatment among children in The Netherlands aged 0 to 18 years was 30 cases per 1000 children (Euser et al. 2010). More than half of the reported cases experienced neglect, and fewer reported physical or sexual abuse (Euser et al. 2010). A recent cross-sectional study of child maltreatment in Viet Nam found that approximately half of all children aged 12 to 18 years reported physical abuse, whereas one third reported neglect and even fewer reported sexual abuse (Nguyen, Dunne, and Le 2010). More than one third of all Vietnamese children reported that they experienced two or more types of child maltreatment (Nguyen, Dunne, and Le 2010). In addition to the short-term effects of child maltreatment, children exposed to abuse and neglect may also experience long-term health and social consequences. For example, exposure to child maltreatment during childhood has been found to be associated with mental health disorders, violence perpetration, and involvement in risky behaviors (e.g., substance use and sexual activity) (Krug et al. 2002; WHO and International Society for Prevention of Child Abuse and Neglect 2006). These behaviors may also lead to chronic diseases in adulthood.

There are several known risk factors for child maltreatment, including, but not limited to, age, sex, parental education, parental employment, and household income. In most countries, children aged less than 1 year have the highest reported child maltreatment fatality rates, with a risk of mortality that is approximately three times higher than for children aged 1 to 4 years (UNICEF Innocenti Research Centre 2003). In addition, children aged 1 to 4 years have a higher risk of fatal child maltreatment than their older peers. The increased risk of maltreatment among the youngest age groups is likely because of their increased vulnerability and dependency on their caregivers (WHO and International Society for Prevention of Child Abuse and Neglect 2006). The rates of nonfatal child maltreatment are also high among young infants, although in some countries (e.g., China and India) children in older age groups may be more vulnerable to nonfatal child abuse (Krug et al. 2002). In addition to age, there are gender differences in the risk and types of child maltreatment. For example, in Viet Nam, females reported a higher prevalence of neglect and emotional abuse and a lower prevalence of physical abuse than males (Nguyen, Dunne, and Le 2010). In India, males reported a higher prevalence of abuse compared with females (Mathur and Rathore 2009). Overall, it has been suggested that females are at higher risk of sexual abuse and males are at higher risk of physical abuse worldwide (WHO and International Society for Prevention of Child Abuse and Neglect 2006). Females may also be at higher risk of death as infants (i.e., infanticide) in some countries, such as India, where males are preferred over females during pregnancy (Diamond-Smith, Luke, and McGarvey 2008). Parental education and employment may also affect a child's risk of victimization from maltreatment. For example, a recent study in The Netherlands found that children had a higher risk of maltreatment if they had parents who were less educated and unemployed (Euser et al. 2010). Similar findings have been reported in other developing and industrialized countries (Krug et al. 2002). In regard to income, findings from the WHO suggest that children in low- or middle-income countries are at higher risk of fatal abuse than those in high-income countries (WHO and International Society for Prevention of Child Abuse and Neglect 2006).

Research and Prevention Strategies

Evidence from the development and implementation of several prevention strategies has shown that parent-centered programs may prevent the occurrence of child maltreatment. A systematic review of review articles published between 2000 and 2008 evaluated several child maltreatment interventions across 12 countries (Mikton and Butchart 2009). This review found that home visitations (e.g., home-based programs providing support education and prevention information), parent education (e.g., center-based programs focused on child-rearing skills, child development knowledge, and child management strategies), abusive head trauma prevention (e.g., hospital-based parent education programs), and multi-component programs (e.g., programs with family support, preschool education, parenting skills, and child care services) were effective at preventing child maltreatment (Mikton and Butchart 2009). For example, home visitation as part of New Zealand's Early Start Project resulted in significant improvements in parenting and child abuse and neglect among families experiencing stress and hardship (Fergusson et al. 2006). In Australia, the Triple P-Positive Parenting Program, focused on parent training and education, resulted in improved parental competence to ensure a safe environment for children (Sanders, Cann, and Markie-Dadds 2003). In the United States, a hospital-based education program that educated parents about infant shaking significantly reduced the incidence of abusive head trauma (Dias et al. 2005). In contrast with these effective strategies, the systematic review found insufficient evidence to determine whether sexual abuse prevention programs, media-based campaigns, or support groups were effective at preventing child maltreatment (Mikton and Butchart 2009).

To plan and implement effective prevention strategies for child maltreatment, epidemiologic studies and data are needed to estimate the incidence of child maltreatment and to identify patterns and important risk and protective factors. Although several countries have estimated fatal and nonfatal child maltreatment rates, these estimates are likely underreported. In-depth investigations of child deaths are often lacking. This has hindered efforts to accurately quantify the number of homicides that occur from maltreatment each year (Krug et al. 2002). In addition, the cause of death may be misclassified on child death certificates (Krug et al. 2002). These reporting limitations also affect data regarding nonfatal child maltreatment. For example, in many countries reporting nonfatal cases of child maltreatment is not mandatory. In addition, children may choose not to report abuse and neglect when it occurs. As such, there is a need for improved data collection and surveillance worldwide to ascertain the true extent of fatal and nonfatal child abuse and neglect and to adequately assess risk factors to develop evidence-based prevention programs. The WHO further recommends that countries that already collect data on maltreatment coordinate data-collection efforts among their agencies to develop a more comprehensive system (WHO and International Society for Prevention of Child Abuse and Neglect 2006).

Legislation and Advocacy

There are several legislative efforts that have been implemented internationally to prevent child maltreatment. These efforts vary by country and have focused mostly on child protection policy and legislation as part of their commitment to the United Nations Convention on the Rights of Children (CRC). The CRC was adopted by the United Nations General Assembly in 1989 to protect the rights of children by providing standards and obligations to ensure children's rights (UNICEF 2008). All countries, with the exception of Somalia and the United States, have ratified the 54 obligations outlined by the CRC. As such, these countries must uphold their commitment to protecting children (Krug et al. 2002). CRC Article 19 describes the obligations specific to child abuse and neglect by requiring all participating countries to take all legislative, administrative, social, and educational measures to protect the child from all forms of physical or mental violence, injury or abuse, and neglect (WHO and International Society for Prevention of Child Abuse and Neglect 2006). In response to these obligations, participating countries must integrate specific measures to develop child protection services. These measures span across several areas of child protection, including laws and regulations, education, training, data management, and the progress of children's health and well-being (Svevo-Cianci, Hart, and Rubinson 2010).

Youth Suicide

Risk and Protective Factors

Worldwide, suicide deaths are more common than interpersonal violence deaths (Krug et al. 2002). Overall data pertaining to suicide tend to be considered an undercount of the real problem because of lack of reporting, misclassification of events, and different definitions (Krug et al. 2002). In the last decade, suicide attempts and suicides among young populations are increasing (Dodig-Curkovic et al. 2010). Suicides tend to increase with age, although in certain countries, such as Canada, it peaks among younger populations (Krug et al. 2002). Suicide accounts for approximately 9% of all mortality among adolescent populations (Wasserman, Cheng, and Jiang 2005) and is the third leading cause of death among this group (Belfer 2008). Globally, suicide is more common among males than females. However, in some low- and middle-income countries, suicide or suicidal ideation is more common among young females, especially in rural areas (Aytur et al. 2008; Hesketh, Ding, and Jenkins 2002; Muula et al. 2007). Younger people also attempt suicide more frequently than older people (Wasserman, Cheng, and Jiang 2005).

Geographically, suicide is not distributed equally. The countries that report the highest rates of suicide among youth are the Russian Federation, the Baltic countries, New Zealand, Kazakhstan, Kyrgyzstan and Belarus, Scandinavian countries, Canada, and Cuba (Wasserman,

Cheng, and Jiang 2005). Countries reporting the lowest rates of suicide among youth include Mediterranean countries of Western Europe, Kuwait, Mexico, and Bahamas (Wasserman, Cheng, and Jiang 2005). A study from Bangladesh indicated that the highest proportion of deaths among women aged 10 to 19 years was due to injuries (39.3%), with suicides accounting for 21.7% (Yusuf et al. 2007).

Suicidal attempts are more difficult to record because only a minority of the population seeks medical attention. In many cases this information is not properly recorded, and in some countries such behaviors are punishable offenses. Age and method of attempt, access to healthcare, and cultural factors also affect reporting (Krug et al. 2002). The ratio of fatal to nonfatal suicidal behavior is considerably higher among younger populations compared with older populations (Wells and Stuart 1981). The mechanisms used for suicide are multiple and depend on access to means. For example, in India the use of poisons is common among young children (Dutta et al. 1998). In the United States, the use of firearms is more common than in other countries (Grossman et al. 2005; Richardson and Hemenway 2010). In China, the use of pesticides is more common (Law and Liu 2008).

A variety of factors are associated with suicidal behaviors among youth, including psychiatric, biological, social, and environmental factors. The most common psychiatric factor for youth suicide is depression and having feelings of hopelessness or helplessness, although more severe disorders such as psychoses can also be associated with increased risks (Beck et al. 1985). These disorders can be accompanied by concomitant alcohol or substance abuse, as shown in a study of adolescents in Hong Kong (Wong et al. 2008). Biological factors include a family history of suicide (Krug et al. 2002). Social factors include abuse in the home or at school (e.g., bullying), academic failures, loss of friends including boyfriends or girlfriends, social isolation, and substance abuse (Greydanus and Calles 2007). Bullying has been linked to increased depression among adolescents, and depression is associated with higher rates of suicide among this population. A study from Chile indicated higher rates of depression among adolescents who had been bullied (Fleming and Jacobsen 2009). A systematic review of 37 studies conducted with children and adolescents showed that bullying was associated with increased risk of suicide (Kim and Leventhal 2008; Law and Liu 2008). Evidence from The Netherlands indicates that having a history of sexual or physical abuse in childhood can increase the risk of suicide in adolescence or later in life (Joiner et al. 2007). Evidence from Australia shows that other social conditions, such as isolation in rural communities and among ethnic minorities, tied with access to lethal means can increase suicide mortality (Dudley et al. 1998). In another study from Nigeria, adolescents living in urban areas, and from polygamous or disrupted families, had higher rates of suicidal behavior (Omigbodun et al. 2008). Other situations, such as having economic difficulties, being unemployed, or lacking religious beliefs or practices, such as in Russia or countries that were under the Soviet Union, have been linked to increased suicides (Krug et al. 2002). In China, a high number of rural, young females who experience acute interpersonal or financial crises frequently attempt suicides using pesticides or other poisons (Law and Liu 2008).

In many societies, being a minority has been identified as a risk factor for suicide. For example, some indigenous youth populations (Ahlm et al. 2010; Berger, Wallace, and Bill 2009; De Leo, Sveticic, and Milner 2011), populations with different sexual preferences (Bouris et al. 2010; Hatzenbuehler 2011; O'Donnell, Meyer, and Schwartz 2011; Voelker 2011), or immigrants who might find themselves isolated in certain communities (Bursztein Lipsicas and Henrik Makinen 2010; Cho and Haslam 2010; Ozdel et al. 2009; van Bergen et al. 2010; van Leeuwen et al. 2010) are at higher risk of suicide.

Research and Prevention Strategies

There are pharmacologic, behavioral, and psychosocial interventions aimed at preventing suicide. These include treatment for depression or other mental disorders. A study from Oxford, United

Kingdom, found that problem-oriented interventions and psychotherapy contributed to reducing the risks of suicide in the short term (Salkovskis, Atha, and Storer 1990). In middle- and low-income countries, mental health problems are less frequently recognized and treated. A recent study in Mexico showed that most suicidal adolescents do not receive treatment (Borges et al. 2010). High-income countries and to a lesser degree middle-income countries provide help through suicide help lines or centers. A review of the effectiveness of those centers was inconclusive as some indicated some preventive effects (Lester 1997). Another study in Germany found increased suicides in some cities providing these services (Möller et al. 1988). More recently, group youth suicides by means of pacts through the Internet have been described in Japan (Kaga, Takeshima, and Matsumoto 2009; Katsumata et al. 2008; Hagihara, Miyazaki, and Tarumi 2010; Naito 2007; Ozawa-de Silva 2008; Ozawa-De Silva 2010), and studies have linked suicidal ideation with the Internet in Korea (Kim et al. 2006). School support and school programs serve as tools not only for identifying and reducing bullying but also for dealing with isolation. As such, schools are an important setting for suicide prevention activities (Krug et al. 2002). Research also indicates that suicides also have high costs for health systems. A study from Thailand showed that the total direct medical cost, due to interpersonal and suicidal injuries, accounted for approximately 4% of Thailand's total health budget. More than 90% of the economic loss was incurred from productivity loss, largely from men (Bundhamcharoen et al. 2008).

Legislation and Advocacy

Legislative approaches to suicide prevention can have an important impact. Many measures are aimed at restricting access to means. In the early 1950s in England, the removal of carbon monoxide from domestic gas led to an immediate reduction in suicide by this means (Kreitman 1976). Similar measures in Switzerland, Japan, The Netherlands, and the United States led to a decrease in these events (Lester and Abe 1989; Lester 1998). In other countries, restrictions to access to firearms have shown reduction in suicide mortality by these means (Lester and Leenaars 1993). In the United States, restrictions of access to firearms by children and adolescents have focused on safe storage practices (Grossman et al. 2005). There is also evidence that with more available means, certain methods of committing suicide can increase. For example, with the increased availability of pesticides in Samoa, suicides by ingestion of these products increased (Diekstra and WHO 1995). In low- and middle-income countries, legislation aimed at restricting or controlling access to poisons is not sufficiently developed. Its potential is promising given that it can help reduce youth unintentional and suicidal injuries alike. More recent WHO efforts have focused on integrating mental health into primary care treatment and improving overall mental care in countries that do not provide adequate services (WHO and World Organization of Family Doctors 2008).

Unintentional Injuries

Road Traffic Injuries

Risk and Protective Factors

Of the 1.3 million deaths that occur globally as a result of traffic injuries, approximately 21% correspond to children according to data reported by the WHO (Peden et al. 2008). Most injuries occur in Asia, but the highest rates are in the Middle East and in Africa. Road traffic injuries are one of the main causes of mortality among children, and their global ranking is similar to that of the United States. Approximately 30% of deaths among populations aged 0 to 19 years are due to traffic injuries. Overall, most deaths occur in low- and middle-income countries compared with those occurring in high-income countries, except for populations aged 15 to 19 years, in whom mortality is greater in high-income countries (Peden et al. 2008). Deaths due to road traffic injuries occur mostly among males (Bener et al. 2010). Although mortality is high, morbidity is even higher. Unfortunately, reliable global data are unavailable. Global estimates of child morbidity calculated on the basis of hospital admissions indicate that more than 25% of injuries treated in emergency departments are the result of road traffic injuries (Bener 2005; Karbakhsh et al. 2008; Savitsky et al. 2007). Most children injured in road traffic injuries are pedestrians, although this proportion varies by country (Naci, Chisholm, and Baket 2009). High-income countries tend to have a greater proportion of population using motor vehicles, and consequently most injuries are associated to their use. Countries with low- or middle-income report a greater proportion of pedestrian injuries among younger populations (Bartels et al. 2010; Feitas, Ribeiro, and Jorge 2007; Hyder, Muzaffar, and Bachani 2008; Rodríguez, Fernández, and Acero-Velázquez 2003). The World Health Organization also shows that overall fatal road traffic injuries among children are more common in middle and low-income countries compared to high-income countries (Figure 14.1).

There are environmental, behavioral, and social factors that modulate the occurrence of road traffic injuries. Physical and cognitive characteristics can put children at higher risks of injury (Pitcairn and Edlmann 2000). In addition, risk-taking behaviors and peer pressure also play an important part (Bina, Graziano, and Bonino 2006; Clarke et al. 2010; Organisation for Economic Co-operation and Development 2006). Likewise, parental supervision also plays a role in increasing or decreasing risks of injury. Of the many risk-taking behaviors, speeding in vehicles is the most common. But in many countries with weak enforcement of laws, the consumption of alcohol while driving among youth greatly increases the risk of death for drivers, occupants, and the community in general (Karam, Kypri, and Salamoun 2007).

Studies have also shown that poverty is associated with injuries, and this is true for high-, middle-, and low-income countries. The conditions of motor vehicles are an additional factor related to injuries and the state and design of the physical environment (e.g., lack of traffic calming devices in residential areas) (Roberts et al. 1995). In countries with more limited resources, the consequences of injuries are further aggravated by poor or insufficient pre-hospital care (Mock et al. 1998).

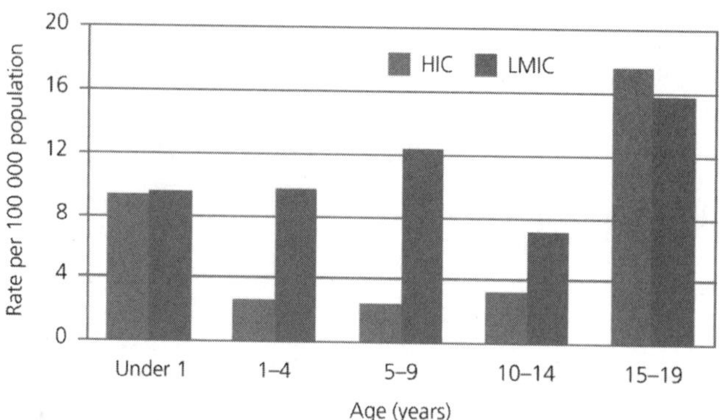

Figure 14.1. Fatal Road Traffic Injury Rates per 100,000 Children by Age and Country Income Level, Worldwide, 2004.

HIC = high-income countries; LMI = low- and middle-income countries.

Source: WHO (2008), Global Burden of Disease: 2004 update, reproduced from the WHO *World Report on Child Injury Prevention* (Peden et al. 2008).

Research and Prevention Strategies

Effective interventions to reduce mortality can be adopted in multiple settings. For example, incorporating energy-absorbing vehicle design characteristics or establishing speed limits can be implemented in any nation. Larger engineering modifications, although in some instances costly, can and have been adapted by many countries even in settings with more limited resources. For example, the city of Bogotá, Colombia, invested considerable amounts of money by separating road users in many throughways, as well as creating considerable infrastructure for pedestrians and bicyclists (Clinton Climate Initiative 2010). Other useful interventions to protect children include the creation of safe play areas, such as those promoted by UNICEF and the Child Friendly Cities (UNICEF Innocenti Research Centre 2010), which are similar in some ways to U.S. programs, such as the Safe Routes to School program (Watson and Dannenberg 2008). The promotion of the use of safety equipment available in most parts of the world includes increasing seat belt use and bicycle helmets. The adoption of these behaviors, however, varies according to the type of population (Babio and Daponte-Codina 2006; Brewin and Peters 2003; Lang 2007; Passmore and Ozanne-Smith, 2006). Finally, improving conspicuity among pedestrians and bicyclists is essential, especially in middle- and low-income countries in light of the high proportion of people who move by these means (Kobusingye, Tumwesigye, and Atuyambe 2004). Many of these strategies are also supported by legislation and can be adapted to virtually any country. However, limited resources (material and human) and lack of funding frequently hamper proper implementation of preventative strategies.

Legislation and Advocacy

There are plenty of legal strategies aimed at controlling or preventing road traffic injuries that have been implemented throughout the world. A recent review by the WHO shows that there are many legislative measures, but these vary considerably between countries and even within countries (WHO 2009). This also applies to the enforcement of such laws. Legislation for the prevention and control of road traffic injuries can be divided into two types: 1) legislation aimed at modifying or regulating behaviors (e.g., for drivers or riders, occupants, or pedestrians, or licensing regulations) and 2) legislation aimed at setting industry or environmental standards (e.g., product safety standards, such as those that apply to motor vehicles or helmets, and norms for the built environment in roadways).

Within the first group, there are helmet-wearing laws, seat belt laws, child restraint device laws, alcohol consumption laws, jaywalking laws, and licensing laws. Compliance with many of these laws that apply to young children depends on the behavior of adults. There is also evidence showing that compliance with regulations is less common among younger populations (parents and youth) (Babio and Daponte-Codina 2006). Bicycle helmet laws are key to prevent traumatic brain injury. The actual use of bike helmets depends not only on the existence of the law but also on its enforcement and existing public awareness. In addition, availability and affordability of products are needed. This is especially important in countries with fewer economic resources. Bicycle helmet use among children is important because their motor skills are still in development. Among younger populations, the use of helmets when riding motorcycles is even more important because of the increased risks of injury that these vehicles entail. In countries where the motor pool is mostly composed of two-wheelers, this strategy is essential. In many countries in Southeast Asia and increasingly in Latin America, the use of motorcycles as a family vehicle is increasing (Peden et al. 2004). This poses new challenges from a legislative and preventative viewpoint. Seat belt use and child restraint use laws are useful but can only be effective with proper enforcement. In poorer countries or among poor populations, the purchasing of child restraint devices is not possible because of the high costs. Lack of awareness about them and of knowledge on how to use these devices are added risk factors. Child restraint laws are not common in most low-income countries (WHO 2009).

In terms of licensing laws, most countries provide full driving benefits for populations aged more than 18 years. However, in certain countries it is legal under some circumstances to begin driving beginning from age 16 years. Licensing laws and graduated licensing programs are a mechanism to control who can or cannot gain driving privileges. New drivers are disproportionately linked to more crashes, and in settings where enforcement is weak, risk of injuries and mortality are greatly increased. In regard to education, the development of roadside skills is an important strategy. Examples of this include the Kerbcraft Pilot Programme of the United Kingdom (Thomson et al. 2008). Other countries, such as The Netherlands, have focused on creating traffic skills learning environments, such as the traffic gardens for children (City of Utrecht 2010). In Norway and South Africa, programs have focused on improving conspicuity of pedestrians (Peden et al. 2008). Legislation aimed at setting product standards varies between countries. Many countries, however, have no comprehensive legislation in place and as a consequence products do not comply with recommended safety standards for children (WHO 2009).

Falls

Risk and Protective Factors

Falls are a common occurrence among children and adolescents. Although they are not the leading cause of childhood mortality, they continue to be recognized as an important global public health issue. In 2004, approximately 47,000 children and youth aged 19 years or less died as the result of fall-related events (Peden et al. 2008). In addition to deaths, falls have a considerable effect on childhood morbidity, with rates of nonfatal injuries exceeding those of fatalities. Although worldwide childhood nonfatal fall rates are lacking, several countries have conducted studies to estimate country or region-specific morbidity rates. For example, falls were the leading cause of hospitalization and outpatient care among Iranian children aged less than 15 years in 2005, particularly those aged 1 to 4 years with a hospitalization incidence of 182 per 100,000 and an outpatient care incidence of 860 per 100,000 (Naghavi et al. 2010). The locations where these nonfatal falls most frequently occurred were the home, sidewalks and streets, and school. Likewise, a prospective study of pediatric injuries conducted in Lebanon found that falls were the leading cause of trauma admissions (40%) among children and youth aged less than 18 years (El-Chemaly et al. 2007). In addition to the immediate injury associated with falls, children may sustain lifelong disabilities. Falls are the leading cause of disability among children (UNICEF 2004). According to *The Injury Chart Book* (Peden, McGee, and Sharma 2002), half of the disability-adjusted life years lost globally to falls occur among children aged 14 years and younger.

There are several characteristics among children and adolescents that can increase their risk of morbidity and mortality from falls. These factors include age and developmental stage, gender, income, and degree of urbanization. In high-income countries, there is no variability in fall incidence by age during childhood and adolescence. However, in low-income countries, children aged less than 1 year have considerably higher rates of injury (Peden et al. 2008). In addition, although all children are at risk of falls, the location where falls occur varies by age. Young children (aged < 1 year) are more likely to fall from furniture and stairs, or from being dropped, whereas older children are more likely to fall from playground equipment or from being pushed or shoved by others (Flavin et al. 2006). As with most injuries, males are more likely than females to sustain a fall injury (Khambalia et al. 2006; Naghavi et al. 2010). It has been suggested that the gender differences in fall injury risk are due to varying behaviors and differential hazard exposures (Peden et al. 2008). In regard to income, the 2008 WHO *World Report on Child Injury*

Prevention reports that low- and middle-income countries, particularly Southeast Asian and Eastern Mediterranean regions, have the highest fall-related death rates among children and youth (Peden et al. 2008). Nonfatal fall rates may also vary by income, although most countries lack these data. A recent study conducted in Iran examined patterns of both fatal and nonfatal injuries, including fall-related injuries by degree of urbanization among children aged less than 15 years. This study found that mortality rates were higher among children living in rural areas for all causes of injury and that outpatient rates for nonfatal injuries were higher among children living in urban areas (Naghavi et al. 2010).

Research and Prevention Strategies

There are several domestic and global strategies that have been used for preventing both fatal and nonfatal fall-related injuries among children and youth. These strategies are age-specific and focus on parents (e.g., improving supervision and educating parents to limit access to hazards), products (e.g., limiting the use of baby walkers), and the environment (e.g., modifying equipment or other fall hazards). For example, improving parental supervision in the home environment may prevent fall-related injuries among young infants and toddlers (Flavin et al. 2006). Given that falls among children in these younger age groups occur most often from furniture or from being dropped in the home, increasing parental awareness and improving accessibility to the child should limit the occurrence of these fall events. There is little evidence that safety education increases fall prevention practices or prevents fall-related injuries in young children. However, a recent meta-analysis of childhood fall prevention activities found that home safety education and interventions that provided subsidized safety devices were effective at increasing the use of stair gates and decreasing the use of baby walkers (Kendrick et al. 2008). In addition, educating parents about safety devices and encouraging them to use these devices to limit access to hazards in the home may prevent young children from falling. For example, the installation of safety gates on stairwells or the addition of safety guards to windows may prevent falls (European Association for Injury Prevention and Safety Promotion 2006; Sengoelge, Hasselberg, and Laflamme 2011).

In addition to fall prevention strategies targeted at young children, there are other strategies that may be more effective for older children and youth. Older children are more likely to fall in playgrounds or during sports. As such, these activities have been targeted for prevention efforts. For example, the modification of playground equipment, such as the improvement of impact-absorbing surfaces, the removal of sharp edges, and the installation of guardrails or other barriers in high areas, may minimize the severity or occurrence of injuries from falls. In New Zealand, the reduction of equipment height to 6 meters or less and the addition of impact-absorbing surfaces resulted in a decreased fall-related injury risk among children (Chalmers et al. 1996). A systematic review of articles published between 1974 and 2001 that focused on playground injuries had similar findings regarding the lower risk of falls after equipment modifications (Norton, Nixon, and Sibert 2004). This review also indicated that injury risks from specific equipment, such as swings, have declined because of the introduction of impact-absorbent seats and fences, whereas injury risks from monkey bars and other climbing equipment have not declined. Aside from environmental factors, this review also suggested that child behavior and the frequency of playground use can influence the risk of fall-related injuries and should be considered when developing fall prevention strategies for playgrounds. In regard to falls during sports and recreational activities, protective equipment can be used to prevent injuries. For example, in South Wales, it has been suggested that wrist guards can reduce the high rate of fractures of the radius resulting from roller skating (Lyons et al. 1999). In the United States, the American Academy of Pediatrics further recommends that children wear helmets and other protective pads when skating (American Academy of Pediatrics Committee on Injury and Poison

Prevention and Committee on Sports Medicine and Fitness 1998). These types of protective equipment can also be worn during other recreational activities to prevent fall-related injuries, such as bicycling, horseback riding, and playing football or other contact sports.

Legislation and Advocacy

Although there are few mandatory regulations for childhood fall prevention, several countries have implemented safety standards for safety products and other equipment to reduce the incidence of fall-related injuries to children. For example, in the United States, the Consumer Product Safety Commission has worked with companies to develop a set of stricter mandatory safety standards on performance and testing with specific warning notices, applicable to all such products sold in the United States (Consumer Product Safety Commission 2010). Safety standards on baby walkers have also been adopted in other countries. For example, Australia (2002) and New Zealand (2001 and 2005) implemented a mandatory standard on baby walkers that complies with the American Standard ASTM F977-03 Consumer Safety Specification for Infant Walkers (American Society for Testing and Materials International 2009). In Canada, the Consumer Product Safety Bureau initiated the voluntary adoption of a safety standard (1989) that later resulted in a ban on baby walker sales (Health Canada Consumer Product Safety 2005). Additional safety standards that have been adopted to prevent the occurrence and severity of childhood fall injuries have focused on playground equipment. In 1981, the U.S. Consumer Product Safety Commission issued the first *Handbook for Public Playground Safety.* Further revisions of this handbook led to the publication of the ASTM F2373 *Standard Consumer Safety Performance Specification for Public Use Play Equipment for Children 6 Months Through 23 Months* in 2005, later revised in 2008 (U.S. Consumer Product Safety Commission 2008). In 1986, New Zealand introduced safety standards (NZS 5828) to regulate the height and surfacing of playground equipment (Standards Association of New Zealand 1986). In addition, the Canadian Standards Association developed voluntary guidelines (CAN/CSA-Z614 *Children's Playspaces and Equipment*) (1990) regarding the design, installation, surface, and inspection of playground equipment in Canada (Canadian Standards Association 1990). In 2004, the European Standards for Playground Equipment (EN1176 and EN1177) were revised and published (The Royal Society for the Prevention of Accidents 2004). Similar to the Canadian guidelines, these standards required modifications to the equipment's height, separation, and surfaces.

Poisoning

Risk and Protective Factors

Approximately 13% of fatal unintentional poisonings in the world occur among children and young populations. Acute poisonings worldwide account for approximately 45,000 deaths annually. The rate of poisonings in middle- and low-income countries is up to four times greater than in high-income countries (Peden et al. 2008). The highest rates of poisonings are reported in Africa, East Asia, and middle- or low-income countries of Europe. In the Americas, poisonings tend to be higher in high-income countries and lower in middle- and low-income countries (Peden et al. 2008). Global fatal poisonings primarily affect children aged less than 1 year. This is somewhat different from the United States, where poisonings are more common among adolescents (Centers for Disease Control and Prevention 2010). In general, males have greater mortality than females, although their rates are similar in adolescence. Nevertheless, there are marked geographic variations, with African countries reporting considerably higher rates and countries in the Middle East reporting lower rates (Peden et al. 2008). Morbidity data are scarce globally, although a few middle-income countries provide information available from poison control centers or hospitals (Presgrave, Camacho, and Villas Boas 2008; Werneck and Hasselmann 2009). Data comparisons are difficult because of the different classification systems used in countries (Peden et al. 2008). Similar data problems exist when hospital admissions data are used. Available data reported from middle- and low-income countries suggest that nonfatal poisonings are more common among children aged 1 to 4 years (Hyder et al. 2009). There are multiple factors associated with poisoning, including the type of substance used, the dose and route of exposure, the age of the person, the presence of other poisons, and other conditions such as nutrition or comorbidities (Figure 14.2).

Data indicate that the most common types of poisons are pharmaceuticals, household cleaning products, recreational drugs, pesticides, and a variety of plant products or animal substances acquired through bites (Chien et al. 2003; Dutta et al. 1998; Fernando and Fernando 1997; Flanagan, Rooney, and Griffiths 2005; Hanssens, Deleu, and Taqi 2001; Rajka et al. 2007). A multi-country study involving Bangladesh, Colombia, Egypt, and Pakistan showed that approximately one third of poisonings occurred because of exposure to medications (Hyder et al. 2009). Higher percentages of poisoning from medications and household chemicals have been reported in countries such as Turkey (Andiran and Sarikayalar 2004). In high-income countries, the incidence of poisonings is lower than in other countries, as is the proportion of poisonings resulting from exposure to medications (Flanagan, Rooney, and Griffiths 2005).

In many countries, the exposure to organic solvents or fuels (e.g., paraffin oil for cooking) has been reported as an important cause of poisoning mortality (Gupta et al. 1998; Hyder et al. 2009). Many of these exposures in low- and middle-income countries are related to poor regulation of product manufacturing and packaging processes (O'Brien et al. 1998). Among adolescents or poor street children, glue sniffing is used to combat hunger or for recreational purposes. Exposure to these chemicals and solvents constitutes a frequent source of intentional and unintentional poisoning in low- and middle-income countries (Anderson and Loomis 2003;

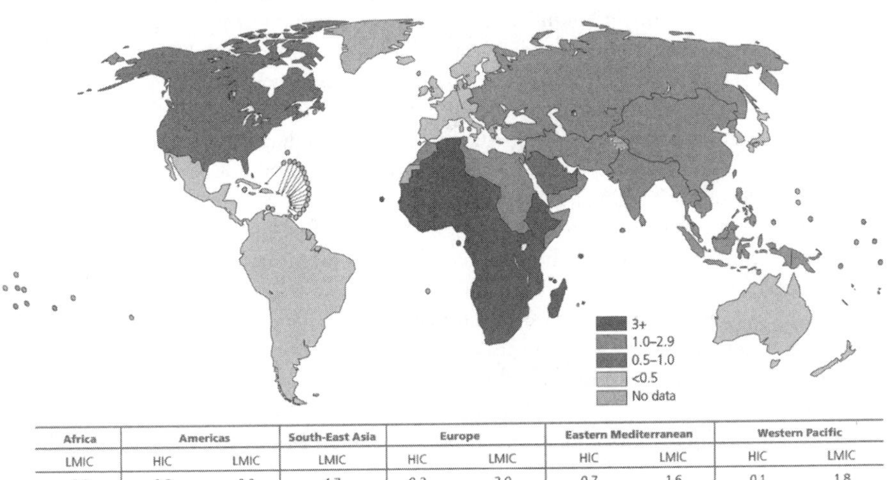

Africa	Americas		South-East Asia	Europe		Eastern Mediterranean		Western Pacific	
LMIC	HIC	LMIC	LMIC	HIC	LMIC	HIC	LMIC	HIC	LMIC
4.0	0.8	0.3	1.7	0.2	2.0	0.7	1.6	0.1	1.8

Figure 14.2. Fatal Rates Due to Poisoning per 100,000 Children[a] by WHO Region and Country Income Level, Worldwide, 2004.

HIC = high-income countries; LMI = low- and middle-income countries.

[a]These data refer to those aged less than 20 years.

Source: WHO (2008), Global Burden of Disease: 2004 update, reproduced from the WHO *World Report on Child Injury Prevention* (Peden et al. 2008).

Meadows and Verghese 1996; Pfeffer and Wilson 2004; Turkbay et al. 2004; Zabedah et al. 2001).

In largely rural areas in several countries, exposure and access to pesticides are common as they relate to occupations. Poor supervision controls, storage practices (e.g., storing poisons in milk or juice bottles), labeling practices, and misuse also contribute to increased exposures and fatalities (Joyce 1997). In some cases, easy access contributes to intentional exposures (Peden et al. 2008). At home, apart from pharmaceuticals, cleaning agents can also be a cause of poisoning. Similar lack of supervision or lack of child-safe product design contributes to increased morbidity and mortality in children (Azizi, Zulkifli, and Kasim 1993; Jolly, Moller, and Volkmer 1993). Another source of poisoning in the home is carbon monoxide exposure. In poor, crowded settings, with poor ventilation, carbon monoxide coming from kitchens can poison children (Turrell and Mathers 2001). Other inorganic substances from the ground or leaking into water wells can poison the population, as is the case with arsenic in water wells in Bangladesh (Ahamed et al. 2006) or fluoride exposures in India (Nayak et al. 2009). In tropical and subtropical areas especially, poisonings due to animal bites or stings are also causes of child poisoning (Peden et al. 2008; Sharma et al. 2005) and follow a seasonal distribution. There are certain social conditions prevalent in poor settings that increase the risks for poisonings. The presence of young parents with high residential mobility and where there is poor supervision increase the likelihood of exposure to poisons according to data from Malaysia or Australia (Azizi, Zulkifli, and Kasim 1993; Jolly, Moller, and Volkmer 1993). In low- and middle-income countries, access to poison control centers might be unavailable or scarce, increasing the likelihood of mortality.

Research and Prevention Strategies

There are proven engineering modifications that reduce the likelihood of poisoning among children. Using less toxic substances is one way to reduce poisonings. Safe packaging and storage practices are also important. In South Africa, a successful program to store paraffin oil used for cooking in child-safe containers reduced mortality by 50% in a period of 14 months (Odendaal et al. 2009; Schwebel et al. 2009; Swart et al. 2008). Early implementation of similar safe storage practices led to great reductions in poisonings in the United States and United Kingdom (Flanagan, Rooney, and Griffiths 2005; U.S. Consumer Product Safety Commission 1970). Unfortunately, many countries do not have similar programs in place. In Australia, other measures have included changing the color of substances to make them less attractive to children (Pearn et al. 1984). In addition to these changes, the use of labels and warnings can partially contribute to reduce poisonings, although these measures alone are less effective with younger children (Peden et al. 2008). Educational interventions have also been developed and include raising awareness, increasing knowledge about poisons, and changing behaviors. An example of an intervention for controlling pesticide poisoning yielded promising results in India (Sam et al. 2008). These interventions are usually effective when combined with other measures, such as environmental or engineering modifications and legislation. However, these combined approaches are usually more common in high-income countries (Peden et al. 2008).

Legislation and Advocacy

Packaging standards for medications have been mandated in many high-income countries, including the United States, Canada, Australia, New Zealand, and the European Union. In 1970 the United States passed the Poisons Prevention Packaging Act (U.S. Consumer Product Safety Commission 1970), which led to a decrease in child mortality due to ingestion of aspirin (Scherz 1971). Other similar policies include the Australian Standard AS1928-2001 entitled "Child-Resistant Packages," the British Standards Institution Standard BS EN 2 8317:1993 entitled

"Child-Resistant Packaging—Requirements and Testing Procedures for Reclosable Packages," and the Canadian Standards Association Standard CSA Z76.1-99 entitled "Reclosable Child-Resistant Packages" (National Drugs and Poisons Schedule Committee 2007). Similar laws, such as the General Product Safety Directives 92/59/EC and 2001/95/EC, have been passed in the European Union (European Union 2009). The use of nonreclosable packages has some advantages, such as better recall from parents about the available number of tablets. However, despite the difficulty for children to open them, they can access these packages (Peden et al. 2008). On a larger scale, the absence of adequate legislative frameworks has contributed to events such as the release of toxic gases from industry in Bhopal, India, which led to thousands of deaths among the population (Peden et al. 2008).

Burns

Risk and Protective Factors

The global annual mortality due to burns according to WHO estimates is approximately 310,000. Approximately one third of burn-related injuries occur among populations aged less than 20 years (Peden et al. 2008). The global mortality rate of burn-related injuries is approximately 3.9 per 100,000, and infants have the highest mortality. This distribution by age among youth is similar to the distribution reported in the United States (Centers for Disease Control and Prevention 2010). Most deaths occur in low- and middle-income countries (Figure 14.3). The majority of these deaths occur in Africa and Southeast Asia. In terms of mechanism of injury, the most common cause of mortality is fire-related burns. In the 70 countries reporting these data, fire-related burns account for 93% of deaths and scalding accounts for 5.4% of deaths. The remaining are due to other mechanisms (e.g., electrical and chemical) (Peden et al. 2008). The high percentage of fire-related deaths is probably due to smoke inhalation. A study in the United States suggests that child mortality is linked mostly to this specific mechanism and most severe in children aged 0 to 3 years (Barrow et al. 2004). A recent study from Iran also suggests that inhalation deaths are related to fire injuries, but among children aged more than 3 years (Maghsoudi and Samnia 2005). In the United States, evidence shows that among children, males have higher rates of mortality (Centers for Disease Control and Prevention 2010). On a global level, evidence suggests that burn-related fatalities are more common among young females, and this increased mortality is particularly evident in the Middle East and Southeast Asia (Peden et al. 2008). Morbidity data are not available on a global level.

Evidence from high-income countries suggests that most hospitalizations are for scald-related injuries (Palmieri et al. 2008; Papp et al. 2008). In middle- and low-income countries, these mechanisms vary considerably. In China, Nigeria, Mexico, Iran, and Israel, scald injuries seem to be more common (Gali, Madziga, and Naaya 2004; Haik et al. 2007; Híjar-Medina et al. 1992; Jiang et al. 2010; Maghsoudi and Samnia 2005) among children, whereas in Kenya fire injuries are more common (Ndiritu, Ngumi, and Nyaim 2006). In most countries, burn injuries occur mostly in urban areas in the home and are frequently linked to cooking activities (Gali, Madziga, and Naaya 2004; Saadat, Naseripour, and Rahimi 2009) (Figure 14.3).

Nonfatal burns have multiple consequences that include permanent disabilities and psychological short- and long-term consequences (Landolt et al. 2009; Pardo, García, and Gómez-Cia 2010). These also create a serious economic burden for affected families in low-income settings. Apart from age, development, and sex, another important risk factor is poverty. Data from Peru and the United States suggest that poorer families have increased risks of burns because of low literacy, crowded environments, and poor supervision of children (Delgado et al. 2002; Liao and Rossignol 2000). The use of unsafe equipment (e.g., cooking equipment and fuels) increases the risk of burns among children. In many countries, the use of fireworks is also a

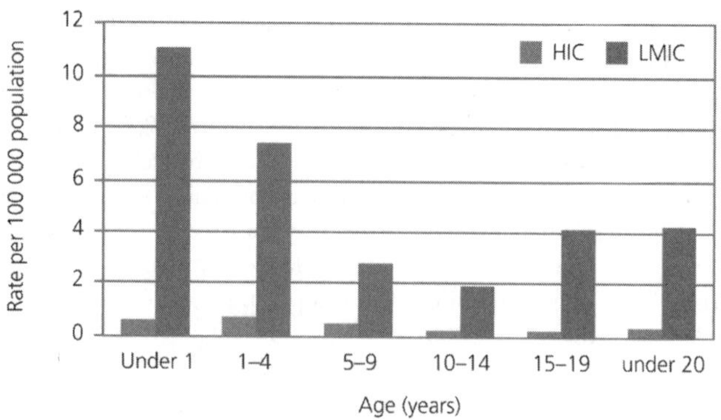

Figure 14.3. Fatal Fire-Related Burn Rates per 100,000 Children by Age and Country Income Level, Worldwide, 2004. HIC = high-income countries; LMI = low- and middle-income countries.

Source: WHO (2008), Global Burden of Disease: 2004 update, reproduced from the WHO *World Report on Child Injury Prevention* (Peden et al. 2008).

cause of pediatric burns and injuries (Al-Qattan and Al-Tamimi 2009; de Faber 2009; Rashid et al. 2011; Vassilia, Eleni, and Dimitrios 2004; Zohar et al. 2004). In some settings, the lack of smoke detectors increases risks of mortality (Jordan, Squires, and Busuttil 1999). Despite this knowledge, there is a need for further evidence of effectiveness in different countries and settings (Arai et al. 2005). In view of these risk factors, it follows that improving literacy among mothers, increasing awareness of risks of burns, reducing crowding, and installing smoke detectors are protective factors.

Research and Prevention Strategies

As with other injuries, interventions aimed at preventing burns can be grouped into environmental or engineering, educational, and legislative measures. In many countries, the use of unsafe lamps and stoves causes fires. Redesigning these is therefore a desirable strategy. Improving wood stoves in Guatemala has reduced both inhalation and burn-related injuries (Peden et al. 2008). In Sri Lanka, the use of safe paraffin lamps has also proven to be an effective strategy for preventing burns in children (Peden et al. 2008). In countries where homes are mostly built with wood, the use of smoke detectors is especially important, such as in the United States (Runyan et al. 2005). Improving construction materials is thus desirable but not always feasible, especially among families with very low incomes or in settings such as shantytowns. In urban settings and multifamily dwellings, the use of sprinklers and fire extinguishers can also contribute to reducing burn injuries (Kay and Baker 2000; Passingham 2010). Because most burn events occur in the home and are linked to cooking activities, many interventions can be done in these settings. Raising cooking facilities off the ground is important because it further separates children from hot fluids or fire. These interventions have not yet been adequately evaluated (Peden et al. 2008). Educational approaches include improving awareness of burn risks and supervision strategies. Parental education about the safe use of materials is also important. Evidence on the effectiveness of these educational strategies is scarce in most countries. In addition to these measures, the existence of adequate facilities for the care of children with burn injuries is important to reduce mortality and permanent sequelae. Such care measures include improving adequate access to care, providing prompt first aid to burns, and making acute care management more accessible for victims. In many middle- and low-income settings, such as in Pakistan, these facilities and tools are not available or are scarce. This invariably increases mortality and disability (Peden et al. 2008). There is also evidence, reported mostly in high-income countries, of the association of smoking and burn injuries in the home. Studies from the United States and New Zealand suggest smokers are at higher risk of burn injuries (Burns 1992; Smith et al. 2009).

Legislation and Advocacy

One of the most efficient ways to prevent burns is to have appropriate legislation aimed at promoting safe practices and creating safe environments. In high-income countries, legislation enforcing the use of smoke detectors has been shown to be effective (Runyan et al. 2005). The reduction of hot water temperature in water heaters is a passive intervention proven to be effective in many settings. Apart from the United States, other countries where such legislation alone or legislation in combination with education has been effective include Canada, New Zealand, and Norway (Peden et al. 2008). Unfortunately, such desirable measures have not been properly put in place in most countries of the world. Playing with lighters has also injured children, who are curious by nature. Legislation enforcing the sale of child-safe lighters was initially passed in the United States, and several European countries followed (Peden et al. 2008). Another effective intervention has been the development and sale of fire-safe cigarettes to prevent home fires associated with smoking in bed or smoking and consuming alcohol in the home (Barillo et al. 2000). The first country in the world to pass this measure was Canada in 2005. The Canadian law was modeled on the first U.S. legislation passed in New York in 2003 and effective since 2004 (Coalition for Fire-Safe Cigarettes 2010). Australia also developed a Standard for Reduced Fire Risk Cigarettes AS4830-2007, entitled "Determination of the Extinction Propensity of Cigarettes in 2007" (Coalition for Fire-Safe Cigarettes 2007). The European Union has approved this measure too, and fire-safe cigarettes will be sold in 27 European Union countries starting in 2011 (EurActiv network 2008). The United States fully implemented these laws as of July 2011 when Wyoming's law became effective. Finally, evidence from many countries has shown that banning fireworks is an effective tool to reduce burn injuries in children. In South Africa, India, Denmark, the United Kingdom, and Iran, efforts to regulate or ban fireworks have been promoted by a combination of educational and legislation strategies (Edwin, Cubison, and Pape 2008; Foged, Lauritsen, and Ipsen 2007; Puri et al. 2009; Saadat, Naseripour, and Rahimi 2009; Smittenberg et al. 2010). Combined strategies provide the greatest effectiveness.

Drowning

Risk and Protective Factors

Drowning is a leading cause of death and disability among children and adolescents worldwide. In 2004, an estimated 175,000 children aged 19 years or younger died as the result of drowning; the majority of these deaths occurred in low- and middle-income countries (Peden et al. 2008). Several region-specific studies have been conducted to assess the global burden of drowning. In the East Asia and Pacific region, drowning is the leading cause of death in late infancy and early and middle childhood. It has been estimated that in this region more children die from drowning than several infectious diseases, including pertussis, measles, diphtheria, plague, cholera, dengue fever, and typhoid (UNICEF 2004). For example, in Bangladesh, more than half of all deaths among children aged 1 to 4 years are caused by drowning (UNICEF 2004). In Vietnam, drowning accounted for more than two thirds of all child injury deaths (UNICEF 2004). A more recent cross-sectional study of injury mortality conducted across 16 countries in Europe found that unintentional drowning and submersion/near drowning was the leading cause of unintentional injury death (Sengoelge, Hasselberg, and Laflamme 2011). The majority of these deaths occurred among children aged 1 to 4 years in Romania, Lithuania, and the Czech Republic (Sengoelge, Hasselberg, and Laflamme 2011) (Figure 14.4).

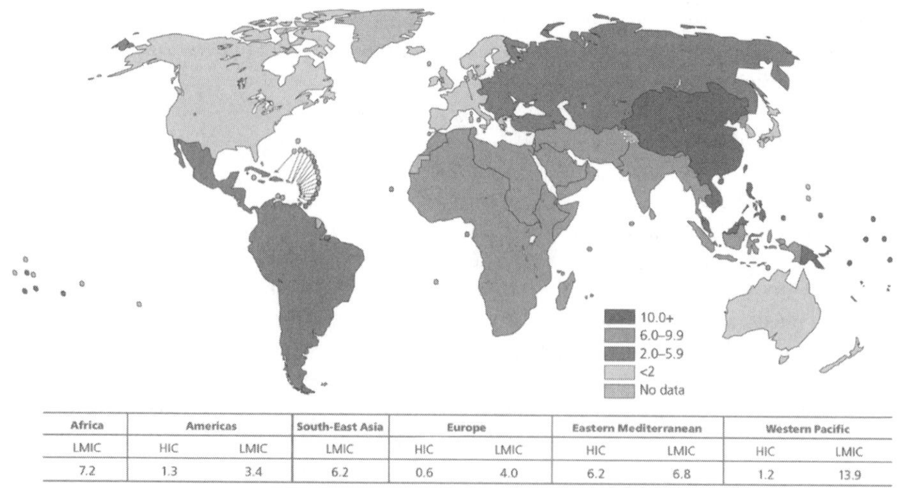

Africa	Americas		South-East Asia	Europe		Eastern Mediterranean		Western Pacific	
LMIC	HIC	LMIC	LMIC	HIC	LMIC	HIC	LMIC	HIC	LMIC
7.2	1.3	3.4	6.2	0.6	4.0	6.2	6.8	1.2	13.9

Figure 14.4. Fatal Drowning Rates per 100,000 Children[a] by WHO Region and Country Income Level, Worldwide, 2004.

HIC = high-income countries; LMI = low- and middle-income countries.

[a]These data refer to those aged less than 20 years.

Source: WHO (2008), Global Burden of Disease: 2004 update, reproduced from the WHO *World Report on Child Injury Prevention* (Peden et al. 2008).

There are several known risk factors for drowning, including, but not limited to, age, sex, parental education, household income, and region or country. In most countries, children aged 1 to 4 years have the highest drowning death rates (Peden et al. 2008). It is believed that the majority of these deaths are due to inadequate supervision (International Lifesaving Federation 2007; Peden et al. 2008). In late adolescence, drowning rates also increase, most likely because of increased substance use and involvement in other risky behaviors during this time period. In addition, males are more likely than females to die or to be hospitalized as a result of drowning across all regions, particularly during early childhood and in later adolescence (Peden et al. 2008). In contrast, findings from the WHO suggest that among infants aged less than 1 year, females have a higher death rate than males (Peden et al. 2008). Although an earlier study found that maternal education was not associated with drowning deaths in Bangladesh (Ahmed, Rahman, and van Ginneken 1999), a more recent case-control study found that children in Bangladesh whose mother had little or no education were at higher risk of drowning than those with at least a secondary education (Rahman et al. 2006). In regard to income and region, the 2008 WHO *World Report on Child Injury Prevention* states that the highest drowning death rates are in the low- and middle-income countries of the Western Pacific region, followed by the African, Eastern Mediterranean, and South-East Asia regions (Peden et al. 2008). These rates may vary by location depending on the proximity to open water. For example, in countries with several natural bodies of water (e.g., rivers, oceans, and lakes), nonresidential drowning rates may be higher than in countries with fewer open water sources.

Research and Prevention Strategies

Drowning is predictable and preventable, as are most injuries. Evidence from several prevention and intervention studies has shown that changes in safety design, environment, and behaviors may prevent the occurrence of drowning. Examples of these strategies were presented at the 2004

UNICEF/The Alliance for Safe Children (Towards a World Safe for Children) Conference on Child Injury (UNICEF 2004). Safety design changes, such as the installation of barriers around water sources and covers on wells, and improved supervision may be effective for children aged less than 4 years (UNICEF 2004). For older infants, it was suggested that the most effective preventive measures focused on behavioral changes through water safety instruction (including first-aid), swimming lessons, and lifeguard training (UNICEF 2004). Similar strategies have been recommended in some countries and adapted in others. For example, in China, it has been suggested that parents and guardians in rural areas receive first-aid training courses to improve their knowledge of how to prevent childhood drowning. In addition, the installation of safety barriers around natural bodies of water may deter children from wandering into unsafe areas (Yang et al. 2007). In Bangladesh, some of these strategies have been implemented. The Centre for Injury Prevention and Research in Bangladesh developed a water safety program for rural villagers. This program provides survival swimming technique instruction for children aged 5 years or more and home safety counseling for improving adult supervision and decreasing water hazards among children aged 4 years or less (Ahmed 2007). Mid-review evaluations of the program's effectiveness found that among the 6000 children who received the swimming survival training, none have drowned or experienced near drowning. Likewise, reductions in drowning deaths were found among households with younger children whose parents received home safety counseling. Another example of a successful drowning prevention program includes Brazil's Dolphin Project (Nunes 2007). This program was developed in Rio de Janeiro in the 1960s to provide children with beach knowledge, including wave and wind information, and knowledge and awareness regarding drowning avoidance and first aid. In addition to the program's impact on the reduction of drowning, it has provided widespread educational impact on the prevention of drowning and has provided participants with knowledge that can be applied to other activities.

To implement the most effective prevention strategies such as those mentioned above, it is important to have sufficient data to identify the risk and protective factors of drowning and to quantify the number of child deaths that occur from drowning each year. Although several risk factors for drowning among children and adolescents have been identified, these factors may vary from country to country. In addition, not all countries have been able to accurately quantify the incidence of drowning-related injuries or death. There is considerable variability in the quality and availability of these data across countries, and as a result, there are limitations in the acquisition and interpretation of epidemiologic data on drowning. As such, there is a need for improved data collection and surveillance worldwide to more adequately assess the risk factors for drowning and to develop targeted prevention programs.

Legislation and Advocacy

An alternate avenue toward the prevention of drowning deaths among children and adolescents is the development of policy and legislation. Although behavioral changes from voluntary participation in educational initiatives or active safety modifications can be effective in preventing drowning events, mandatory changes from legislation regarding individual behaviors, safety designs, and environmental factors may be more effective. A major step in this direction was the adoption of a common definition of drowning as determined after the 2002 World Congress on Drowning. Drowning is thus defined as the process of experiencing respiratory impairment from submersion/immersion in liquid (Van Beeck et al. 2005; WHO 2010). Drowning outcomes are classified as death, morbidity, or no morbidity. In addition to this, other legislation has focused on specific environments. For example, in Australia, pool fencing legislation was passed in 1992 to reduce drowning deaths by requiring swimming pools to be isolated from residential areas with three-sided fencing (if built before 1992) or four-sided fencing (if built after 1992) or enclosed by a wall with door or window access and locks (Stevenson et al. 2003). These swimming pools are required to be inspected continuously to ensure that they comply with the legislation. Similar legislation has been adapted in other developed countries, including New Zealand and the United States. Additional regulatory efforts that may be effective at preventing drowning deaths and near-drowning events include mandatory wearing of personal flotation devices and swimming instruction (Peden et al. 2008).

Children at Work

Risk and Protective Factors

Child labor is a key global issue associated with poverty, poor educational opportunities, gender inequality, parental unemployment, beliefs about the advantages of child work, lack of schools, socioeconomic inequalities, discrimination, wars and conflicts, and the absence of policies prohibiting child labor (Pinzón-Rondón et al. 2009). Child labor is also associated with a wide range of health risks, among which intentional and unintentional injuries rank high (Global Fund for Children 2002; Roggero et al. 2007; The Global Occupational Health Network 2005). Estimates from the International Labor Office (ILO) state that there are 351.7 million economically active children in the world, of whom 210.8 million are aged 5 to 14 years and 140.9 million are aged 15 to 17 years. Approximately 170 million of these children are involved in hazardous work (111 million aged 5–14 years and 59 million aged 15–17 years; The Global Occupational Health Network 2005). Most children and youth work in hazardous occupations and conditions that threaten their health and lives. Approximately 96% of child workers live in middle- or low-income countries, including Africa, Asia, and Latin America. In high-income countries, there are sectors of the population also subjected to child labor practices. Most child workers begin at young ages, work long hours, and are exposed to hazardous conditions. Their schedules usually hamper school attendance. In addition, they frequently receive low or no wages and have to contribute their salaries for their families' sustenance. Most young workers do so within the informal sector of the economy, and by far the largest activities they conduct are within the agricultural sector (Roggero et al. 2007). Children working in this sector usually start early in life and frequently do so as part of a family team (Gamlin and Hesketh 2007). In the Philippines, reports suggest that children harvesting sugarcane start as early as 7 years of age and are exposed to hazardous instruments (Gamlin and Hesketh 2007). In the United States, approximately one third of boys working on farms have driven tractors by the age of 9 years (Wilk 1993). Exposures to these environments, tasks, and working tools pose a high risk for injury and permanent disability. Many tools are designed for adults and not children, who are still developing (Gamlin and Hesketh 2007). Agricultural work accounts for approximately 70% of all work done by children in the world, whereas the rest is done in manufacturing, street trading, domestic work, and mining industries (Hesketh, Gamlin, and Jenkins 2006). A study conducted in Honduras found that children working in the agricultural sector were more exposed to injury than children working in other industries. In regard to the nature of injuries, 87% of fractures, 78% of sprains, and 67% of less severe wounds occurred among children working in the agricultural sector, making it the most hazardous sector of work (Gamlin and Hesketh 2007). Occupational injuries from all work-related hazards is decreasing in more developed countries, where workers are also working and living longer (European Environment and Health Information System 2007). Simultaneously, the number of occupational injuries is increasing in low- and middle-income countries. The proportion of occupational injuries is 17% of all work-related deaths, varying in each region. Data are lowest in high-income countries (5%) and the highest in Asian countries (34%) (Hamalainen, Takala, and Saarela 2007). In poorer countries such as Ethiopia, approximately 9% of children aged 8 years had worked for money or goods and 50% combined work and school activities. In a related study published by the United Nations

Development Programme, a survey of children indicated that three quarters of working children supplemented their household income and more than one quarter said they had missed school because of work. Among those who had worked, 5% had been seriously injured (U.N. Development Programme 2004). Although many children find benefits from working, such as economic returns, skill-learning opportunities, more independence, and higher self-esteem, child labor practices tend to be linked with less opportunities for education (Hesketh, Gamlin, and Jenkins 2006). As a consequence, child workers grow up to be low-wage-earning adults (Roggero et al. 2007).

In urban settings, the ILO has recognized that street work is one of the most hazardous and exploitative forms of child labor and common in places such as Bolivia, Chile, Ecuador, El Salvador, Nicaragua, Panama, Paraguay, and throughout Latin America (Pinzón-Rondón et al. 2009). Most children beg for money, although older ones sell items, perform, or clean cars. They work approximately 40 hours per week during the daytime, and those who worked at night did so for an average of 7 hours (Pinzón-Rondón et al. 2009). Approximately 40% of children working in cities of Latin America were injured, and most injuries were scratches (19.5%), cuts or lacerations (16.4%), burns (8.6%), traffic-related (8.9%), sprains (4.6%), and amputations (0.3%). Approximately one fifth had suffered moderate to severe injuries (Pinzón-Rondón et al. 2009). Factors related to work injuries include exposures to hazardous substances (e.g., asbestos, silica dusts, pesticides, and radon), ionizing radiation, nonionizing radiation, and noise. In addition, there are individual risk factors, such as age, sex, shift work, overwork and stress, and violence at work. Work hazards affect children more seriously than adults, resulting in both physical and psychologic consequences (Hamalainen, Takala, and Saarela 2007).

Research and Prevention Strategies

Research on the health impact of work on children has been limited and sometimes inconsistent. Work-related morbidity and mortality cannot be easily calculated because of lack of reliable information or coding mechanisms, poor reporting from informal economic activities, and cultural differences (Hamalainen, Takala, and Saarela 2007). Graitcer and Lerer were able to estimate work-related injury and mortality globally. They concluded that in all regions the occupational mortality rate among children matched the adult occupational mortality rate, indicating that children may be working in conditions that are as hazardous as, or even more hazardous than, those of adults (Graitcer and Lerer 1998). Work can also expose children to physical and social environments conducive to high-risk sexual behavior (Roggero et al. 2007). In agricultural settings, many educational strategies have been used for child safety and labor. However, two reviews show that most interventions have not been adequately evaluated, lack methodological rigor, and focus mostly on educational approaches rather than combining environmental, engineering, or legal approaches (DeRoo and Rautiainen 2000; Hartling et al. 2004). Research in urban Latin American settings indicates that predictors of occupational injuries are hours of daytime and nighttime work, child's age, minority status, and being male (Pinzón-Rondón et al. 2009).

Legislation and Advocacy

Governments and communities can combat the causes of inappropriate child labor, such as the shortage of good schools and day care, lack of social and health care services, and limited occupational choices for parents. Parental unemployment or underemployment forces children to work; thus, policies should be aimed at providing more employment for parents and better education for children (Pinzón-Rondón et al. 2009). Specific legislation addressing child labor states that children aged less than 15 years are not allowed to work and those aged less than 18 years should not work in dangerous occupations (Pinzón-Rondón et al. 2009). The enforcement of such legislation in remote and isolated areas, where agricultural practices are common, is difficult. Lack of worker training and mismanagement of hazardous substances or inappropriate use of tools cannot be controlled in these settings. This is compounded by low literacy rates among some subpopulations (Gamlin and Hesketh 2007). In urban settings, such as in the United States, employers provide basic occupational safety and health training, but many employers are frequently not aware of the type of jobs that are prohibited to young workers (The Global Occupational Health Network 2005). Many low-income countries have set goals to eliminate child labor and passed comprehensive legislation toward this goal. These laws in some cases have been complemented with effective programs such as the Bolsa Família program in Brazil that provides money to poor families to help them get children out of jobs and into educational settings (Ministry of Social Development and Combat of Hunger, Brazil 2011). This program however has been more effective in rural areas of the country (The Economist 2010).

There are important measures worldwide, such as the United Nations Convention on the Rights of the Child. This was the first international convention to recognize the right of the child to be protected from work that is likely to be "harmful to the child's health or physical, mental, spiritual, moral, or social development and not solely focus on the age of the worker" (Hesketh, Gamlin, and Jenkins 2006). More recently, the WHO Global Strategy on Occupational Health for All and the WHO Global Plan of Action on Workers' Health 2008–2017 recognize child workers and young employees as high-risk groups and recommend the elimination of hazardous forms of labor (European Environment and Health Information System 2007). In addition, the ILO Convention No. 182 (Global Fund for Children 2002) seeks to progressively eliminate all forms of child labor that might increase health risks among children while focusing on the elimination of the worst forms of child labor. This convention has been ratified by 163 countries worldwide (European Environment and Health Information System 2007).

The Need for Global Prevention Efforts

This short review of injuries among children and adolescents provides a small glimpse of the magnitude of a problem that affects millions worldwide. Young populations are more vulnerable and the most frequently and severely affected by injuries both violence-related and unintentional. Efforts toward improving research and prevention activities in the injury field should follow local interests and priorities but should also follow common principles of quality and transferability of knowledge that can benefit all. Each one of the topics addressed has its own characteristics, but all of these problems affect younger populations. Prevention efforts focused toward younger populations are key to breaking cycles of violence and to avoiding the social and economic downhill spiral that many families experience when confronted with injuries in general. Lessons learned in the United States are important because of their great potential to translate into effective public health measures worldwide. Conversely, lessons learned elsewhere are also important for Americans to learn about, to enhance prevention efforts and reduce injuries domestically. Every nation has limitations in its ability to prevent or control injuries and violence, to provide care, and to contribute to the rehabilitation of injured persons. In nations where the problem is larger, such burden is greater and has wider social implications. It is therefore crucial that training and knowledge of prevention and control of injuries be transferred. Knowledge transfer is urgently needed and will likely benefit those who carry the greatest burden.

Worldwide, there is substantial evidence concerning strategies, programs, or interventions that work and those that do not. However, the translation and implementation of such strategies will vary considerably between and even within countries. The reasons for this are multiple. There are different physical, social, cultural, economic, and legal environments. For example, in the area of road safety there are several interventions that have been tried in high-income countries but could well be implemented in middle- and low-income countries (Forjuoh and Li 1996). Interventions that are sensitive to these different environments are more likely to be effective (Mackay et al. 2006; Schopper, Lormand, and Waxweiler 2006).

Although there are interventions from high-income countries that can be implemented in settings with more limited resources, the inverse is also true. There are multiple problems related to child injuries that can more easily be studied and understood in countries with less income because the patterns of injury are different or the problems are more prevalent. With higher prevalence or different patterns of injury, new evidence can be generated and injury risks further identified. It is essential that interventions, programs, and strategies for injury prevention and control be evaluated. Equally as important is the need to understand the local contexts in which such interventions, programs, or strategies can be applied. Success will depend on the local context and the community involvement in injury prevention. Lessons can be learned in both directions between high-income and middle- and low-income countries. As such, injuries must be understood in a global context and not as isolated national problems, but implemented within a local context.

References

Ahamed S, Sengupta MK, Mukjerjee, SC, et al. 2006. An eight-year study report on arsenic contamination in groundwater and health effects in Eruani village, Bangladesh and an approach for its mitigation. *J Health Popul Nutr.* 24:129–141.

Ahlm K, Hassler S, Sjolander P, Eriksson A. 2010. Unnatural deaths in reindeer-herding Sami families in Sweden, 1961-2001. *Int J Circumpolar Health.* 69:129–137.

Ahmed MK. 2007. *The Bangladesh Experience: A Developing Country's Perspective on Child Drowning Prevention.* World Conference on Drowning Prevention. Porto, PT: International Life Saving Federation (ILS).

Ahmed MK, Rahman M, van Ginneken J. 1999. Epidemiology of child deaths due to drowning in Matlab, Bangladesh. *Int J Epidemiol.* 28:306–311.

Al-Qattan MM, Al-Tamimi AS. 2009. Localized hand burns with or without concurrent blast injuries from fireworks. *Burns.* 35:425–429.

American Academy of Pediatrics Committee on Injury and Poison Prevention and Committee on Sports Medicine and Fitness. 1998. Inline skating injuries in children and adolescents. *Pediatrics.* 101:720–722.

American Society for Testing and Materials International. 2009. *ASTM F977-09 Standard Consumer Safety Specification for Infant Walkers.* Available at: http://www.astm.org/Standards/F977.htm. Accessed July 18, 2011.

Anderson CE, Loomis GA. 2003. Recognition and prevention of inhalant abuse. *Am Fam Physician.* 68:869–874.

Andiran N, Sarikayalar F. 2004. Pattern of acute poisonings in childhood in Ankara: what has changed in twenty years? *Turk J Pediatr.* 46:147–152.

Arai L, Roen K, Roberts H, Popay J. 2005. It might work in Oklahoma but will it work in Oakhampton? Context and implementation in the effectiveness literature on domestic smoke detectors. *Inj Prev.* 11:148–151.

Aytur SA, Rodriguez DA, Evenson KR, Catellier DJ. 2008. Urban containment policies and physical activity a time-series analysis of metropolitan areas, 1990-2002. *Am J Prev Med.* 34:320–332.

Azizi BH, Zulkifli HI, Kasim MS. 1993. Risk factors for accidental poisoning in urban Malaysian children. *Ann Trop Paediatr.* 13:183–188.

Babio GO, Daponte-Codina A. 2006. Factors associated with seatbelt, helmet, and child safety seat use in a spanish high-risk injury area. *J Trauma.* 60:620–626.

Barillo DJ, Brigham PA, Kayden, DA, et al. 2000. The fire-safe cigarette: a burn prevention tool. *J Burn Care Rehabil.* 21:162–170.

Barrow RE, Spies M, Barrow LN, Herndon DN. 2004. Influence of demographics and inhalation injury on burn mortality in children. *Burns.* 30:72–77.

Bartels D, Bhalla K, Shahraz S, et al. 2010. Incidence of road injuries in Mexico: country report. *Int J Inj Contr Saf Promot.* 1–8.

Beck AT, Steer RA, Kovacs M, Garrison B. 1985. Hopelessness and eventual suicide: a 10-year prospective study of patients hospitalized with suicidal ideation. *Am J Psychiatry.* 142:559–563.

Belfer ML. 2008. Child and adolescent mental disorders: the magnitude of the problem across the globe. *J Child Psychol Psychiatry.* 49:226–236.

Bener A. 2005. The neglected epidemic: road traffic accidents in a developing country, State of Qatar. *Int J Inj Contr Saf Promot.* 12:45–47.

Bener AS, Hussain J, Gaffar A, et al. 2010. Trends in childhood trauma mortality in the fast economically developing State of Qatar. *World J Pediatr.*

Berger LR, Wallace LJ, Bill NM. 2009. Injuries and injury prevention among indigenous children and young people. *Pediatr Clin North Am.* 56:1519–1537.

Bina M, Graziano F, Bonino S. 2006. Risky driving and lifestyles in adolescence. *Accid Anal Prev.* 38:472–481.

Borges G, Benjet C, Medina-Mora ME, et al. 2010. Service use among Mexico City adolescents with suicidality. *J Affect Disord.* 120:32–39.

Bouris A, Guilamo-Ramos V, Pickard A, et al. 2010. A systematic review of parental influences on the health and well-being of lesbian, gay, and bisexual youth: time for a new public health research and practice agenda. *J Prim Prev.* 31:273–309.

Brewin M, Peters T. 2003. An investigation of child restraint/seatbelt usage in motor vehicles by Maori in Northland New Zealand. *Inj Prev.* 9:85–86.

Bundhamcharoen K, Odton P, Mugem S, et al. 2008. Costs of injuries due to interpersonal and self-directed violence in Thailand, 2005. *J Med Assoc Thai.* (Suppl 2):S110–S118.

Burns DM. 1992. Positive evidence on effectiveness of selected smoking prevention programs in the United States. *J Natl Cancer Inst Monogr.* 17–20.

Bursztein Lipsicas C, Henrik Makinen I. 2010. Immigration and suicidality in the young. *Can J Psychiatry.* 55:274–281.

Canadian Standards Association. 1990. *Children's Playspaces and Equipment Playground Safety Standards.* Ottawa: Canadian Standards Association.

Centers for Disease Control and Prevention. 2010. *WISQARS Fatal Injury Reports 2007, United States.* Available at: http://webappa.cdc.gov/sasweb/ncipc/mortrate10_sy.html. Accessed July 6, 2011.

Chalmers DJ, Marshall SW, Langley JD, et al. 1996. Height and surfacing as risk factors for injury in falls from playground equipment: a case-control study. *Inj Prev.* 2:98–104.

Chien C, Marriott JL, Ashby K, Ozanne-Smith J. 2003. Unintentional ingestion of over the counter medications in children less than 5 years old. *J Paediatr Child Health.* 39:264–269.

Cho YB, Haslam N. 2010. Suicidal ideation and distress among immigrant adolescents: the role of acculturation, life stress, and social support. *J Youth Adolesc.* 39:370–379.

City of Utrecht. 2010. *Educatieve Verkeerstuin.* Available at: http://www.utrecht.nl/smartsite.dws?id=52435. Accessed July 6, 2011.

Clarke DD, Ward P, Bartle C, Truman W. 2010. Killer crashes: fatal road traffic accidents in the UK. *Accid Anal Prev.* 42:764–770.

Clinton Climate Initiative. 2010. *Bogotá's CicloRuta Is One of the Most Comprehensive Cycling Systems in the World.* Available at: http://www.c40cities.org/bestpractices/transport/bogota_cycling.jsp. Accessed July 6, 2011.

Coalition for Fire-Safe Cigarettes. 2007. *OZ RFR Cig Standard Finally a Reality.* Available at: http://www.firesafecigarettes.org/itemDetail.

asp?categoryID=103&itemID=1502&URL=In the news/International/Australia. Accessed July 6, 2011.

Coalition for Fire-Safe Cigarettes. 2010. *States That Have Passed Fire-Safe Cigarette Laws.* Available at: http://www.firesafecigarettes.org/categoryList.asp?categoryID=77&URL=Legislative updates/Adoptions. Accessed July 6, 2011.

de Faber JT. 2009. Fireworks injuries treated by Dutch ophthalmologists New Year 2008/'09. *Ned Tijdschr Geneeskd.* 153:A507.

De Leo D, Sveticic J, Milner A. 2011. Suicide in indigenous people in Queensland, Australia: trends and methods, 1994-2007. *Aust N Z J Psychiatry.* 45:532–538.

Delgado J, Ramirez-Cardich ME, Gilman RH, et al. 2002. Risk factors for burns in children: crowding, poverty, and poor maternal education. *Inj Prev.* 8:38–41.

DeRoo LA, Rautiainen RH. 2000. A systematic review of farm safety interventions. *Am J Prev Med.* 18(4 Suppl):51–62.

Diamond-Smith N, Luke N, McGarvey S. 2008. 'Too many girls, too much dowry': son preference and daughter aversion in rural Tamil Nadu, India. *Cult Health Sex.* 10:697–708.

Dias MS, Smith K, DeGuehery K, et al. 2005. Preventing abusive head trauma among infants and young children: a hospital-based, parent education program. *Pediatrics.* 115:e470–477.

Diekstra RFW, World Health Organization. 1995. *Preventive Strategies on Suicide.* Leiden; New York: E.J. Brill.

Dodig-Curkovic K, Curkovic M, Radic J, et al. 2010. Suicidal behavior and suicide among children and adolescents-risk factors and epidemiological characteristics. *Coll Antropol.* 34:771–777.

Dudley MJ, Kelk NJ, Florio TM, et al. 1998. Suicide among young Australians, 1964–1993: an interstate comparison of metropolitan and rural trends. *Med J Aust.* 169:77–80.

Dutta AK, Seth A, Goyal PK, et al. 1998. Poisoning in children: Indian scenario. *Indian J Pediatr.* 65:365–370.

Edwin AF, Cubison TC, Pape SA. 2008. The impact of recent legislation on paediatric fireworks injuries in the Newcastle upon Tyne region. *Burns.* 34:953–964.

El-Chemaly SY, Akkary G, Atoul M, et al. 2007. Hospital admissions after paediatric trauma in a developing country: from falls to landmines. *Int J Inj Contr Saf Promot.* 14:131–134.

EurActiv network. 2008. *Europe Lights Up to Fire-Safety Rules for Cigarettes.* Available at: http://www.euractiv.com/en/health/europe-lights-fire-safety-rules-cigarettes/article-174979. Accessed July 6, 2011.

European Association for Injury Prevention and Safety Promotion 2006. *Child Safety Good Practice Guide.* Amsterdam: European Association for Injury Prevention and Safety Promotion (EUROSAFE).

European Environment and Health Information System. 2007. *Work Injuries in Children and Young People.* Copenhagen: World Health Organization.

European Union. 2009. *The General Product Safety Directive (GPSD).* Available at: http://ec.europa.eu/consumers/safety/prod_legis/index_en.htm. Accessed July 6, 2011.

Euser EM, van Ijzendoorn MH, Prinzie P, Bakermans-Kranenburg MJ. 2010. Prevalence of child maltreatment in The Netherlands. *Child Maltreat.* 15:5–17.

Feitas JP, Ribeiro LA, Jorge MT. 2007. Pediatric victims of traffic accidents admitted to a university hospital: epidemiological and clinical aspects. *Cad Saude Publica.* 23:3055–3060.

Fergusson DM, Grant H, Horwood LJ, Ridder EM. 2006. Randomized trial of the Early Start program of home visitation: parent and family outcomes. *Pediatrics.* 117:781–786.

Fernando R, Fernando DN. 1997. Childhood poisoning in Sri Lanka. *Indian J Pediatr.* 64:457–460.

Flanagan RJ, Rooney C, Griffiths C. 2005. Fatal poisoning in childhood, England & Wales 1968–2000. *Forensic Sci Int.* 148:121–129.

Flavin MP, Dostaler SM, Simpson K, et al. 2006. Stages of development and injury patterns in the early years: a population-based analysis. *BMC Public Health.* 6:187.

Fleming LC, Jacobsen KH. 2009. Bullying and symptoms of depression in Chilean middle school students. *J Sch Health.* 79:130–137.

Foged T, Lauritsen J, Ipsen T. 2007. Firework injuries in Denmark in the period 1995/1996 to 2006/2007. *Ugeskr Laeger.* 169:4271–4275.

Forjuoh SN, Li G. 1996. A review of successful transport and home injury interventions to guide developing countries. *Soc Sci Med.* 43:1551–1560.

Gali BM, Madziga AG, Naaya HU. 2004. Epidemiology of childhood burns in Maiduguri north-eastern Nigeria. *Niger J Med.* 13:144–147.

Gamlin J, Hesketh T. 2007. Child work in agriculture: acute and chronic health hazards. *Child Youth Environ.* 17:1–23.

Global Fund for Children. 2002. *Hazardous and Harmful Child Labor.* Washington, DC: Global Fund for Children.

Graticer PL, Lerer LB. 1998. *Child Labor and Health: Quantifying the Global Health Impacts of Child Labors.* Washington, DC: World Bank.

Greydanus DE, Calles J Jr. 2007. Suicide in children and adolescents. *Prim Care.* 34:259–273; abstract vi.

Grossman DC, Mueller BA, Riedy C, et al. 2005. Gun storage practices and risk of youth suicide and unintentional firearm injuries. *JAMA.* 293:707–714.

Gupta S, Govil YC, Misra PK, et al. 1998. Trends in poisoning in children: experience at a large referral teaching hospital. *Natl Med J India.* 11:166–168.

Hagihara A, Miyazaki S, Tarumi K. 2010. Internet use and suicide among younger age groups between 1989 and 2008 in Japan. *Acta Psychiatr Scand.* 121:485; author reply 485–486.

Haik J, Liran A, Tessone A, et al. 2007. Burns in Israel: demographic, etiologic and clinical trends, 1997–2003. *Isr Med Assoc J.* 9:659–662.

Hamalainen P, Takala J, Saarela KL. 2007. Global estimates of fatal work-related diseases. *Am J Ind Med.* 50:28–41.

Hanssens Y, Deleu D, Taqi A. 2001. Etiologic and demographic characteristics of poisoning: a prospective hospital-based study in Oman. *J Toxicol Clin Toxicol.* 39:371–380.

Hartling L, Brison RJ, Crumley ET, et al. 2004. A systematic review of interventions to prevent childhood farm injuries. *Pediatrics.* 114:e483–496.

Hatzenbuehler ML. 2011. The social environment and suicide attempts in lesbian, gay, and bisexual youth. *Pediatrics.* 127:896–903.

Health Canada Consumer Product Safety. 2005. *Regulatory Review and Recommendation Regarding Baby Walkers Pursuant to the Hazardous Products Act.* Available at: http://www.hc-sc.gc.ca/cps-spc/pubs/cons/walker-review-marchette/purpose-objectif-eng.php. Accessed July 6, 2011.

Hesketh T, Ding QJ, Jenkins R. 2002. Suicide ideation in Chinese adolescents. *Soc Psychiatry Psychiatr Epidemiol.* 37:230–235.

Hesketh T, Gamlin J, Woodhead M. 2006. Policy in child labour. *Arch Dis Child.* 91:721–723.

Híjar-Medina MC, Tapia-Yañez JR, Lozano-Ascencio R, López-López MV. 1992. Home accidents in children less than 10 years of age: causes and consequences. *Salud Publica Mex.* 34:615–625.

Hyder AA, Muzaffar SS, Bachani AM. 2008. Road traffic injuries in urban Africa and Asia: a policy gap in child and adolescent health. *Public Health.* 122:1104–1110.

Hyder AA, Sugerman DE, Puvanachandra P, et al. 2009. Global childhood unintentional injury surveillance in four cities in developing countries: a pilot study. *Bull World Health Organ.* 87:345–352.

International Lifesaving Federation. 2007. *World Drowning Report.* Leuven: International Lifesaving Federation.

Jiang X, Zhang Y, Wang Y, et al. 2010. An analysis of 6215 hospitalized unintentional injuries among children aged 0-14 in northwest China. *Accid Anal Prev.* 42:320–326.

Joiner TE Jr, Sachs-Ericsson NJ, Wingate LR, et al. 2007. Childhood physical and sexual abuse and lifetime number of suicide attempts: a persistent and theoretically important relationship. *Behav Res Ther.* 45:539–547.

Jolly DL, Moller JN, Volkmer RE. 1993. The socio-economic context of child injury in Australia. *J Paediatr Child Health.* 29:438–444.

Jordan LB, Squires TJ, Busuttil A. 1999. Incidence trends in house fire fatalities in eastern Scotland. *J Clin Forensic Med.* 6:233–237.

Joyce S. 1997. Growing pains in South America. *Environ Health Perspect.* 105:794–799.

Kaga M, Takeshima T, Matsumoto T. 2009. Suicide and its prevention in Japan. *Leg Med (Tokyo).* (Suppl 1):S18–S21.

Karam E, Kypri K, Salamoun M. 2007. Alcohol use among college students: an international perspective. *Curr Opin Psychiatry.* 20:213–221.

Karbakhsh M, Zargar M, Zarei MR, Khaji K. 2008. Childhood injuries in Tehran: a review of 1281 cases. *Turk J Pediatr.* 50:317–325.

Katsumata Y, Matsumoto T, Kitani M, Takeshima T. 2008. Electronic media use and suicidal ideation in Japanese adolescents. *Psychiatry Clin Neurosci.* 62:744–746.

Kay RL Jr, Baker SP. 2000. Let's emphasize fire sprinklers as an injury prevention technology. *Inj Prev.* 6:72–73.

Kendrick D, Watson MC, Mulvaney CA, et al. 2008. Preventing childhood falls at home: meta-analysis and meta-regression. *Am J Prev Med.* 35:370–379.

Khambalia A, Joshi P, Brussoni, M, et al. 2006. Risk factors for unintentional injuries due to falls in children aged 0-6 years: a systematic review. *Inj Prev.* 12:378–381.

Kim K, Ryu E, Chon MY, et al. 2006. Internet addiction in Korean adolescents and its relation to depression and suicidal ideation: a questionnaire survey. *Int J Nurs Stud.* 43:185–192.

Kim YS, Leventhal B. 2008. Bullying and suicide. A review. *Int J Adolesc Med Health.* 20:133–154.

Kobusingye O, Tumwesigye NM, Atuyambe L. 2004. *Protecting Vulnerable Road Users Through Visibility Improvement: A Pilot Study.* Colombo: Road Traffic Injuries Research Network.

Kreitman N. 1976. The coal gas story. United Kingdom suicide rates, 1960–71. *Br J Prev Soc Med.* 30:86–93.

Krug E, Dahlberg LL, Mercy JA, et al, editors. 2002. *World Report on Violence and Health.* Geneva: World Health Organization.

Landolt MA, Buehlmann C, Maag T, Schiesti C. 2009. Brief report: quality of life is impaired in pediatric burn survivors with posttraumatic stress disorder. *J Pediatr Psychol.* 34:14–21.

Lang IA. 2007. Demographic, socioeconomic, and attitudinal associations with children's cycle-helmet use in the absence of legislation. *Inj Prev.* 13:355–358.

Law S, Liu P. 2008. Suicide in China: unique demographic patterns and relationship to depressive disorder. *Curr Psychiatry Rep.* 10:80–86.

Lester D. 1997. The effectiveness of suicide prevention centers: a review. *Suicide Life Threat Behav.* 27:304–310.

Lester D. 1998. Preventing suicide by restricting access to methods for suicide. *Arch Suicide Res.* 4:7–24.

Lester D, Abe K. 1989. The effect of restricting access to lethal methods for suicide: a study of suicide by domestic gas in Japan. *Acta Psychiatr Scand.* 80:180–182.

Lester D, Leenaars A. 1993. Suicide rates in Canada before and after tightening firearm control laws. *Psychol Rep.* 72(3 Pt 1):787–790.

Liao CC, Rossignol AM. 2000. Landmarks in burn prevention. *Burns.* 26:422–434.

Lyons RA, Delahunty AM, Kraus D, et al. 1999. Children's fractures: a population based study. *Inj Prev.* 5:129–132.

Mackay M, Vincenten J, Brussoni M, Towner L. 2006. Child Safety Good Practice Guide: Good Investments in Unintentional Child Injury Prevention and Safety Promotion. Amsterdam: European Child Safety Alliance, Eurosafe.

Maghsoudi H, Samnia N. 2005. Etiology and outcome of pediatric burns in Tabriz, Iran. *Burns.* 31:721–725.

Mathur M, Rathore P. 2009. Incidence, type and intensity of abuse in street children in India. *Child Abuse Negl.* 33:907–913.

Meadows R, Verghese A. 1996. Medical complications of glue sniffing. *South Med J.* 89:455–462.

Mikton C, Butchart A. 2009. Child maltreatment prevention: a systematic review of reviews. *Bull World Health Organ.* 87:353–361.

Ministry of Social Development and Combat of Hunger, Brazil. 2011. *Bolsa Familia.* Available at: http://www.mds.gov.br/bolsafamilia. Accessed October 17 2011.

Mock CN, Jurkovich GJ, nii-Amon-Kotei D, et al. 1998. Trauma mortality patterns in three nations at different economic levels: implications for global trauma system development. *J Trauma.* 44:804–814.

Möller H-J, Schmidtke A, Welz R, et al. 1988. *Current Issues of Suicidology.* Berlin; New York, Springer-Verlag.

Muula AS, Kazembe LN, Rudatsikira E, Siziya S. 2007. Suicidal ideation and associated factors among in-school adolescents in Zambia. *Tanzan Health Res Bull.* 9:202–206.

Naci H, Chisholm D, Baket TD. 2009. Distribution of road traffic deaths by road user group: a global comparison. *Inj Prev.* 15:55–59.

Naghavi M, Pourmalek F, Shahraz, S, et al. 2010. The burden of injuries in Iranian children in 2005. *Popul Health Metr.* 8:5.

Naito A. 2007. Internet suicide in Japan: implications for child and adolescent mental health. *Clin Child Psychol Psychiatry.* 12:583–597.

National Drugs and Poisons Schedule Committee. 2007. *Packaging, Labelling and Regulation of Paints, Tinters, and Related Products.* Canberra: Department of Health and Ageing.

Nayak B, Roy MM, Das B, et al. 2009. Health effects of groundwater fluoride contamination. *Clin Toxicol (Phila).* 47:292–295.

Ndiritu S, Ngumi ZW, Nyaim O. 2006. Burns: the epidemiological pattern, risk and safety awareness at Kenyatta National Hospital, Nairobi. *East Afr Med J.* 83:455–460.

Nguyen HT, Dunne MP, Le AV. 2010. Multiple types of child maltreatment and adolescent mental health in Viet Nam. *Bull World Health Organ.* 88:22–30.

Norton C, Nixon J, Sibert JR. 2004. Playground injuries to children. *Arch Dis Child.* 89:103–108.

Nunes RDS. 2007. The Dolphin Project Since 1963, the Largest Drowning Prevention Program in Brazil - 150,000 Children Trained. World Conference on Drowning Prevention. Porto: PT, International Lifesaving Federation (ILS).

O'Brien KL, Selanikio JD, Hecdivert C, et al. 1998. Epidemic of pediatric deaths from acute renal failure caused by diethylene glycol poisoning. Acute Renal Failure Investigation Team. *JAMA.* 279:1175–1180.

Odendaal W, van Niekerk A, Jordaan D, Seedat M. 2009. The impact of a home visitation programme on household hazards associated with unintentional childhood injuries: a randomised controlled trial. *Accid Anal Prev.* 41:183–190.

O'Donnell S, Meyer IH, Schwartz S. 2011. Increased risk of suicide attempts among black and latino lesbians, gay men, and bisexuals. *Am J Public Health.* 101:1055–1059.

Omigbodun O, Dogra N, Esan O, Adedokun B. 2008. Prevalence and correlates of suicidal behaviour among adolescents in southwest Nigeria. *Int J Soc Psychiatry.* 54:34–46.

Organisation for Economic Co-operation and Development. 2006. *Young Drivers: The Road to Safety.* Paris: Organisation for Economic Co-operation and Development.

Ozawa-de Silva C. 2008. Too lonely to die alone: Internet suicide pacts and existential suffering in Japan. *Cult Med Psychiatry.* 32:516–551.

Ozawa-De Silva C. 2010. Shared death: self, sociality and internet group suicide in Japan. *Transcult Psychiatry.* 47:392–418.

Ozdel O, Varma G, Atesci FC, et al. 2009. Characteristics of suicidal behavior in a Turkish sample. *Crisis.* 30:90–93.

Palmieri TL, Alderson TS, Ison D, et al. 2008. Pediatric soup scald burn injury: etiology and prevention. *J Burn Care Res.* 29:114–118.

Papp A, Rytkonen T, Koljonen V, Vuola J. 2008. Paediatric ICU burns in Finland 1994-2004. *Burns.* 34:339–344.

Pardo GD, García IM, Gómez-Cia T. 2010. Psychological effects observed in child burn patients during the acute phase of hospitalization and comparison with pediatric patients awaiting surgery. *J Burn Care Res.* 31:569–578.

Passingham A. 2010. A common sense approach to sprinklers. *Health Estate.* 64:59–62.

Passmore J, Ozanne-Smith J. 2006. Seatbelt use amongst taxi drivers in Beijing, China. *Int J Inj Contr Saf Promot.* 13:187–189.

Pearn J, Nixon J, Ansford A, Corcoran A. 1984. Accidental poisoning in childhood: five year urban population study with 15 year analysis of fatality. *Br Med J (Clin Res Ed).* 288:44–46.

Peden M, McGee KS, Sharma G. 2002. Fall-related injuries. In: *The Injury Chart Book.* Geneva: World Health Organization. 2003. 1–76.

Peden M, Oyegbite K, Ozanne-Smith J, et al, editors. 2008. *World Report on Child Injury Prevention.* Geneva, Switzerland: World Health Organization.

Peden M, Scurfield R, Sleet D, et al, editors. 2004. *World Report on Road Traffic Injury Prevention.* Geneva: World Health Organization.

Pfeffer K, Wilson B. 2004. Children's perceptions of dangerous substances. *Percept Mot Skills.* 98:700–710.

Philippakis A, Hemenway D, Alexe DM, et al. 2004. A quantification of preventable unintentional childhood injury mortality in the United States. *Inj Prev.* 10:79–82.

Pinzón-Rondón AM, Koblinsky SA, Hofferth SL, et al. 2009. Work-related injuries among child street-laborers in Latin America: prevalence and predictors. *Rev Panam Salud Publica.* 26:235–243.

Pitcairn TK, Edlmann T. 2000. Individual differences in road crossing ability in young children and adults. *Br J Psychol.* 91(Pt 3):391–410.

Presgrave R de F, Camacho LA, Villas Boas MH. 2008. A profile of unintentional poisoning caused by household cleaning products, disinfectants and pesticides. *Cad Saude Publica.* 24:2901–2908.

Puri V, Mahendru S, Rana R, Deshpande M. 2009. Firework injuries: a ten-year study. *J Plast Reconstr Aesthet Surg.* 62:1103–1111.

Rahman A, Giashuddin SM, Svanström L, Rahman F. 2006. Drowning—a major but neglected child health problem in rural Bangladesh: implications for low income countries. *Int J Inj Contr Saf Promot.* 13:101–105.

Rajka T, Heyerdahl F, Hovda KE, et al. 2007. Acute child poisonings in Oslo: a 2-year prospective study. *Acta Paediatr.* 96:1355–1359.

Rashid RA, Heidary F, Hussein A, et al. 2011. Ocular burns and related injuries due to fireworks during the Aidil Fitri celebration on the East Coast of the Peninsular Malaysia. *Burns.* 37:170–173.

Richardson EG, Hemenway D. 2010. Homicide, suicide, and unintentional firearm fatality: comparing the United States with other high-income countries, 2003. *J Trauma.* 70:238–243.

Roberts I, Norton R, Jackson R, et al. 1995. Effect of environmental factors on risk of injury of child pedestrians by motor vehicles: a case-control study. *BMJ.* 310:91–94.

Rodríguez DY, Fernández FJ, Acero-Velázquez H. 2003. Road traffic injuries in Colombia. *Inj Control Saf Promot.* 10:29–35.

Roggero P, Mangiaterra V, Bustreo F, Rosati F. 2007. The health impact of child labor in developing countries: evidence from cross-country data. *Am J Public Health.* 97:271–275.

Runyan CW, Johnson RM, Yang J, et al. 2005. Risk and protective factors for fires, burns, and carbon monoxide poisoning in U.S. households. *Am J Prev Med.* 28:102–108.

Saadat S, Naseripour M, Rahimi B. 2009. Safety preparedness of urban community for New Year fireworks in Tehran. *Burns.* 35:719–722.

Salkovskis PM, Atha C, Storer D. 1990. Cognitive-behavioural problem solving in the treatment of patients who repeatedly attempt suicide. A controlled trial. *Br J Psychiatry.* 157:871–876.

Sam KG, Andrade HH, Pradhan L, et al. 2008. Effectiveness of an educational program to promote pesticide safety among pesticide handlers of South India. *Int Arch Occup Environ Health.* 81:787–795.

Sanders MR, Cann W, Markie-Dadds C. 2003. The Triple-P Positive Parenting Programme: a universal population-level approach to the prevention of child abuse. *Child Abuse Review.* 12:155–171.

Savitsky B, Aharonson-Daniel L, Giveon A, et al. 2007. Variability in pediatric injury patterns by age and ethnic groups in Israel. *Ethn Health.* 12:129–139.

Scherz RG. 1971. Prevention of childhood aspirin poisoning. Clinical trials with three child-resistant containers. *N Engl J Med.* 285:1361–1362.

Schopper D, Lormand JD, Waxweiler R. 2006. Developing National Policies to Prevent Violence and Injuries: A Guideline for Policy-Makers and Planners. Geneva: World Health Organization. Available at: http://www.who.int/violence_injury_prevention/publications/39919_oms_br_2.pdf. Accessed August 14, 2010.

Schwebel DC, Swart D, Simpson J, et al. 2009. An intervention to reduce kerosene-related burns and poisonings in low-income South African communities. *Health Psychol.* 28:493–500.

Sengoelge M, Hasselberg M, Laflamme L. 2011. Child home injury mortality in Europe: a 16-country analysis. *Eur J Public Health.* 21:166–170.

Sharma N, Chauhan S, Faruqi S, et al. 2005. Snake envenomation in a north Indian hospital. *Emerg Med J.* 22:118–120.

Smith J, Bullen C, Laugesen M, Glover M. 2009. Cigarette fires and burns in a population of New Zealand smokers. *Tob Control.* 18:29–33.

Smittenberg MN, Lungelow D, Rode H, et al. 2010. Can fireworks-related injuries to children during festivities be prevented? *S Afr Med J.* 100:525–528.

Standards Association of New Zealand. 1986. *Standard Specification for Playgrounds and Playground Equipment (NZS 5828).* Wellington: Standards Association of New Zealand.

Stevenson MR, Rimajova M, Edgecombe D, Vickery K. 2003. Childhood drowning: barriers surrounding private swimming pools. *Pediatrics.* 111:E115–E119.

Svevo-Cianci KA, Hart SN, Rubinson C. 2010. Protecting children from violence and maltreatment: a qualitative comparative analysis assessing the implementation of U.N. CRC Article 19. *Child Abuse Negl.* 34:45–56.

Swart L, van Niekerk A, Seedat M, Jordaan E. 2008. Paraprofessional home visitation program to prevent childhood unintentional injuries in low-income communities: a cluster randomized controlled trial. *Inj Prev.* 14:164–169.

The Economist. How To Get Children Out of Jobs and Into School. *The Economist* (London), July 29, 2010. Available at: http://www.economist.com/node/16690887. Accessed October 17 2011.

The Global Occupational Health Network. 2005. Child labour and adolescent workers. 1–5. Issue 9, Summer 2005.

The Royal Society for the Prevention of Accidents. 2004. *EN1176 Playground Equipment Standard.* Birmingham: The Royal Society for the Prevention of Accidents.

Thomson J, Whelan K, Stephenson C, et al. 2008. *Kerbcraft Training Manual.* London: Department of Transport.

Turkbay T, Sarici SU, Kismet E, et al. 2004. Blood lead levels in glue sniffers. *Biol Trace Elem Res.* 98:45–49.

Turrell G, Mathers C. 2001. Socioeconomic inequalities in all-cause and specific–cause mortality in Australia: 1985-1987 and 1995-1997. *Int J Epidemiol.* 30:231–239.

U.N. Development Programme. 2004. Children and poverty. *In Focus.* Page 6, March 2004.

U.S. Consumer Product Safety Commission. 1970. Poison Prevention Packaging Act. U. S. Congress.

U.S. Consumer Product Safety Commission. 2008. *Public Playground Safety Handbook.* Washington, DC: United States Consumer Product Safety Commission.

U.S. Consumer Product Safety Commission. 2010. Revocation of regulations banning certain baby walkers. *Fed Regist.* 75:35279–35280.

UNICEF. 2004. *Towards a World Safe for Children.* UNICEF/The Alliance for Safe Children Conference on Child Injury. Bangkok: UNICEF.

UNICEF. 2008. *Convention on the Rights of the Child.* Available at: http://www.unicef.org/crc/. Accessed July 6, 2011.

UNICEF Innocenti Research Centre. 2003. *A League Table of Child Maltreatment Deaths in Rich Nations.* Innocenti Report Card. Torino: Innocenti Research Centre. 5.

UNICEF Innocenti Research Centre. 2010. *What Is a Child Friendly City?* Available at: http://www.childfriendlycities.org/en/overview/what-is-a-child-friendly-city. Accessed July 6, 2011.

Van Beeck EF, Branche CM, Szpilman D, et al. 2005. A new definition of drowning: towards documentation and prevention of a global public health problem. *Bull World Health Organ.* 83:853–856.

van Bergen DD, Eikelenboom M, Smit JH, et al. 2010. Suicidal behavior and ethnicity of young females in Rotterdam, The Netherlands: rates and risk factors. *Ethn Health.* 15:515–530.

van Leeuwen N, Rodgers R, Regner I, Chabrol H. 2010. The role of acculturation in suicidal ideation among second-generation immigrant adolescents in France. *Transcult Psychiatry.* 47:812–832.

Vassilia K, Eleni P, Dimitrios T. 2004. Firework-related childhood injuries in Greece: a national problem. *Burns.* 30:151–153.

Voelker R. 2011. Community a factor in suicide attempts by lesbian, gay, and bisexual teens. *JAMA.* 305:1951.

Wasserman D, Cheng Q, Jiang GX. 2005. Global suicide rates among young people aged 15-19. *World Psychiatry.* 4:114–120.

Watson M, Dannenberg AL. 2008. Investment in safe routes to school projects: public health benefits for the larger community. *Prev Chronic Dis.* 5:A90.

Wells CF, Stuart IR. 1981. *Self-destructive Behavior in Children and Adolescents.* New York: Van Nostrand Reinhold.

Werneck GL, Hasselmann MH. 2009. Profile of hospital admissions due to acute poisoning among children under 6 years of age in the metropolitan region of Rio de Janeiro, Brazil. *Rev Assoc Med Bras.* 55:302–307.

Wilk VA. 1993. Health hazards to children in agriculture. *Am J Ind Med.* 24:283–290.

Wong JP, Stewart SM, Claassen C, et al. 2008. Repeat suicide attempts in Hong Kong community adolescents. *Soc Sci Med.* 66:232–241.

World Health Organization. 2009. *Global Status Report on Road Safety.* Geneva: World Health Organization.

World Health Organization. 2010. *Drowning.* Available at: http://www.who.int/violence_injury_prevention/other_injury/drowning/en/index.html. Accessed July, 2010,

World Health Organization and International Society for Prevention of Child Abuse and Neglect. 2006. *Preventing Child Maltreatment: A Guide to Taking Action and Generating Evidence.* Geneva: World Health Organization.

World Health Organization and World Organization of Family Doctors. 2008. *Integrating Mental Health into Primary Care: A Global Perspective.* Geneva: World Health Organization.

Yang L, Nong QQ, Li CL, et al. 2007. Risk factors for childhood drowning in rural regions of a developing country: a case-control study. *Inj Prev.* 13:178–182.

Yusuf HR, Akhter HH, Chowdhury ME, Rochat RW. 2007. Causes of death among women aged 10-50 years in Bangladesh, 1996-1997. *J Health Popul Nutr.* 25:302–311.

Zabedah MY, Razak M, Zakiah I, Zuraidah AB. 2001. Profile of solvent abusers (glue sniffers) in East Malaysia. *Malays J Pathol.* 23:105–109.

Zohar Z, Waksman I, Stolero J, et al. 2004. Injury from fireworks and firecrackers during holidays. *Harefuah.* 143:698–701, 768.

Chapter 15

Moving Child and Adolescent Injury Prevention and Control Research Into Practice: A Framework for Translation

Michael Yonas, DrPH, MPH,[1] Shannon Frattaroli, PhD, MPH,[2] Karen D. Liller, PhD,[3] Ann Christiansen, MPH,[4,5] Andrea Carlson Gielen, ScD, ScM, CHES,[2] Stephen Hargarten, MD, MPH,[4,5] and Lenora M. Olson, PhD[6]

Injuries, both unintentional and intentional, are among the ten leading causes of mortality and morbidity in children aged 1 to 15 years. It is estimated that more than 875,000 children aged less than 18 years die annually as a result of all injuries, more than 90% of which are unintentional (World Health Organization 2003). In addition to the loss in mortality, for every child who dies, thousands of children are forced to live with the consequences of injury-induced disability (Hyder, Puvanachandra, and Tran 2008; World Health Organization and UNICEF 2005). The resulting need for short- and long-term care has substantial social, emotional, and financial consequences for the family, community, and society, in addition to the devastating impact on the injured child.

For more than 50 years, researchers have used rigorous epidemiologic methods to examine the devastating impact of injuries on population health (World Health Organization 2003). As are other areas within public health, the field of injury prevention and control is an applied field with a clear connection between research and practice. As a result, evidence-based interventions to prevent injuries have been adopted into practice for workplace violence (Peek-Asa and Casteel 2010), child and adolescent transportation safety (Simons-Morton and Winston 2006), underage drinking (Spoth, Greenberg, and Turrisi 2008), and unintentional childhood injury prevention, such as falls, poisonings, and chokings (Saul et al. 2008; Weaver et al. 2008).

Translating scientific evidence into practice is receiving increasing attention within the health sciences. The National Institutes of Health (NIH) and the Centers for Disease Control and Prevention in the United States, and the Canadian Institutes of Health Research are investing in the infrastructure to support translation science and translational research projects (Woolf 2008). With the growing attention on the science of translation (Centers for Disease Control and Prevention [CDC] and National Center for Injury Prevention and Control 2008; Wandersman et al. 2008) and the increasing emphasis on the need to implement interventions that will save both lives and money (Cohen, Neumann, and Weinstein 2008; Woolf 2008), child and adolescent injury researchers have an opportunity to advance the understanding of how evidence can most effectively

[1]Department of Family Medicine, University of Pittsburgh, Pennsylvania.

[2]The Johns Hopkins Bloomberg School of Public Health, Center for Injury Research and Policy, Baltimore, Maryland.

[3]University of South Florida Graduate School and the College of Public Health, Tampa, Florida.

[4]Department of Emergency Medicine, Medical College of Wisconsin, Milwaukee, Wisconsin.

[5]Injury Research Center, Medical College of Wisconsin, Milwaukee, Wisconsin.

[6]Intermountain Injury Control Research Center, Department of Pediatrics, University of Utah, Salt Lake City, Utah.

translate and influence decisions about programs and policies to prevent and control injuries. Given the applied orientation of injury prevention and control, and the historic connection between evidence and practice, our field has the potential to make important contributions to the current dialogue on the science of translating health research into practice.

The development of a robust translational research agenda within injury prevention and control requires a paradigm shift. Published studies currently offer empirically based evidence of the effectiveness of injury interventions (Sogolow, Sleet, and Saul 2007; Zaza, Briss, and Harris 2005). However, there are often limited or no data provided on how to effectively translate evidence-based interventions into programs and policies. The lack of data on translating evidence into programs or policies makes it easier for scientists to assume effective interventions will automatically be adopted by those who run programs and make policy decisions (Koh et al. 2010). To cultivate a focus on translational research among the next generation of researchers, training programs must emphasize knowledge discovery and intervention testing with increased emphasis on understanding and applying the skills needed to translate research results beyond traditional peer-reviewed publications (Gielen et al. 2006). As a result, bringing translational science fully into the field of child and adolescent injury prevention and control will require *actions* to translate science into programs and policies, and *studies* of the translation processes to guide future efforts.

In this chapter, we offer a conceptual approach to the science and practice of translational research that is specific to child and adolescent injury prevention and control. First, we discuss existing definitions commonly used. We then present two frameworks from the clinical translation literature that we adapted for the field of child and adolescent injury prevention and control. Finally, by using two examples of injuries common in children and adolescents—motor vehicle injuries and intentional firearm injuries—we apply the adapted tools, discuss areas where translational research is needed, and consider the implications for the field of child and adolescent injury prevention and control. Our primary goal is to encourage dialogue about how to incorporate translation considerations into future research efforts. A secondary goal is to provide a framework and guidance for child and adolescent injury prevention and control scientists seeking to tailor and incorporate translational research and translation activities into their work.

Translational Science in the Context of Injury Prevention and Control

Defining Translational Science

Translational science is scientific research that is motivated by the need for practical applications that help people. Consistent with currently published definitions, we consider translation and translational research to be the process of systematically moving empirically based interventions into widespread practice through programs, policies, or clinical initiatives (Sussman et al. 2006; Woolf 2008). The Centers for Disease Control and Prevention's *Knowledge to Action* work group defines three activities associated with the process of conducting translational research: dissemination, implementation, and diffusion (CDC and National Center for Injury Prevention and Control, Division of Violence Prevention 2008; Sogolow, Sleet, and Saul 2007). *Dissemination* is the intentional spreading of information—product, practice, program, policy, research findings, or results—to relevant stakeholders (e.g., policymakers, community leaders, and clinical administrators) to improve the public's health. *Implementation* is a purposeful set of activities designed to put a program or policy to use, and includes decisions to use an innovation, commit needed resources, and ensure the relevant processes are in place. *Diffusion* is the process through which program staff, policymakers, or other stakeholders move an innovation into widespread use. Strategies to influence diffusion may include dissemination and implementation initiatives, social marketing, laws and regulations, and organization-level policies (CDC and National Center for Injury Prevention and Control, Division of Violence

Prevention 2008). Thus, translating and expanding opportunity for the practical application of scientific results is complex and involves many different processes, institutions, and individuals.

Translational Research Models

In recent years, several agencies and individuals have offered conceptual models of translational research (Brekke, Ell, and Palinkas 2007; Woolf 2008). The Clinical and Translational Science Awards program of the NIH offers a well-known model for translational research in the health sciences (Woolf 2008). However, the clinical orientation of the NIH model often limits its utility for many injury prevention and control interventions. To address this limitation and to acknowledge the evolving nature of the translational research field, we adapted the NIH translational research stages to better align with the orientation of injury prevention and control by including academic, practice-based, community, and policy applications (Table 15.1).

We then applied these revised stages of the translation process to a recently published model of clinical translation. In our adapted model (Figure 15.1) from Westfall, Mold, and Fagnan (2007), the application of translational science occurs across the same four distinct but interrelated stages that characterize the NIH approach to translation but includes the broader program and policy venues where many injury interventions occur. In the field of injury prevention and control, "interventions" or "countermeasures" may be considered analogous to medical treatments. For example, the interventions may be a device or product (e.g., car seat), a program or policy to motivate individuals to use the device or product (e.g., seat belt laws), or a mandatory standard (e.g., a mandatory motor vehicle safety standard). In whatever case we apply the word "intervention," translational research uses a systematic research process to prove its efficacy.

Although this is a linear model, it is important to realize that translational research is an iterative process, allowing researchers to return to a prior stage to respond to challenges discovered in the current stage.

The process of taking available information and developing effective countermeasures (e.g., product, program, or policy intervention) defines the T1 stage and includes efforts to develop interventions based on biomechanical or epidemiologic discoveries. Translational science during this stage focuses on the logistics and decisions associated with developing an intervention on the basis of available data on the nature of and risks associated with a particular problem or the biomechanics of a countermeasure. It is here that studies of the intervention's efficacy in controlled settings take place. Building on information about the intervention that resulted from T1 activities occurs during the T2 stage of the translation process. T2 research includes studying the processes of disseminating and implementing an intervention using efficacy trials and effectiveness studies to inform evidence-based guidelines for T2 actions. Thus, the aim in the T2 stage is to understand how target recipients of the intervention receive, respond to, and take up an intervention and what approaches facilitate uptake. T2 activities tend to be small in scale because the clinical, program, or policy intervention is untested. If positive evaluation results are found during the T2 stage, then the translation process moves to diffusing the intervention on a larger scale.

T3 activities aim to diffuse information regarding evidence-based interventions with the decision makers, policymakers, and community leaders who serve populations who would benefit from effective interventions. The studies that occur during this phase are larger than T2 studies. Assessing the impact of a diffusion strategy designed to encourage uptake of an effective intervention is an example of T3 research.

With the intervention working to scale, T4 research is conducted to monitor and test variations in adoption among communities and to document the evolution of intervention implementation that often occurs when communities take up a new program or policy. T4 studies are also used to address shortcomings in the implementation process and to identify recommended adaptations to improve the scope and effectiveness of the intervention. Findings

Table 15.1. Comparison of Clinical and Injury Prevention and Control Models for Translational Process and Research

	Clinical		Injury Prevention and Control	
	Process of Translation	Translational Research	Process of Translation	Translational Research
T1	Move laboratory discoveries to human clinical research; "bench to bedside" efficacy trial studies	Research to facilitate institutional review board processes, improve the efficiency of subject recruiting, and examine safety issues usually among a small group of patients in one setting or hospital	Move epidemiologic discoveries from data to intervention, using formative, process, and impact evaluation in efficacy studies	Understand processes associated with intervention development and management using a small or limited number of participants Demonstrate the effectiveness of products, programs, and policies
T2	Move clinical research into clinical practice (translation to patients)	Study the delivery of intervention to a larger group of patients	Move evidence-based intervention into organizational and community settings, using efficacy studies	Study the dissemination and implementation of interventions into nonresearch settings using larger and more diverse samples
T3	Move clinical research into clinical practice (translation to practice)	Study dissemination and implementation of intervention to clinical infrastructure using randomized, controlled, multicenter trials on large patient groups	Scale-up effective intervention to larger population, using effectiveness trials for injury prevention and control	Diffusion research to the public
T4	Refine intervention and intervention delivery based on fidelity monitoring	Policy research: What is the best method to reach clinicians and patients with a nationwide policy to understand and use new treatment (patient and practice)?	Refine intervention based on ongoing fidelity monitoring	Fidelity assessment, ongoing refinement, and policy research

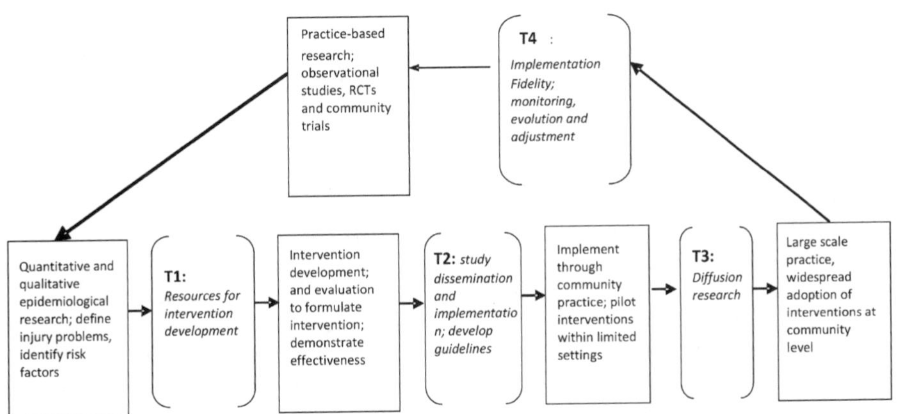

Figure 15.1. Injury Prevention and Control Translational Research Model (modified from Westfall, Mold, and Fagnan 2007).

from T4 research lead to additional translational science research and practice-based studies to inform evidence-based modifications to interventions that are specific to community needs.

Effective translational science incorporates all four stages of the model. Although each stage answers important research questions, the combination of the four stages brings quantitative and qualitative findings, as well as epidemiologic data of intervention research, into practice in clinical, community, and policy settings.

Application to Motor Vehicle and Firearm Injuries

To further illustrate the adapted translation stages, we apply the framework described above to motor vehicle and firearm injuries. We include both published examples of research for each stage, when available, and examples of research questions for those stages where we were unable to identify a published example.

Motor Vehicle Crashes

Motor vehicle crash–related injury is a leading cause of death and disability for those aged 1 to 19 years in the United States (Anderson et al. 2004; Simons-Morton and Winston 2006). Motor vehicle crash–related injuries account for more than 1500 deaths annually among children and some 3820 deaths among 15- to 20-year-old drivers and passengers (National Highway Traffic Safety Administration 2004). Nonfatal crashes are more common than fatal crashes, injuring more than 220,000 children annually (National Highway Traffic Safety Administration 2004). Children and adolescents are also at elevated risk as passengers and pedestrians for motor vehicle–related injury (Chen et al. 2005; National SAFE KIDS Campaign 2004).

Reductions in motor vehicle–related deaths and injuries have been described as one of the great public health achievements of the 20th century (Adekoya 2009). Despite an increase in the overall use of motor vehicles, the annual death rate per vehicle mile traveled decreased 90% from 1925 to 1997 (Adekoya 2009). These dramatic improvements in the presence of increased exposure are the result of engineering improvements (vehicle safety standards), environmental changes (improved roadways), advances in emergency medical systems (enhanced 911 systems), and behavioral (enhanced enforcement campaigns) and policy changes (zero tolerance laws), also including increased use of safety belts and car safety seats (Adekoya 2009; Martin, Green, and Gielen 2007).

Effective motor vehicle crash injury prevention and intervention efforts require a variety of integrated approaches, including technology, legislation, policy, regulation, interdisciplinary outreach, enforcement, and education for adolescents, parents, and organizations (Gielen et al. 2006; Simons-Morton and Winston 2006). Although many of the successes in the reduction of motor vehicle crashes took place before translation science was developed, we can ascertain how these achievements occurred by using the lens of translation science to review these changes.

Table 15.2 summarizes select research in the four phases of translational research (T1–T4) for motor vehicle–related injuries to young children. It is understood that to decrease motor vehicle–related injuries in children multifaceted strategies are essential, including education/behavioral changes, legislative and policy implementation and enforcement, and engineering and environmental improvements. Table 15.2 focuses mostly on the legislative strategies for illustrative purposes only.

In 2008, the restraint use for children aged less than 4 years was estimated to be 90% (National Highway Traffic Safety Administration 2009). Despite significant progress, persistent challenges remain. For example, despite such progress, child restraint systems are still often used incorrectly.

Intentional Firearm Injuries

Although motor vehicle injury research has been ongoing since the 1960s, firearm injury prevention research began two decades later (Baker, Teret, and Dietz 1980). During the 1980s, the United States experienced a dramatic increase in intentional firearm injuries. In response, the injury paradigm expanded to include firearms as public health researchers brought a new perspective to this problem (Blumstein and Rosenfeld 1998). Youth violence, encompassing children and adolescents, is the second leading cause of death for young people aged 10 and 24 years, with an average of 16 deaths per day in 2007 (CDC and National Center for Injury Prevention and Control 2010). Among those aged 10 to 24 years, homicide is the leading cause of death for African Americans, the second leading cause of death for Hispanics, and the third leading cause of death for Asian/Pacific Islanders and American Indians and Alaska Natives (CDC and National Center for Injury Prevention and Control 2010). Among young people aged 10 to 24 years who succumbed to violence, 84% were killed with a firearm (CDC and National Center for Injury Prevention and Control 2010).

As with motor vehicle crash injuries, the solutions offered to address firearm injuries include attention to all four phases of translational research. Table 15.3 summarizes select examples of research in each of the four phases as applied to intentional firearm injuries and the specific risks associated with Saturday night special handguns.

On the topic of Saturday night specials, the literature includes examples of translational research that explore the processes of communicating information beyond the research community (Wallack 1999) and implementing the regulations promulgated as a result of Saturday night special legislation (Fennell 1992). These within-state studies reflect the initial stages of the translational research process (T1 and T2). To our knowledge, translational research concerning the diffusion of Saturday night special access policies to other states and the fidelity of these policies as the intervention spread has yet to occur.

Discussion

Advancing a new generation of translation practices and translational research in the area of child and adolescent injury prevention and control will require new ways of thinking, teaching, and mentoring. In addition, it is essential to cultivate long-term collaboration and commitment among injury prevention and control researchers, practitioners, policymakers, and communities to ensure that evidence-based strategies are implemented and that the lessons from implementation are studied and disseminated through evidenced-based translation processes. Without attention to these matters, the ability of injury professionals to prevent and control injuries will fall short of their full and necessary potential.

Table 15.2. Motor Vehicle–Related Injuries Among Young Children

	Translational Process	Translational Research
T1	*Research Informing Translation:* Through biomechanics, properly restrained children sustain less severe injuries in motor vehicle crashes (National Safety Council 1984; Simons-Morton and Winston 2006; Stapp 1986). *Translation Action:* Develop strategies to increase the percentage of child passengers who are restrained when riding in motor vehicles.	*Example of T1 Research:* What factors affected the translation of these research findings into the resulting interventions?
T2	*Translation Action:* In 1978, Tennessee passes the first law in the United States requiring parents of children aged < 4 years to use restraint systems when transporting children in motor vehicles (Centers for Disease Control and Prevention 2006; Williams 1979). Legislation and community education are aimed at parents, children, health professionals, and law enforcement (Zaza et al. 2001)	*Examples of T2 Research:* Understand the processes through which the research was communicated to stakeholders and decision makers. Identify the factors that influenced stakeholders' decisions to implement interventions to promote the use of child restraints.
T3	*Research Informing Translation:* Educational interventions to increase proper restraint show limited results (Reisinger and Williams 1978; Zaza et al. 2001). Laws mandating restraint use are promising (Williams 1979). *Translation Actions:* By 1980, 23 states had initiated legislation requiring children aged 0–5 years to be restrained in federally approved child safety seats (Meyer 1981). In 1985, all 50 states and the District of Columbia had enacted child passenger restraint laws (Wagenaar and Webster 1986).	*Examples of T3 Research:* How did the legislation diffuse from the initial early adopter states to 23 and then 50 states? What were the mechanisms for diffusing information about the law and compliance to the public? What diffusion strategies were effective?
T4	*Research Informing Translation:* Evaluation of Tennessee law shows that child restraint use increased by 20%, but the rate of children traveling in arms remains the same (Williams and Wells 1981; Zaza et al. 2001). *Translation Action:* Interventions encourage enforcement of laws through citations. *Research Informing Translation:* Research shows that laws are correlated with a substantial increase in restraint use and a decrease in children injured or killed in motor vehicle crashes (Wagenaar and Webster 1986; Zaza et al. 2001). *Translation Action:* Interventions promote correct installation and use of child safety seats.	*Examples of T4 Research:* Issuing citations for noncompliance with the child restraint law in Tennessee is correlated with a reduction in motor vehicle fatalities among children (Decker et al. 1984). Children's Safety Center work on car seat installations (Children's Safety Center 2010). Will these findings be applicable in global settings? What will need to be changed in global settings to accommodate enhanced policies and laws that favor child restraint use?

Table 15.3. Firearm Injuries

	Translational Process	Translational Research
T1	*Research Informing Translation:* Saturday night special handguns are disproportionately represented in crime gun traces (Wintemute 1994). Many Saturday night special handgun manufacturers are located in California (Wintemute 1994). *Translation Action:* Raise awareness about the risks associated with Saturday night special handguns and the concentration of manufacturers in Southern California.	*Example of T1 Research:* Evaluation of a statewide violence prevention campaign in California that included efforts to disseminate information about the risks associated with Saturday night specials to stakeholders and the presence of manufacturers in the state (Wallack 1999).
T2	*Research Informing Translation:* Legal research establishing limited authority of California localities to restrict the manufacture, sale, or possession of handguns, despite state-level preemption (Berkley Media Studies Group; Gorovitz 1996). *Translation Action:* Localities and states enact policies to reduce access to Saturday night special handguns (e.g., California enacts a law outlawing the manufacture and sale of Saturday night special handguns, and Maryland enacts a law prohibiting the sale of Saturday night special handguns).	*Example of T2 Research:* Research documenting how stakeholders organized and advocated for policies to reduce access to Saturday night special handguns provides insight into how support for state and local policies evolved in California (Wallack 1999). Research examining the regulatory implementation of Maryland's law suggests ways in which the implementation compromised the intent of the law (Fennell 1992).
T3	*Research Informing Translation:* Compilation of local California ordinances addressing manufacture, sale, or possession of Saturday night special handguns. *Translation Action:* States pass laws prohibiting the manufacture, sale, or possession of Saturday night special handguns.	*Example of T3 Research:* How did this policy intervention diffuse from the initial early adopter states? What were the mechanisms for diffusing information about the law to the public? What diffusion strategies were effective?
T4	*Research Informing Translation:* Evaluation of Saturday night special law in Maryland is associated with a reduction in gun homicide (Webster, Vernick, and Hepburn 2002). *Translation Action:* Advocates organize against efforts to repeal Saturday night special laws.	*Example of T4 Research:* What factors are influencing the law's success? How can the implementation of this law be improved? How can what is learned in the United States about the efficacy of these laws be translated into global settings?

Identifying Opportunities for Translation and Translation Research

The motor vehicle and firearm examples provide examples of translated and translational research and demonstrate the value of such efforts to realizing population-level injury prevention and control accomplishments achieved to date. We offer this framework and revised translation stages as tools for systematically assessing the state of the evidence on particular injury problems. By assessing the current research from a translation perspective, the readiness of the evidence for implementation through policies, programs, or clinical practice can be easily identified. Through a more systematic inventory of the existing injury prevention and control evidence, our field can make important gains in strategically reducing the implementing of evidence into practice timeline.

Translation as an Opportunity to Raise the Profile of Child and Adolescent Injury Prevention and Control

We also view translation science as an opportunity for injury to gain greater recognition as a health issue. Despite the high injury-related morbidity and mortality, health is largely understood as the absence of disease. This is true across populations, even though injuries are the leading cause of death for children and adolescents. By advancing translation and translational research, we can inform the ongoing dialogue about effective translation processes. Our field has enjoyed success in identifying effective countermeasures for injury. This is evident in the success of child restraint use (especially among infants and young children) and seat belt use. We are well positioned to use those proven interventions to test implementation, dissemination, and diffusion strategies in pursuit of evidence that will lead to effective uptake by policymakers, community leaders, and clinicians, and should further decrease injuries in children and adolescents. Although these approaches are in their infancy, the potential for informing future evidence-based practice and research is huge. We look forward to building our continued understanding and application of translational processes and research related to injury prevention for children and adolescents.

Conclusions

In this chapter, we have used a common organizing translational research framework. The analysis of injury-related problems by translational phase serves as a valuable tool for framing translation across the diverse and evolving field of injury prevention and control. The proposed framework serves as a reminder of the complexity of the research agenda and the importance of purposefully assessing how best to apply research findings to practice. Our goal is to generate interdisciplinary discussion and common understanding to further the rapid translation of injury prevention and control evidence into policy and practice across all age groups. Given the exceptional public health burden of injuries, it is the responsibility of governments worldwide, nongovernment organizations, and the private sector to promote and support a translation agenda for injury prevention and control. As William Haddon (1999) stated, "we must recognize the conceptual transitions in which we are participating and the difference between descriptive and etiologic approaches, and that the payoffs for society and in scientific understanding lie chiefly in the latter. We must also recognize that this area and approach must be considered as part of any overall approach to human ecosystems, and we can no longer afford to deal in terms of concepts of the past."

References

Adekoya N. 2009. *Motor Vehicle-Related Death Rates—United States, 1999-2005.* (Report, statistical data.) Vol. 58. Available at: http://find.galegroup.com/gtx/infomark.do?&contentSet=

IAC-Documents&type=retrieve&tabID=T004&prodId=AONE&docId=A196383467&source=gale&srcprod=AONE&userGroupName=upitt_main&version=1.

Anderson RN, Miniño AM, Fingerhut LA, et al. 2004. Deaths: injuries 2001. *Natl Vital Stat Rep.* 52:1–86.

Baker SP, Teret SP, Dietz PE. 1980. Firearms and the public health. *J Public Health Policy.* 1:224–229.

Berkley Media Studies Group. Reporting on Violence. 2010. *Prevention Approaches: Limiting the Availability of Handguns* [cited 11/2 2010]. Available at: http://www.bmsg.org/pcvp/HANDG.SHTML. Accessed July 7, 2011.

Blumstein A, Rosenfeld R. 1998. Explaining recent trends in U.S. homicide rates. *J Crim Law Crimonol.* 88:1175–1216.

Brekke JS, Ell K, Palinkas LA. 2007. Translational science at the National Institute of Mental Health: can social work take its rightful place? *Res Soc Work Pract.* 17:123–133.

Centers for Disease Control and Prevention. 2006. Nonfatal injuries and restraint use among child passengers—United States, 2004. *MMWR Morb Mortal Wkly Rep.* 55:624–627.

Centers for Disease Control and Prevention, and National Center for Injury Prevention and Control. 2008. *National Center for Injury Prevention and Control Translation Research Guidance in Centers for Disease Control and Prevention* [database online] [cited September 15, 2010]. Available at: http://www.cdc.gov/ncipc/res-opps/translation.htm. Accessed July 7, 2011.

Centers for Disease Control and Prevention, and National Center for Injury Prevention and Control, Division of Violence Prevention. 2008. *Youth Violence Prevention Scientific Information: Translation in Centers for Disease Control and Prevention* [database online] [cited June 11, 2009]. Available at: http://www.cdc.gov/ncipc/dvp/YVP/YVP-translation.htm. Accessed July 7, 2011.

Centers for Disease Control and Prevention, and National Center for Injury Prevention and Control. 2010. *Web-Based Injury Statistics Query and Reporting System (WISQARS) in Centers for Disease Control and Prevention* [database online] [cited June 14 2010]. Available at: http://www.cdc.gov/injury/wisqars/index.html. Accessed July 7, 2011.

Chen IG, Elliott MR, Durbin DR, Winston FK. 2005. Teen drivers and the risk of injury to child passengers in motor vehicle crashes. *Inj Prev.* 11:12–17.

Children's Safety Center. 2010. [database online] [cited September 19, 2010]. Available at: http://www.childrenssafetycenter.org/. Accessed July 7, 2011.

Cohen JT, Neumann PJ, Weinstein MC. 2008. Does preventive care save money? Health economics and the presidential candidates. *N Engl J Med.* 358:661–663.

Decker MD, Dewey MJ, Hutcheson RH Jr, Schaffner W. 1984. The use and efficacy of child restraint devices: the Tennessee experience, 1982 and 1983. *JAMA.* 252:2571–2575.

Fennell M. 1992. Missing the mark in Maryland: how poor drafting and implementation vitiated a model state gun control law. *Hamline J Pub Law Policy.* 13:37–71.

Gielen AC, Sleet DA, DiClemente RJ, editors. 2006. Injury and Violence Prevention: Behavioral Science Theories, Methods, and Applications. San Francisco, CA: Jossey-Bass.

Gorovitz E. 1996. California dreamin': the myth of state preemption of local firearm regulation. *University of San Francisco Law Review.* 30:395.

Haddon W. 1999. The changing approach to the epidemiology, prevention, and amelioration of trauma: the transition to approaches etiologically rather than descriptively based. *Inj Prev.* 5:231–235.

Hyder AA, Puvanachandra P, Tran NH. 2008. Child and adolescent injuries: a new agenda for child health. *Inj Prev.* 14:67.

Koh KH, Oppenheimer SC, Massin-Short S, et al. 2010. Translating research evidence into practice to reduce health disparities: a social determinants approach. *Am J Public Health.* 100:S72–S80.

Martin JB, Green LW, Gielen AC. 2007. Potential lessons from public health and health promotion for the prevention of child abuse. *J Prev Interv Community.* 34:205–222.

Meyer RJ. 1981. *Save That Child: Children and Automobile Restraints.* Vol. 71. Washington, DC: American Public Health Association. Available at: http://search.ebscohost.com/login.aspx?direct=true&db=aph&AN=4947904&site=ehost-live.

National Highway Traffic Safety Administration. 2004. *Traffic Safety Facts 2003: A Compilation of Motor Vehicle Crash Data From the Fatality Analysis Reporting System and the General Estimates System.* Washington, DC: National Center for Statistics and Analysis, U.S. Department of Transportation, DOT HS 809 775.

National Highway Traffic Safety Administration. 2009. *Child Restraint Use in 2008—Demographic Results.* Washington DC: National Highway Traffic Safety Administration, DOT HS 811 148.

National SAFE KIDS Campaign. 2004. *Trends in Unintentional Childhood Injury Fact Sheet in National SAFE KIDS Campaign* [database online] [cited October 24, 2010]. Available at: http://www.preventinjury.org/PDFs/TRENDS_IN_UNINTENTIONAL_CHILDHOOD_INJURY.pdf. Accessed July 7, 2011.

National Safety Council. 1984. *Accident Facts.* National Safety Council. Statistics Department. Itasca, IL: National Safety Council.

Peek-Asa C, Casteel CH. 2010. Documenting the need for translational research: an example from workplace violence prevention. *Inj Prev.* 16:50–52.

Reisinger KS, Williams AF. 1978. Evaluation of programs designed to increase the protection of infants in cars. *Pediatrics.* 62:280.

Saul J, Wandersman A, Flaspohler P, et al. 2008. Research and action for bridging science and practice in prevention. *Am J Community Psychol.* 41:165–407.

Simons-Morton BG, Winston FK. 2006. Translational research in child and adolescent transportation safety. *Eval Health Prof.* 29:33–64.

Sogolow ED, Sleet DA, Saul JS. 2007. Dissemination, implementation, and widespread use of injury prevention interventions. In: Haas EN, editor. *Handbook of Injury and Violence Prevention.* New York, NY: Springer. 493–510.

Spoth R, Greenberg M, Turrisi R. 2008. Preventive interventions addressing underage drinking: state of the evidence and steps toward public health impact. *Pediatrics.* 121(Suppl 4):S311–S336.

Stapp JP. 1986. Historical overview, human and chimpanzee tolerance to linear decelerative force. In: Sances A, Thomas DJ, Ewing CL, Larson SJ, Unterharnscheidt F, editors. *Mechanisms of Head and Spine Trauma.* Goshen, NY: Aloray Publishing Inc. 1–46.

Sussman S, Valente TW, Rohrbach LA, et al. 2006. Translation in the health professions. *Eval Health Prof.* 29:7–32.

Wagenaar AC, Webster DW. 1986. Preventing injuries to children through compulsory automobile safety seat use. *Pediatrics.* 78:662.

Wallack L. 1999. The California violence prevention initiative: advancing policy to ban Saturday night specials. *Health Educ Behav.* 26:841–857.

Wandersman A, Duffy J, Flaspohler P, et al. 2008. Bridging the gap between prevention research and practice: the interactive systems framework for dissemination and implementation *Am J Commun Psychol.* 41:171–181.

Weaver NL, Williams J, Jacobsen HA, et al. 2008. Translation of an evidence-based tailored childhood injury prevention program. *J Public Health Manag Pract.* 14:177.

Webster DW, Vernick JS, Hepburn LM. 2002. Effects of Maryland's law banning "Saturday night special" handguns on homicides. *Am J Epidemiol.* 155:406–412.

Westfall JM, Mold J, Fagnan L. 2007. Practice-based research—"blue highways" on the NIH roadmap. *JAMA.* 297:403–406.

Williams AF. 1979. Evaluation of the Tennessee child restraint law. *Am J Public Health.* 69:455–458.

Williams AF, Wells JK. 1981. The Tennessee child restraint law in its third year. *Am J Public Health.* 71:163–165.

Wintemute GJ. 1994. *Ring of Fire: The Handgun Makers of Southern California.* Sacramento, CA: Violence Prevention Research Program, University of California, Davis.

Woolf SH. 2008. The meaning of translational research and why it matters. *JAMA.* 299:211–213.

World Health Organization. 2003. *Department of Injuries and Violence Prevention Annual Report: 2002.* Geneva, Switzerland: World Health Organization.

World Health Organization and UNICEF. 2005. *Child and Adolescent Injury Prevention: A Global Call to Action.* Geneva: World Health Organization.

Zaza S, Briss PA, Harris KW. 2005. *The Guide to Community Preventive Services: What Works to Promote Health?* Task Force on Community Preventive Services (U.S.). New York: Oxford University.

Zaza S, Sleet DA, Thompson RS, et al. 2001. Reviews of evidence regarding interventions to increase use of child safety seats. *Am J Prev Med.* 21:31–47.

Chapter 16

Conclusions and Recommendations

Karen D. Liller, PhD[1]

Through this text, we hope to inform academicians, students, and practitioners of up-to-date research, practice, and advocacy efforts related to child and adolescent injury prevention, and what is important for the future.

As stated in the first edition of the text, the synergistic and complementary roles of research, practice, and advocacy have been effective, as evidenced by several injury prevention wins, such as the incorporation of child safety seats, seat belts, graduated licensing, and prevention of poisonings into society. But more can be done, and innovative approaches still need to take place with motor vehicle injuries, recreational injuries, residential injuries, school injuries, agricultural injuries, workplace injuries, youth violence, child abuse and neglect, injuries related to firearms, and the increase in the number of poisonings, to name a few. We now must add to the list global injuries and the role for translational research and practice.

What questions need to be pursued and answered in the future pertaining to children's injuries? For research, a common theme across injury topics is the need for better surveillance data across the globe. Although we have made great advances in the United States, the data obtained internationally arise from disparate sources with varying definitions and level of completeness. Research also needs to continue on the most appropriate role for education and parental supervision and advocacy because these elements remain important as children age. This is seen in many areas, including motor vehicle injury prevention and safe work environments for adolescents. Comprehensive evaluations of interventions need to be developed and implemented using more sophisticated research designs. Research in injury prevention for children and adolescents needs to be developmentally based and to incorporate as much as possible the community participatory research model where communities are directly involved with research endeavors. Finally, we must learn those mechanisms and processes that will best allow us to translate research into action locally, statewide, and globally. This will take resources, and advocacy must be present so these resources are found and used effectively.

In terms of practice, it is very important that practitioners and researchers work in concert. Representatives from education, media, marketing, advocacy groups, business, engineering, law enforcement, and others should be at the table using ecologic interventions that are rigorously tested for efficacy and effectiveness.

As in the previous edition of the text, knowledge of the costs related to injury is extremely important to incorporate in our prevention efforts. Legislative committees often want to know how much money interventions will cost the state or community and exactly what are the cost benefits to society as a whole. What will society be willing to pay for these efforts? Focusing only on those injuries that lead to death will not lead to the most effective use of resources for prevention strategies.

A most important role for child and adolescent injury prevention is advocacy. Knowing how to work with the media and legislators and understanding the role of coalitions are vital. The American Public Health Association continues to provide several helpful educational materials on

[1]University of South Florida Graduate School and the College of Public Health, Tampa, Florida.

these topics (see http://www.apha.org/advocacy/tips). Being known to legislators and testifying on legislative committees, writing editorials and press releases, conducting press conferences, using media advocacy to promote injury policies, and joining community coalitions are just a few of the ways that injury prevention advocates can make their voices heard.

Injury prevention education needs to continue and be included in grades pre-K to 12 and in higher learning. Core competencies for violence and injury prevention have been developed for injury prevention practitioners (Runyan and Stidham 2009). The school system and other educational institutions have vital roles here as important community leaders in injury prevention efforts. However, these competencies and understandings must be updated on an ongoing basis because "booster" sessions are often necessary to keep the information current in the minds of the audiences.

The Centers for Disease Control and Prevention's National Center for Injury Prevention and Control (2011) has been important to the growth of injury prevention efforts throughout the country. Their 2009–2018 Injury Research Agenda corresponds well with many of the research, practice, and advocacy measures already described in the text (http://www.cdc.gov/injury/ResearchAgenda). Cross-cutting priorities in the report include preventing injury and violence worldwide, evaluating the effectiveness of interventions to reduce excessive alcohol use and alcohol dependency, and understanding and reducing health disparities. In addition, the injury data resource, the Web-based Injury Statistics Query and Reporting System (http://www.cdc.gov/injury/wisqars/index.html), has been updated to include an injury mapping model (with cost estimates) for states and counties (2010). Also, a new and user-friendly module provides cost estimates for injury deaths (including violent deaths) and nonfatal injuries where the patient was treated and released from a hospital or an emergency department.

Finally, there is now a real need to pursue intervention efforts in developing countries. Road injuries alone pose major threats to life across the globe, killing 1.2 million people (with new figures showing 1.3 million) and injuring up to 50 million more per year (World Health Organization 2009). It is predicted that if things remain at status quo, road traffic injuries will become the fifth leading cause of death worldwide by 2030. On November 18, 2009, Michael Bloomberg announced he would donate $125 million to prevent death and injuries caused by road traffic crashes worldwide (World Health Organization 2010). Strategies will include enhancing professional and front-line worker training; improving infrastructure projects through road safety assessments; monitoring and evaluating traffic-related deaths, injuries, and policy effectiveness; helping the public and not-for-profit sectors propose, pass, and implement effective road safety laws, regulations, and policies; incorporating sustainable transport and reduced emissions in urban planning; and creating global resources for advocacy (World Health Organization 2009). Soon after this information was released, the First Global Ministerial Conference on Road Safety took place in Moscow, and a proclamation for a Decade of Action of Road Safety 2011–2020 was signed. The Decade of Action for Road Safety began May 11, 2011, and includes a global plan, a symbol/logo, training aids, and more (United Nations Road Safety Collaboration 2011). Also, in 2010 a group of six partners received funding from Bloomberg Philanthropies to work toward enhancing road safety in ten low- and middle-income countries (Peyden 2010). These countries include Brazil, Cambodia, China, Egypt, India, Kenya, Mexico, Russian Federation, Turkey, and Vietnam. We look forward to learning more about the success of this project, known as the "Road Safety in 10 Countries Project," during the next 5 years, as well as the several global efforts to reduce the toll of transportation injuries on morbidity and mortality.

I hope the second edition of this text has enhanced the reader's understanding of child and adolescent injury prevention, and that readers are inspired to begin or build their own present efforts along with developing strategic and comprehensive plans for the future. We will be successful by focusing on the "faces of injury" so that our efforts have real meaning in saving the lives of children and adolescents throughout the world.

References

Centers for Disease Prevention and Control. 2011. *Injury and Violence Prevention and Control.* Atlanta, GA: Centers for Disease Control and Prevention. Available at: http://www.cdc.gov/injury/index.html. Accessed February 25, 2011.

Peyden M. 2010. Road safety in 10 countries. *Inj Prev.* 16:433.

Runyan CW, Stidham SS. 2009. Core competencies for injury and violence prevention. *Inj Prev.* 15:141.

United Nations Road Safety Collaboration. 2011. *Decade of Action for Road Safety, 2011–2020.* Geneva, Switzerland: World Health Organization. Available at: http://www.who.int/roadsafety/decade_of_action/en/index.html. Accessed February 24, 2011.

World Health Organization (WHO). 2009. *Global Status Report on Road Safety: Time for Action.* Geneva, Switzerland: WHO. Available at: www.who.int/violence_injury_prevention/road_safety_status/2009. Accessed September 10, 2010.

World Health Organization (WHO). 2010. *Michael Bloomberg Commits $125 Million to Reduce Deaths and Injuries on World's Roads.* Geneva, Switzerland: WHO. Available at: http://www.who.int/roadsafety/ministerial_conference/announcement_bloomberg.pdf. Accessed November 28, 2010.

Appendix A

Selected Historical Timeline for Injury Prevention and Control

Les Fisher, MPH[1] *and Andrés Villaveces, MD, PhD, MPH*[2]

This timeline shows the continued growth of our field. Other timelines are available from various injury prevention organizations. The purpose of the timeline below is to update the timeline published in the first edition of the text so that the events that shaped the field of injury prevention and control are highlighted.[3]

Historical Timeline

1912	U.S. Congress creates the Children's Bureau.
1913	U.S. Congress charters National Safety Council.
1920	President Woodrow Wilson issues the first National Fire Prevention Day proclamation.
1921	National Safety Council first publishes Accident Facts (annual U.S. injury data projections).
1924	Cadillac offers first car with safety windshield glass equipment as a standard.
1932	Maryland is the first U.S. state to introduce mandatory car inspections.
1937	E.S. Godfrey publishes one of the first U.S. statements on the need for public health involvement in "accident" prevention, in the *American Journal of Public Health.* As American Public Health Association (APHA) President, Godfrey requests Congress to establish a national accident prevention program.
1942	In *War Medicine,* Hugh De Haven publishes his research on survival of falls and reports that it is not fate that someone dies or is injured but width of seat belt and distance from front of airplane.
1943	APHA Committee on Administrative Practice appoints a Subcommittee on "Accident" Prevention.
1945	APHA Subcommittee on "Accident" Prevention develops program guidelines for accident prevention.
1946	U.S. Public Health Service establishes home accident prevention program staffer.
1949	John E. Gordon formalizes concept that epidemiology could be used as a theoretic foundation for accident prevention.

[1]Archivist, Injury Control and Emergency Health Services Section of the American Public Health Association and Safety/Leadership Consultant.

[2]Department of Epidemiology, University of North Carolina Injury Prevention Research Center, University of North Carolina at Chapel Hill.

[3]Special thanks to the Children's Safety Network for their contributions. For detailed reviews, references, and more information for these and other landmarks, see Mr. Fisher's Archivist Attics in newsletter commentaries (at http:// HYPERLINK "http://www.icehs.org" www.icehs.org and at http://extranet.icehs.org). Additional information can be found in his Shaping the Millennium: A History of Child and Home Injury Prevention With Applications to Leadership Systems, a copyrighted historiography, with related archives posted for parts 1–7, at: http://www.apha.org/membergroups/sections/aphasections/icehs/ecommunity.

1950 American Academy of Pediatrics forms Committee on "Accident" Prevention and Poison Control.
1955 R.A. McFarland publishes Epidemiological Principles Applicable to the Study and Prevention of Child Accidents in the *American Journal of Public Health.*
1956 First annual Stapp conference on the biomechanics of crashes.
1957 APHA policy statement urges health agencies to assume an active role in all types of "accident" prevention programs.
1959 Insurance Institute for Highway Safety founded.
1960 APHA publishes public policy statement recommending that "accident" prevention be recognized as a major public health problem.
The Public Health Service funds hundreds of accident prevention staff and diverse program sections within the Division of State Services.
1961 APHA publishes *Accident Prevention: The Role of Physicians and Public Health Workers.*
Operations Research, Bethesda, Maryland, recommends a comprehensive, well-funded accident control program.
Journal of Trauma begins publication.
James J. Gibson publishes theory that injuries are caused by energy exchange.
1963 William Haddon, Jr. publishes "injury matrix" concept article.
1964 Injury Prevention training offered in 11 schools of Public Health.
1965 Ralph Nader publishes *Unsafe at Any Speed.*
1966 National Highway Safety Bureau (later named the "National Highway Traffic Safety Administration") is established to set car safety standards in 1968.
National Research Council report is published: *Accidental Death and Disability: The Neglected Disease of Modern Society.*
1968 Congress passes the Federal Gun Control Act.
American Trauma Association is established.
Lap belts in all seated occupants are installed by the four major manufacturers of U.S. automobiles.
1969 *Accident Analysis and Prevention* and the *Journal of Safety Research* begin publication.
1970 The Federal Poison Prevention Packaging Act is passed.
National Institutes on Alcohol Abuse and Alcoholism is established.
National Institute for Occupational Safety and Health is established.
1972 The Federal Flammable Clothing Act is passed.
Consumer Product Safety Commission is established.
1973 Emergency Medical Services Act passes U.S. Congress.
National Center on Child Abuse and Neglect is established.
1974 General Motors produces first air bag.
Congress mandates 55 mph national maximum speed limit.
National Association of Governor's Highway Traffic Safety Representatives is established.
1976 National Emergency Medical Services/Poison Control Center law passes with limited funding.
1978 U.S. state of Tennessee first worldwide to mandate child passenger safety law.
U.S. Remove Intoxicated Drivers is established.
1979 Federal Division of Maternal and Child Health of the U.S. Department of Health and Human Services is established (designated as a Bureau later).
Promoting Health/Preventing Disease: Objectives for the Nation is published.
Centers for Disease Control and Prevention (CDC) establishes a violence epidemiology branch to track incidence of interpersonal violence.
1980 First population-based and emergency department-based injury surveillance system is implemented in two states.
Mothers Against Drunk Driving is established.

American Academy of Pediatrics publishes *Handbook on Accident Prevention.*

1981 First National Conference on Injury Control, sponsored by the Johns Hopkins University and CDC.

1982 CDC publishes *Injury Control Implementation Plan for State and Local Governments.*

1983 Maternal and Child Health Bureau publishes *Developing Childhood Injury Prevention Programs: An Administrative Guide for Maternal and Child Health (Title V) Programs.*

1984 Congress establishes the Emergency Medical Services for Children program.

New York State enacts first U.S. seat belt law.

Contra Costa County, California, adopts fencing ordinance for new swimming pools.

1985 Every state has passed legislation requiring the use of child safety seats.

Injury in America: A Continuing Public Health Problem is published by the Committee on Trauma Research.

Surgeon General's workshop on "Violence and Public Health."

1986 CDC awards five academic centers $2 million to address research on injuries.

Maternal and Child Health Bureau awards demonstration funding to address violence prevention.

Minimum Drinking Age is passed by Congress.

1987 Launch of the National Safe Kids Campaign.

First Injury in America Conference (a partnership with CDC and National Highway Traffic Safety Administration).

1988 *Injury Control,* a follow-up to *Injury in America,* is published.

CDC establishes the National Center for Injury Prevention and Control.

Surgeon General's workshop on drunk driving.

The Future of Public Health is released by the Institute of Medicine.

1989 *Release of Cost of Injury,* a report to Congress.

Injury Prevention: Meeting the Challenge is published as a supplement to the *American Journal of Preventive Medicine.*

1990 *Healthy People 2000: National Health Promotion and Disease Prevention Objectives* report is published.

External Cause of Injury coding (E-coding) is mandated by six states.

1991 World Health Organization (WHO) Helmet initiative begins.

Rosenberg JL, Fenley MA. *Violence in America: A Public Health Approach.* New York: Oxford University Press.

1992 California Wellness Foundation begins a 5-year Violence Prevention Initiative.

1993 President Clinton declares violence to be a public health emergency.

Injury Control in the 1990s: A National Plan for Action is published.

1995 The journal *Injury Prevention* begins publication.

1997 E-coding mandated in 17 states.

Institute of Medicine National Committee on Injury Prevention and Control holds public meeting in Washington, DC.

1998 CDC's Tenth Anniversary of the National Center for Injury Prevention and Control (with a timeline).

1999 Bonnie RJ, Fulco CE, Liverman CT, editors. *Reducing the Burden of Injury: Advancing Prevention and Treatment.* Published (with a timeline) by the Committee on Injury Prevention and Control, Division of Health Promotion and Disease Prevention, Institute of Medicine.

National Violent Injury Statistics System is funded, a precursor of the National Violent Death Reporting System (NVDRS).

2000 California is the first state to pass a booster seat law for children.

CDC publishes *Best Practices of Youth Violence Prevention: A Sourcebook for Community Action.*

U.S. Consumer Product Safety Commission expands the National Electronic Injury Surveillance System to include an All Injury Program.

2001 Funding of National Poison Control Center Enhancement Act.

National Strategies for Suicide Prevention: Goals and Objectives for Action is published by the U.S. Department of Health and Human Services.

School health guidelines to prevent unintentional injuries and violence. Published by *MMWR.* Dec. 7, 2001, No. RR-22.

First congressional appropriations for child maltreatment are approved.

2002 Goldsmith SK, Pellmar TC, Kleinman AM, Bunney WE, eds. *Reducing Suicide.* Published by Committee on Pathophysiology and Prevention of Adolescent Suicides. A National Imperative. Institute of Medicine of the National Academies.

World Report on Violence and Health is published by WHO, Geneva, Switzerland.

U.S. National Electronic Injury Surveillance System-Cooperative Adverse Drug Events Surveillance System is created.

Congress makes its first appropriation to the CDC for NVDRS, which was funded in six states: Massachusetts, Maryland, New Jersey, Oregon, South Carolina, and Virginia.

2003 Baldessarini RJ, Tondo L. Suicide risk and treatments for patients with bipolar disorder. *JAMA.* 2003; 290:1467–1473; Editorial, Ibid, 1517–1519. Linkage between Rx drugs and intentional injury is published.

Child Abuse Prevention and Treatment Act enacted as amended by the Keeping Children and Families Safe Act of 2003, Department of Health and Human Services.

2004 *Forging a Poison Prevention and Control System.* Committee on Poison Prevention and Control. Board on Health Promotion and Disease Prevention. Published by Institute of Medicine of the National Academies of Sciences, Washington, DC.

President Bush signs Suicide Prevention Law, November 2004.

Firearms and Violence is published by National Academy of Sciences, Washington, DC.

World Report on Road Traffic Injury Prevention is published by WHO, Geneva, Switzerland.

Creation of the Violence Prevention Alliance. WHO, CDC, and a global consortium of organizations.

The NVDRS is expanded to include 17 states.

2005 Asia's tsunamis and follow-up public health/injury control responses.

Core Competencies for Injury and Violence Prevention are defined.

TEACH-VIP Training and Capacity Building Initiative is published by WHO, Geneva, Switzerland.

Child and Adolescent Injury Prevention: A Global Call to Action is published by WHO, UNICEF.

2006 United Nations Secretary General's Report on Violence against Children.

Child and Adolescent Injury Prevention: A WHO Plan of Action is published by WHO, Geneva, Switzerland.

Preventing Child Maltreatment: A Guide to Taking Action and Generating Evidence is published by WHO and International Society for the Prevention of Child Abuse and Neglect.

CDC launches Choose Respect, the first national communication initiative designed to prevent unhealthy relationship behaviors and dating abuse.

2007 CDC publishes a study that estimates the cost of violence in the United States exceeds $70 billion each year.

Youth and Road Safety is published by WHO, Geneva, Switzerland.

The National Violence Prevention Network is formally established to increase federal funding for NVDRS to expand the program to all 50 states by 2011.

2008 *World Report on Child Injury Prevention* is published by WHO, Geneva, Switzerland.
20th Anniversary of the National Center for Injury Prevention and Control at CDC.

2009 First Global Ministerial Conference on Road Safety, Moscow, Russia.
Special issue of the *Bulletin of the World Health Organization* focusing on childhood injuries and violence. Volume 87, Number 5, May 2009, 325–404.

2010 TEACH-VIP E-Learning, WHO, and Educational Development Center developed.

2011 Sleet DA, Dahlberg LL, Basavaraju, SV, et al. 2011. Injury prevention, violence prevention, and trauma care: building the scientific base. MMWR 60(Suppl.): 78–85. Published in supplement *Public Health Then and Now: Celebrating 50 Years of MMWR at CDC* (http://www.cdc.gov/mmwr/pdf/other/su6004.pdf).

2011 The United Nations launches The Decade of Action for Road Safety 2011–2020.

Appendix B

Resources

Updates by Si-won Jang

The resources listed here were derived from many sources. Although the list is not meant to be exhaustive, these resources should assist the reader in learning more about injury prevention resources and materials.

I. Funding Resources

Various funding opportunities are available to support injury prevention and control research and programs. Visit these Web sites to learn more about a variety of funding opportunities:

• Centers for Disease Control and Prevention Funding Opportunities
http://www.cdc.gov/od/pgo/funding/grants/grantmain.shtm
• Centers for Disease Control and Prevention's National Center for Injury Prevention and Control
http://www.cdc.gov/ncipc/ncipchm.htm
• Community of Science, Inc.
http://www.cos.com
• Directory of Charitable Grantmakers
http://www.foundations.org
• FundsnetServices.com
http://www.fundsnetservices.com
• Grants.gov
http://www.grants.gov
• National Institutes of Health Grants Database
http://grants.nih.gov/grants/oer.htm
• Robert Wood Johnson Foundation
http://www.rwjf.org
• Shaping America's Youth Funding Opportunities
http://www.shapingamericasyouth.org/programs.aspx?page=featured
• Small Business Innovative Research
http://www.sba.gov/category/navigation-structure/loans-grants/grants
• The Foundation Center
http://www.fdncenter.org
• The Joyce Foundation
http://www.joycefdn.org
• U.S. Department of Health and Human Services' Grants Forecast
http://www.acf.hhs.gov/hhsgrantsforecast

II. Research Centers and Organizations of Interest

Note: Information for many of these organizations was directly quoted from their Web sites.

A. Centers for Disease Control and Prevention–Funded Injury Control Research Centers (as of 2011)

The Centers for Disease Control and Prevention's National Center for Injury Prevention and Control funds 11 injury control research centers around the country to conduct research and serve as both training centers for public health professionals and information centers for the public.

- Brown School's Center for Violence and Injury Prevention
http://cvip.wustl.edu/Pages/Home.aspx
- Center for Injury Research and Policy in Columbus, Ohio
http://www.nationwidechildrens.org/injury-research-and-policy
- Colorado Injury Control Research Center
http://psy.psych.colostate.edu/CICRC
- Emory Center for Injury Control
http://www.emorycenterforinjurycontrol.org
- Injury Research Center at the Medical College of Wisconsin
http://www.mcw.edu/injuryresearchcenter.htm
- San Francisco Injury Center for Research and Prevention
http://www.surgery.ucsf.edu/sfic
- The Johns Hopkins Center for Injury Research and Policy
http://www.jhsph.edu/InjuryCenter
- The Mount Sinai Injury Control Research Center
http://www.mssm.edu/research/programs/injury-control-research-center
- University of Iowa Injury Prevention Research Center
http://www.public-health.uiowa.edu/IPRC
- University of North Carolina Injury Prevention Research Center
http://www.iprc.unc.edu
- West Virginia University Injury Control Research Center
http://www.hsc.wvu.edu/icrc/index.html

B. Other Research Centers

- Alberta Centre for Injury Control and Research (Canada)
http://acicr.ca
- Center for the Prevention of School Violence
http://www.ncdjjdp.org/cpsv
- Harborview Injury Prevention Research Center
http://depts.washington.edu/hiprc
- Harvard Injury Prevention Research Center
http://www.hsph.harvard.edu/hicrc
- Injury Prevention Center at the Connecticut Children's Medical Center
http://www.connecticutchildrens.org/body_dept.cfm?id=93
- Kentucky Injury Prevention and Research Center
http://www.kiprc.uky.edu
- Monash University Accident Research Centre (Australia)
http://www.monash.edu.au/muarc
- Southern California Injury Prevention Research Center
http://www.ph.ucla.edu/sciprc
- The Center for Injury Prevention Policy and Practice at San Diego State University
http://www.cippp.org

• The University of Alabama Injury Control Research Center
http://www.uab.edu/icrc
• University of Michigan Transportation Research Institute
http://www.umtri.umich.edu/news.php
• University of Minnesota Center for Violence Prevention and Control
http://www1.umn.edu/cvpc
• University of New South Wales, Injury Risk Management Research Centre (Australia)
http://www.irmrc.unsw.edu.au
• University of Otago Injury Prevention and Research Unit (New Zealand)
http://www.otago.ac.nz/ipru
• UT Health Science Center Injury Prevention Program
http://www.injury.uthscsa.edu

C. Organizations of Interest

• AAA Foundation for Traffic Safety
http://www.aaafoundation.org
The AAA Foundation for Traffic Safety is a not-for-profit, publicly supported charitable educational and research organization. Its mission is to identify problems, foster research that seeks solutions, and disseminate information and educational materials that promote good traffic safety practices.
• Advancement of Automotive Medicine
http://www.carcrash.org
The Association for the Advancement of Automotive Medicine is a professional multidisciplinary organization dedicated entirely to motor vehicle crash injury prevention and control.
• American Academy of Pediatrics: Section on Injury, Violence, and Poison Prevention
http://www.aap.org/sections/ipp
The Section on Injury, Violence, and Poison Prevention educates the general pediatrician and pediatric subspecialist on the prevention of injuries, violence, and poisonings. In addition, the Section consults to the American Academy of Pediatrics (AAP) Board of Directors on related issues and works with the AAP Committee on Injury, Violence, and Poison Prevention to provide comments on official AAP policy in this area.
• American Association of Poison Control Centers
http://www.aapcc.org
The American Association of Poison Control Centers is a nonprofit, national organization founded in 1958 that represents the poison control centers of the United States and the interests of poison prevention and treatment of poisoning.
• American Association of Suicidology
http://www.suicidology.org
The American Association of Suicidology (AAS) is a membership organization for all those involved in suicide prevention and intervention, or touched by suicide. The goal of the AAS is to understand and prevent suicide through research, education, and training; the development of standards and resources; and survivor support services.
• American Burn Association
http://www.ameriburn.org
The American Burn Association and its members dedicate their efforts and resources to promoting and supporting burn-related research, education, care, rehabilitation, and prevention. Members include physicians, nurses, occupational and physical therapists, researchers, social workers, firefighters, and hospitals with burn centers.

- American Foundation for Suicide Prevention
http://www.afsp.org
The Suicide Prevention Action Network USA (SPAN USA) has merged with American Foundation for Suicide Prevention (AFSP) in 2009 to create a public policy program within the Foundation. This program is dedicated to preventing suicide through public education and awareness, community engagement, and federal, state and local grassroots advocacy.
- American Public Health Association–Injury Control and Emergency Health Services Section
http://www.icehs.org
The American Public Health Association–Injury Control and Emergency Health Services Section provides a forum through which to establish and strengthen relationships with colleagues working to advance the field of injury control, violence prevention, emergency health services, and emergency preparedness.
- American Spinal Injury Association
http://www.asia-spinalinjury.org
The American Spinal Injury Association (ASIA) has developed an Internet Web site to provide information and education about spinal cord injury to ASIA members and to the general public. Among its objectives, ASIA aims to foster research that strives to prevent spinal cord injury, improve care, reduce consequent disability, and find a cure for both acute and chronic spinal cord injury.
- American Trauma Society
http://www.amtrauma.org
The American Trauma Society is dedicated to the prevention of trauma and improvement of trauma care. Their goals include fostering legislative and financial support for trauma care, trauma systems development, and injury prevention; creating a greater awareness of trauma and trauma care throughout the community; and instilling a greater awareness of trauma and trauma care throughout the community.
- Bicycle Helmet Safety Institute
http://www.bhsi.org
The Bicycle Helmet Safety Institute is a small, active, nonprofit, consumer-funded program for bicycle helmet information. Through their Web site, the Bike Helmet Safety Institute tries to explain the technology of helmets to consumers and promote better helmets through improved standards.
- Brain Injury Association of America
http://www.biausa.org
Founded in 1980, the Brain Injury Association of America (BIAA) is a national organization serving and representing individuals, families, and professionals who are touched by a life-altering, often devastating, traumatic brain injury. The BIAA provides information, education, and support to assist the 3.17 million Americans currently living with traumatic brain injury and their families.
- The Burn and Shock Trauma Institute of Loyola Institute
http://www.stritch.luc.edu/burn_shock/
The Burn and Shock Trauma Institute of Loyola University is a community of scientists and clinicians devoted to the study of traumatic injury. This is a multidisciplinary research institute, whose programs include both clinical and laboratory research relevant to trauma injury and burns. In the laboratories, scientists investigate the body's reaction to injury and infection, with the hope that their research findings may someday lead to innovative therapies for trauma and burn patients.
- California Injury Prevention Network
http://www.injurypreventionnetwork.org
The California Injury Prevention Network (CIPN) is a group of individuals and organizations working to advance childhood injury prevention programs and efforts throughout California. The CIPN Web site provides a unique collection of resources for both new and experienced

professionals in childhood injury prevention. The CIPN promotes professional growth and leadership skills via online tools, resources, and training opportunities.

• Canadian Hospitals Injury Reporting and Prevention Program, Child Injury Division (Canada)
http://www.phac-aspc.gc.ca/injury-bles/chirpp/index-eng.php
Canadian Hospitals Injury Reporting and Prevention Program is a computerized information system that collects and analyzes data on injuries to people (mainly children) who are seen at the emergency departments of ten pediatric hospitals and four general hospitals in Canada.

• CDC Injury and Violence Prevention and Control
http://www.cdc.gov/injury
The National Center for Injury Prevention and Control, as part of the Centers for Disease Control and Prevention, works to prevent injuries and violence and reduce their consequences.

• Child Passenger Safety
http://childcarsafety.adcouncil.org
The Child Passenger Safety Web site provides resources for parents, including video instructions for child safety seats, information about car seat inspection centers, and child passenger safety tips linked with the National Highway Traffic Safety Administration.

• The Children's Hospital of Philadelphia–Kohl's Injury Prevention Program
http://www.chop.edu/service/injury-prevention-program/injury-prevention-information
The Kohl's Injury Prevention Program at The Children's Hospital of Philadelphia is dedicated to preventing injuries in children through educating families about safety and offering safety devices to increase safety practices in the community.

• Children's Safety Network
http://www.childrenssafetynetwork.org
The Children's Safety Network (CSN) is a national resource center for the prevention of childhood injuries and violence. The CSN offers expertise on a wide range of injury topics to State and Territorial Maternal and Child Health and Injury and Violence Prevention programs.

• Center for Advanced Public Safety
http://care.cs.ua.edu
The CARE Research and Development Laboratory recently became the Center for Advanced Public Safety (CAPS) by a decree from the University of Alabama Board of Trustees. The mission of CAPS is to create innovative solutions through information technology research and software development to enhance the public safety and security of our state and homeland.

• Emergency Medical Services for Children National Resource Center
http://www.childrensnational.org/EMSC
The Emergency Medical Services for Children (EMSC) National Resource Center was established in 1991 to help improve the pediatric emergency care infrastructure throughout the United States and its territories. The services they provided are designed to proactively assist EMSC grantees, program partners, and family advocates in their efforts to improve all aspects of children's emergency medical care.

• European Association for Injury Prevention and Safety Promotion
http://www.eurosafe.eu.com/csi/eurosafe.nsf/html/homepage/$file/index.htm
The European Association for Injury Prevention and Safety Promotion (EuroSafe) builds on the foundation of the former ECOSA, bringing together the various injury areas and profiling the overall burden of injury and the challenges of safety promotion within national and European policies.

• Futures Without Violence
http://www.futureswithoutviolence.org/
Futures Without Violence, formerly Family Violence Prevention Fund, works to prevent and end violence against women and children around the world. They train professionals such as doctors, nurses, athletic coaches, and judges on improving responses to violence and abuse. They also work

with advocates, policy makers and others to build sustainable community leadership and educate people everywhere about the importance of respect and healthy relationships.

• FIA Foundation (United Kingdom)
http://www.fiafoundation.org
The FIA Foundation is an independent U.K.-registered charity that manages and supports an international program of activities promoting road safety, environmental protection, and sustainable mobility, as well as funding specialist motor sport safety research. The Make Roads Safe (http://www.makeroadssafe.org) campaign is one of the initiatives coordinated by the FIA Foundation to promote road safety.

• Foundation for Spinal Cord Injury Prevention, Care & Cure
http://www.fscip.org
The Foundation for Spinal Cord Injury Prevention, Care & Cure is a nonprofit educational group dedicated to the prevention, care, and cure of spinal cord injuries through public awareness, education, and funding research.

• Governors Highway Safety Association
http://www.ghsa.org
The Governors Highway Safety Association (GHSA) represents the state and territorial highway safety offices that implement programs to address behavioral highway safety issues, including occupant protection, impaired driving, and speeding. The GHSA provides leadership and representation for the states to improve traffic safety, influence national policy, and enhance program management.

• Home Safety Council
http://www.homesafetycouncil.org
The Home Safety Council (HSC) is a national nonprofit organization solely dedicated to preventing home-related injuries. Through national programs, partnerships, and the support of volunteers, the HSC educates people of all ages to be safer in and around their homes.

• Honouring Life Network (Canada)
http://www.honouringlife.ca
The Honouring Life Network is a project of the National Aboriginal Health Organization. The Web site offers culturally relevant information and resources on suicide prevention to help Aboriginal youths and youth workers dealing with a problem that has reached crisis proportions in some First Nations, Inuit, and Métis communities in Canada.

• Indian Health Service American Indian and Alaska Native Suicide Prevention Web site
http://www.ihs.gov/NonMedicalPrograms/nspn
The purpose of the Indian Health Service's Community Suicide Prevention Web site is to provide American Indian and Alaska Native communities with culturally appropriate information about best and promising practices, training opportunities, and other relevant information regarding suicide prevention and intervention. The goal of the Web site is to provide Native communities with the tools and information to create, or adapt to, their own suicide prevention programs.

• Indian Health Service Injury Prevention Program
http://www.ihs.gov/MedicalPrograms/InjuryPrevention/index.cfm
The mission of the Indian Health Service Injury Prevention Program is to raise the health status of American Indians and Alaska Natives to the highest possible level by decreasing the incidence of severe injuries and death to the lowest possible level and increasing the ability of tribes to address their injury problems. Their Web site provides information on injury prevention programs, training courses, and related articles and publications.

• Injury Free Coalition for Kids
http://www.injuryfree.org

The Injury Free Coalition for Kids is composed of hospital-based, community-oriented programs, whose efforts are anchored in research, education, and advocacy. Currently, the coalition includes 42 sites located in 40 cities, each housed in the trauma centers of their participating institutions.

• Insurance Institute for Highway Safety
http://www.highwaysafety.org
The Insurance Institute for Highway Safety is an independent, nonprofit, scientific, and educational organization dedicated to reducing the losses—deaths, injuries, and property damage—from crashes on the nation's highways. The institute is wholly supported by auto insurers.

• International Bullying Prevention Association
http://www.stopbullyingworld.org
The mission of the International Bullying Prevention Association is to support and enhance quality research-based bullying prevention principles and practices to achieve a safe school climate, healthy work environment, good citizenship, and civic responsibility.

•International Collaborative Effort on Injury Statistics
http://www.cdc.gov/nchs/injury/advice.htm
The International Collaborative Effort on Injury Statistics is one of several international activities sponsored by the Centers for Disease Control and Prevention's National Center for Health Statistics. The goal is to provide a forum for international exchange and collaboration among injury researchers who develop and promote international standards in injury data collection and analysis.

• International Society for Child and Adolescent Injury Prevention
http://www.iscaip.net
In 1993, the International Society for Child and Adolescent Injury Prevention was created with a goal to promote a significant reduction in the number and severity of injuries to children and adolescents through international collaboration. Both unintentional injury and violence are addressed by the Society. The objectives of the Society are to (1) provide a multidisciplinary forum for global dialogue; (2) assist in providing advocacy at national and international levels; (3) foster national and international injury prevention initiatives; (4) stimulate the translation of research findings into programs and policies; and (5) facilitate collaborative and interdisciplinary international research.

• International Traffic Medicine Association
http://www.trafficmedicine.org
Founded in 1960 as the International Association for Accident and Traffic Medicine, the International Traffic Medicine Association works to promote and develop the study of traffic medicine in all transport modes.

• Means Matter
http://www.hsph.harvard.edu/means-matter
The Means Matter Campaign was launched by the Harvard Injury Control Research Center and is funded by The Joyce Foundation and the David Bohnett Foundation. The mission of the Means Matter Campaign is to increase the proportion of suicide prevention groups that promote ways to reduce suicidal persons' access to lethal means of suicide.

• National Alliance for Safe Schools
http://www.safeschools.org
The National Alliance for Safe Schools was founded in 1977 as a not-for-profit corporation whose purpose is to provide technical assistance, staff training, school safety assessments, safe school plans, and emergency response training to individual school and school district personnel.

• National Center for Statistics and Analysis of the National Highway Traffic Safety Administration—State Data Program & Crash Outcome Data Evaluation System
http://www.nhtsa.gov/Data/State+Data+Program+&+CODES
The State Data Program (SDP) supports NHTSA's efforts to identify traffic safety problems, help develop and implement vehicle and driver countermeasures, evaluate motor vehicle standards, and

to study crash avoidance issues, crashworthiness issues, and regulations. The Crash Outcome Data Evaluation System (CODES) is a collaborative approach to generating medical and financial outcome information relating to motor vehicle crashes and using this outcome-based data as the basis for decisions related to highway traffic safety.

• National Center on Shaken Baby Syndrome
http://www.dontshake.com
The National Center on Shaken Baby Syndrome focuses their efforts in two areas: professional training for those who work with shaken baby syndrome/abusive head trauma cases and prevention education for parents and those who work to prevent child abuse.

• National Children's Center for Rural and Agricultural Health and Safety
http://research.marshfieldclinic.org/children
The center is dedicated to enhancing the health and safety of all children exposed to hazards associated with agricultural work and rural environments.

• National Fire Protection Association
http://www.nfpa.org
The mission of the international nonprofit National Fire Protection Association, established in 1896, is to reduce the worldwide burden of fire and other hazards on the quality of life by providing and advocating consensus codes and standards, research, training, and education.

• National Highway Traffic Safety Administration
http://www.nhtsa.gov
The National Highway Traffic Safety Administration (NHTSA) was established by the Highway Safety Act of 1970 to carry out safety programs previously administered by the National Highway Safety Bureau. Dedicated to achieving the highest standards of excellence in motor vehicle and highway safety, the NHTSA works daily to help prevent crashes and their attendant costs, both human and financial.

• National Maternal and Child Health Center for Child Death Review
http://www.childdeathreview.org
The National Center for Child Death Review is a resource center for state and local Child Death Review programs, funded by the Maternal and Child Health Bureau. It promotes supports and enhances child death review methodology and activities at the state, community, and national levels.

• National Organizations for Youth Safety
http://www.noys.org
National Organizations for Youth Safety (NOYS) is a collaborative network of national organizations and federal agencies that serve youths and focus on youth safety and health. NOYS was created in 1994 as a coalition of national nonprofit organizations and federal agencies to promote collaboration of youth member and youth-serving organizations and agencies. Through this network, NOYS influences more than 80 million young people, aged 5 to 24 years, and adult advisors.

• National Program for Playground Safety
http://www.uni.edu/playground
The mission of the National Program for Playground Safety is to help the public create safe and developmentally appropriate play environments for children.

• National Safety Council
http://www.nsc.org
The National Safety Council's mission is to save lives by preventing injuries and deaths at work, in homes and communities, and on the roads, through leadership, research, education, and advocacy.

• National Youth Sports Safety Foundation
http://www.health.gov/nhic/nhicscripts/Entry.cfm?HRCode=HR2693

The National Youth Sports Safety Foundation is a national nonprofit, educational organization dedicated to reducing the number and severity of injuries that youths sustain in sports and fitness activities.

• Operation Lifesaver
http://www.oli.org
Operation Lifesaver is a nonprofit, international continuing public education program first established in 1972 to end collisions, deaths, and injuries at places where roadways cross train tracks and on railroad rights-of-way.

• Partnership Against Domestic Violence
http://www.padv.org
Partnership Against Domestic Violence works to end domestic violence by offering safety and shelter for battered women and their children; restoring power, self-sufficiency, and control to domestic violence survivors; and educating the public on the dynamics of domestic violence.

• Pedestrian and Bicycle Information Center
http://www.bicyclinginfo.org
The Pedestrian and Bicycle Information Center (PBIC) provides information about health and safety, engineering, advocacy, education, enforcement, access, and mobility for pedestrians (including transit users) and bicyclists. The PBIC serves anyone interested in pedestrian and bicycle issues, including planners, engineers, private citizens, advocates, educators, police enforcement, and the health community.

• Prevent Child Abuse America
http://www.preventchildabuse.org
Since 1972, Prevent Child Abuse America (PCA America) has been focused on building awareness, providing education, and inspiring hope to everyone involved in the effort to prevent the abuse and neglect of our nation's children. Based in Chicago, PCA America has chapters in 47 states and more than 400 Healthy Families America sites in 41 states.

• Preventing Violence Through Education, Networking, and Technical Assistance
http://http://www.prevent.unc.edu
The mission of the Preventing Violence through Education, Networking, and Technical Assistance (PREVENT) program is to enhance national capacity of practitioners, leaders, and their organizations to prevent violence through effective education, networks, and technical assistance.

• Research Centre for Injury Studies (Australia)
http://http://www.nisu.flinders.edu.au/index.php
The Research Centre's mission is to contribute to reducing the burden of human injury and adding to knowledge of its nature, causes, effects, and control. To do this, staff of the Centre undertake research, surveillance, analysis, consultation, and teaching, and disseminate information on injury control and related matters to public health and other practitioners, academics, government, and the community.

• Safe Communities America
http://www.safecommunitiesamerica.org
Founded in 1913, and chartered by the U.S. Congress in 1953, the National Safety Council is a not-for-profit, public service, mission-based organization committed to educating and influencing people to prevent accidental injury and death. Safe Communities America, a program of The National Safety Council, is the Safe Communities Affiliate Support Center and a Certifying Center for the World Health Organization Collaborating Center.

• Safe Communities Canada
http://www.safecommunities.ca
Safe Communities Canada is a national charitable organization dedicated to helping communities across the country build the capacity and resources they will need as they commit to mounting

coordinated, collaborative programs designed to reduce the pain and cost of injury and promote a culture of safety for all their citizens.

• SafeKids Worldwide

http://www.safekids.org/worldwide/?gclid=CMK_1KuA3qkCFYfs7Qode2EEaQSafe Kids Worldwide is a global network of organizations with a mission of preventing unintentional childhood injury, a leading cause of death and disability for children ages 14 and under.

• SafetyBeltSafe U.S.A.

http://www.carseat.org

SafetyBeltSafe U.S.A. is a national, nonprofit organization dedicated to child passenger safety. Their mission is to help reduce the number of serious and fatal traffic injuries suffered by children by promoting the correct, consistent use of safety seats and safety belts.

• SafetyLit.org

http://www.safetylit.org

The purpose of SafetyLit is to provide SafetyLit users with information to allow users to identify and find material that has been published about injury prevention and safety promotion topics. Their weekly *SafetyLit Update Bulletin* provides abstracts of English language reports from researchers who work in the more than 30 professional disciplines relevant to preventing unintentional injuries, violence, and self-harm. The database exceeded 100,000 items in June 2009.

• Safe Ride News

http://www.saferidenews.com

The goals of Safe Ride News publications are to help save lives and prevent injury to children in traffic. Safe Ride News does this primarily by developing accurate and up-to-date information on injury prevention for professionals, advocates, and parents. They also advocate for improved standards, laws, and programs related to childhood injury prevention by supporting and collaborating with other organizations and agencies working in this field.

•Safe States Alliance

http://safestates.org

The Safe States Alliance (formerly the State and Territorial Injury Prevention Directors Association) is a national nonprofit membership organization whose mission is to serve as the national voice in support of state and local injury and violence prevention professionals engaged in building a safer, healthier America.

• Society for the Advancement for Violence and Injury Research

http://www.savirweb.org

The mission of the Society for the Advancement for Violence and Injury Research is to promote scholarly activity in the prevention, control, acute care, and rehabilitation of intentional and unintentional injury.

• Striving to Reduce Youth Violence Everywhere

http://www.safeyouth.gov

Striving to Reduce Youth Violence Everywhere (STRYVE) is a national initiative led by the Centers for Disease Control and Prevention to prevent youth violence before it starts among young people aged 10 to 24 years. STRYVE's vision is safe and healthy youths who can achieve their full potential as connected and contributing members of thriving, violence-free families, schools, and communities.

• Suicide Prevention Resource Center

http://www.sprc.org

The Suicide Prevention Resource Center is a national resource center offering training; information; resources; a best practices registry; information for states, tribes, and campuses; and a comprehensive library dedicated to suicide prevention. It provides prevention support, training, and resources to assist organizations and individuals to develop suicide prevention programs, interventions, and policies, and to advance the National Strategy for Suicide Prevention.

• Temple University Fall Prevention Project
http://www.temple.edu/older_adult
Fall Prevention in Older Adults is a federally funded grant project. The project objective is to inform and educate older adults about the causes of falls in older adults, and the assessment, rehabilitative, and health promotion measures that can be taken to reduce the risk of falls.
• ThinkFirst National Injury Prevention Foundation (formally known as the National Health and Spinal Cord Injury Prevention Program)
http://www.thinkfirst.org
ThinkFirst programs educate young people about their personal vulnerability and the importance of making safe choices. Their mission is to lead injury prevention through education, research, and policy.
• U.S. Consumer Product Safety Commission
http://www.cpsc.gov/about/about.html
The U.S. Consumer Product Safety Commission (CPSC) is charged with protecting the public from unreasonable risks of serious injury or death from thousands of types of consumer products under the agency's jurisdiction. The CPSC is committed to protecting consumers and families from products that pose a fire, electrical, chemical, or mechanical hazard or that can injure children.
• Violence and Injury Control Through Education, Networking, and Training on the World Wide Web
http://www.ibiblio.org/vincentweb
This free introductory course on injury prevention and control contains material from the June 6, 1997, video conference "Getting Started in Injury Control and Violence Prevention," presented in a Web-based format that expands on and supplements the televised program.
• World Health Organization's Department of Violence and Injury Prevention
http://www.who.int/violence_injury_prevention/en
The World Health Organization's Department of Violence and Injury Prevention works to prevent injuries and violence, to mitigate their consequences, and to enhance the quality of life for persons with disabilities irrespective of the causes.
• World Health Organization's Helmet Initiative (WhoHelmets.org)
http://www.whohelmets.org
The World Health Organization's Helmet Initiative promotes the use of helmets as a strategy for preventing head injuries caused by bicycle or motorcycle crash or fall.

III. Data Sources of Interest

• CDC WONDER
http://wonder.cdc.gov
CDC WONDER, developed by the Centers for Disease Control and Prevention (CDC), is an integrated information and communication system for public health. It provides access to statistical research data published by the CDC, as well as reference materials, reports, and guidelines on health-related topics, including public-use data sets about mortality (deaths), cancer incidence, HIV and AIDS, tuberculosis, vaccinations, natality (births), and census data.
• Fatality Analysis Reporting System
http://www.nhtsa.gov/FARS
The Fatality Analysis Reporting System (FARS) includes information about motor vehicle traffic crashes that result in fatality to a vehicle occupant or nonmotorist as the result of injuries in a traffic crash that occurred within 30 days of the crash. FARS contains data on all fatal traffic crashes within the 50 states, the District of Columbia, and Puerto Rico. The data system was conceived, designed, and developed by the National Center for Statistics and Analysis to assist the traffic safety

community in identifying traffic safety problems, developing and implementing vehicle and driver countermeasures, and evaluating motor vehicle safety standards and highway safety initiatives.

• Morbidity and Mortality Weekly Report
http://www.cdc.gov/mmwr
The *Morbidity and Mortality Weekly Report (MMWR)* series prepared by the Centers for Disease Control and Prevention (CDC) provide scientific publication of timely, reliable, authoritative, accurate, objective, and useful public health information and recommendations. *MMWR* readership predominantly consists of physicians, nurses, public health practitioners, epidemiologists and other scientists, researchers, educators, and laboratorians. The data in the weekly *MMWR* are provisional, based on weekly reports to the CDC by state health departments.

• National Automotive Sampling System
http://www.nhtsa.gov/NASS
The National Automotive Sampling System is composed of two systems: the Crashworthiness Data System (CDS) and the General Estimates System (GES). These are based on cases selected from a sample of police crash reports. CDS data focus on passenger vehicle crashes and are used to investigate injury mechanisms to identify potential improvements in vehicle design. GES data focus on the bigger overall crash picture and are used for problem size assessments and tracking trends.

• National Center for Injury Prevention and Control
http://www.cdc.gov/injury
The National Center for Injury Prevention and Control works to reduce morbidity, disability, mortality, and costs associated with injuries. The site offers links to injury data in a variety of formats, including vital statistics, the National Electronic Injury Surveillance System All Injury Program (which includes data on all emergency department injuries, not just those related to consumer products), and international data information. The Web-based Injury Statistics Query and Reporting System (WISQARS) is the Injury Center's interactive, online database that provides customized injury-related mortality data and nonfatal injury data.

• The National Electronic Injury Surveillance System
http://www.cpsc.gov/library/neiss.html
The National Electronic Injury Surveillance System is composed of a sample of hospitals that are statistically representative of hospital emergency departments nationwide. From the data collected, estimates can be made of the numbers of injuries associated with consumer products and treated in hospital emergency departments. Data are collected on a broad range of injury-related issues, covering hundreds of product categories, and provide national estimates of the number and severity of product-related injuries.

• Youth Risk Behavior Surveillance System
http://www.cdc.gov/HealthyYouth/yrbs/index.htm
The Youth Risk Behavior Surveillance System (YRBSS) monitors priority health-risk behaviors and the prevalence of obesity and asthma among youths and young adults. The YRBSS includes a national school-based survey conducted by the Centers for Disease Control and Prevention and state, territorial, tribal, and district surveys conducted by state, territorial, and local education and health agencies and tribal governments.

The following data files can be accessed by contacting the U.S. Consumer Product Safety Commission (CPSC; info@cpsc.gov).

• Death Certificate File
Death certificates in which consumer products are involved are provided to the CPSC through state health departments. The Clearinghouse provides summaries of these, with victim information removed.

• In-Depth Investigations File
The In-Depth Investigations file contains CPSC summaries of reports of investigations into events surrounding product-related injuries or incidents. According to the victim/witness

interviews, the reports provide details about incident sequence, human behavior, and product involvement.

• Injury/Potential Injury Incident File

The Injury/Potential Injury Incident File contains summaries, indexed by consumer product, of hotline reports, product-related newspaper accounts, reports from medical examiners, and letters to the CPSC.

IV. Selected Journals of Interest

The journals listed in this section publish articles relating primarily to injury. However, there are many journals that do not focus on injury but publish articles related to the field. A fairly comprehensive list is available at the SafetyLit Web site (http://www.safetylit.org/week/journals.php).

• *Accident Analysis and Prevention*
Elsevier Science
http://www.sciencedirect.com/science/journal/00014575
• *Aggressive Behavior*
Wiley-Liss
http://www.interscience.wiley.com/jpages/0096-140X
• *Aggression and Violent Behavior*
Elsevier Science
http://www.sciencedirect.com/science/journal/13591789
• *Archives of Suicide Research*
Taylor & Francis Group
http://www.tandf.co.uk/journals/titles/13811118.asp
• *Australasian Journal of Disaster and Trauma Studies*
Massey University, New Zealand
http://www.massey.ac.nz/~trauma
• *Brain Injury*
Informa Healthcare
http://informahealthcare.com/bij
• *Burns*
Elsevier Science
http://www.sciencedirect.com/science/journal/03054179
• *Child Abuse and Neglect*
Elsevier Science
http://www.elsevier.com/wps/find/journaldescription.cws_home/586/description#description
• *Crime and Delinquency*
Sage Publishing
http://cad.sagepub.com
• *Disaster Management and Response*
Mosby
http://www.sciencedirect.com/science/journal/15402487
• *Fire Safety Journal*
Elsevier Science
http://www.elsevier.com/wps/find/journaldescription.cws_home/405896/description
• *Homicide Studies*
Sage Publishing
http://hsx.sagepub.com
• *Injury Control and Safety Promotion*

Taylor & Francis
http://www.tandf.co.uk/journals/titles/17457300.asp
• *Injury Prevention*
BMJ Publishing Group
http://ip.bmjjournals.com
• *International Journal of the Care of the Injured*
Elsevier Science
http://www.elsevier.com/wps/find/journaldescription.cws_home/30428/description#description
• *Journal of Burn Care and Research*
Lippincott, Williams & Wilkins
http://www.burncarerehab.com/pt/re/jburncr/ home.htm
• *Journal of Family Violence*
Kluwer
http://www.springerlink.com/content/1573-2851
• *Journal of Interpersonal Violence*
Sage Publishing
http://jiv.sagepub.com
• *Journal of Safety Research*
Elsevier Science
http://www.sciencedirect.com/science/journal/00224375
• *Journal of School Violence*
Taylor & Francis Group
http://tandfonline.com/loi/wjsv20
• *Safety Science*
Elsevier Science
http://www.elsevier.com/wps/find/journaldescription.cws_home/505657/description#description
• *Suicide and Life-Threatening Behavior*
Wiley-Blackwell
http://onlinelibrary.wiley.com/journal/10.1111/(ISSN)1943-278X
• *Traffic Injury Prevention*
Taylor & Francis Group
http://www.tandf.co.uk/journals/titles/15389588.asp
• *Trauma, Violence, and Abuse*
Sage Publishing
http://tva.sagepub.com
• *Violence Against Women*
Sage Publishing
http://vaw.sagepub.com
• *Violence and Victims*
Springer Publishing
http://www.springerpub.com/product/08866708

VI. Related Listservs

• EPIDEMIOL-L. Epidemiology list server.
LISTPROC@CC.UMON TREAL.CA
• SAFETY list discusses safety issues, with a focus on educational institutions.
LISTSERV@UVMVM.UVM.EDU
• TRAUMA-LIST is based, moderated, and archived at TRAUMA.ORG to provide a receptacle for educational materials, sources of information, details of forthcoming events, and eventually

original articles, contributions, and articles relating to the field of trauma care. To subscribe to the trauma-list, refer to http://www.trauma.org/archive/traumalist.html.

• Suicide Prevention Resource Center Listserv
Contact info@sprc.org to subscribe.

V. Sample Social Network Sites

In addition to the Web sites listed above, social network sites provide more ways to interact with injury researchers, practitioners, and in some cases the public.

• The Children's Safety Network Communities is a social network site for state and territorial Maternal and Child Health staff and Injury and Violence Prevention staff to connect and collaborate.
http://csncommunities.ning.com

• Members of the International Society for Child and Adolescent Injury Prevention (ISCAIP) can join the Yahoo ISCAIP discussion group.
http://health.groups.yahoo.com/group/ISCAIP

• The Centers for Disease Control and Prevention Heads Up Brain Injury Awareness initiative has its Facebook site to share information with individuals who are interested in brain injury.
http://http://www.facebook.com/cdcheadsup

• The Facebook site of Safe Kids USA provides safety tips and checklists for parents, safety videos, safety quizzes, and other hands-on, useful, and interactive information to help keep kids safe from unintentional injury.
http://www.facebook.com/SafeKidsUSA

• ChildPassengerSafety Twitter posts information related to child seat safety for its followers.
http://twitter.com/childseatsafety

Appendix C

Leading Causes of Death and Nonfatal Injury

The Ten Leading Causes of Death: United States, 2007, All Races, Both Sexes

	Age Groups										
Rank	**<1 y**	**1–4 y**	**5–9 y**	**10–14 y**	**15–24 y**	**25–34 y**	**35–44 y**	**45–54 y**	**55–64 y**	**≥65 y**	**All Ages**
1	Congenital Anomalies 5785	Unintentional Injury 1588	Unintentional Injury 965	Unintentional Injury 1229	Unintentional Injury 15,897	Unintentional Injury 14,977	Unintentional Injury 16,931	Malignant Neoplasms 50,167	Malignant Neoplasms 103,171	Heart Disease 496,095	Heart Disease 616,067
2	Short Gestation 4857	Congenital Anomalies 546	Malignant Neoplasms 480	Malignant Neoplasms 479	Homicide 5551	Suicide 5278	Malignant Neoplasms 13,288	Heart Disease 37,434	Heart Disease 65,527	Malignant Neoplasms 389,730	Malignant Neoplasms 562,875
3	SIDS 2453	Homicide 398	Congenital Anomalies 196	Homicide 213	Suicide 4140	Homicide 4758	Heart Disease 11,839	Unintentional Injury 20,315	Chronic Lower Respiratory Disease 12,777	Cerebrovascular 115,961	Cerebrovascular 135,952
4	Maternal Pregnancy Complications 1769	Malignant Neoplasms 364	Homicide 133	Suicide 180	Malignant Neoplasms 1653	Malignant Neoplasms 3463	Suicide 6722	Liver Disease 8212	Unintentional Injury 12,193	Chronic Lower Respiratory Disease 109,562	Chronic Lower Respiratory Disease 127,924
5	Unintentional Injury 1285	Heart Disease 173	Heart Disease 110	Congenital Anomalies 178	Heart Disease 1084	Heart Disease 3223	HIV 3572	Suicide 7778	Diabetes Mellitus 11,304	Alzheimer's Disease 73,797	Unintentional Injury 123,706

(*continued on next page*)

(continued)

	Age Groups										
Rank	**<1 y**	**1–4 y**	**5–9 y**	**10–14 y**	**15–24 y**	**25–34 y**	**35–44 y**	**45–54 y**	**55–64 y**	**⩾65 y**	**All Ages**
6	Placenta Cord Membranes 1135	Influenza and Pneumonia 109	Chronic Lower Respiratory Disease 54	Heart Disease 131	Congenital Anomalies 402	HIV 1091	Homicide 3052	Cerebrovascular 6385	Cerebrovascular 10,500	Diabetes Mellitus 51,528	Alzheimer's Disease 74,632
7	Bacterial Sepsis 820	Septicemia 78	Influenza and Pneumonia 48	Chronic Lower Respiratory Disease 64	Cerebrovascular 195	Diabetes Mellitus 610	Liver Disease 2570	Diabetes Mellitus 5753	Liver Disease 8004	Influenza and Pneumonia 45,941	Diabetes Mellitus 71,382
8	Respiratory Distress 789	Perinatal Period 70	Benign Neoplasms 41	Influenza and Pneumonia 55	Diabetes Mellitus 168	Cerebrovascular 505	Cerebrovascular 2133	HIV 4156	Suicide 5069	Nephritis 38,484	Influenza and Pneumonia 52,717
9	Circulatory System Disease 624	Benign Neoplasms 59	Cerebrovascular 38	Cerebrovascular 45	Influenza and Pneumonia 163	Congenital Anomalies 417	Diabetes Mellitus 1984	Chronic Lower Respiratory Disease 4153	Nephritis 4440	Unintentional Injury 38,292	Nephritis 46,448
10	Neonatal Hemorrhage 597	Chronic Lower Respiratory Disease 57	Septicemia 36	Benign Neoplasms 43	Three Tied 160	Liver Disease 384	Septicemia 910	Viral Hepatitis 2815	Septicemia 4231	Septicemia 26,362	Septicemia 34,828

SIDS = sudden infant death syndrome.

WISQARS. Produced by the Office of Statistics and Programming, National Center for Injury Prevention and Control, Centers for Disease Control and Prevention. Data source: National Center for Health Statistics, National Vital Statistics System, Centers for Disease Control and Prevention.

The Ten Leading Causes of Nonfatal Injury: All Cases, United States, 2009, All Races, Both Sexes, Disposition

	Age Groups										
Rank	**<1 y**	**1–4 y**	**5–9 y**	**10–14 y**	**15–24 y**	**25–34 y**	**35–44 y**	**45–54 y**	**55–64 y**	**≥65 y**	**All Ages**
1	Unintentional Fall 147,280	Unintentional Fall 955,381	Unintentional Fall 631,381	Unintentional Fall 615,145	Unintentional Struck by/ Against 1,027,646	Unintentio-nal Fall 791,629	Unintentio-nal Fall 794,906	Unintentional Fall 928,315	Unintentional Fall 781,827	Unintentional Fall 2,202,024	Unintentional Fall 8,765,597
2	Unintentional Struck by/ Against 31,360	Unintentional Struck by/ Against 372,402	Unintentional Struck by/ Against 406,045	Unintentional Struck by/ Against 574,267	Unintentional Fall 917,167	Unintentio-nal Overexertio-n 654,125	Unintentio-nal Overexertio-n 564,548	Unintentional Overexertion 444,515	Unintentional Struck by/ Against 232,696	Unintentional Struck by/ Against 242,014	Unintentional Struck by/ Against 4,435,906
3	Unintentional Other Bite/ Sting 10,922	Unintentional Other Bite/ Sting 137,352	Unintentional Cut/Pierce 104,940	Unintentional Overexertion 276,076	Unintentional MV Occupant 741,159	Unintentio-nal Struck by/ Against 643,495	Unintentio-nal Struck by/ Against 495,060	Unintentional Struck by/ Against 410,712	Unintentional Overexertion 217,605	Unintentional Overexertion 180,152	Unintentional Overexertion 3,207,877
4	Unintentional Foreign Body 8860	Unintentional Foreign Body 126,060	Unintentional Other Bite/ Sting 92,885	Unintentional Cut/Pierce 118,440	Unintentional Overexertion 703,809	Unintentio-nal MV Occupant 553,680	Unintentio-nal MV Occupant 419,564	Unintentional MV Occupant 363,518	Unintentional MV Occupant 216,997	Unintentional MV Occupant 174,999	Unintentional MV Occupant 2,643,652
5	Unintentional Fire/Bum 7846	Unintentional Cut/Pierce 84,095	Unintentional Pedal Cyclist 84,590	Unintentional Pedal Cyclist 118,095	Other Assault* Struck by/ Against 451,123	Unintentio-nal Cut/ Pierce 382,187	Unintentio-nal Cut/ Pierce 308,801	Unintentional Cut/Pierce 271,617	Unintentional Cut/Pierce 171,584	Unintentional Cut/Pierce 127,735	Unintentional Cut/Pierce 1,997,752
6	Unintentional Other Specified 7036	Unintentional Overexertion 83,056	Unintentional Overexertion 77,742	Unintentional Unknown/ Unspecified 98,282	Unintentional Cut/Pierce 422,182	Other Assault* Struck by/ Against 301,791	Other Assault* Struck by/ Against 194,859	Unintentional Other Specified 179,577	Unintentional Other Bite/ Sting 81,881	Unintentional Other Bite/ Sting 86,559	Other Assault* Struck by/ Against 1,252,243

(continued on next page)

(continued)

	Age Groups									
Rank	**<1 y**	**1–4 y**	**5–9 y**	**10–14 y**	**15–24 y**	**25–34 y**	**35–44 y**	**45–54 y**	**55–64 y**	**≥65 y**	**All Ages**
7	Unintentional Overexertion 6249	Unintentional Other Specified 62,861	Unintentional MV Occupant 58,049	Unintentional MV Occupant 75,701	Unintentional Other Specified 191,694	Unintentio-nal Other Bite/ Sting 158,668	Unintentio-nal Other Specified 164,558	Unintentional Poisoning 159,067	Unintentional Other Specified 77,309	Unintentional Poisoning 65,707	Unintentional Other Bite/ Sting 1,067,922
8	Unintentional Inhalation/ Suffocation 6057	Unintentional Fire/Burn 49,896	Unintentional Foreign Body 55,185	Other Assault* Struck by/ Against 73,360	Unintentional Other Bite/ Sting 178,506	Unintentio-nal Other Specified 153,741	Unintentio-nal Other Bite/Sting 129,701	Other Assault* Struck by/ Against 141,586	Unintentional Poisoning 75,542	Unintentional Other Transport 62,519	Unintentional Other Specified 924,345
9	Unintentional Cut/Pierce 6049	Unintentional Unknown/ Unspecified 48,454	Unintentional Dog Bite 43,512	Unintentional Other Bite/ Sting 59,912	Unintentional Unknown/ Unspecified 176,499	Unintentio-nal Unknown/ Unspecified 113,738	Unintentio-nal Poisoning 124,292	Unintentional Other Bite/ Sting 131,536	Unintentional Other Transport 46,573	Unintentional Unknown/ Unspecified 59,185	Unintentional Unknown/ Unspecified 755,175
10	Unintentional MV Occupant 4942	Unintentional Poisoning 41,265	Unintentional Other Transport 39,732	Unintentional Other Transport 55,176	Unintentional Other Transport 123,824	Unintentio-nal Poisoning 101,454	Unintentio-nal Unknown/ Unspecified 94,310	Unintentional Unknown/ Unspecified 81,378	Other Assault* Struck by/ Against 45,992	Unintentional Other Specified 48,972	Unintentional Poisoning 708,318

MV = motor vehicle.

*The "Other Assault" category includes all assaults that are *not* classified as sexual assault. It represents the majority of assaults.

Produced by the Office of Statistics and Programming, National Center for Injury Prevention and Control, Centers for Disease Control and Prevention. Data source: National Electronic Injury Surveillance System All Injury Program, operated by the Consumer Product Safety Commission.

INDEX

Page numbers in *italics* denotes a figure/table

A

C

E

G

H

I

N

Q

R

S

T

U

V

W

Y

Z